# Current Progress in Hepatology

# Current Progress in Hepatology

Edited by Tiffany Brown

hayle medical

New York

Hayle Medical,
750 Third Avenue, 9th Floor,
New York, NY 10017, USA

Visit us on the World Wide Web at:
www.haylemedical.com



ISBN: 978-1-63241-633-9

The publisher's policy is to use permanent paper from mills that operate a sustainable forestry policy. Furthermore, the publisher ensures that the text paper and cover boards used have met acceptable environmental accreditation standards.



Printed in China.

**Cataloging-in-Publication Data**

Current progress in hepatology / edited by Tiffany Brown.
p. cm.
Includes bibliographical references and index.
ISBN 978-1-63241-633-9
1. Hepatology. 2. Gastroenterology. 3. Digestive organs--Diseases. I. Brown, Tiffany.
RC845 .C87 2019
616.362--dc23

# Contents

# Preface

I am honored to present to you this unique book which encompasses the most up-to-date data in the field. I was extremely pleased to get this opportunity of editing the work of experts from across the globe. I have also written papers in this field and researched the various aspects revolving around the progress of the discipline. I have tried to unify my knowledge along with that of stalwarts from every corner of the world, to produce a text which not only benefits the readers but also facilitates the growth of the field.

Hepatology is a branch of medicine concerned with the study of the gallbladder, liver, biliary tree and pancreas, and their associated disorders. The management of diseases related to viral hepatitis and alcohol is an important domain of hepatology. Nearly 2 billion people have been infected with hepatitis B virus at some stage in their life, while around 350 million people are carriers. Hepatitis B and C viruses are associated with up to 80% of liver cancers. Such widespread infection is increasingly being countered by strict screening before blood transfusion and widespread vaccination. The scope of hepatology is wide and specialists in this domain may be involved in a number of diverse regimes, from drug overdose and liver disease to cancers and liver transplant. This book provides comprehensive insights into the field of hepatology. From theories to research to practical applications, case studies related to all contemporary topics of relevance to this field have been included in this book. It includes contributions of experts and scientists, which will provide innovative insights into this field.

Finally, I would like to thank all the contributing authors for their valuable time and contributions. This book would not have been possible without their efforts. I would also like to thank my friends and family for their constant support.

**Editor**

1

# Modern Prospection for Hepatic Arterial Infusion Chemotherapy in Malignancies with Liver Metastases

**Yi-Hsin Liang,[1,2] Yu-Yun Shao,[2,3] Jia-Yi Chen,[2] Po-Chin Liang,[4] Ann-Lii Cheng,[2,3,5] and Zhong-Zhe Lin[2,5]**

[1] *Department of Hemato-Oncology, E-Da Hospital, No. 1, Yi-da Road, Jiaosu Village, Yanchao, Kaohsiung 82445, Taiwan*
[2] *Department of Oncology, National Taiwan University Hospital, No. 7, Chung-Shan South Road, Taipei City 10002, Taiwan*
[3] *Graduate Institute of Oncology, College of Medicine, National Taiwan University, No. 1, Section 1, Ren-Ai Road, Taipei City 10051, Taiwan*
[4] *Department of Medical Imaging, National Taiwan University Hospital, No. 7, Chung-Shan South Road, Taipei City 10002, Taiwan*
[5] *Department of Internal Medicine, National Taiwan University Hospital, No. 7, Chung-Shan South Road, Taipei City 10002, Taiwan*

Correspondence should be addressed to Zhong-Zhe Lin; zzlin7460@ntu.edu.tw

Academic Editor: Jorge Ortiz

Malignancy with liver metastasis plays an important role in daily oncology practice, especially for primary cancers of the gastrointestinal tract and hepatopancreatobiliary system. On account of the dual vascular supply system and the fact that most metastatic liver tumors are supplied by the hepatic artery, hepatic artery infusion chemotherapy (HAIC) is an appealing method for the treatment of liver metastases. Herein, we summarize recent study results reported in the literature regarding the use of HAIC for metastatic liver tumors, with special focus on colorectal cancer.

## 1. Introduction

Malignancy with liver metastasis plays an important role in daily oncology practice, especially for primary cancers of the gastrointestinal (GI) tract and hepatopancreatobiliary system [1]. The liver is commonly the first site of distant metastasis. For example, about three-quarters of patients with stage IV colorectal cancer (CRC) have liver metastases [2]. Many of these patients have metastatic disease confined to the liver only. It has been demonstrated that for patients with such limited distant metastases, locoregional therapy such as surgery may be helpful [3, 4]. However, usually the liver metastases are too advanced to be resected by hepatectomy. Fewer than 15% of these patients receive hepatectomy to a curative extent [5].

On account of the dual vascular supply system and the fact that most metastatic liver tumors are supplied by the hepatic artery [6, 7], hepatic artery infusion chemotherapy (HAIC) is an appealing method for the treatment of liver metastases. HAIC has several advantages over intravenous chemotherapy. First, chemotherapeutic agents can be delivered more specifically to malignant cells. Normal hepatocytes that mostly rely on the portal venous system are thus exposed to fewer chemotherapeutic agents. Second, many chemotherapy agents used in HAIC have a high first-pass hepatic clearance effect, such as 5-fluorouracil (5-FU) and floxuridine (FUDR), a prodrug of 5-FU. Over 90% of FUDR and 19%–50% of 5-FU are cleared by the liver when they are administered by HAIC [8]. Systemic exposure to chemotherapeutic agents is thus decreased.

These two mechanisms enable HAIC to provide a higher exposure of chemotherapy to malignant cells with minimized toxicities. The higher drug level may also overcome drug resistance. For example, intravenous (IV) anthracyclines are generally considered ineffective for CRC. HAIC with pirarubicin, an anthracycline that is an analogue of doxorubicin, has been demonstrated to have a fair efficacy in CRC patients with liver metastases [9–11].

The equipment and skills related to HAIC have been in development for more than 5 decades. With advances in implantable catheters and ports, external infusion pumps can be avoided to decrease catheter-related complications. Catheter implantation is generally performed via the femoral, axillary, or subclavian arteries under fluoroscopic guidance [12–15]. The angiography should be carefully reviewed before and after catheter implantation to identify any anomalous vasculature. The tips of HAIC catheters are fixed at the gastroduodenal artery or proper hepatic artery. The HAIC ports are then immobilized subcutaneously. Finally, a perfusion scan is usually performed for HAIC catheters to detect any unexpected shunting to other organs.

Adverse reactions to HAIC can be divided into catheter-related complications and chemotherapy-related complications. Common catheter-related complications include catheter displacement, hepatic artery occlusion, and catheter-related infection [16–18]. The complication rates for these issues have been reported to be lower than 7% in recent studies, compared to 22–35% in earlier studies. The most common chemotherapy-related complication is gastrointestinal symptoms. Nausea and vomiting can occur in 25–35% patients [17, 19]. Hepatobiliary toxicity, including elevation of serum hepatic transaminase levels, and hyperbilirubinemia are also important problems [20–23].

Although the rationale for the use of HAIC for metastatic liver tumors is appealing, the actual benefit of HAIC is not wholly clear. The lack of large randomized clinical trials makes it difficult to examine the overall survival benefits. However, results from previous studies are accumulating gradually and could provide some hints as to the actual efficacy of HAIC for metastatic liver tumors. Herein, we summarize recent study results reported in the literature with regards to the use of HAIC for metastatic liver tumors, with special focus on CRC.

## 2. Colorectal Cancer

*2.1. HAIC Combined with Systemic Chemotherapy.* CRC is the third most prevalent malignant disease around the world [24, 25]. Despite screening and early surgery, many patients eventually suffer from metastatic disease. The liver is the most frequent metastatic site of CRC. CRC with liver metastasis becomes an important issue for treatment of metastatic CRC, and HAIC potentially provides good local control with a response rate (RR) ranging from 34% to 92% (Table 1) when combined with systemic chemotherapy.

Mancini et al. conducted a clinical trial that enrolled 123 CRC patients with unresectable liver metastasis [27]. The patients were randomized into two arms. In arm one, patients received intravenous 5-FU chemotherapy and infusional cisplatin via HAIC. In arm two, patients received intravenous 5-FU chemotherapy and bolus cisplatin via HAIC. There was no significant difference in response between the two arms, and thus, treatment response was presented as a combination of all patients in the two arms. The overall RR was 52%, which included a 17% complete response rate. The median overall survival (OS) was 18 months and 28 months for all patients and responders, respectively. Kemeny et al. conducted a clinical trial that enrolled 49 patients with CRC who had unresectable liver-confined metastasis only [31]. The patients received intravenous oxaliplatin and irinotecan (CPT-11) combined with FUDR via HAIC. The overall RR was 92%, which included a 8% complete response rate [31]. The median OS was 50.8 months for chemotherapy-naïve patients and 35 months for previously-treated patients.

Although these studies did not incorporate targeted therapy agents, the reported response rates are comparable to current standards using combination therapy with targeted and cytotoxic chemotherapy. However, whether the addition of HAIC to current standard treatment, which generally provides a high response rate of 47%–64%, is useful remains unclear [32–35]. Recently, targeted therapy has also been used with HAIC in some small series. Bouchahda et al. demonstrated that HAIC could be combined with intravenous cetuximab in two patients in a retrospective study [36]. Further research with different combinations of novel targeted therapy is warranted.

*2.2. Reversing Inoperable Disease to Operable Disease.* For patients with CRC and liver-only metastatic disease, complete resection provides the chance of a cure. When liver metastatic disease develops, complete resection can provide a potential cure for CRC patients. However, only 10–15% of these patients are eligible for such surgery upon diagnosis [5]. Because of the high response rate, HAIC may reverse inoperable liver metastatic disease to an operable status.

Kemeny et al. conducted a clinical trial examining the use of intravenous oxaliplatin and CPT-11 combined with FUDR via HAIC for patients with CRC-related unresectable liver-confined metastasis only [31]. Initially, 98% of these resectable cases had bilobar metastatic lesions, and 73% of them had >5 hepatic lesions. The overall RR was high at 92%. Twenty-three (47%) patients eventually received hepatectomy to a curative extent. Yamaguchi et al. conducted a clinical trial that enrolled 22 patients who had CRC and unresectable liver metastasis to receive intravenous CPT-11 with oral tegafur/uracil in combination with 5-FU via HAIC [26]. The definition of unresectability included (1) tumors involved all liver segments, (2) inadequate liver reservation after resection, and (3) tumors involved all main hepatic veins or both inflow pedicles. The overall RR was 86.4%, and eventually 14 patients (63.6%) underwent complete resection of liver tumors.

Other than 5-FU, oxaliplatin and CPT-11 have also been tested in HAIC. Ducreux et al. conducted a clinical trial that enrolled 28 patients who had CRC-related inoperable liver-confined metastatic diseases only [37]. Twenty-one of these patients had received previous intravenous 5-FU therapy. The patients then received intravenous 5-FU and leucovorin (LV) with oxaliplatin infused via HAIC. The RR was 64%, and the median overall survival (OS) was 27 months. Approximately 18% of patients' diseases became operable following therapy. The same group then further applied this regimen in a second-line setting [38]. Boige et al. conducted a clinical trial that enrolled 44 patients who had CRC-related inoperable

Table 1: Selective studies of combining HAIC with systemic chemotherapy for colorectal cancer.

| Authors | Year | Setting | Treatment | Line | Inclusion population | Patient no. (treat[a]) | Median OS (months) | RR | Note |
|---|---|---|---|---|---|---|---|---|---|
| Yamaguchi et al. [26] | 2011 | Pro, phase I/II | HAIC → 5-FU<br>IV → CPT-11 + LV<br>Oral tegafur/uracil | First line | Unresectable hepatic mets | Phase 1: 12 (12)<br>Phase 2: 22 (22) | Not reach | 86.4% | RCR: 63.6% |
| Mancini et al. [27] | 2003 | Pro, Ran | Arm1: HAIC → continuous cisplatin<br>IV → 5-FU<br>Arm2: HAIC → bolus cisplatin<br>IV → 5-FU | First line | Unresectable hepatic mets | 58 (58)<br>65 (65) | 18 | 52% | |
| Goéré et al. [28] | 2010 | Ret | HAIC → oxaliplatin<br>IV → 5-FU + LV | First line: 18<br>Second line: 69 | Unresectable hepatic mets | 87 (87) | NM | 55% | 5-year survival: 56% |
| Gallagher et al. [29] | 2007 | Ret | HAIC → FUDR + Dexa<br>IV → CPT-11 | Failed oxaliplatin | Unresectable hepatic mets | 39 (39) | 18 | 44% | |
| Pilati et al. [30] | 2009 | Ret | Arm1: HAIC → FUDR + LV<br>Arm2: HAIC → FUDR + LV<br>IV → 5-FU + LV | NM | Unresectable hepatic mets | 72 (72)<br>81 (81) | 18<br>19.1 | 52.7%<br>50.6% | |

Selected studies that enroll patients with colorectal cancer to receive systemic chemotherapy in combination with HAIC are listed here. Studies designed for patients with colorectal cancer-related liver-confined metastatic disease were listed in Table 2.
*With statistical significance.
[a]Actual patients' number who received treatment.
Abbreviations—OS: overall survival, RR: response rate, Pro: prospective, Ran: randomized, Ret: retrospective, NM: not mentioned, HAIC: hepatic artery infusion chemotherapy, IV: intravenous, FUDR: floxuridine, LV: leucovorin, Dexa: dexamethasone, CPT-11: irinotecan, Mets: metastasis, and RCR: resectability conversion rate.

liver-confined metastatic diseases only and in whom first-line chemotherapy failed [38]. Treatment of twenty-eight of these patients with 5-FU, oxaliplatin, and CPT-11 had previously failed. For only one patient, 5-FU alone failed, and in the others both 5-FU and either CPT-11 or oxaliplatin treatment failed. The RR was 62% and the median overall survival (OS) was 16 months. Similarly, 18% of patients' disease became operable following therapy.

For HAIC, the hepatic resectability conversion rate is worthy of emphasis. The current standard treatment, combined targeted and cytotoxic chemotherapy, usually generates a less than 10% hepatic resectability conversion rate according to post hoc analysis [32, 35, 39]. Folprecht et al. conducted the CELIM study that enrolled 114 patients who had CRC and inoperable liver-confined metastatic diseases who received intravenous cetuximab and combination cytotoxic chemotherapy [40]. Overall, 38% of patients eventually received curative hepatectomy. It is worthy of note that 32% of patients with paired images before and after surgery in CELIM trial were considered operable prior to chemotherapy when the images were reviewed centrally. Although there has been no large-scale phase III trial to prove the concept that HAIC might improve the liver resectability conversion rate, the above results are promising, with high response rates and good conversion rates of reversing inoperable disease to operable disease. The outcome is even more encouraging considering that these studies did not incorporate novel targeted agents, such as bevacizumab and cetuximab.

*2.3. Liver-Confined Disease.* Some patients who receive local therapy for early CRC may suffer from recurrence, with liver metastasis as the only disease site (liver-confined disease). Although systemic chemotherapy is the standard treatment for metastatic CRC, some of these patients had had their primary cancer treated previously and suffered from liver-confined metastatic disease. For these patients, it is reasonable to develop a local therapy with an enhanced efficacy against liver metastases. The mechanism of HAIC suits this purpose.

HAIC exhibits a high RR, ranging from 22% to 92%, albeit with an unclear effect on overall survival in this setting (Table 2). In the CALGB 9481 trial, 135 CRC patients with inoperable liver-confined disease were randomly assigned to receive FUDR via HAIC or intravenous bolus 5-FU and LV [41]. Patients who received HAIC compared to patients who received IV chemotherapy had a significantly higher RR (47% versus 24%, $P = 0.012$) and a longer median OS (24.4 months versus 20.0 months; $P = 0.003$). Patients treated with HAIC had a significantly longer time to hepatic progression compared to patients who received IV chemotherapy (9.8 months versus 7.3 months; $P = 0.034$), but a significantly shorter time to extrahepatic progression (7.7 months versus 14.8 months; $P = 0.029$).

Besides FUDR or 5-FU, mitomycin-C (Mit-C) has also been used in HAIC [47, 49]. Kemeny et al. randomly assigned 63 CRC patients with inoperable liver-confined disease to receive high-dose Mit-C and FUDR/LV via HAIC [47].

Table 2: Selective studies of HAIC for liver-confined metastatic disease from colorectal cancer.

| Authors/ Year | Setting | Treatment | Line | Inclusion population | Patient no. (treat)[a] | Median OS (months) | RR | Note |
|---|---|---|---|---|---|---|---|---|
| Kemeny et al. 2006 [41] | Pro, Ran | Arm1: HAIC → FUDR + LV + Dexa<br>Arm2: IV → 5-FU + LV | First line | Unresectable liver confined | 68 (59)<br>67 (58) | 24.4*<br>20 | 47%*<br>24% | QOL improvement |
| Fiorentini et al. 2006 [42] | Pro, phase III | Arm1: HAIC → 5-FU + LV<br>Arm2: HAIC → 5-FU + LV<br>IV → 5-FU + LV | First line | Unresectable liver confined | 40 (36)<br>42 (40) | 14<br>20 | 41.7%<br>47.5% | |
| Fallik et al. 2003 [11] | Pro, phase II | HAIC → pirarubicin<br>IV → 5-FU + LV | First line | Unresectable liver confined | 75 (69) | 20 | 34.4% | |
| Kerr et al. 2003 [43] | Pro, Ran | Arm1: HAIC → 5-FU + LV<br>Arm2: IV → 5-FU + LV | First line | Unresectable liver confined | 145 (95)<br>145 (126) | 14.7<br>14.8 | 22%<br>19% | |
| Allen-Mersh et al. 2000 [44] | Pro, Ran | Arm1: HAIC → FUDR<br>IV → 5-FU + LV<br>Arm2: IV → 5-FU | First line | Unresectable liver confined | 41 (39)<br>43 (42) | NM | 45%<br>23% | No QOL difference |
| Lorenz et al. 2000 [45] | Pro, Ran | Arm1: HAIC → 5-FU + LV<br>Arm2: IV → 5-FU + LV<br>Arm3: HAIC → FUDR | First line | Unresectable liver confined | 57 (40)<br>57 (71)[b]<br>54 (37) | 18.7<br>17.6<br>12.7 | 45%<br>19.7%<br>43.2% | |
| Kemeny et al. 2009 [31] | Pro, phase I | HAIC → FUDR + Dexa<br>IV → oxaliplatin + CPT-11 | First line: 23<br>Second line: 26 | Unresectable liver confined | 49 (49) | First line: 50.8<br>Second line: 35 | 92% | RCR: 47% |
| Ducreux et al. 2005 [37] | Pro | HAIC → Oxaliplatin<br>IV → 5-FU + LV | First line: 7<br>Second line: 21 | Unresectable liver confined | 28 (26) | 27 | 64% | RCR: 18% |
| Kemeny et al. 2005 [46] | Pro, phase I | Arm1: HAIC → FUDR + DEXA<br>IV → oxaliplatin + CPT-11<br>Arm2: HAIC → FUDR + DEXA<br>IV → oxaliplatin + 5-FU + LV | First line: 4<br>After first line: 32 | Unresectable liver confined | 36 (36) | 36<br>22 | 90%<br>87% | |
| Kemeny et al. 2009 [31] | Pro, phase I | HAIC → FUDR + Dexa<br>IV → Oxaliplatin + CPT-11 | First line: 23<br>Second line: 26 | Unresectable liver confined | 49 (49) | First line: 50.8<br>Second line: 35 | 92% | RCR: 47% |
| Kemeny et al. 2005 [47] | Pro, phase II | HAIC → FUDR + Dexa + Mit-C | First line: 26<br>Second line: 37 | Unresectable liver confined | 63 (63) | First line: 23<br>Second line: 20 | First line: 73%<br>Second line: 70% | |
| Lorenz et al. 2001 [48] | Pro, phase II | HAIC → 5-FU + LV | First line: 40<br>Second line: 10 | Unresectable liver confined | 50 (50) | 22.3 | 56% | |

Table 2: Continued.

| Authors/ Year | Setting | Treatment | Line | Inclusion population | Patient no. (treat)[a] | Median OS (months) | RR | Note |
|---|---|---|---|---|---|---|---|---|
| Boige et al. 2008 [38] | Pro | HAIC → oxaliplatin<br>IV → 5-FU + LV | After first line | Unresectable liver confined | 44 (43) | 16 | 62% | RCR: 18% |
| Fazio et al. 2003 [49] | Ret | HAIC → cisplatin + Mit-C + 5-FU | After first line | Hepatic mets predominent[c] | 45 (44) | NM | 35% | |
| Kemeny et al. 2001 [50] | Pro, phase I | HAIC → FUDR + DEXA<br>IV → CPT-11 | After first line | Unresectable liver confined | 46 (46) | 17.2 | 74% | |
| Van Riel et al. 2000 [51] | Ret | HAIC → 5-FU | All | Hepatic mets predominent[c] | 145 (145) | 14.3 m | 34% | Hepatic artery thrombosis (48%) |
| Fujimoto et al. 2009 [52] | Ret | HAIC → 5-FU | NM | Unresectable liver confined | 72 (72) | 18 | 38% | |
| Sameshima et al. 2007 [53] | Ret | HAIC → 5-FU | NM | Unresectable liver confined | 42 (42) | 29.1 | 57% | |

Selected studies that enroll patients with colorectal cancer-related liver-confined metastatic disease are listed here. Studies designed for patients with colorectal cancer to receive systemic chemotherapy in combination with HAIC are listed in Table 1.
*With statistical significance.
[a]Actual patients' number who received treatment.
[b]Patients who did not receive treatment in arm1 and arm3 received treatment as arm2.
[c]Trial enrolled patients with liver-confined disease or "minimal" extrahepatic disease.
Abbreviations—OS: overall survival, RR: response rate, Pro: prospective, Ran: randomized, Ret: retrospective, NM: not mentioned, HAIC: hepatic artery infusion chemotherapy, IV: intravenous, FUDR: floxuridine, LV: leucovorin, Dexa: dexamethasone, Mit-C: mitomycin C, CPT-11: irinotecan, QOL: quality of life, Mets: metastasis, and RCR: resectability conversion rate.

The RR was 73% in the chemotherapy naïve patients and 70% in previously-treated patients. However, the expense was a high biliary toxicity. Elevation of the serum bilirubin level >3 mg/dL occurred in 22.5% patients. Half of the patients suffered from at least a doubling of the serum hepatic transaminase level. Besides, biliary sclerosis was noted in 6 patients (9.5%) and liver bilomas in 5 (7.9%) patients.

Fallik et al. enrolled 75 patients with CRC and inoperable liver-confined metastatic diseases in a phase II trial [11]. All patients received intravenous 5-FU and LV in combination with HAIC using pirarubicin, an anthracycline analog. The overall RR was 31.9% and the median OS was 19 months. Most important was that grade 4 neutropenia was reported for 27 cycles (23%). The toxicity profile seemed acceptable in this trial and no cardiac toxicity was reported.

Several small studies in the literature have addressed the use of HAIC in liver-confined disease of CRC. The study designs and results were heterogeneous across these trials. Therefore, Mocellin et al. conducted a meta-analysis to compare HAIC and intravenous chemotherapy for liver-confined metastatic diseases of CRC [54, 55]. Ten randomized controlled trials, including a total of 1277 patients, were enrolled in the analysis. All studies used 5-FU or FUDR as single agents via HAIC or intravenous chemotherapy. Although the RR was significantly higher in patients receiving HAIC than in patients receiving intravenous chemotherapy (42.9% versus 18.4%, $P < 0.001$), the median OS was not significantly longer (15.9 months versus 12.4 months, $P = 0.240$).

The result of this meta-analysis should be interpreted cautiously. The analyzed ten clinical trials were mostly conducted a decade ago and used 5-FU only in intravenous chemotherapy, which is clearly inadequate as compared with present therapies. This explains the inferior OS outcome of 12 months only in either treatment arm and the uncertainty regarding the interpretation of this meta-analysis result. On the contrary, many patients who were allocated into the HAIC arms in these trials did not receive HAIC mainly due to catheter-related complications. Some of them were allowed to cross over into intravenous chemotherapy arms but still analyzed as HAIC in an intent-to-treat manner. All these reasons suggest difficulty in interpretation of this meta-analysis.

According to current evidence, HAIC demonstrates better locoregional control for CRC patents with liver-confined disease, at the expense of poor extrahepatic disease progression. Although there was a survival benefit for HAIC-treated patients reported in the CALGB 9481 study, this OS benefit became nonsignificant when ten studies were enrolled into a meta-analysis. Evidence as to whether HAIC provides a better survival benefit than systemic therapy is thus still lacking, and further large-scale clinical trials are warranted. Except for 5-FU and FUDR, some other cytotoxic agents such as Mit-C and pirarubicin are also applied via HAIC. As we know, anthracycline drugs were thought to be ineffective in the treatment of CRC. However, anthracycline analogs demonstrated potential efficacy in CRC via HAIC because of their special mechanism, which provides a greater drug selection for the treatment of CRC.

*2.4. HAIC after Curative Hepatectomy.* With improvement in surgical techniques, more and more CRC patients with liver-confined metastasis receive surgery for both the primary CRC and liver tumors with a curative intent. Prevention of disease recurrence is crucial in these patients. Some physicians use a local treatment, HAIC, in this adjuvant setting.

Kemeny et al. enrolled 156 CRC patients who received complete resection of liver metastatic disease [56, 57]. These patients were randomized into groups receiving either intravenous 5-FU alone or in combination with HAIC using FUDR. In an updated result after a median follow-up duration of 10.3 years, patients who received combination therapy with HAIC had a significantly longer progression-free survival than patients who received intravenous therapy alone (31.3 months versus 17.2 months, $P = 0.02$) [57]. Although the OS was not significantly different, the trend still favored combination therapy with HAIC (68.4 months versus 58.8 months, $P = 0.10$).

Oxaliplatin is the current standard for adjuvant treatment of stage III CRC [58]. When the efficacy of newer agents for the treatment of CRC has been proven, they have been tested for HAIC. Alberts et al. conducted a phase II trial that enrolled 76 patients with CRC who had liver-confined metastasis [59]. After curative surgery for both the primary tumor and liver metastases, patients received adjuvant intra-venous oxaliplatin and oral capecitabine alternated with HAIC FUDR plus dexamethasone. Although 3 treatment-related deaths were reported, the median disease-free survival was 32.7 months and only 30 patients developed recurrent malignancies after median follow-up time of 4.8 years.

In addition to oxaliplatin, CPT-11 has also shown a fair efficacy for stage 4 CRC and thus was also examined in combination with HAIC. Kemeny et al. conducted a phase I/II trial that enrolled 96 patients with CRC who had liver-confined metastasis [60]. After curative surgery, patients received adjuvant intravenous CPT-11 combined with HAIC FUDR plus dexamethasone. With a median follow-up time of 26 months, the 2-year survival rate was 89%, and 1.5-year hepatic disease-free survival rate was 88%.

In the targeted therapy era, a combination of HAIC with novel targeted agents was also tested in some series. Kemeny et al. randomly assigned 73 CRC patients with resected liver-confined disease to receive curative hepatectomy [61]. All patients received intravenous oxaliplatin or CPT-11 plus infusional 5-FU in combination with FUDR plus dexamethasone via HAIC. Patients were randomized into two arms, receiving intravenous bevacizumab or not. The 4-year recurrence-free survival rate was 46% and 37% for the no bevacizumab arm and the bevacizumab arm ($P = 0.4$), respectively, after a median follow-up duration of 30 months.

There have recently been some convincing results showing a lower recurrence rate for HAIC in combination with systemic therapy after curative hepatectomy. Systemic chemotherapy after curative surgery for liver metastatic disease is still the standard treatment, and HAIC might provide enhanced locoregional control for the liver. Further large-scale phase III trials are warranted.

## 3. Other Malignancies

*3.1. Gastric Cancer.* The prognosis of gastric cancer with liver metastases is extremely poor, with median OS of only 2–6 months if untreated [62]. The standard treatment is combination systemic chemotherapy including platinum analogs and 5-FU. For better palliation, some case series reported the efficacy of HAIC as a liver-directed therapy. Tarazov reported the results of HAIC using 5-FU and doxorubicin in 12 patients with unresectable gastric cancer-related bilobar liver metastases [62]. The RR was 25% and the median OS was 23 months. One patient had 60 months of stable disease after 7 courses of HAIC treatment. Kumada et al. conducted a phase II trial that tested HAIC with 5-FU, epirubicin, and Mit-C in 63 patients with gastric cancer who had unresectable liver metastasis [63]. Only 36 patients were documented to have liver-confined metastatic diseases. The response rate was 55.6%, with three complete responders. For patients with liver-confined disease, the median OS was 13 months.

As a treatment for synchronous multiple liver metastases from gastric cancer after palliative gastrectomy to maintain quality of life, Ojima et al. retrospectively analyzed 18 patients who received HAIC with 5-FU [64]. The RR was 83% with a response duration of 7.6 months. The median OS was 19.2 months.

According to the limited data above, HAIC potentially provides high response rates in patients with liver metastases of gastric cancer. The median OS in these small groups of patients seemed longer given that the best survival in patients receiving systemic chemotherapy has been reported to be 13.8 months [65]. Therefore, HAIC might have the potential to be a feasible local treatment for gastric cancer with unresectable liver metastases.

*3.2. Uveal Melanoma.* Uveal melanoma usually hematogenously spreads into the liver in up to 95% patients [66]. Once liver metastases occur, the life expectancy is less than 5 months. Because no systemic therapy is proved to have definite efficacy for metastatic uveal melanoma, regional therapy to control liver metastases and delay extrahepatic spread becomes one of the treatment choices. Melichar et al. performed HAIC with the combination of cisplatin, vinblastine, and dacarbazine in 10 liver metastatic uveal melanoma patients [67]. Two patients had partial response, and four patients achieved stable disease. Those who had clinical benefit survived for more than one year. Becker et al. conducted a phase II prospective clinical trial that enrolled 48 patients with metastatic uveal melanoma [66]. HAIC with fotemustine was given to the 23 patients who had liver metastases alone. Intravenous fotemustine was given to the 25 patients who had metastases other than liver. All patients received subcutaneous interleukin-2 and interferon $\alpha$. The overall RR was significantly higher for patients who received HAIC than those patients who received intravenous chemotherapy (21.7% versus 8.0%). However, the median OS was similar (369 days versus 349 days).

With the therapeutic activity demonstrated above, HAIC might play a role to control liver-confined metastatic uveal melanoma. Comparing with the cumulating results from chemoembolization in uveal melanoma with liver metastases, the evidence for the better efficacy of HAIC is still scarce and needs more studies [68].

*3.3. Pancreatic Cancer.* The prognosis of pancreatic cancer is extremely poor because of the low resection rate at diagnosis, rapid progression, and frequent metastasis even after curative surgery. Despite the advances of cancer therapy generally, the survival of patients with pancreatic cancer did not improve significantly in the past decades. Liver is the most common site of metastasis, and thus, HAIC was examined as a strategy for palliation or prevention of liver metastasis. For unresectable pancreatic cancer without metastasis, HAIC was also examined as a primary treatment modality for primary tumors from pancreatic body and tails [69].

Homma et al. also enrolled 16 patients with pancreatic cancer-related liver metastases who received cisplatin and 5-FU via HAIC [70]. The RR was 68.8% with median survival 16.25 months.

There were few studies focusing on HAIC in the adjuvant setting. Hashimoto et al. conducted a retrospective analysis that enrolled 42 patients with pancreatic cancer who received curative pancreatectomy and subsequent 5-FU via HAIC [71]. Hepatic recurrence rate was 7.1% with a median 19-month followup.

From the above studies, HAIC for pancreatic cancer is a way for local treatment. Besides, HAIC also provides potential benefit to reduce recurrence after pancreatectomy, compared to the 36% recurrent rate reported by CONKO-001 study using systemic gemcitabine alone [72]. The cost of relative high complication rate remains the problem. Common complications include high probability of hepatic arterial stenosis (19.6%) and liver abscess (3.6%). Due to the limitation of various HAIC techniques and different vasculatures of each patient, large prospective trial is required for further investigation.

*3.4. Biliary Tree Cancer.* Due to limited effective therapy for unresectable and metastatic biliary tract cancers, HAIC was also applied in several studies. These studies of biliary tract cancer were heterogeneous in patient population, and most studies included more than one cancer type. Inaba et al. conducted a phase I/II trial for patients with unresectable intrahepatic cholangiocarcinoma [73]. HAIC with gemcitabine was applied in 13 patients. One patient had partial response and 8 patients had stable disease. The response rate was 7.7%. In addition to gemcitabine, cisplatin and epirubicin combination were also examined. Cantore et al. conducted a phase II study that enrolled 25 patients with metastatic intrahepatic cholangiocarcinoma and 5 patients with gallbladder carcinoma to receive intravenous 5-FU and HAIC with cisplatin and epirubicin [74]. Overall RR was 40% including 1 patient who achieved complete remission. Median OS was 13.2 months. Mambrini et al. conducted a phase II trial that enrolled 20 patients with unresectable metastatic intra- or extra-hepatic biliary tree cancers to receive oral capecitabine and HAIC using cisplatin and epirubicin [75]. The overall RR was 31.5%, and median OS was 18 months.

From the evidence of these phase II studies, combination HAIC with oral or intravenous chemotherapy seems to be a safe and effective treatment modality. With the advance of intervention radiology and radiotherapy techniques, multimodality treatment incorporating radiation, drug-eluting beads, and chemoembolization were also developing in combination with HAIC [76, 77]. Further comparison of different treatments modality and large scale phase III trials are needed.

*3.5. Neuroendocrine Tumor.* Gastroenteropancreatic neuroendocrine tumors often metastasize to liver and contribute substantially to one of the most important noncolorectal causes of liver metastases [78]. Due to limited patients numbers, HAIC for unresectable liver metastases from neuroendocrine tumors has mostly been studied retrospectively.

Christante et al. collected 77 patients with extensive liver metastases with disease progression after octreotide treatment [79]. Fifty-nine patients received four cycles of 5-FU via HAIC with the addition of selective chemoembolization at the end of third and fourth cycles. However, 18 patients received HAIC alone due to the concern of hepatotoxicity. Overall response rate was 80%, and median progression-free survival was 19 months, and all the responders were treated with combination of HAIC and chemoembolization.

Most of the HAIC studies in neuroendocrine tumors were conducted in combination with chemoembolization. Due to the limitation of scarce retrospective studies with HAIC treatment alone, the efficacy of HAIC for neuroendocrine tumors seems to be difficult to clearly be identified based on current evidences. Further studies are warranted.

## 4. Conclusion

In this article, we presented the current lines of evidence of HAIC as a treatment of liver metastases. HAIC provides a good locoregional control to liver tumors. Most of evidences mainly came from studies of CRC. For patients with CRC and inoperable liver metastasis, HAIC has potentials to enhance the treatment response of the liver metastases when combined with systemic chemotherapy. For CRC patients who had failed previous intravenous chemotherapies, HAIC still provides fair efficacy of control to liver tumors. Patients with initially considered inoperable liver metastases could have a chance to receive surgery if HAIC converts the tumors back to operable status. However, the evidence to support if HAIC could totally replace the intravenous chemotherapies is still not strong enough across previous trials. Therefore, current standard for liver metastatic CRC is still intravenous chemotherapy, and HAIC could be provided as local control focusing on liver. As for CRC patients with initially operable liver metastatic tumors who received curative operation, HAIC in combination with intravenous chemotherapies demonstrated good competence to reduce liver recurrent and to subsequently prolong the overall survival. Some new agents could be used in HAIC in combination to systemic agents, such as pirarubicin, which is initially considered ineffective for CRC. With the emergent novel agents and targeted agents in the 21 century, more studies are needed for different combinations with HAIC.

HAIC is also applied for other malignant diseases with liver metastases, especially for those malignancies which have poor response to systemic chemotherapy, such as melanoma or pancreatic cancer. Although the results for large-scale prospective phase III trials are warranted, HAIC seems to become an attractive procedure for hepatic metastatic diseases in the future.

## Abbreviations

CRC: Colorectal cancer
HAIC: Hepatic artery infusion chemotherapy
OS: Overall survival
5-FU: 5-Fluorouracil
FUDR: Floxuridine
RR: Response rate
CPT-11: Irinotecan
LV: Leucovorin
TACE: Transarterial chemoembolization
MIT-C: Mitomycin C
IV: Intravenous
GI: Gastrointestinal.

## Acknowledgment

This study was supported by a Grant from the National Science Council in Taiwan (NSC 101-2314-B-002-164).

## References

[1] J. P. Ayoub, K. R. Hess, M. C. Abbruzzese, R. Lenzi, M. N. Raber, and J. L. Abbruzzese, "Unknown primary tumors metastatic to liver," *Journal of Clinical Oncology*, vol. 16, no. 6, pp. 2105–2112, 1998.

[2] S. Manfredi, C. Lepage, C. Hatem, O. Coatmeur, J. Faivre, and A. M. Bouvier, "Epidemiology and management of liver metastases from colorectal cancer," *Annals of Surgery*, vol. 244, no. 2, pp. 254–259, 2006.

[3] J. S. Tomlinson, W. R. Jarnagin, R. P. DeMatteo et al., "Actual 10-year survival after resection of colorectal liver metastases defines cure," *Journal of Clinical Oncology*, vol. 25, no. 29, pp. 4575–4580, 2007.

[4] T. Ruers and R. P. Bleichrodt, "Treatment of liver metastases, an update on the possibilities and results," *European Journal of Cancer*, vol. 38, no. 7, pp. 1023–1033, 2002.

[5] R. Stangl, A. Altendorf-Hofmann, R. M. Charnley, and J. Scheele, "Factors influencing the natural history of colorectal liver metastases," *Lancet*, vol. 343, no. 8910, pp. 1405–1410, 1994.

[6] J. A. Ridge, J. R. Bading, and A. S. Gelbard, "Perfusion of colorectal hepatic metastases. Relative distribution of flow from the hepatic artery and portal vein," *Cancer*, vol. 59, no. 9, pp. 1547–1553, 1987.

[7] N. B. Ackerman, "Experimental studies on the circulation dynamics of intrahepatic tumor blood supply," *Cancer*, vol. 29, no. 2, pp. 435–439, 1972.

[8] W. D. Ensminger, A. Rosowsky, and V. Raso, "A clinical-pharmacological evaluation of hepatic arterial infusions of 5-fluoro-2′deoxyuridine and 5-fluorouracil," *Cancer Research*, vol. 38, no. 11, pp. 3784–3792, 1978.

[9] J. N. Munck, P. Rougier, G. G. Chabot et al., "Phase I and pharmacological study of intraarterial hepatic administration of pirarubicin in patients with advanced hepatic metastases," *European Journal of Cancer A*, vol. 30, no. 3, pp. 289–293, 1994.

[10] P. Rougier, J. N. Munck, D. Elias et al., "Intra-arterial hepatic chemotherapy with pirarubicin. Preclinical and clinical studies," *American Journal of Clinical Oncology*, vol. 13, supplement 1, pp. S1–S4, 1990.

[11] D. Fallik, M. Ychou, J. Jacob et al., "Hepatic arterial infusion using pirarubicin combined with systemic chemotherapy: a phase II study in patients with nonresectable liver metastases from colorectal cancer," *Annals of Oncology*, vol. 14, no. 6, pp. 856–863, 2003.

[12] N. Hayashi, T. Sakai, M. Kitagawa, T. Kimoto, and Y. Ishii, "Percutaneous long-term arterial access with implantable ports direct subclavian approach with US," *European Journal of Radiology*, vol. 26, no. 3, pp. 304–308, 1998.

[13] M. Yoshikawa, M. Ebara, T. Nakano, A. Minoyama, N. Sugiura, and M. Ohto, "Percutaneous transaxillary catheter insertion for hepatic artery infusion chemotherapy," *American Journal of Roentgenology*, vol. 158, no. 4, pp. 885–886, 1992.

[14] R. M. Barone, J. E. Byfield, and P. B. Goldfarb, "Intra-arterial chemotherapy using an implantable infusion pump and liver irradiation for the treatment of hepatic metastases," *Cancer*, vol. 50, no. 5, pp. 850–862, 1982.

[15] H. Buchwald, T. B. Grage, and P. P. Vassilopoulos, "Intraarterial infusion chemotherapy for hepatic carcinoma using a totally implantable infusion pump," *Cancer*, vol. 45, no. 5, pp. 866–869, 1980.

[16] P. J. Allen, A. Nissan, A. I. Picon et al., "Technical complications and durability of hepatic artery infusion pumps for unresectable colorectal liver metastases: an institutional experience of 544 consecutive cases," *Journal of the American College of Surgeons*, vol. 201, no. 1, pp. 57–65, 2005.

[17] K. T. Barnett and M. P. Malafa, "Complications of hepatic artery infusion: a review of 4580 reported cases," *International Journal of Gastrointestinal Cancer*, vol. 30, no. 3, pp. 147–160, 2001.

[18] Y. Arai, Y. Inaba, Y. Takeuchi, and Y. Ariyoshi, "Intermittent hepatic arterial infusion of high-dose 5FU on a weekly schedule for liver metastases from colorectal cancer," *Cancer Chemotherapy and Pharmacology*, vol. 40, no. 6, pp. 526–530, 1997.

[19] O. Kanat, A. Gewirtz, and N. Kemeny, "What is the potential role of hepatic arterial infusion chemo-therapy in the current armamentorium against colorectal cancer," *Journal of Gastrointestinal Oncology*, vol. 3, pp. 130–138, 2012.

[20] Y. Y. Shao, C. C. Huang, P. C. Liang, and Z. Z. Lin, "Hepatic arterial infusion of chemotherapy for advanced hepatocellular carcinoma," *Asia-Pacific Journal of Clinical Oncology*, vol. 6, no. 2, pp. 80–88, 2010.

[21] A. D. Cohen and N. E. Kemeny, "An update on hepatic arterial infusion chemotherapy for colorectal cancer," *Oncologist*, vol. 8, no. 6, pp. 553–566, 2003.

[22] H. Toyoda, S. Nakano, T. Kumada et al., "The efficacy of continuous local arterial infusion of 5-fluorouracil and cisplatin through an implanted reservoir for severe advanced hepatocellular carcinoma," *Oncology*, vol. 52, no. 4, pp. 295–299, 1995.

[23] A. Minoyama, M. Yoshikawa, M. Ebara, H. Saisho, N. Sugiura, and M. Ohto, "Study of repeated arterial infusion chemotherapy with a subcutaneously implanted reservoir for advanced hepatocellular carcinoma," *Journal of Gastroenterology*, vol. 30, no. 3, pp. 356–366, 1995.

[24] A. Jemal, M. M. Center, C. DeSantis, and E. M. Ward, "Global patterns of cancer incidence and mortality rates and trends," *Cancer Epidemiology Biomarkers and Prevention*, vol. 19, no. 8, pp. 1893–1907, 2010.

[25] J. Ferlay, H. R. Shin, F. Bray, D. Forman, C. Mathers, and D. M. Parkin, "Estimates of worldwide burden of cancer in 2008: GLOBOCAN 2008," *International Journal of Cancer*, vol. 127, no. 12, pp. 2893–2917, 2010.

[26] T. Yamaguchi, H. Matsumoto, M. Yasutome, T. Mori, and K. Takahashi, "Phase I/II study of irinotecan, UFT and leucovorin with hepatic arterial infusion using 5-FU in colorectal cancer patients with unresectable liver metastases," *Cancer Chemotherapy and Pharmacology*, vol. 67, no. 3, pp. 629–635, 2011.

[27] R. Mancini, M. Tedesco, C. Garufi et al., "Hepatic arterial infusion (HAI) of cisplatin and systemic fluorouracil in the treatment of unresectable colorectal liver metastases," *Anticancer Research C*, vol. 23, no. 2, pp. 1837–1841, 2003.

[28] D. Goéré, I. Deshaies, T. De Baere et al., "Prolonged survival of initially unresectable hepatic colorectal cancer patients treated with hepatic arterial infusion of oxaliplatin followed by radical surgery of metastases," *Annals of Surgery*, vol. 251, no. 4, pp. 686–691, 2010.

[29] D. J. Gallagher, M. Capanu, G. Raggio, and N. Kemeny, "Hepatic arterial infusion plus systemic irinotecan in patients with unresectable hepatic metastases from colorectal cancer previously treated with systemic oxaliplatin: a retrospective analysis," *Annals of Oncology*, vol. 18, no. 12, pp. 1995–1999, 2007.

[30] P. Pilati, E. Mammano, S. Mocellin, E. Tessari, M. Lise, and D. Nitti, "Hepatic arterial infusion for unresectable colorectal liver metastases combined or not with systemic chemotherapy," *Anticancer Research*, vol. 29, no. 10, pp. 4139–4144, 2009.

[31] N. E. Kemeny, F. D. Huitzil Melendez, M. Capanu et al., "Conversion to resectability using hepatic artery infusion plus systemic chemotherapy for the treatment of unresectable liver metastases from colorectal carcinoma," *Journal of Clinical Oncology*, vol. 27, no. 21, pp. 3465–3471, 2009.

[32] C. Bokemeyer, I. Bondarenko, J. T. Hartmann et al., "Efficacy according to biomarker status of cetuximab plus FOLFOX-4 as first-line treatment for metastatic colorectal cancer: the OPUS study," *Annals of Oncology*, vol. 22, no. 7, pp. 1535–1546, 2011.

[33] T. S. Maughan, R. A. Adams, C. G. Smith et al., "Addition of cetuximab to oxaliplatin-based first-line combination chemotherapy for treatment of advanced colorectal cancer: results of the randomised phase 3 MRC COIN trial," *The Lancet*, vol. 377, no. 9783, pp. 2103–2114, 2011.

[34] K. M. Tveit, T. Guren, B. Glimelius et al., "Phase III trial of cetuximab with continuous or intermittent fluorouracil, leucovorin, and oxaliplatin (Nordic FLOX) versus FLOX alone in first-line treatment of metastatic colorectal cancer: the NORDIC-VII study," *Journal of Clinical Oncology*, vol. 30, pp. 1755–1762, 2012.

[35] E. Van Cutsem, C. H. Köhne, I. Láng et al., "Cetuximab plus irinotecan, fluorouracil, and leucovorin as first-line treatment for metastatic colorectal cancer: updated analysis of overall survival according to tumor KRAS and BRAF mutation status," *Journal of Clinical Oncology*, vol. 29, no. 15, pp. 2011–2019, 2011.

[36] M. Bouchahda, R. Adam, S. Giacchetti et al., "Rescue chemotherapy using multidrug chronomodulated hepatic arterial infusion for patients with heavily pretreated metastatic colorectal cancer," *Cancer*, vol. 115, no. 21, pp. 4990–4999, 2009.

[37] M. Ducreux, M. Ychou, A. Laplanche et al., "Hepatic arterial oxaliplatin infusion plus intravenous chemotherapy in colorectal cancer with inoperable hepatic metastases: a trial of the Gastrointestinal Group of the Fédération Nationale des Centres de Lutte Contre le Cancer," *Journal of Clinical Oncology*, vol. 23, no. 22, pp. 4881–4887, 2005.

[38] V. Boige, D. Malka, D. Elias et al., "Hepatic arterial infusion of oxaliplatin and intravenous LV5FU2 in unresectable liver metastases from colorectal cancer after systemic chemotherapy failure," *Annals of Surgical Oncology*, vol. 15, no. 1, pp. 219–226, 2008.

[39] L. B. Saltz, S. Clarke, E. Díaz-Rubio et al., "Bevacizumab in combination with oxaliplatin-based chemotherapy as first-line therapy in metastatic colorectal cancer: a randomized phase III study," *Journal of Clinical Oncology*, vol. 26, no. 18, pp. 2013–2019, 2008.

[40] G. Folprecht, T. Gruenberger, W. O. Bechstein et al., "Tumour response and secondary resectability of colorectal liver metastases following neoadjuvant chemotherapy with cetuximab: the CELIM randomised phase 2 trial," *The Lancet Oncology*, vol. 11, no. 1, pp. 38–47, 2010.

[41] N. E. Kemeny, D. Niedzwiecki, D. R. Hollis et al., "Hepatic arterial infusion versus systemic therapy for hepatic metastases from colorectal cancer: a randomized trial of efficacy, quality of life, and molecular markers (CALGB 9481)," *Journal of Clinical Oncology*, vol. 24, no. 9, pp. 1395–1403, 2006.

[42] G. Fiorentini, M. Cantore, S. Rossi et al., "Hepatic arterial chemotherapy in combination with systemic chemotherapy compared with hepatic arterial chemotherapy alone for liver metastases from colorectal cancer: results of a multi-centric randomized study," *In Vivo A*, vol. 20, no. 6, pp. 707–710, 2006.

[43] D. J. Kerr, C. S. McArdle, J. Ledermann et al., "Intrahepatic arterial versus intravenous fluorouracil and folinic acid for colorectal cancer liver metastases: a multicentre randomised trial," *Lancet*, vol. 361, no. 9355, pp. 368–373, 2003.

[44] T. G. Allen-Mersh, C. Glover, C. Fordy, P. Mathur, and H. Quinn, "Randomized trial of regional plus systemic fluorinated pyrimidine compared with systemic fluorinated pyrimidine in treatment of colorectal liver metastases," *European Journal of Surgical Oncology*, vol. 26, no. 5, pp. 468–473, 2000.

[45] M. Lorenz and H. H. Müller, "Randomized, multicenter trial of fluorouracil plus leucovorin administered either via hepatic arterial or intravenous infusion versus fluorodeoxyuridine

administered via hepatic arterial infusion in patients with non-resectable liver metastases from colorectal carcinoma," *Journal of Clinical Oncology*, vol. 18, no. 2, pp. 243–254, 2000.

[46] N. Kemeny, W. Jarnagin, P. Paty et al., "Phase I trial of systemic oxaliplatin combination chemotherapy with hepatic arterial infusion in patients with unresectable liver metastases from colorectal cancer," *Journal of Clinical Oncology*, vol. 23, no. 22, pp. 4888–4896, 2005.

[47] N. Kemeny, A. Eid, J. Stockman et al., "Hepatic arterial infusion of Floxuridine and dexamethasone plus high-dose Mitomycin C for patients with unresectable hepatic metastases from colorectal carcinoma," *Journal of Surgical Oncology*, vol. 91, no. 2, pp. 97–101, 2005.

[48] M. Lorenz, H. H. Mueller, E. Mattes et al., "Phase II study of weekly 24-hour intra-arterial high-dose infusion of 5-fluorouracil and folinic acid for liver metastasses from colorectal carcinomas," *Annals of Oncology*, vol. 12, no. 3, pp. 321–325, 2001.

[49] N. Fazio, F. Orsi, R. F. Grasso et al., "Hepatic intra-arterial chemotherapy using a percutaneous catheter in pretreated patients with metastatic colorectal carcinoma," *Anticancer Research D*, vol. 23, no. 6, pp. 5023–5030, 2003.

[50] N. E. Kemeny, M. Gonen, D. Sullivan et al., "Phase I study of hepatic arterial infusion of floxuridine and dexamethasone with systemic irinotecan for unresectable hepatic metastases from colorectal cancer," *Journal of Clinical Oncology*, vol. 19, no. 10, pp. 2687–2695, 2001.

[51] J. M. G. H. Van Riel, C. J. Van Groeningen, S. H. M. Albers et al., "Hepatic arterial 5-fluorouracil in patients with liver metastases of colorectal cancer: single-centre experience in 145 patients," *Annals of Oncology*, vol. 11, no. 12, pp. 1563–1570, 2000.

[52] Y. Fujimoto, T. Akasu, S. Yamamoto, S. Fujita, and Y. Moriya, "Long-term results of hepatectomy after hepatic arterial infusion chemotherapy for initially unresectable hepatic colorectal metastases," *Journal of Gastrointestinal Surgery*, vol. 13, no. 9, pp. 1643–1650, 2009.

[53] S. Sameshima, H. Horikoshi, K. Motegi et al., "Outcomes of hepatic artery infusion therapy for hepatic metastases from colorectal carcinoma after radiological placement of infusion catheters," *European Journal of Surgical Oncology*, vol. 33, no. 6, pp. 741–745, 2007.

[54] S. Mocellin, S. Pasquali, and D. Nitti, "Fluoropyrimidine-HAI (hepatic arterial infusion) versus systemic chemotherapy (SCT) for unresectable liver metastases from colorectal cancer," *Cochrane Database of Systematic Reviews*, no. 3, Article ID CD007823, 2009.

[55] S. Mocellin, P. Pilati, M. Lise, and D. Nitti, "Meta-analysis of hepatic arterial infusion for unresectable liver metastases from colorectal cancer: the end of an era?" *Journal of Clinical Oncology*, vol. 25, no. 35, pp. 5649–5654, 2007.

[56] N. Kemeny, Y. Huang, and A. M. Cohen, "Hepatic arterial infusion of chemotherapy after resection of hepatic metastases from colorectal cancer," *New England Journal of Medicine*, vol. 341, pp. 2039–2048, 1999.

[57] N. E. Kemeny and M. Gonen, "Hepatic arterial infusion after liver resection," *New England Journal of Medicine*, vol. 352, no. 7, pp. 734–735, 2005.

[58] T. André, C. Boni, L. Mounedji-Boudiaf et al., "Oxaliplatin, fluorouracil, and leucovorin as adjuvant treatment for colon cancer," *New England Journal of Medicine*, vol. 350, no. 23, pp. 2343–2351, 2004.

[59] S. R. Alberts, M. S. Roh, M. R. Mahoney et al., "Alternating systemic and hepatic artery infusion therapy for resected liver metastases from colorectal cancer: a North Central Cancer Treatment Group (NCCTG)/ National Surgical Adjuvant Breast and Bowel Project (NSABP) phase II intergroup trial, N9945/CI-66," *Journal of Clinical Oncology*, vol. 28, no. 5, pp. 853–858, 2010.

[60] N. Kemeny, W. Jarnagin, M. Gonen et al., "Phase I/II study of hepatic arterial therapy with floxuridine and dexamethasone in combination with intravenous irinotecan as adjuvant treatment after resection of hepatic metastases from colorectal cancer," *Journal of Clinical Oncology*, vol. 21, no. 17, pp. 3303–3309, 2003.

[61] N. E. Kemeny, W. R. Jarnagin, M. Capanu et al., "Randomized phase II trial of adjuvant hepatic arterial infusion and systemic chemotherapy with or without bevacizumab in patients with resected hepatic metastases from colorectal cancer," *Journal of Clinical Oncology*, vol. 29, no. 7, pp. 884–889, 2011.

[62] P. G. Tarazov, "Transcatheter therapy of gastric cancer metastatic to the liver: preliminary results," *Journal of Gastroenterology*, vol. 35, no. 12, pp. 907–911, 2000.

[63] T. Kumada, Y. Arai, K. Itoh et al., "Phase II study of combined administration of 5-fluorouracil, epirubicin and mitomycin-C by hepatic artery infusion in patients with liver metastases of gastric cancer," *Oncology*, vol. 57, no. 3, pp. 216–223, 1999.

[64] H. Ojima, S. Ootake, T. Yokobori et al., "Treatment of multiple liver metastasis from gastric carcinoma," *World Journal of Surgical Oncology*, vol. 5, article 70, 2007.

[65] Y. J. Bang, E. Van Cutsem, and A. Feyereislova, "Trastuzumab in combination with chemotherapy versus chemotherapy alone for treatment of HER2-positive advanced gastric or gastro-oesophageal junction cancer (ToGA): a phase 3, open-label, randomised controlled trial," *The Lancet*, vol. 376, no. 9749, pp. 687–697, 2010.

[66] J. C. Becker, P. Terheyden, E. Kämpgen et al., "Treatment of disseminated ocular melanoma with sequential fotemustine, interferon $\alpha$, and interleukin 2," *British Journal of Cancer*, vol. 87, no. 8, pp. 840–845, 2002.

[67] B. Melichar, Z. Voboril, M. Lojík, and A. Krajina, "Liver metastases from uveal melanoma: clinical experience of hepatic arterial infusion of cisplatin, vinblastine and dacarbazine," *Hepato-Gastroenterology*, vol. 56, no. 93, pp. 1157–1162, 2009.

[68] T. Vogl, K. Eichler, S. Zangos et al., "Preliminary experience with transarterial chemoembolization (TACE) in liver metastases of uveal malignant melanoma: local tumor control and survival," *Journal of Cancer Research and Clinical Oncology*, vol. 133, no. 3, pp. 177–184, 2007.

[69] G. H. Han, Z. X. Yin, X. J. Meng et al., "Prospective randomized clinical trial of two drug delivery pathway in the treatment of inoperable advanced pancreatic carcinoma," *Chinese Journal of Digestive Diseases*, vol. 7, no. 1, pp. 45–48, 2006.

[70] H. Homma, T. Doi, S. Mezawa et al., "A novel arterial infusion chemotherapy for the treatment of patients with advanced pancreatic carcinoma after vascular supply distribution via superselective embolization," *Cancer*, vol. 89, no. 2, pp. 303–313, 2000.

[71] A. Hashimoto, H. Nishiofuku, T. Tanaka et al., "Safety and optimal management of hepatic arterial infusion chemotherapy after pancreatectomy for pancreatobiliary cancer," *American Journal of Roentgenology*, vol. 198, pp. 923–930, 2012.

[72] H. Oettle, S. Post, P. Neuhaus et al., "Adjuvant chemotherapy with gemcitabine vs observation in patients undergoing curative-intent resection of pancreatic cancer: a randomized controlled trial," *Journal of the American Medical Association*, vol. 297, no. 3, pp. 267–277, 2007.

[73] Y. Inaba, Y. Arai, H. Yamaura et al., "Phase I/II study of hepatic arterial infusion chemotherapy with gemcitabine in patients with unresectable intrahepatic cholangiocarcinoma (JIVROSG-0301)," *American Journal of Clinical Oncology*, vol. 34, no. 1, pp. 58–62, 2011.

[74] M. Cantore, A. Mambrini, G. Fiorentini et al., "Phase II study of hepatic intraarterial epirubicin and cisplatin, with systemic 5-fluorouracil in patients with unresectable biliary tract tumors," *Cancer*, vol. 103, no. 7, pp. 1402–1407, 2005.

[75] A. Mambrini, A. Guglielmi, P. Pacetti et al., "Capecitabine plus hepatic intra-arterial epirubicin and cisplatin in unresectable biliary cancer: a phase II study," *Anticancer Research C*, vol. 27, no. 4, pp. 3009–3013, 2007.

[76] S. Matsumoto, H. Kiyosue, E. Komatsu et al., "Radiotherapy combined with transarterial infusion chemotherapy and concurrent infusion of a vasoconstrictor agent for nonresectable advanced hepatic hilar duct carcinoma," *Cancer*, vol. 100, no. 11, pp. 2422–2429, 2004.

[77] S. C. Schiffman, T. Metzger, G. Dubel et al., "Precision hepatic arterial irinotecan therapy in the treatment of unresectable intrahepatic cholangiocellular carcinoma: optimal tolerance and prolonged overall survival," *Annals of Surgical Oncology*, vol. 18, no. 2, pp. 431–438, 2011.

[78] A. Benevento, L. Boni, L. Frediani, A. Ferrari, and R. Dionigi, "Result of liver resection as treatment for metastases from noncolorectal cancer," *Journal of Surgical Oncology*, vol. 74, pp. 24–29, 2000.

[79] D. Christante, S. Pommier, B. Givi, and R. Pommier, "Hepatic artery chemoinfusion with chemoembolization for neuroendocrine cancer with progressive hepatic metastases despite octreotide therapy," *Surgery*, vol. 144, no. 6, pp. 885–894, 2008.

2

# Growing Up: Not an Easy Transition—Perspectives of Patients and Parents regarding Transfer from a Pediatric Liver Transplant Center to Adult Care

**Sona Chandra,[1] Shannon Luetkemeyer,[2] Rene Romero,[2,3] and Nitika Arora Gupta[2,3]**

[1]*Department of Biomedical Engineering, Georgia Institute of Technology, Atlanta, GA 30332, USA*
[2]*Children's Healthcare of Atlanta, Transplant Services, Atlanta, GA 30322, USA*
[3]*Department of Pediatrics, Emory University School of Medicine, Health Science Research Building (HSRB), Suite No. E200, Office No. 216, Atlanta, GA 30322, USA*

Correspondence should be addressed to Nitika Arora Gupta; narorag@emory.edu

Academic Editor: Daisuke Morioka

The transition from pediatric to adult care is a critical time when children with chronic illness sustain high morbidity and mortality. Transition services need to be focused on the adolescents' needs, which may differ from those perceived by healthcare providers. In this study, a survey of 31 patients with chronic liver disease and/or liver transplant who were "transferred" to adult services within the last 3 years was conducted. Patients were asked about their current health status and their perceptions of the overall transfer process. The mean age at transfer was 19.81 (18–21) years. Almost half the patients (47%) were not seen at the adult facility until 2–6 months after leaving the Children's hospital and 20% were not seen until 6–12 months. About 20% had their first contact with adult services through an emergency room visit. About 19% reported being out of medication during transition. Of the transplanted patients, 19% were being evaluated for a retransplant. The majority (82%) felt that an increased emphasis on promoting independence and "letting go" both by parents and by pediatric care providers was critical in their transition to independence and adult care services. This study provides thought-provoking insights, which are critical in designing the ideal transition program for children with chronic diseases.

## 1. Introduction

With improved outcomes of postliver transplantation, a large number of pediatric liver transplant recipients are reaching adulthood [1]. The posttransplantation five-year graft/survival rate for pediatric liver transplant recipients currently ranges from 67% to 82% [2, 3]. Therefore, the need to prepare pediatric liver transplant recipients for the transfer to adult-centered transplant care has increasingly become an important area of investigation.

According to the American Society for Adolescent Medicine, the transfer process should include a planned movement of adolescents with chronic medical conditions that addresses their medical as well as psychological needs as they shift from pediatric to adult-oriented healthcare systems [4, 5]. There are a number of barriers that a young adult transplant patient faces, with the most important one being the development of a sense of autonomy and independence [6]. The suggested level of autonomy before transferring to adult care includes the patient's adequate demonstration of knowledge of the disease and transplant as well as a thorough understanding of the impact on his or her overall health [2]. In addition, the patient should be able to complete his or her medication regimen, refill medications independently, make and attend appointments, and recognize how and when to seek medical attention [7]. Furthermore, avoiding risky behaviors such as poor diet, unsafe sexual activity, drug and alcohol abuse, and bad hygiene is essential to the success of a patient [8]. A fully independent, self-governing, and autonomous adult patient at the time of transfer is a common goal of pediatric healthcare providers.

Patients who have undergone liver transplantation in their childhood are more likely to display a delayed sense of independence and are at risk for medication nonadherence [2]. A recent study revealed that nonadherence ranged from 17% to 53% [9, 10]. Nonadherence can have severe consequences including poor graft survival rates, increased need for clinical visits, and rejection episodes [7].

As pediatric patients approach the age for the transfer to adult care, it is increasingly important for healthcare professionals to effectively equip their adolescent patients with the knowledge and support to cope with the transfer. This study is aimed at assessing the patient/parent perspectives of the transfer process 1–3 years after their transfer to adult care in order to develop a more effective transition program. In addition, the survey asked for suggestions for the improvement of facilities and the changes pediatric caregivers can make to facilitate the above. This information can help caregivers and healthcare providers shape their services to better target patient needs and ultimately encourage independence and autonomy amongst adult patients.

## 2. Materials and Methods

*2.1. Patients and Methods.* Transplant patients, who have previously been transferred from pediatric care at Children's Healthcare of Atlanta to adult care at various different facilities, completed a survey designed to assess the issues they faced during the transition and their suggestions regarding the transfer process. This study was conducted prior to the establishment of a formal transition program at Children's Healthcare of Atlanta and was aimed at patients who had undergone a "simple transfer" process from Children's Healthcare of Atlanta to adult services in the past 3 years. The study was performed as a quality improvement service and data were analyzed retrospectively. It was reviewed and approved for an exemption by the Institutional Review Board of Emory University. All patients who were between 1 and 3 years after transfer to the adult facility were contacted for a survey over the phone. If the patients were unavailable, the survey was conducted with the parents, only if the parents were involved with the care of the child and accompanied them to clinic visits at the Children's hospital. Patients who had been diagnosed with chronic liver disease but had not undergone a transplant were included in this study because they were followed by the same medical team hence facing a similar "transfer" process. Additionally, the challenges faced during the transfer to adult care were very similar to the challenges faced by transplant patients [11]. A nurse navigator who was familiar with the patients and had been closely involved with their care while in the pediatric facility conducted the survey.

*2.2. Survey.* The survey was designed to assess the effectiveness of each patient's transfer via certain key markers of health outcome such as (i) ER visits; (ii) time until the patient's first labs are drawn in the adult care; (iii) liver function tests; (iv) number of rejection episodes; and (v) the evaluation for a new transplant. In addition, the survey asked for any suggestions these patients or parents may have had regarding the transition process such as (vi) additional education on the part of healthcare professionals, (vii) parent involvement and management of their children, and (viii) changes that could be implemented to evolve the current transition process.

Phone survey respondents were primarily given questions with multiple choice answers assessing the basics of their transfer process including, for example, how much medication they were given at the time of transfer as well as the number of emergency room episodes that occurred in the interim period. The respondent additionally had the option of submitting an alternate, "free-form" answer that was not listed for each question. There were three questions which assessed the patient's transfer experience and any suggestions that respondents may have regarding the transfer process (Tables 1–3). The suggestion part of the survey gave several different options for each question so that each person surveyed was able to choose the answer(s) that best reflected their perspective on the transition. The patient or parent surveyed additionally had the option of inputting their own suggestion if it was not listed.

The survey included questions about the patient's medication access and availability for refill because they are important indications of the effectiveness of the transfer. Adherence to immunosuppressant medications is a critical factor in the transfer process as poor medication adherence is associated with an increased risk of poor long-term health outcomes, including increased graft loss and rejection [10, 12].

## 3. Results

*3.1. Patient Demographics.* All patients were within the range of 18–23 years (median age: 20). Majority of them were Caucasians (57%), with 33% being African American and 10% being Hispanic. Females were predominant in this group (70%). Of the 31 survey respondents, 39% were patients, and the remaining 61% were parents of patients. There were 4 patients (or parents) who did not have a working phone number and were unable to be contacted. Hence, our response rate was 31/35 (88.5%).

*3.2. Patient Diagnosis and Transplant Information.* The primary diagnosis for liver transplant and chronic liver disease was reported by the patients and parents and is detailed in Figure 1(a). The largest percentage of surveyed patients had autoimmune hepatitis with the second largest group being biliary atresia. The majority of the patients surveyed had received a liver transplant (67%) with two (6%) receiving both a liver and kidney transplant. The rest of the patients had chronic liver disease of varying etiology (27%) and had not been evaluated for a transplant at the time of transfer (Figure 1(b)).

*3.3. Time Lag between the Last Visit with the Children's Hospital and First Visit with the Adult Facility.* The time elapsed between the last visit at the Children's hospital and the first visit at the adult facility is an important predictor of nonadherence with clinic visits and the possibility of being lost to follow-up [10, 12]. At the time of the survey, it was our center's practice to recommend follow-up with the adult practice within 3 months of transfer from Children's Healthcare of Atlanta. A small number of young adults (17%)

TABLE 1: What can be done to make the transition to adult care easier?

| Suggestion | Parents $n = 19$ | Patients $n = 12$ | Total $n = 31$ |
|---|---|---|---|
| Educate about their disease | 14 | 4 | 18 |
| Educate about insurance | 13 | 4 | 17 |
| Educate about college with transplant | 13 | 3 | 16 |
| Educate about drugs/alcohol/sex | 13 | 4 | 17 |
| Educate about medication | 14 | 4 | 18 |
| Educate about nutrition after transplant | 12 | 3 | 15 |
| Educate about total body care (hygiene, yearly exams, etc.) | 13 | 7 | 20 |
| Educate about support system | 13 | 4 | 17 |
| Make the kids listen | 1 | 1 | 2 |
| Give specific instructions about new place | 0 | 1 | 1 |
| Meet other transitioned teens | 1 | 0 | 1 |
| Teen clinic | 1 | 0 | 1 |
| Nothing | 4 | 3 | 7 |

TABLE 2: How can parents be prepared and help prepare patients for the transition?

| Suggestion | Parents $n = 19$ | Patients $n = 12$ | Total $n = 31$ |
|---|---|---|---|
| Parent support Groups | 16 | 3 | 19 |
| Parents setting boundaries with children with chronic illness | 2 | 1 | 3 |
| Parents/caregivers letting kids grow and do self-care | 8 | 5 | 13 |
| Parents should not be involved in care | 0 | 4 | 4 |
| Review how adult care center works | 1 | 0 | 1 |
| Parents need to be more involved | 2 | 2 | 4 |

TABLE 3: What should be changed to help with transition of care?

| Suggestion | Parents $n = 19$ | Patients $n = 12$ | Total $n = 31$ |
|---|---|---|---|
| Earlier education about facility | 10 | 4 | 14 |
| Let kids learn and not remind them so often | 4 | 6 | 10 |
| Educate about insurance and what to do if you lose it | 1 | 1 | 2 |
| Educate about how to deal with pregnancy | 1 | 0 | 1 |
| Nothing | 1 | 2 | 3 |

were seen within one month of leaving the Children's hospital facilities. The majority of patients (47%) were seen at the new facility 2–6 months after their last scheduled appointment with the Children's hospital. Furthermore, about 20% of the young adults were not seen until between 6 and 12 months and 13% were not seen until after a year (Figure 2(a)). This was regardless of the adult facility they were transferred to.

We also assessed the time until the new facility was first contacted to make/confirm an initial appointment after transfer because this is reflective of the efficiency of the transfer, with 26% of patients contacting between 2 and 4 weeks, 13% between 2 and 3 months, 22% of patients between 4 and 6 months, and 25% not contacting until after six months. Some patients (13%) did not contact the adult facility to make an appointment.

*3.4. Medication Supply at the Time of Transfer.* Through our survey, we wanted to gain insight regarding the patients' adherence to their prescribed medication regimen. In order to accomplish this, we asked direct questions relating to the amount of medication they had at the time of transfer (Figure 3(a)). Interestingly, most patients (68%) had more than 4 months' supply of medication at the time of transfer, with 6.4% having just under 4 months' worth and 9.7% having 2-3 months' supply of medications (Figure 3(a)). This, however, could possibly be a reflection of the pediatric transplant center's prescribing practices rather than the patients themselves. Prior to seeing the adult caregivers, 68% of patients did not run out of medications. Some of the surveyed patients (19%) did run out of medication. The remaining 13% were unable to answer questions or were unsure of the amount of medication in their possession at the time of transfer (Figure 3(b)).

A patient's ability to refill their medication as needed is highly indicative of their autonomy. A majority of the patients (81%) reported that they did not need to refill their medication (Figure 3(c)). The majority of the patients did not run out of their medications (Figure 3(d)). Of the patients who did run out of medication, 67% were able to refill their prescription at some location (50% at the Children's hospital pharmacy, 25% at ER, and 25% other) within 1–7 days. The remaining 33%, representing 6% of the total patients, were not taking their medication.

*3.5. First Contact with the Adult Facility.* Having assessed the medication supply of the patients at the time of transfer and the time lag before they were seen at the adult facility, we wanted to evaluate the health status during the transition prior to first contact with the adult care providers. Interestingly, we found that 23% of the patients had a visit to the emergency room prior to seeing the adult care providers in the outpatient setting. Out of these, the majority (5/7; 77%) had 1-2 visits and 2/7 (29%) had 3–5 visits to the emergency room (Figure 4(a)). After leaving the Children's hospital, almost half of the patients (47%) did not get labs done until more than 3 months after transfer. Only a quarter of the patients reported labs being done within 1–4 weeks after transfer. The remaining 28% had their labs done between 2 and 3 months (Figure 4(b)).

*3.6. Status of Liver Function.* While the timing of getting labs drawn was an important indicator of patient compliance or responsibility, it was also critical to assess the actual status of the disease or disease severity. At the time of the survey,

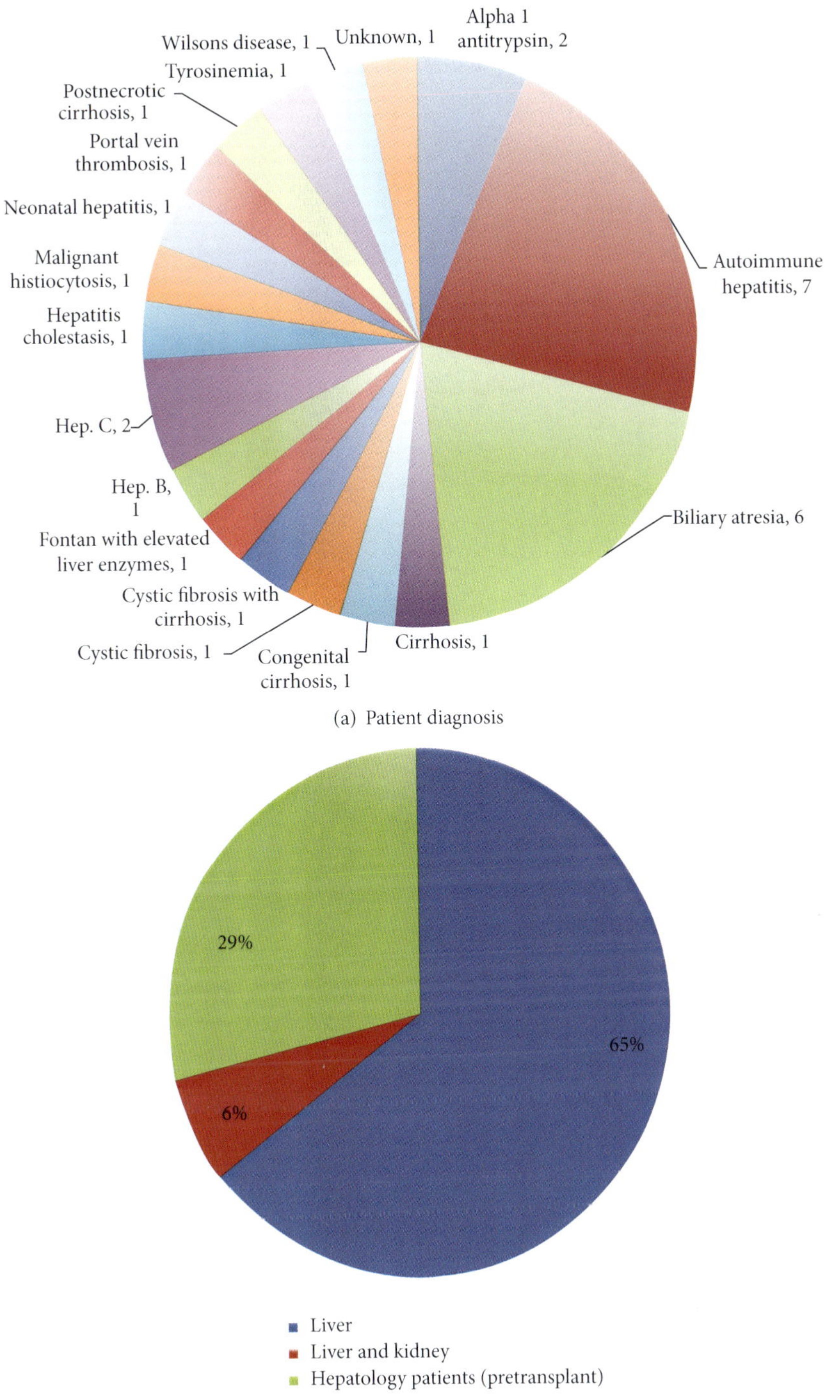


(a) Patient diagnosis



(b) Transplant information

FIGURE 1: Patient diagnosis and transplant information. (a) Patient diagnoses were distributed over a large spectrum and were representative of the larger population of children requiring a liver transplant. (b) Distribution of patients with isolated liver transplantation, liver-kidney combined transplantation, and preliver transplantation.

more than one-third of the patients (39%) reported having abnormal liver function tests (Figure 5(a)), with 10% being diagnosed with acute rejection soon after being transferred from the pediatric facility. Most however had normal liver function and had not had a rejection episode (Figures 5(a) and 5(b)). About 19% of the patients were being evaluated for a new transplant. None of the patients with chronic liver disease were undergoing a transplant evaluation at the time of transfer (Figure 5(c)).

*3.7. Patient and Parent Suggestions for Transition Clinics.* At the time of this survey, the liver transplant service did

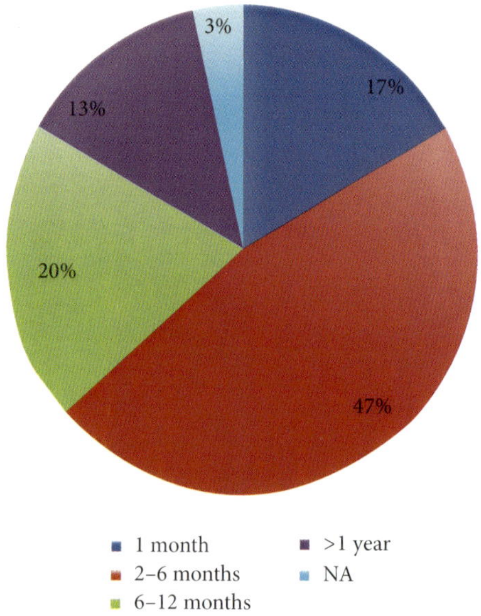


(a) Time elapsed (during transition period)

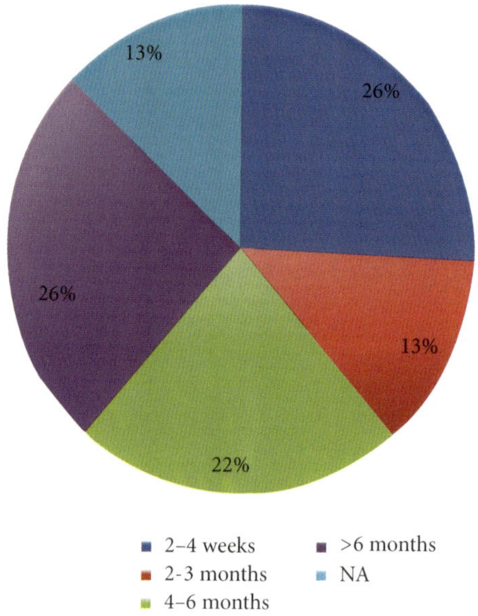


(b) Time until first contact with adult hospital

FIGURE 2: Time lag between the last visit with the Children's hospital and first visit with the adult facility. (a) Time between the last visit at the Children's hospital and the first visit with the adult care facility. (b) Time until first contact with Emory University to make/confirm a clinic appointment.

not have a formal transition process. In order to establish an effective transition clinic, we wanted to assess patient needs and perspectives. We asked the patients who had transferred from the Children's Hospital to the adult services what they felt were the important components to make the transition to adult services smoother and of higher utility. More than half of the survey respondents were the parents. The difference between the suggestions and perceptions of patients and parents was striking. Education about the disease, transition process, insurance, and medications were all deemed extremely important by the parents but by only about quarter of the patients. About half of the patients did feel they needed to be educated about their disease with emphasis on the total body care (Table 1).

When asked about how parents and patients could be better prepared to ensure a smooth transition, a majority of the patients and the parents agreed on one thing: patients needed to be "let go" and empowered in order to assume self-care and independence. 25% of the patients felt that parents needed to be "less" involved in the care of the patients and very few of the parents and patients (10% and 16%, resp.) felt that there needed to be more involvement of the parents. About 50% of the patients felt that they should receive fewer reminders about their healthcare regimen and that the parent should trust them to be capable of self-care (Table 2).

Most parents felt that a parent support group would help them in learning how to empower their children and let them assume independent care, which can be incredibly difficult after several years of taking care of a child with a chronic illness (Table 2). The parents also reported that they would have preferred earlier education about the adult facilities, rather than information at the time of transfer.

It was interesting to note that one-third of the patients/parents felt that repeated reminders should not be given and were actually counterproductive to a good outcome. Of concern was the fact that there was a lack of interest reported from both the patients and parents with regard to education about insurance and what to do in the face of loss of insurance (Table 3).

## 4. Discussion

Liver transplantation is now an accepted treatment for several end stage liver diseases. The survival rate of patients with pediatric transplantation is at an all-time high as the posttransplantation five-year graft/survival rate for pediatric liver transplant recipients currently ranges from 67% to 82% [2, 3, 13, 14]. However, it is also clear by UNOS data that graft loss increases dramatically from ages of 16–30 years [15–17]. Since most pediatric and adult centers operate in their own freestanding hospitals, the process of transfer from pediatric to adult services has been deemed as one of the primary reasons for this graft loss [9, 10, 17]. Adolescents have not been prepared for or are unable to maneuver the demands of the adult healthcare system and hence find themselves lost in the maze leading to increased noncompliance, nonadherence, and eventual graft loss [18].

Our study set out to evaluate patient and parent perspectives of the transfer process in order to determine the key factors, which were critical to the establishment of a successful transition program. We wanted to assess this process from the patients' and parents' viewpoint, instead of exclusively basing it on what was deemed important by caregivers. This study provided us with some interesting

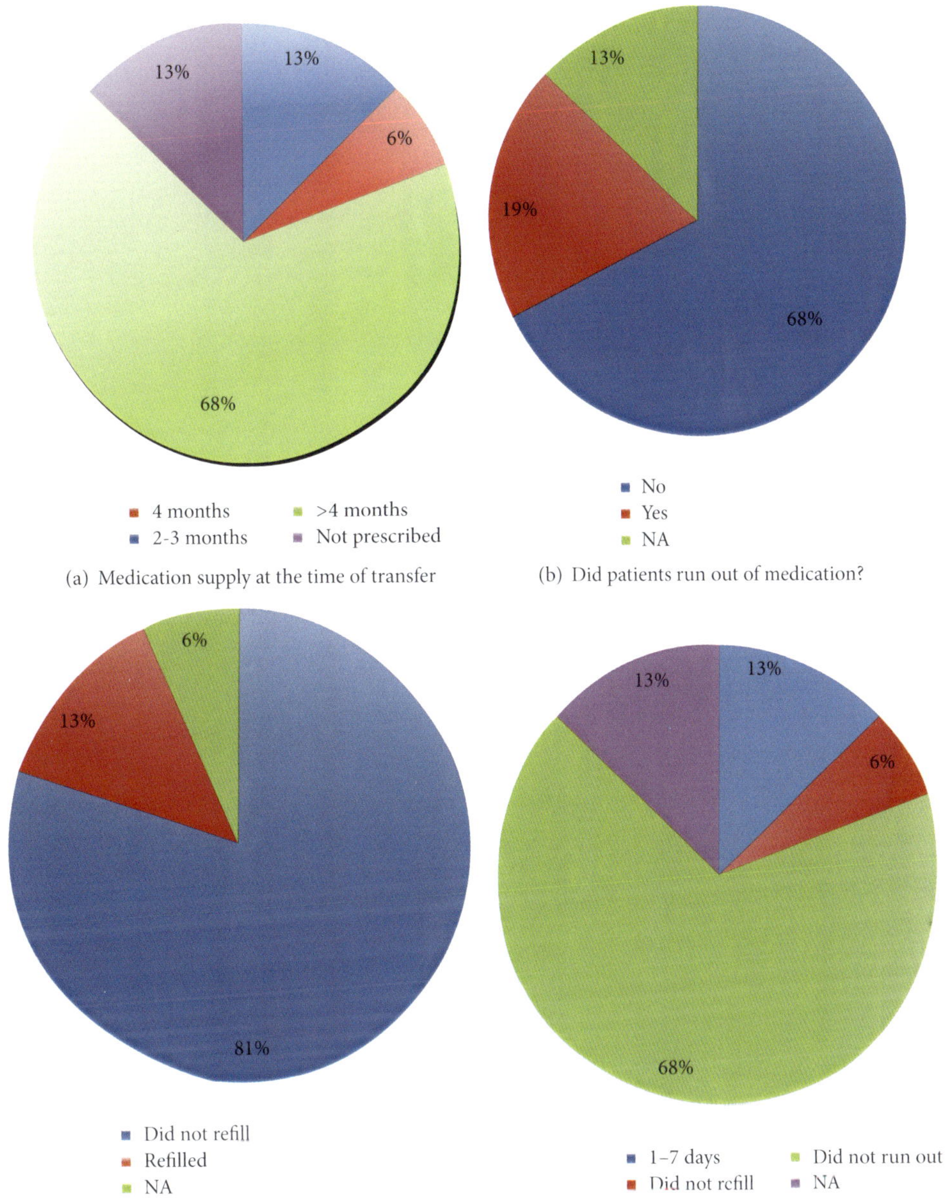


(a) Medication supply at the time of transfer

(b) Did patients run out of medication?

(c) Percent of patients who refilled medication when running out of it

(d) Time until refill

FIGURE 3: Medication supply at the time of transfer. (a) Amount of medication obtained at the time of transfer. (b) Patients who ran out of medications prior to being seen by the adult care facility. (c) Number of patients who refilled their medication prior to being seen by the adult care facility. (d) Time lag between refills.

perspectives, which enabled us to institute key components in the structure of our transition clinics, details of which are discussed below. These insights have applicability to all transition clinics catering to children with a wide variety of chronic diseases.

Most care providers worldwide attempt to provide enough medication refills to the patients prior to transfer [19]. In this study, we found that there was still a significant number who ran out of their medications and did not attempt to refill their prescription, which can be detrimental to the overall health outcomes. Similarly, since graft loss is high during this stressful time of transition, at the time of transfer, it was best to conduct more frequent labs, with the first labs and clinic visit being within one month of transfer, at the adult center [1]. Most of our patients did not make the first contact with the adult services until after 3 months of transfer, with a quarter of patients waiting more than 6–12 months, during which they had emergency room visits. This resulted in a "limbo period" in which the patients were technically "not owned" by any service and were not under the care of any provider, as is evident by the rejection episodes and graft dysfunction. This is a critical period and underlines the importance of instituting measures to bridge this gap.

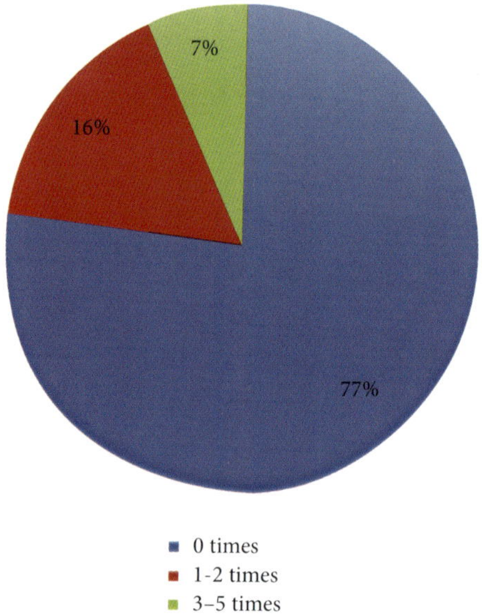


(a) Number of ER visits prior to the visit to the adult facility

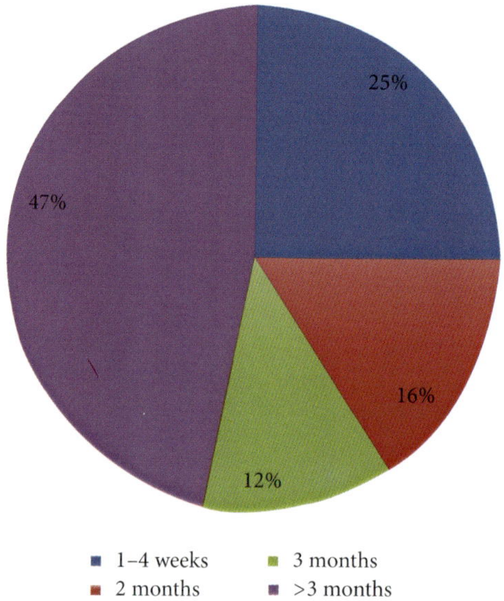


(b) Time until labs drawn at the adult care facility

FIGURE 4: First contact with the adult facility. (a) Number of emergency room visits prior to being seen in the adult facility. (b) Time between last labs at the Children's hospital and when first drawn at the adult facility.

In addition, clinic appointments for the adult care facility are best scheduled prior to transfer since a percentage of patients are likely to show up in the emergency room in critical condition. However, this does not always solve the problem, as it has been reported that patients do not show up for appointments even if they are scheduled beforehand [6, 9, 10, 20]. In order to alleviate some of the anxiety associated with the first visit, we have instituted joint clinics with the adult care providers with the goal that this will alleviate anxiety associated with the first visit and hence encourage the patient to be compliant and work towards building a relationship new care team.

Changes in medication prescription and scheduling of appointments and joint clinics with the adult care providers are structural issues that can be resolved by the medical providers. More difficult are the conceptual and ideological issues associated with pediatric medical teams, who have not only provided care to the children from sometimes as early as infancy and neonatal period, but have also bonded with them to the extent of being part of the "enabling team" along with their parents. The parents and patients both felt that there should be earlier teaching towards independent care and ownership. Neither the parents nor the providers followed the philosophy of "letting go." One example of that was the repeated phone calls and reminders made by the pediatric care team for missed clinic and laboratory appointments.

Based on these recommendations, we changed the structure of a visit within our transition clinics to have a greater focus on self-empowerment and education about adult facilities. Instead of an entire care team seeing the patients during clinic, after the patient is 18 years old, the physician and the nurse saw patients exclusively, as occurs in adult clinics, without the parents being present. They were given the opportunity to voice their concerns and ask for any other care provider who they felt was necessary for them to see, such as the nutritionist, pharmacist, psychologist, and social worker. Updated "the parents" separately. For patients 14–16 years of age, the parents were asked to step out of the room for personal questions only. Between the ages of 16 and 18 years, the physician first saw the patients individually, and the appointment was concluded with the parent in the room. All patients were expected to make their own future appointments and given training to call in their own refills. The transition program was renamed Adolescent Program, "I own It" (AP 101), which emphasized self-care, empowerment, education, and independence.

We also instituted parent support groups, which included sessions on insurance, college courses, and jobs with benefits. This education was also provided to the patients, since it was concerning to see that very few felt education about their insurance was an important issue in the United States, where healthcare is not government provided [21].

As with any retrospective data collection, there were some limitations to this study. Markers of health outcomes (LFTs, rejection episodes, new transplant evaluation, etc.) as well as indicators of adherence, such as medication supply at the time of transfer and the first visit at the adult facility, were based on the responses of patients or parents. This method of data collection is subject to such limitations as lapses in memory or recall bias, which may have resulted in relatively inaccurate responses. While ideally a patient's health outcomes could be drawn from medical records, in this case it was extremely difficult to obtain access to those records considering that this study included patients who had been transferred to a number of different healthcare facilities both within and outside of the state of Georgia. As a result, we chose to rely

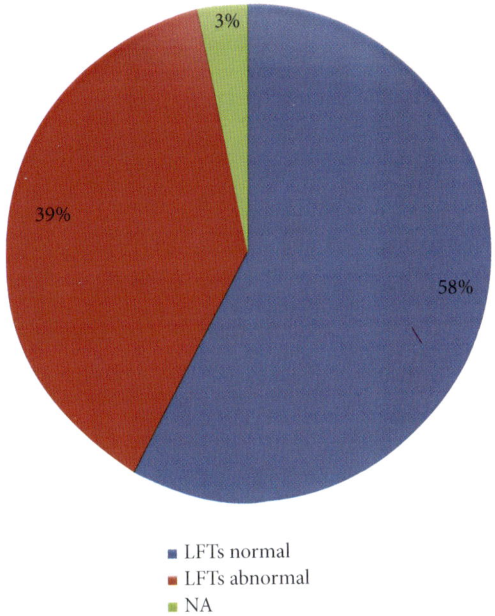


(a) Liver function test (LFT) results

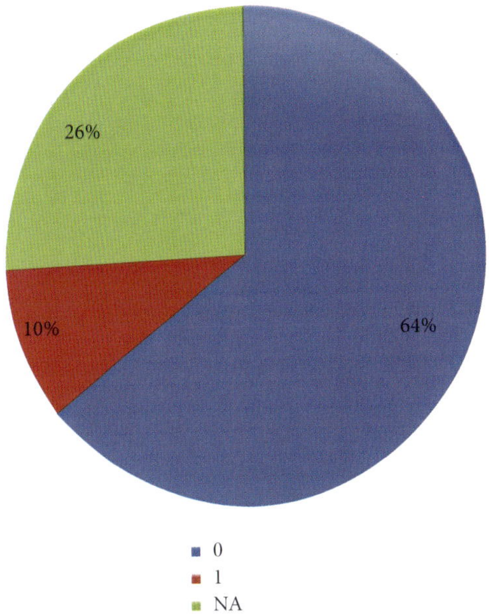


(b) Number of rejection episodes

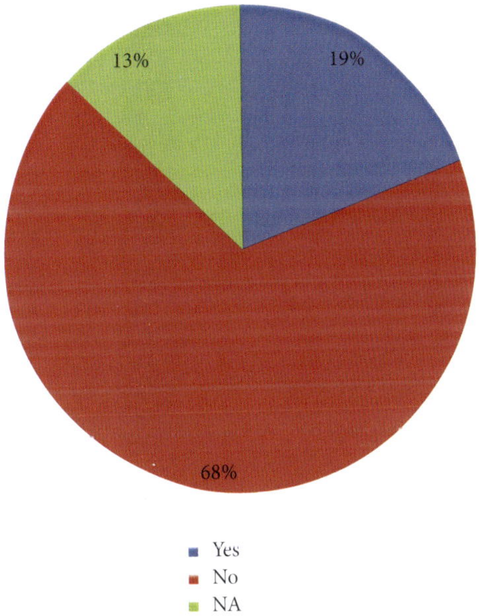


(c) Number of patients evaluated for a new transplant

FIGURE 5: Status of liver function. (a) Status of the liver function tests. (b) Number of rejection episodes. (c) Number of patients evaluated for a new transplant.

on the responses given by the patient or parent. Furthermore, there could be a difference in the accuracy of information provided by a parent or a patient. However, we felt that this gave us a different perspective which also added valuable information.

The study group we chose was limited by its size of 31 survey subjects composed of 12 patients and 18 parents of patients, none of which were patient/parent dyads. We chose a cut-off of 1–3 years since the time of transfer in order to limit the amount of recall bias in the responses. Furthermore, we limited the study to liver transplant recipients and chronic liver disease patients since the same care team managed both, and the education provided to each patient was similar. We could have increased our sample size by introducing kidney and heart transplant patients but chose not to do so to avoid introduction of individual provider and care team practice styles, which may have skewed the data. Additionally, since the outcomes and longevity of the grafts between the solid organs are different [22], we wanted to ensure a uniform study group. Hence, though the study group is small, its strength is that it is homogenous in terms of the disease process and the medical team practices and hence provides valuable information, which was utilized in the organization of the transition services.

## 5. Conclusion

This study provided us with valuable input from the patients who had experienced both the pediatric and adult care in the recent past and were in a unique position to provide genuine and workable solutions towards the establishment of a successful transition process. Implementation of these simple strategies has a global application for children with chronic disease transitioning to the adult services and will go a long way in ensuring safety and good outcomes for young adults.

## Acknowledgment

The authors would like to acknowledge the funding support received from Carlos and Marguerite Mason Trust for this work and subsequent establishment of a transition program.

## References

[1] P. R. Atkison, B. C. Ross, S. Williams et al., "Long-term results of pediatric liver transplantation in a combined pediatric and adult transplant program," *Canadian Medical Association Journal*, vol. 166, no. 13, pp. 1663–1671, 2002.

[2] L. E. Bell, S. M. Bartosh, C. L. Davis et al., "Adolescent transition to adult care in solid organ transplantation: a consensus conference report," *American Journal of Transplantation*, vol. 8, no. 11, pp. 2230–2242, 2008.

[3] E. M. Fredericks, "Nonadherence and the transition to adulthood," *Liver Transplantation*, vol. 15, no. 2, pp. S63–S69, 2009.

[4] R. W. M. Blum, D. Garell, C. H. Hodgman et al., "Transition from child-centered to adult health-care systems for adolescents with chronic conditions: a position paper of the Society for Adolescent Medicine," *Journal of Adolescent Health*, vol. 14, no. 7, pp. 570–576, 1993.

[5] R. Viner, "Transition from paediatric to adult care: bridging the gaps or passing the buck?" *Archives of Disease in Childhood*, vol. 81, no. 3, pp. 271–275, 1999.

[6] C. LaRosa, C. Glah, H. J. Baluarte, and K. E. C. Meyers, "Solid-organ transplantation in childhood: transitioning to adult health care," *Pediatrics*, vol. 127, no. 4, pp. 742–753, 2011.

[7] E. M. Fredericks, M. J. Lopez, J. C. Magee, V. Shieck, and L. Opipari-Arrigan, "Psychological functioning, nonadherence and health outcomes after pediatric liver transplantation," *American Journal of Transplantation*, vol. 7, no. 8, pp. 1974–1983, 2007.

[8] E. Shemesh, R. A. Annunziato, R. Arnon, T. Miloh, and N. Kerkar, "Adherence to medical recommendations and transition to adult services in pediatric transplant recipients," *Current Opinion in Organ Transplantation*, vol. 15, no. 3, pp. 288–292, 2010.

[9] F. Dobbels, R. Van Damme-Lombaert, J. Vanhaecke, and S. De Geest, "Growing pains: non-adherence with the immunosuppressive regimen in adolescent transplant recipients," *Pediatric Transplantation*, vol. 9, no. 3, pp. 381–390, 2005.

[10] R. A. Annunziato, S. Emre, B. Shneider, C. Barton, C. A. Dugan, and E. Shemesh, "Adherence and medical outcomes in pediatric liver transplant recipients who transition to adult services," *Pediatric Transplantation*, vol. 11, no. 6, pp. 608–614, 2007.

[11] P. Vajro, L. Ferrante, S. Lenta, C. Mandato, and M. Persico, "Management of adults with paediatric-onset chronic liver disease: strategic issues for transition care," *Digestive and Liver Disease*, vol. 46, no. 4, pp. 295–301, 2014.

[12] A. R. Watson, "Non-compliance and transfer from paediatric to adult transplant unit," *Pediatric Nephrology*, vol. 14, no. 6, pp. 469–472, 2000.

[13] A. Jain, G. Mazariegos, R. Kashyap et al., "Pediatric liver transplantation in 808 consecutive children: 20-years experience from a single center," *Transplantation Proceedings*, vol. 34, no. 5, pp. 1955–1957, 2002.

[14] R. M. Ghobrial, D. G. Farmer, F. Amersi, and R. W. Busuttil, "Advances in pediatric liver and intestingal transplantation," *The American Journal of Surgery*, vol. 180, no. 5, pp. 328–334, 2000.

[15] E. Sieders, P. M. J. G. Peeters, E. M. TenVergert et al., "Analysis of survival and morbidity after pediatric liver transplantation with full-size and technical-variant grafts," *Transplantation*, vol. 68, no. 4, pp. 540–545, 1999.

[16] I. R. Diamond, A. Fecteau, J. M. Millis et al., "Impact of graft type on outcome in pediatric liver transplantation: a report from Studies of Pediatric Liver Transplantation (SPLIT)," *Annals of Surgery*, vol. 246, no. 2, pp. 301–310, 2007.

[17] P. L. Abt, R. Rapaport-Kelz, N. M. Desai et al., "Survival among pediatric liver transplant recipients: impact of segmental grafts," *Liver Transplantation*, vol. 10, no. 10, pp. 1287–1293, 2004.

[18] J. P. Dommergues, A. Letierce, L. Gravereau, F. Plainguet, O. Bernard, and D. Debray, "Current lifestyle of young adults after liver transplantation during childhood," *American Journal of Transplantation*, vol. 10, no. 7, pp. 1643–1651, 2010.

[19] D. A. Kelly, J. C. Bucuvalas, E. M. Alonso et al., "Long-term medical management of the pediatric patient after liver transplantation: 2013 practice guideline by the American Association for the Study of Liver Diseases and the American Society of Transplantation," *Liver Transplantation*, vol. 19, no. 8, pp. 798–825, 2013.

[20] S. V. McDiarmid, "Management of the pediatric liver transplant patient," *Liver Transplantation*, vol. 7, no. 11, pp. S77–S86, 2001.

[21] L. M. Willoughby, S. Fukami, S. Bunnapradist et al., "Health insurance considerations for adolescent transplant recipients as they transition to adulthood," *Pediatric Transplantation*, vol. 11, no. 2, pp. 127–131, 2007.

[22] D. Bloomm R, L. R. Goldberg, A. Y. Wang, T. W. Faust, and R. M. Kotloff, "An overview of solid organ transplantation," *Clinics in Chest Medicine*, vol. 26, no. 4, pp. 529–543, 2005.

# Outcome following Resection of Biliary Cystadenoma

**M. Pitchaimuthu, G. Aidoo-Micah, C. Coldham, R. Sutcliffe, J. K. Roberts, P. Muiesan, J. Isaac, D. Mirza, and R. Marudanayagam**

*Liver and HPB Unit, Queen Elizabeth Hospital, University Hospitals Birmingham NHS Foundation Trust, Birmingham B15 2TH, UK*

Correspondence should be addressed to M. Pitchaimuthu; drmpitchaimuthu@yahoo.com

Academic Editor: Pierluigi Toniutto

*Background.* Biliary cystadenomas (BCAs) are rare, benign, potentially malignant cystic lesions of the liver, accounting for less than 5% of cystic liver tumours. We report the outcome following resection of biliary cystadenoma from a single tertiary centre. *Methods.* Data of patients who had resection of BCA between January 1993 and July 2014 were obtained from liver surgical database. Patient demographics, clinicopathological characteristics, operative data, and postoperative outcome were analysed. *Results.* 29 patients had surgery for BCA. Male : female ratio was 1 : 28. Clinical presentation was abdominal pain (74%), jaundice (20%), abdominal mass (14%), and deranged liver function tests (3%). Cyst characteristics included septations (48%), wall thickening (31%), wall irregularity (38%), papillary projections (10%), and mural nodule (3%). Surgical procedures included atypical liver resection (52%), left hemihepatectomy (34%), right hemihepatectomy (10%), and left lateral segmentectomy (3%). Median length of stay was 7 (IQ 6.5–8.5) days. Two patients developed postoperative bile leak. No patients had malignancy on final histology. Median follow-up was 13 (IQ 6.5–15.7) years. One patient developed delayed biliary stricture and one died of cholangiocarcinoma 11 years later. *Conclusion.* Biliary cystadenomas can be resected safely with significantly low morbidity. Malignant transformation and recurrence are rare. Complete surgical resection provides a cure.

## 1. Introduction

Biliary cystadenomas (BCAs) are rare, benign, but potentially malignant unilocular or multilocular cystic lesions of the biliary system occurring most commonly in women [1–5]. It commonly arises from the liver, but BCAs of extra hepatic biliary tract and gall bladder have been reported [2, 6–9]. BCAs account for approximately 5% of all hepatic cystic lesions [10].

First publication on BCA was in 1887 and the first resection was performed in 1892 [11]. With the widespread availability of modern imaging techniques and developments in safe liver surgery, the number of reported cases increased in 1990s [12]. Diagnosis of BCA was complicated by the presence of wide variety of cystic lesions in the liver, including simple cysts, parasitic cysts, degenerated metastatic tumours, mucin-producing metastatic tumours, congenital cystic dilatations, cystic hemangioma, lymphangioma, hepatic foregut cysts, mesenchymal hamartoma, and teratoma [5, 13–15]

Due to its premalignant nature and lack of reliability of imaging and preoperative aspiration cytology in differentiating BCA from cystadenocarcinoma, all lesions suspected of BCA should be surgically removed with negative margin [14–21]. We aim to describe and analyse the outcome following resection of BCA from a single tertiary centre.

## 2. Methods

A retrospective analysis of all patients who had resection of BCA was carried out from a prospectively maintained liver surgical and pathological database over a period of 21 years (January 1993 to July 2014). Patients' demographics, clinical presentation, preoperative imaging, operative data and postoperative outcome were analysed. Cystic lesions of the liver were evaluated with ultrasound scan, CT scan, and MRI liver (in selected cases). Cyst characteristics were analysed with respect to number of cysts (single/multiple), locularity (unilocular or multilocular), presence of cyst wall thickening, irregularity, papillary projections, and mural nodule. Cystic lesions showing wall thickening, irregularity, internal septations, presence of nodules, papillary projections, and communication with biliary system were offered surgical resection. Nonanatomical/segmental resection was performed if feasible, but large BCAs and lesions confined to few segments were treated with formal right or left hepatectomy or left lateral segmentectomy. Postoperative complications were recorded according to Dindo et al. classification [22]. Histopathological information regarding completeness of excision, resection margin, and evidence of dysplasia/malignancy were collated. Patients who had partial excision of cyst wall for suspected simple cyst and subsequently found to have BCA were subjected to formal resection. All patients were followed up in the clinic within 6 weeks of surgery and were reviewed in the clinic if necessary thereafter. Patients latest follow-up details were collected from the hospital based computer system and where there was no information available, patient's general practitioners were contacted regarding patients current clinical status.

## 3. Statistical Analysis

Continuous variables were presented as median with interquartile range and the categorical variables were presented in percentages. Survival was calculated using Kaplan-Meier method. SPSS version 22.0 (SPSS, Chicago, IL) was used to perform statistical analysis.

## 4. Results

187 patients with cystic liver lesions underwent surgery during the study period. Of these, 29 patients were found to have BCA. Median age was 62 (IQ 48–74) years and all were women except one. The main clinical presentation was abdominal pain (74%) followed by jaundice (20%), abdominal mass (14%), and deranged liver function tests (LFTs) (3%). Patients who presented with deranged LFTs mainly had elevated transaminases with normal bilirubin. One patient was incidentally found to have a cystic lesion in the liver on ultrasound scan performed for irritable bowel syndrome like symptoms.

On preoperative imaging, single cyst was seen in majority of the patients (76%). Approximately half of the cysts were unilocular ($n$ = 15). Cysts were centrally located in 48% of the cases. Cyst characteristics were as follows: wall thickening (31%), wall irregularity (38%), papillary projections (10%), and mural nodule (3%). Twenty-six (89%) patients were suspected of having BCA on preoperative imaging while the remaining 3 patients were suspected to have simple liver cysts. None of the patients had preoperative cyst fluid cytology, as we believe that negative result will not preclude surgery.

Surgical procedures performed were as follows: nonanatomical liver resection (52%), left hemihepatectomy (34%), right hemihepatectomy (10%), and left lateral segmentectomy (3%). Three patients had formal reresection following histological confirmation of BCA after deroofing of suspected simple liver cysts. Median length of stay was 7 (IQ 6.5–8.5) days. Two patients developed postoperative bile leak. One patient had a low volume bile leak, which was treated conservatively. The other patient developed bile leak following deroofing of suspected simple liver cyst and required an endoscopic biliary stenting to control the high volume bile leak. This patient subsequently had a formal resection following histological confirmation of BCA. Two and three patients each developed wound and chest infection, all of which were treated with antibiotics. There was no perioperative mortality.

On pathological examination, the median size of the cyst was 12 (IQ 8.5–18) cm. On histology, 22 patients had typical ovarian/mesenchymal stroma diagnostic of BCA and 6 patients had no mesenchymal stroma but were positively stained for mucin. Three patients had features of papillary tufting (IPNB) with 2 of them also having the presence of ovarian stroma. Two patients showed calcification in addition to ovarian stroma. None of these patients had evidence of malignancy on final histology.

Median follow-up was 13 (IQ 6.5–15.7) years. One patient developed delayed biliary stricture three years after surgery. This was initially treated with percutaneous transhepatic cholangiogram (PTC) guided dilatation but eventually required Roux-en-Y hepaticojejunostomy, 7 years from the primary surgery. None of our patients developed recurrence of BCA during follow-up. One patient died 11 years later due to development of inoperable cholangiocarcinoma at a different site.

## 5. Discussion

Biliary cystadenomas (BCAs) are potentially malignant, rare benign cystic lesions of the biliary system of unknown aetiology [10, 23]. The incidence of BCA is from one in 20,000 to 100,000 people, while the occurrence of cystadenocarcinoma is approximately one in 10 million patients [17]. Even though the previously published literature quoted the incidence of BCAs to be around 5% of cystic hepatic tumours, the true incidence is still unclear [12, 15, 24]. The controversy is due to lack of established criteria for preoperative diagnosis of unilocular BCAs [6, 12, 14, 16]. Due to its potential for malignant transformation and tendency to recur, there is a great concern in treating this tumour with techniques other than formal resection [3–5].

Aetiology of BCA is unclear and both congenital and acquired origins have been proposed. Presence of hamartomatous structures supports the theory of congenital origin [25]. Cruickshank et al. proposed a theory of acquired lesion and reported the development of BCAs as a reactive process to focal injury [3, 26]. It was also suggested that this might have arisen from ectopic embryonal tissue destined to form gall bladder or from ectopic embryonic rest of primitive foregut sequestered within the liver [3, 24, 27, 28]. Presence of endocrine cells in BCAs and cystadenocarcinomas also suggest the origin from peribiliary glands [29].

Biliary cystadenomas are composed of communicating variable sized locules usually containing clear fluid.

The locules are lined by simple, predominantly columnar epithelium resembling biliary epithelium with cytoplasmic mucin [23]. Edmondson initially defined BCAs in 1958 as multilocular lesions with ovarian-like stroma, but subsequently BCAs without ovarian stroma were reported [5]. Due to this uncertainty WHO, which initially classified these lesions as biliary cystadenoma/adenocarcinoma in 2000, redefined these lesions as either mucinous cystic neoplasm (MCN) or intraductal papillary neoplasm of bile duct (IPN-B) depending on the presence of ovarian stroma and papillary growth within the bile duct, respectively [30–32]. WHO further classified these IPNBs into IPN with low- or intermediate-grade intraepithelial neoplasia, IPN with high-grade intraepithelial neoplasia, and IPN with an associated invasive carcinoma [33]. The majority of biliary cystadenomas do not communicate with the bile ducts, but luminal communication may be occasionally observed [34].

The epithelium may show varying degrees of dysplasia. High-grade dysplasia or invasive carcinoma suggest transformation to cystadenocarcinoma [23]. Devaney et al. proposed three subsets of cystadenocarcinoma based on the pathology material submitted to their institutional laboratories for primary diagnosis or consultation: (1) cystadenocarcinoma originating from a benign cystadenoma with ovarian-like stroma occurs exclusively in women; (2) de novo cystadenocarcinoma occurs almost only in men; and (3) cystadenocarcinoma occurs in women but does not contain an ovarian-like stroma [5].

The development of cystadenocarcinomas is unclear, whether they are de novo cancers or develop from preexisting BCAs. However, it is generally believed that they arise from BCAs as many cystadenocarcinomas contain areas of BCAs in the same sample [3, 24, 28, 35]. A malignant transformation rate of up to 30% has been reported, and biliary cystadenocarcinoma accounts for 0.41% of malignant hepatic epithelial tumours [15, 16, 18, 19, 36, 37]. Elements of BCA were present in 1/3 of biliary cystadenocarcinomas [5, 24]. Wheeler and Edmondson reported malignant change in 23% of the resected BCAs [24]. In our study none of the patients had malignant change in the final histology of resected BCAs. But there were no case-control or cohort studies to define the exact risk of malignant transformation of untreated biliary cystadenoma to cystadenocarcinoma. In the present study also it is unclear, as our patient developed cholangiocarcinoma rather than cystadenocarcinoma many years after the resection of BCA.

Majority of the BCAs present with vague abdominal complaints secondary to extrinsic compression of stomach, duodenum, or biliary tree [5, 24, 38]. In our series, about three quarters of the patients presented with vague abdominal pain. But BCAs have also been identified in asymptomatic patients during imaging or surgical exploration for unrelated clinical conditions [39].

Even with improved imaging techniques, it is still challenging to differentiate BCAs from other cystic lesions of the liver. Differential diagnosis for BCAs includes simple liver cysts, parasitic cysts, haematomas or posttraumatic cysts, liver abscesses, congenital cysts, polycystic disease, Caroli's disease, and neoplastic lesions such as biliary cystadenocarcinoma, undifferentiated embryonal sarcoma, cystic metastasis, metastatic pancreatic or ovarian cystadenocarcinoma, biliary papilloma (IPNB), cystic primary hepatocellular carcinoma, cystic cholangiocarcinoma, and hepatobiliary mesenchymal tumours [2, 32, 40, 41].

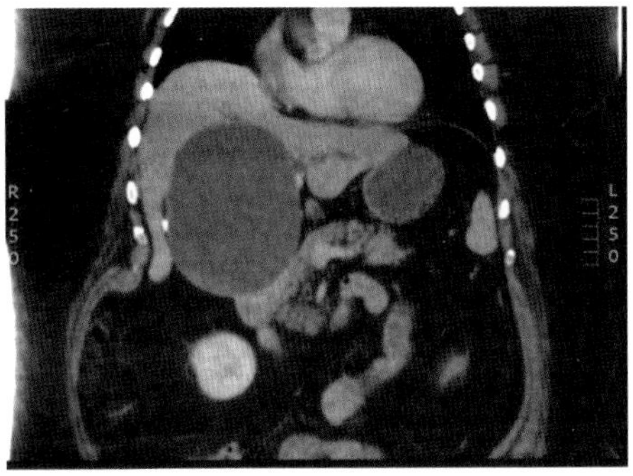

Figure 1: CT scan showing unilocular biliary cystadenoma without any septations but with calcification in the wall.

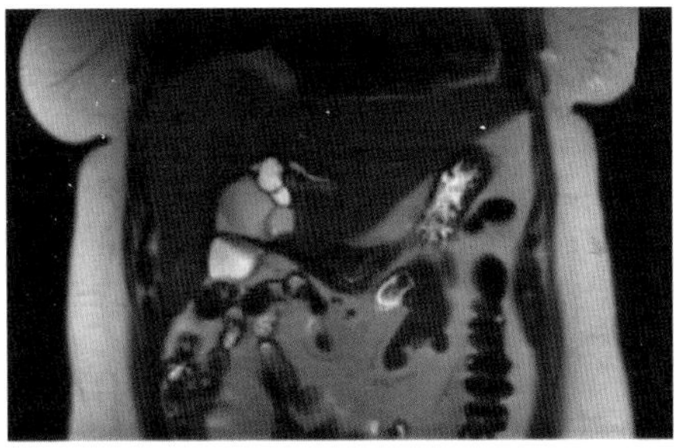

Figure 2: MRI picture showing septated biliary cystadenoma with nodule.

Ultrasound scan, CT (Figure 1), MRI (Figure 2), MRCP, ERCP, intraoperative cholangiography, and choledochoscopy all have been described in the literature for the preoperative work-up of BCA [42–46]. Preoperative radiological diagnostic accuracy may be as low as 30%, so a high index of suspicion is required in the diagnosis of BCA [47].

Although radiologic features such as papillary projections, internal septations, wall thickness, irregularities, and mural nodules suggest the possibility of a BCA, all of these except papillary projections may be observed in simple cysts as well albeit at a lower frequency [48, 49].

Preoperative cyst fluid aspiration for diagnosis has been advocated in the published literature. Cyst fluid CA19-9 and CEA levels can be helpful to enhance the accuracy of diagnosis of BCAs and cystadenocarcinomas from other cystic lesions [10, 17, 50]. However, it is not accurate in differentiating BCAs from cystadenocarcinoma, as inadequate sampling may miss the microscopic foci of carcinoma in a cystadenoma [50–52]. Preoperative differentiation of BCAs from cystadenocarcinoma is extremely difficult and can only be done after pathological examination [1, 3, 24, 28, 39, 41].

FNA and needle biopsy may risk dissemination of tumour cells and it is not generally recommended, especially when surgery is planned [10, 52].

Improper preoperative diagnosis can lead to incorrect and unnecessary procedures such as percutaneous aspiration, ethanol injection, deroofing, and omentoplasty [20]. In our series, 3 patients were diagnosed as simple cysts on imaging but on histological examination were found to be BCAs. These patients had second surgical intervention to remove the lesion with clear margins.

Lewis et al. and Madariaga et al. recommended surgical resection as the treatment of choice for all multiloculated hepatic cystic lesions [16, 53]. If BCA is suspected on imaging, surgery is indicated even if the patient is asymptomatic [1, 24, 28, 39, 52, 54]. The extent of resection remains to be determined, as partial resection with occasional ablation of the residual cyst using electrocautery or argon beam coagulation and/or omentopexy, lobectomy, wedge resection, and enucleation have all been reported [16, 17, 28, 29, 55–57]. Pinson et al. have reported cyst enucleation without late recurrence and mortality [57]. This procedure is a valid alternative where resection is difficult or is likely to be associated with morbidity [10, 14]. In our series, majority of the patients had nonanatomical liver resections. Patients with large BCAs and lesions confined to few segments were treated with formal hepatectomy.

Other limited procedures like aspiration, fenestration, internal drainage, sclerotherapy, and partial resection are associated with extremely high recurrence ranging from 90 to 100%, compared to 0 to 10% with formal resection [4, 14, 16, 20, 52, 55, 58–61]. In our series, all of our patients had formal resection with no recurrence after a median follow-up of 13 (IQ 6.5–15.7) years. Due to its premalignant nature, low radiological diagnostic accuracy, and high recurrence with improper treatment, formal liver resection is recommended.

The prognosis of patients with biliary cystadenoma is good if total excision of the lesion is performed [3, 5, 14, 20, 24, 52]. In the present study the 10-year survival was 90%. Only one patient died of late development of cholangiocarcinoma and 2 other patients died of other causes after 8 and 9 years following resection, respectively.

We conclude that biliary cystadenomas are rare and can be resected safely with significantly low morbidity. Malignant change and recurrence are rare. Complete surgical resection provides a cure.

## Abbreviations

BCA: Biliary cystadenoma
MCN: Mucinous cystic neoplasm
IPNB: Intraductal papillary neoplasm of bile duct.

## Authors' Contribution

M. Pitchaimuthu and R. Marudanayagam initiated the study; M. Pitchaimuthu and G. Aidoo-Micah collected the data; M. Pitchaimuthu and R. Marudanayagam are responsible for data interpretation and paper preparation and submission; all co-authors have actively contributed to the paper reviewing and approved the final paper.

## References

[1] J. Stanley, I. Vujic, S. I. Schabel, R. P. Gobien, and H. D. Reines, "Evaluation of biliary cystadenoma and cystadenocarcinoma," *Gastrointestinal Radiology*, vol. 8, no. 1, pp. 245–248, 1983.

[2] E. Palacios, M. Shannon, C. Solomon, and M. Guzman, "Biliary cystadenoma: ultrasound, CT, and MRI," *Gastrointestinal Radiology*, vol. 15, no. 4, pp. 313–316, 1990.

[3] K. G. Ishak, G. W. Willis, S. D. Cummins, and A. A. Bullock, "Biliary cystadenoma and cystadenocarcinoma: report of 14 cases and review of the literature," *Cancer*, vol. 39, no. 1, pp. 322–338, 1977.

[4] S. S. Florman and D. P. Slakey, "Giant biliary cystadenoma: case report and literature review," *American Surgeon*, vol. 67, no. 8, pp. 727–732, 2001.

[5] K. Devaney, Z. D. Goodman, and K. G. Ishak, "Hepatobiliary cystadenoma and cystadenocarcinoma: a light microscopic and immunohistochemical study of 70 patients," *American Journal of Surgical Pathology*, vol. 18, no. 11, pp. 1078–1091, 1994.

[6] S. G. Delis, Z. Touloumis, A. Bakoyiannis et al., "Intrahepatic biliary cystadenoma: a need for radical resection," *European Journal of Gastroenterology and Hepatology*, vol. 20, no. 1, pp. 10–14, 2008.

[7] K. Kim, J. Choi, Y. Park, W. Lee, and B. Kim, "Biliary cystadenoma of the liver," *Journal of Hepato-Biliary-Pancreatic Surgery*, vol. 5, no. 3, pp. 348–352, 1998.

[8] M. A. Marcial, S. C. Hauser, E. S. Cibas, and J. Braver, "Intrahepatic biliary cystadenoma. Clinical, radiological, and pathological findings," *Digestive Diseases and Sciences*, vol. 31, no. 8, pp. 884–888, 1986.

[9] P. C. Buetow, J. L. Buck, L. Pantongrag-Brown et al., "Biliary cystadenoma and cystadenocarcinoma: clinical-imaging-pathologic correlations with emphasis on the importance of ovarian stroma," *Radiology*, vol. 196, no. 3, pp. 805–810, 1995.

[10] E. Dixon, F. R. Sutherland, P. Mitchell, G. McKinnon, and V. Nayak, "Cystadenomas of the liver: a spectrum of disease," *Canadian Journal of Surgery*, vol. 44, no. 5, pp. 371–376, 2001.

[11] S. W. Henson Jr., H. K. Gray, and M. B. Dockerty, "Benign tumors of the liver. VI. Multilocular cystadenomas," *Surgery, Gynecology, and Obstetrics*, vol. 104, no. 5, pp. 551–554, 1957.

[12] A. Emre, K. R. Serin, I. Özden et al., "Intrahepatic biliary cystic neoplasms: surgical results of 9 patients and literature review," *World Journal of Gastroenterology*, vol. 17, no. 3, pp. 361–365, 2011.

[13] M. F. Hansman, J. A. Ryan Jr., J. H. Holmes IV et al., "Management and long-term follow-up of hepatic cysts," *The American Journal of Surgery*, vol. 181, no. 5, pp. 404–410, 2001.

[14] K. T. Thomas, D. Welch, A. Trueblood et al., "Effective treatment of biliary cystadenoma," *Annals of Surgery*, vol. 241, no. 5, pp. 769–775, 2005.

[15] P. Del Poggio and M. Buonocore, "Cystic tumors of the liver: a practical approach," *World Journal of Gastroenterology*, vol. 14, no. 23, pp. 3616–3620, 2008.

[16] W. D. Lewis, R. L. Jenkins, R. L. Rossi et al., "Surgical treatment of biliary cystadenoma. A report of 15 cases," *Archives of Surgery*, vol. 123, no. 5, pp. 563–568, 1988.

[17] A. Koffron, S. Rao, M. Ferrario, and M. Abecassis, "Intrahepatic biliary cystadenoma: role of cyst fluid analysis and surgical management in the laparoscopic era," *Surgery*, vol. 136, no. 4, pp. 926–936, 2004.

[18] B. J. Ammori, B. L. Jenkins, P. C. M. Lim, K. R. Prasad, S. G. Pollard, and J. P. A. Lodge, "Surgical strategy for cystic diseases of the liver in a western hepatobiliary center," *World Journal of Surgery*, vol. 26, no. 4, pp. 462–469, 2002.

[19] E. Kubota, K. Katsumi, M. Iida et al., "Biliary cystadenocarcinoma followed up as benign cystadenoma for 10 years," *Journal of Gastroenterology*, vol. 38, no. 3, pp. 278–282, 2003.

[20] D. P. Vogt, J. M. Henderson, and E. Chmielewski, "Cystadenoma and cystadenocarcinoma of the liver: a single center experience," *Journal of the American College of Surgeons*, vol. 200, no. 5, pp. 727–733, 2005.

[21] Y. Matsuoka, K. Hayashi, and M. Yano, "Case report: malignant transformation of biliary cystadenoma with mesenchymal stroma: documentation by CT," *Clinical Radiology*, vol. 52, no. 4, pp. 318–321, 1997.

[22] P. A. Clavien, J. Barkun, M. L. De Oliveira et al., "The clavien-dindo classification of surgical complications: five-year experience," *Annals of Surgery*, vol. 250, no. 2, pp. 187–196, 2009.

[23] S. Kakar and L. J. Burgart, "Tumours of the biliary system," *Current Diagnostic Pathology*, vol. 11, no. 1, pp. 34–43, 2005.

[24] D. A. Wheeler and H. A. Edmondson, "Cystadenoma with Mesenchymal Stroma (CMS) in the liver and bile ducts. A clinicopathologic study of 17 cases, 4 with malignant change," *Cancer*, vol. 56, no. 6, pp. 1434–1445, 1985.

[25] P. Devine and A. A. Ucci, "Biliary cystadenocarcinoma arising in a congenital cyst," *Human Pathology*, vol. 16, no. 1, pp. 92–94, 1985.

[26] A. H. Cruickshank and S. M. Sparshott, "Malignancy in natural and experimental hepatic cysts: experiments with aflatoxin in rats and the malignant transformation of cysts in human livers," *The Journal of Pathology*, vol. 104, no. 3, pp. 185–190, 1971.

[27] C. Subramony, G. A. Herrera, and E. A. Turbat-Herrera, "Hepatobiliary cystadenoma. A study of five cases with reference to histogenesis," *Archives of Pathology & Laboratory Medicine*, vol. 117, no. 10, pp 1036–1042, 1993.

[28] G. L. Woods, "Biliary cystadenocarcinoma: case report of hepatic malignancy originating in benign cystadenoma," *Cancer*, vol. 47, no. 12, pp. 2936–2940, 1981.

[29] T. Terada, Y. Kitamura, T. Ohta, and Y. Nakanuma, "Endocrine cells in hepatobiliary cystadenomas and cystadenocarcinomas," *Virchows Archiv*, vol. 430, no. 1, pp. 37–40, 1997.

[30] S. R. Hamilton and L. A. Aaltonen, "Pathology and genetics. Tumors of the digestive system," in *IARC WHO Classification of Tumours*, vol. 2, 2000.

[31] Y. Nakanuma, M. P. Curado, S. Franceschi, G. Gores, V. Paradis, and B. Sripa, "WHO classification of tumours of the digestive system," *World Health Organization Classification of Tumours*, vol. 3, pp. 217–224, 2010.

[32] M. Ohtsuka, H. Shimizu, A. Kato et al., "Intraductal papillary neoplasms of the bile duct," *International Journal of Hepatology*, vol. 2014, Article ID 459091, 10 pages, 2014.

[33] Y. Nakanuma, M. P. Curabo, S. Franceschi et al., "Intrahepatic cholangiocarcinoma," in *WHO Classification of Tumours of the Digestive System*, F. Bosman, F. Carneiro, R. H. Hruban, and N. D. Theise, Eds., pp. 217–227, IARC, Lyon, France, 4th edition, 2010.

[34] S. Ahanatha Pillai, V. Velayutham, S. Perumal et al., "Biliary cystadenomas: a case for complete resection," *HPB Surgery*, vol. 2012, Article ID 501705, 6 pages, 2012.

[35] T. Nakajima, I. Sugano, O. Matsuzaki et al., "Biliary cystadenocarcinoma of the liver. A clinicopathologic and histochemical evaluation of nine cases," *Cancer*, vol. 69, no. 10, pp. 2426–2432, 1992.

[36] R. A. Willis, "Carcinoma arising in congenital cysts of the liver," *The Journal of Pathology and Bacteriology*, vol. 55, no. 4, pp. 492–495, 1943.

[37] P. R. Craig Jr. and H. A. Edmonson, *Tumors of the Liver and Intrahepatic Bile Ducts*, Atlas of Tumour Pathology, fascicle 26, Armed Forces Institute of Pathology, Washington, DC, USA, 2nd edition, 1989.

[38] V. van Roekel, W. J. Marx, W. Baskin, and R. L. Greenlaw, "Cystadenoma of the liver," *Journal of Clinical Gastroenterology*, vol. 4, no. 2, pp. 167–172, 1982.

[39] P. Fiamingo, M. Veroux, U. Cillo, S. Basso, A. Buffone, and D. F. D'Amico, "Incidental cystadenoma after laparoscopic treatment of hepatic cysts: which strategy?" *Surgical Laparoscopy, Endoscopy and Percutaneous Techniques*, vol. 14, no. 5, pp. 282–284, 2004.

[40] N. A. C. S. Wong, I. D. R. Arnott, I. Pope et al., "Hepatobiliary cystadenoma with mesenchymal stroma may mimic biliary smooth muscle neoplasms," *Histopathology*, vol. 39, no. 4, pp. 434–436, 2001.

[41] M. P. Frick and S. B. Feinberg, "Biliary cystadenoma," *American Journal of Roentgenology*, vol. 139, no. 2, pp. 393–395, 1982.

[42] M. P. Federle, R. A. Filly, and A. A. Moss, "Cystic hepatic neoplasms: complementary roles of CT and sonography," *American Journal of Roentgenology*, vol. 136, no. 2, pp. 345–348, 1981.

[43] W. F. Short, A. Nedwich, H. A. Levy, and J. M. Howard, "Biliary cystadenoma. Report of a case and review of the literature," *Archives of Surgery*, vol. 102, no. 1, pp. 78–80, 1971.

[44] M. Lewin, N. Mourra, I. Honigman et al., "Assessment of MRI and MRCP in diagnosis of biliary cystadenoma and cystadenocarcinoma," *European Radiology*, vol. 16, no. 2, pp. 407–413, 2006.

[45] W. van Steenbergen, E. Ponette, G. Marchal et al., "Cystadenoma of the common bile duct demonstrated by endoscopic retrograde cholangiography: an uncommon cause of extrahepatic obstruction," *American Journal of Gastroenterology*, vol. 79, no. 6, pp. 466–470, 1984.

[46] E. J. Udoff, D. P. Harrington, S. L. Kaufman, and J. L. Cameron, "Cystadenoma of the common bile duct demonstrated by percutaneous transhepatic cholangiography," *The American Surgeon*, vol. 45, no. 10, pp. 662–664, 1979.

[47] B. I. Choi, J. H. Lim, M. C. Han et al., "Biliary cystadenoma and cystadenocarcinoma: CT and sonographic findings," *Radiology*, vol. 171, no. 1, pp. 57–61, 1989.

[48] P. C. Buetow and R. B. Midkiff, "MR imaging of the liver. Primary malignant neoplasms in the adult," *Magnetic Resonance Imaging Clinics of North America*, vol. 5, no. 2, pp. 289–318, 1997.

[49] H. K. Choi, J. K. Lee, K. H. Lee et al., "Differential diagnosis for intrahepatic biliary cystadenoma and hepatic simple cyst: significance of cystic fluid analysis and radiologic findings," *Journal of Clinical Gastroenterology*, vol. 44, no. 4, pp. 289–293, 2010.

[50] M. M. Pinto and A. D. Kaye, "Fine needle aspiration of cystic liver lesions. Cytologic examination and carcinoembryonic antigen assay of cyst contents," *Acta Cytologica*, vol. 33, no. 6, pp. 852–856, 1989.

[51] R. Logroño, B. A. Rampy, and P. A. Adegboyega, "Fine needle aspiration cytology of hepatobiliary cystadenoma with mesenchymal stroma," *Cancer*, vol. 96, no. 1, pp. 37–42, 2002.

[52] S. Hai, K. Hirohashi, T. Uenishi et al., "Surgical management of cystic hepatic neoplasms," *Journal of Gastroenterology*, vol. 38, no. 8, pp. 759–764, 2003.

[53] J. R. Madariaga, S. Iwatsuki, T. E. Starzl, S. Todo, R. Selby, and G. Zetti, "Hepatic resection for cystic lesions of the liver," *Annals of Surgery*, vol. 218, no. 5, pp. 610–614, 1993.

[54] D. T. Kehagias, B. V. Smirniotis, A. C. Pafiti, A. E. Kalovidouris, and L. J. Vlahos, "Quiz case of the month. Biliary cystadenoma," *European Radiology*, vol. 9, no. 4, pp. 755–756, 1999.

[55] S. Lei and J. M. Howard, "Biliary cystadenocarcinoma arising from benign cystadenoma," *Archives of Surgery*, vol. 127, no. 12, p. 1478, 1992.

[56] K. A. Forde, M. Wolff, S. L. Fuld, and J. B. Price, "Hepatic lobectomy for biliary cystadenoma," *American Surgeon*, vol. 40, no. 11, pp. 647–650, 1974.

[57] C. W. Pinson, J. L. Munson, R. L. Rossi, and J. W. Braasch, "Enucleation of intrahepatic biliary cystadenomas," *Surgery Gynecology and Obstetrics*, vol. 168, no. 6, pp. 535–537, 1989.

[58] Y. M. Tan, L. L. Ooi, K. C. Soo, and P. O. P. Mack, "Does laparoscopic fenestration provide long-term alleviation for symptomatic cystic disease of the liver?" *ANZ Journal of Surgery*, vol. 72, no. 10, pp. 743–745, 2002.

[59] C. J. Cahill and M. E. Bailey, "Biliary cystadenoma," *American Journal of Roentgenology*, vol. 140, no. 3, p. 630, 1983.

[60] A. Taketomi, R. Tamada, K. Takenaka, R. Kawano, T. Maeda, and K. Sugimachi, "A case of biliary cystadenoma with obstructive jaundice," *Oncology Reports*, vol. 5, no. 4, pp. 833–835, 1998.

[61] M. E. Forrest, K. J. Cho, J. J. Shields, J. D. Wicks, T. M. Silver, and T. L. McCormick, "Biliary cystadenomas: sonographic-angiographic-pathologic correlations," *American Journal of Roentgenology*, vol. 135, no. 4, pp. 723–727, 1980.

# 4

# Targeting Interleukin-4 Receptor Alpha by Hybrid Peptide for Novel Biliary Tract Cancer Therapy

**Kahori Seto,[1,2] Junichi Shoda,[3] Tomohisa Horibe,[2] Eiji Warabi,[4] Masayuki Kohno,[2] Toru Yanagawa,[1] Hiroki Bukawa,[1] Yasuni Nakanuma,[5] and Koji Kawakami[2]**

[1] *Department of Oral and Maxillofacial Surgery, Clinical Sciences, University of Tsukuba, Ibaraki 305-8575, Japan*
[2] *Department of Pharmacoepidemiology, Graduate School of Medicine and Public Health, Kyoto University, Yoshida Konoe-cho, Sakyo-ku, Kyoto 606-8501, Japan*
[3] *Medical Science, Faculty of Medicine, University of Tsukuba, Ibaraki 305-8575, Japan*
[4] *Division of Biomedical Science, Faculty of Medicine, University of Tsukuba, Ibaraki 305-8575, Japan*
[5] *Department of Human Pathology, Graduate School of Medical Science, Kanazawa University, Kanazawa 920-1192, Japan*

Correspondence should be addressed to Koji Kawakami; kawakami.koji.4e@kyoto-u.ac.jp

Academic Editor: Chawalit Pairojkul

It is known that the interleukin-4 receptor $\alpha$ (IL-4R$\alpha$) is highly expressed on the surface of various human solid tumors. We previously designed novel IL-4R$\alpha$-lytic hybrid peptide composed of binding peptide to IL-4R$\alpha$ and cell-lytic peptide and reported that the designed IL-4R$\alpha$-lytic hybrid peptide exhibited cytotoxic and antitumor activity both *in vitro* and *in vivo* against the human pancreatic cancer cells expressing IL-4R$\alpha$. Here, we evaluated the antitumor activity of the IL-4R$\alpha$-lytic hybrid peptide as a novel molecular targeted therapy for human biliary tract cancer (BTC). The IL-4R$\alpha$-lytic hybrid peptide showed cytotoxic activity in six BTC cell lines with a concentration that killed 50% of all cells ($IC_{50}$) as low as 5 $\mu$M. We also showed that IL-4R$\alpha$-lytic hybrid peptide in combination with gemcitabine exhibited synergistic cytotoxic activity *in vitro*. In addition, intravenous administration of IL-4R$\alpha$-lytic hybrid peptide significantly inhibited tumor growth in a xenograft model of human BTC *in vivo*. Taken together, these results indicated that the IL-4R$\alpha$-lytic hybrid peptide is a potent agent that might provide a novel therapy for patients with BTC.

## 1. Introduction

Biliary tract cancer such as gallbladder cancer and extrahepatic bile duct cancer as well as intrahepatic bile duct cancer (one of the primary liver cancers) is likely to undergo metastasis to the peritoneum (peritoneal dissemination) or the liver at early stages and is often resistant to conventional chemotherapy and radiotherapy. These cancers have been thus viewed as intractable cancers unlikely to be cured completely. In Japan, the incidence of biliary tract cancer and intrahepatic bile duct cancer is about 10 out of every 100,000 people [1]. As for intrahepatic bile duct cancer, both the incidence and death rate have been rising in Japan in recent years, resembling the trend observed in western countries [2, 3]. In Japan, gemcitabine and S-1 have recently begun to be used for anticancer chemotherapy, and these drugs are expected to prolong the survival period of patients as compared to existing anticancer drugs [4]. However, because of frequent adverse events of the hematological system arising from these drugs and because of compromised hepatic function often noted in patients with intrahepatic bile duct cancer due to accompanying liver cirrhosis and in those with extrahepatic bile duct cancer or gallbladder cancer due to accompanying obstructive cholestasis, treatment with these drugs has to be discontinued or stopped. To improve the outcome of treatment of these cancers, it is very important to identify the tumor biological factors involved in the progression (e.g., infiltration and metastasis) of the cancers and to develop new valid means of auxiliary treatment targeted at these factors.

Based on the immunohistochemical analysis showing that cultured BTC cell lines and cancerous epithelia in BTC tissue expressed receptors for interleukin-4 (IL-4) *in situ* at high densities, we previously tested the antitumor effects of IL-4-PE, a cytotoxin composed of an interleukin-4 (IL-4) targeting moiety and a truncated form of *Pseudomonas* exotoxin, on human BTC cells [5]. The results showed a significant regression of established BTC tumors and a significant prolongation of the survival of animals with the disseminated tumors [5, 6]. IL-4-PE was previously tested in the clinic for the treatment of human solid tumors [7–10]. However, against expectation of these promising results, the clinical application of IL-4-PE faced many challenges, including nonspecific toxicities and immunogenicity [11].

To overcome these issues, we have recently developed a "hybrid peptide," composed of target-binding and cytotoxic sequences containing cationic-rich D- and L-amino acids to form amphipathic partial $\alpha$-helices that disrupt the cancer cell membrane selectively and are stable when combined with a cancer-targeting moiety [12]. Peptide drugs are relatively easily synthesized using either recombinant or solid-phase chemical synthesis techniques and the production costs are generally affordable when compared to antibody-based therapeutics [12]. The hybrid peptides targeting EGFR, transferrin receptor, Hsp90, neuropilin-1, and interleukin-4 receptor $\alpha$ (IL-4R$\alpha$) have shown cytotoxic activity *in vitro* and antitumor activity *in vivo* against human solid tumors [12–17]. The IL-4R$\alpha$-lytic hybrid peptide is composed of an IL-4R$\alpha$-binding moiety and a cellular-membrane-lytic moiety [17]. Although the biological significance of IL-4R$\alpha$ expression of cancer cells remains unclear, this receptor is a candidate applicable for molecular targeted cancer therapy.

Here, we describe the cytotoxic activity by IL-4R$\alpha$-lytic hybrid peptide toward BTC cell lines which overexpress IL-4R$\alpha$ *in vitro*. We also show the synergetic effect of IL-4R$\alpha$-lytic hybrid peptide with gemcitabine against BTC cells *in vitro* and that this hybrid peptide induces the significant regression of established human xenograft BTC tumor model in mouse *in vivo*.

## 2. Materials and Methods

*2.1. Cell Lines and Culture Conditions.* The experiments were performed on 4 human cholangiocarcinoma cell lines, KMBC [18] from Dr. M. Kojiro (Kurume University School of Medicine, Kurume, Japan), Sk-ChA-1 [19] from Dr. A. Knuth (Johannes Gutenberg University, Mainz, Germany), CCKS-1 [20] from Dr. Y. Nakanuma (Kanazawa University Graduate School, Kanazawa, Japan), and KKU-100 [21, 22] from Dr. B. Sripa (Khon Kaen University, Thailand), and on 2 human gallbladder carcinoma cell lines: TGBC-1-TKB and TGBC-44-TKB [23] from Dr. T. Todoroki (University of Tsukuba, Ibaraki, Japan). All BTC cells were cultured in RPMI 1640 medium containing 10% heat-inactivated fetal calf serum (Invitrogen, Carlsbad, CA, USA) in a humidified atmosphere with 5% $CO_2$ at 37°C.

*2.2. Peptides.* IL-4R$\alpha$-lytic hybrid peptide, KQLIRFLKRL-DRNGGGKL**L**LK**L**L**KK**LLK**L**LKKK (bold and underlined letters correspond to D-amino acids), and lytic peptide, KL**L**LK**L**L**KK**LLK**L**LKKK, were synthesized by Invitrogen (Carlsbad, CA, USA). Peptides were dissolved in water and buffered to pH 7.4 as described previously [17].

*2.3. Immunoblot Analysis.* Immunoblot analysis was carried out as described previously [5]. Briefly, whole-cell extracts were obtained using buffer containing 1% (v/v) Triton X-100, 0.1% (w/v) SDS, and 0.5% (w/v) sodium deoxycholate, separated by SDS/PAGE, and transferred onto a PVDF membrane. IL-4R$\alpha$ antibody was used at dilution 1 : 100 (Santa Cruz Biotechnology, CA, USA) and $\beta$-actin was used as the internal control (R&D Systems, Minneapolis, MN, USA). After treatment with horseradish peroxidase-conjugated anti-mouse IgG antibody, proteins were visualized on Hyperfirm using an enhanced chemiluminescence/western blotting system (GE Healthcare, Piscataway, NJ, USA).

*2.4. Cell Viability Assay.* Cell viability assay was performed as described previously [12]. Briefly, cells were seeded into 96-well plates at $3 \times 10^3$ cells per well in 90 $\mu$L medium and incubated at 37°C for 24 hours. Each peptide (IL-4R$\alpha$-lytic hybrid peptide and lytic peptide) was diluted in 10 $\mu$L culture medium and added to the cells. The concentration range of peptide we used was from 0 to 20 $\mu$M. After 72 hours of incubation, the cell viability assay using WST-8 solution (Nacalai Tesque, Kyoto, Japan) was performed.

*2.5. Combination Assay of Peptide and Gemcitabine.* The *in vitro* cytotoxic activity of IL-4R$\alpha$-lytic hybrid peptide and gemcitabine was measured as cell viability assay. The synergistic effect of IL-4R$\alpha$-lytic hybrid peptide and gemcitabine was assessed at a concentration ratio of 1 : 1, using the combination index (CI), where CI $< 1$, CI $= 1$, and CI $> 1$ indicate synergistic, addictive, and antagonistic effects, respectively. The CI value was calculated as described previously [24].

*2.6. Antitumor Activity of IL-4R$\alpha$-Lytic Hybrid Peptide in Xenografted Tumor Model of Human BTC.* Animal experiments were carried out in accordance with the guidelines of Tsukuba University. $1 \times 10^6$ TGBC-44-TKB cells resuspended in 150 $\mu$L phosphate-buffered saline were inoculated subcutaneously into the flank region of 4- to 6-week-old athymic female nude mice weighing 17–20 g. When the tumor reached 20–60 mm$^3$ in volume, the animals were assigned randomly to 3 groups: saline (control) and IL-4R$\alpha$-lytic hybrid peptide (2 or 5 mg/kg) injected intravenously (50 $\mu$L/injection) three times a week for a total of nine times. Each group had 6 animals ($n = 6$). Tumors were measured with a caliper and the tumor volume (in mm$^3$) was calculated using the formula length $\times$ width$^2$ $\times 0.5$.

*2.7. Statistics.* Values were given as mean $\pm$ SD (standard deviation), and the differences were analyzed using a one-way ANOVA with Dunnett's test. Differences were considered to be statistically significant at $P < 0.05$.

Table 1: Cytotoxic activity of IL-4Rα-lytic hybrid peptide against BTC.

| Cell line | $IC_{50}$ (μM) | | $IC_{50}$ ratio |
|---|---|---|---|
| | Lytic peptide alone | IL-4Rα-lytic peptide | (Lytic/IL-4Rα-lytic ) |
| TGBC-1-TKB | 16.99 ± 1.28 | 2.17 ± 0.54 | 7.83 |
| TGBC-44-TKB | 21.37 ± 4.91 | 3.27 ± 0.51 | 6.53 |
| CCKS-1 | 15.83 ± 0.02 | 2.73 ± 1.26 | 5.80 |
| KKU-100 | 18.93 ± 3.85 | 2.99 ± 1.01 | 6.34 |
| KMBC | 18.50 ± 1.65 | 3.25 ± 1.36 | 5.69 |
| SK-1 | 13.44 ± 0.42 | 4.47 ± 0.40 | 3.00 |

$IC_{50}$ values (peptide concentration inducing 50% inhibition of control cell growth) are represented as mean ± SD from triplicate determinations.

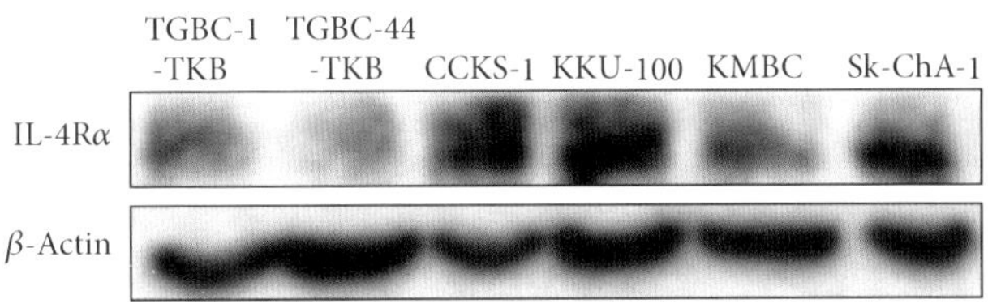


Figure 1: Expression levels of IL-4Rα in BTC cells. Cell lysates were prepared from six BTC cell lines. β-Actin was used as an internal control.

Table 2: Combination therapy of hybrid peptide and GEM.

| | $IC_{50}$ | CI |
|---|---|---|
| IL-4R hybrid peptide (μM) | 4.47 | |
| Gemcitabine (nM) | 12.2 | |
| IL-4R hybrid peptide (μM) + gemcitabine 0.3 nM | 4.29 | 0.95 |
| IL-4R hybrid peptide (μM) + gemcitabine 3 nM | 3.25 | 0.75 |

CI (combination index) < 1, CI = 1, and CI > 1 indicate synergistic, addictive, and antagonistic effect, respectively.

## 3. Results

*3.1. Expression of IL-4Rα in BTC Cell Lines.* Immunoblot analysis demonstrated that IL-4Rα protein is expressed in all cultured BTC cell lines used in this study. As shown in Figure 1, the expression levels of IL-4Rα protein were the highest in intrahepatic cholangiocarcinoma cell lines (CCKS-1 and KKU-100) among tested cell lines. On the other hand, it was also confirmed that gallbladder carcinoma cell lines (TGBC-1-TKB and TGBC-44-TKB) and extrahepatic cholangiocarcinoma cell lines (KMBC and Sk-ChA-1) expressed IL-4Rα, although the expression levels were lower than those of CCKS-1 and KKU-100 cells.

*3.2. Cytotoxic Activity of IL-4Rα-Lytic Hybrid Peptide in BTC Cell Lines.* To assess the *in vitro* cytotoxic activity of IL-4Rα-lytic hybrid peptide to BTC cell lines, the WST assay was performed using BTC cell lines treated with IL-4Rα-lytic hybrid peptide and lytic peptide (Figure 2). TGBC-1-TKB, TGBC-44-TKB, CCKS-1, KKU-100, and KMBC were sensitive to IL-4Rα-lytic hybrid peptide; the concentration that killed 50% of all cells ($IC_{50}$) was less than 3.5 μM. Sk-ChA-1 was also sensitive to IL-4Rα-lytic hybrid peptide with an $IC_{50}$ of less than 4.5 μM. In contrast, optimal cell killing was not induced in these cells by lytic peptide. The cytotoxic activity of the hybrid peptide was strongly enhanced when compared with that of the lytic peptide. The cytotoxic activity of IL-4Rα-lytic hybrid peptide increased 3.0–7.8-fold stronger than that of lytic peptide in BTC cell lines (Table 1).

*3.3. Synergistic Cytotoxicity of IL-4Rα-Lytic Hybrid Peptide and Gemcitabine in BTC Cells.* Gemcitabine alone mediated a dose-dependent cytotoxicity with $IC_{50}$ of 12 nM in Sk-ChA-1. When it combined with IL-4Rα-lytic hybrid peptide, cytotoxicity in Sk-ChA-1 was greatly enhanced (Figure 3). $IC_{50}$ of IL-4Rα-lytic hybrid peptide was 4.29 and 3.25 μM by adding 0.3 and 3 nM of gemcitabine, respectively (Table 2). The combination index was <1 at all concentrations of gemcitabine. The same phenomenon was also observed in TGBC-44-TKB (data not shown).

*3.4. In Vivo Antitumor Activity by IL-4Rα-Lytic Hybrid Peptide in a Human BTC Xenograft Model.* Following the observation that IL-4Rα-lytic hybrid peptide was remarkably cytotoxic to BTC cell lines *in vitro* (Figure 2), the antitumor activity of the hybrid peptide was assessed in a xenograft model of human BTC. TGBC-44-TKB cells were inoculated subcutaneously into athymic nude mice and then the animals were treated with IL-4Rα-lytic hybrid peptide by intravenous injection. As shown in Figure 4, tumors grew aggressively in control mice injected with saline alone, reaching a volume of 1285 $mm^3$ by day 22. In contrast, mice treated with IL-4Rα-lytic hybrid peptide showed significant tumor regression at both dosages: mean tumor volumes were 1025 $mm^3$ (2 mg/kg) and 594 $mm^3$ (5 mg/kg) on day 22. The tumor volume was inhibited significantly at a dose of 5 mg/kg ($P < 0.05$). No other abnormalities, such as loss of appetite and body weight, were observed in mice injected with IL-4Rα-lytic hybrid peptide (data not shown). The number of leukocytes (the mean ($\times 10^3$) and SD values) after the experiments is as follows: control group: 5.1 ± 2.1, 2 mg/kg group: 5.6 ± 4.0, and 5 mg/kg group: 6.6 ± 4.7, and there are no significant differences in each group. Histological analysis also showed no side effects in tissue from the major organs, including liver and kidney, which were obtained from mice treated with intravenous administration of IL-4Rα-lytic hybrid peptide

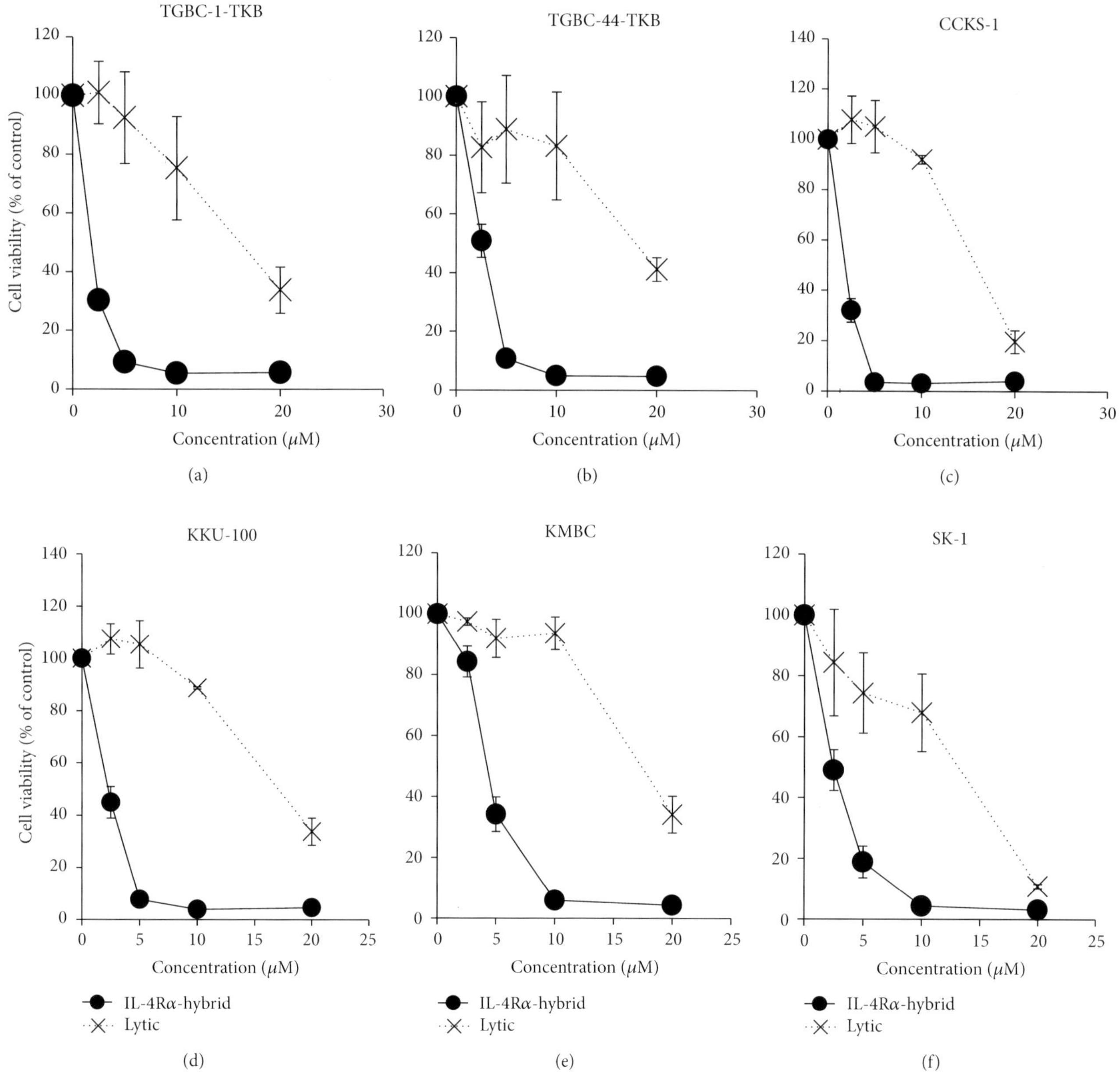


FIGURE 2: Cytotoxic activity of IL-4Rα-lytic hybrid peptide. Six BTC cell lines were cultured with various concentrations of IL-4Rα-lytic hybrid peptide or lytic peptide (0–20 μM) for 72 h, and cytotoxic activity was assessed using WST-8 reagent. The results are represented as mean ± SD (bars) of triplicate determinations, and the assay was repeated three times.

(data not shown). These results demonstrated that IL-4Rα-lytic hybrid peptide induced an effective antitumor activity in a mouse xenograft model of BTC.

## 4. Discussion

Therapeutic options for BTC are unsatisfactory, and the survival outcome is therefore poor. Effective therapeutic approaches against this aggressive disease are urgently needed. We previously demonstrated that human BTC tissue specimens expressed high levels of IL-4 receptor compared to normal gallbladders [5]. These observations were also confirmed in cultured human BTC cell lines that expressed IL-4R by immunoblot analysis. Immunohistochemical analysis showed overexpression of IL-4R in a large proportion (50–63%) of human BTC tissue specimens. Following the results of preclinical study for treatment of BTC with IL-4-PE [5], the efficacy of IL-4Rα-lytic hybrid peptide against human BTC was evaluated in preclinical models in this study.

Using the approach of selective receptor targeting, we have tested the efficacy of IL-4Rα-lytic hybrid peptide on

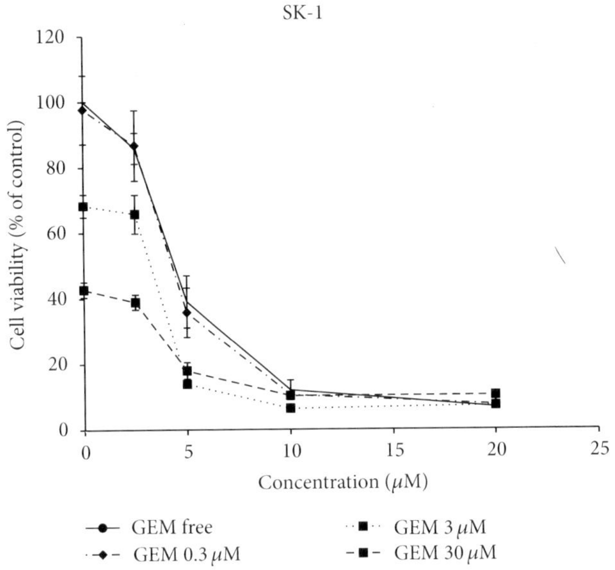


FIGURE 3: Cytotoxic activity by combination therapy of IL-4Rα-lytic hybrid peptide with gemcitabine. SK-1 was incubated with various concentrations of IL-4Rα-lytic hybrid peptide (0–20 μM) and gemcitabine (0–30 nM). The results are represented as mean ± SD (bars) of triplicate determinations, and the assay was repeated three times.

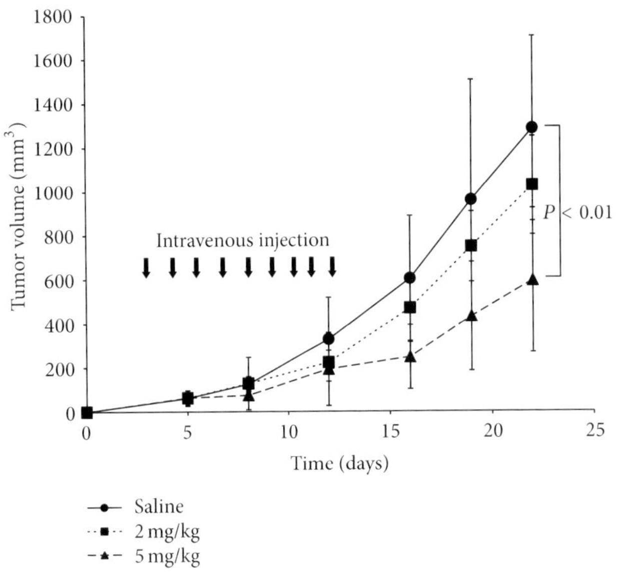


FIGURE 4: Antitumor activity of IL-4Rα-lytic hybrid peptide in tumor xenograft model *in vivo*. TGBC-44-TKB were implanted subcutaneously into athymic nude mice. Intravenous injection of saline and IL-4Rα-lytic hybrid peptide (2 mg/kg or 5 mg/kg) is indicated by the arrows. Data are expressed as mean ± SD ($n = 6$ animals in each group).

BTC cells. The overexpression of IL-4Rα in BTC cell lines sensitized them to the cytotoxic effect of this peptide, which correlated with the level of IL-4Rα expression. The *in vitro* cytotoxicity of this peptide was assessed for 6 cultured BTC cell lines (Figure 1). KMBC and CCKS-1 cell lines showing higher levels of IL-4Rα expression showed higher sensitivity ($IC_{50}$ of IL-4Rα-lytic hybrid peptide toward these cancer cells was approximately 2 μM, shown in Table 1). However the degree of the effect of IL-4Rα-lytic hybrid peptide against each BTC cell line is hardly different. These observations indicate that abundant IL 4Rα expression in BTC tumors will facilitate efficient targeting by this hybrid peptide. We previously reported that IL-4Rα-lytic had effective cytotoxic activity toward cancer cells expressing IL-4Rα and that enhancement of the IL-4Rα-lytic peptide-induced cytotoxicity correlates well with the expression levels of IL-4Rα [17]. We also previously showed the specificity of this hybrid peptide between normal and cancer cells by binding assay [25]. Moreover, it was demonstrated that intravenous administration of this hybrid peptide at 5 mg/kg dramatically inhibited the growth of TGBC44-TKB tumors *in vivo* (Figure 4). Histologic analysis also showed no abnormal changes in the tissue of major organs obtained from mice treated with the hybrid peptide (data not shown).

In this study, IL-4Rα-lytic hybrid peptide in combination with gemcitabine exhibited synergistic cytotoxic activity *in vitro* (Figure 3). Gemcitabine (Gemzar) is a widely accepted first-line therapy for advanced BTC, although the median survival time is not favorable [26]. Most studies using a single agent showed a low response rate and little effect on patient survival in advanced adenocarcinoma. It has recently been reported that cisplatin plus gemcitabine is associated with a significant survival advantage as compared with gemcitabine alone [4]. Moreover, several clinical trials using a combined approach of molecular target therapy with gemcitabine and other drugs have been initiated [27, 28]. Previously, IL-4-PE was shown to exert a synergistic effect with gemcitabine against the *in vitro* and *in vivo* pancreatic cancer models [28]. The results of this study support our observations of gemcitabine synergizing with IL-4Rα-lytic hybrid peptide on BTC cells, although the precise mechanism of the synergistic effect of gemcitabine with this hybrid peptide still remains obscure. It is known that gemcitabine inhibits DNA synthesis through inhibition of ribonucleotide reductase and depletion of deoxynucleotide pools [29]. It is suggested that the inhibition effect by gemcitabine in cancer cells might be exerted synergetically with the disintegration activity toward cancer cell membrane by IL-4Rα-lytic hybrid peptide [12, 17]. Thus, it is possible that gemcitabine enhances cell death induced by IL-4Rα-lytic hybrid peptide. Considering cancer cell death, the combination therapy of these drugs, which act through different mechanisms, may be a beneficial treatment option for patients with BTC.

## 5. Conclusions

Our current data describe that IL-4Rα is overexpressed in BTC cell lines *in vitro*, and BTC cells which overexpress the receptor can be successfully targeted with IL-4Rα-lytic hybrid peptide both *in vitro* and *in vivo*. IL-4Rα-lytic hybrid peptide induces regression of the established mouse model of BTC tumor. Thus, the findings of this study will assist and are available for elucidation of novel and effective BTC therapy targeting IL-4R$\alpha$ by IL-4R$\alpha$-lytic hybrid peptide.

## Acknowledgments

The authors thank Nana Ohkubo (Department of Clinical Sciences and Molecular Cellular Physiology, Tsukuba University) for technical assistance or advice with tissue culturing and *in vivo* experiments. This work was supported in part by Grants-in-Aid for Scientific Research from the Ministry of Education, Culture, Sports, Science and Technology, Japan (nos. 23390318, 24390323, 25282212, 25293278, and 24390449).

## References

[1] "Japan VSo. Tokyo (Japan): Japanese Ministry of Health and Welfare: Statistics Assoc.," 1998.

[2] T. Patel, "Increasing incidence and mortality of primary intrahepatic cholangiocarcinoma in the United States," *Hepatology*, vol. 33, no. 6, pp. 1353–1357, 2001.

[3] S. D. Taylor-Robinson, M. B. Toledano, S. Arora et al., "Increase in mortality rates from intrahepatic cholangiocarcinoma in England and Wales 1968–1998," *Gut*, vol. 48, no. 6, pp. 816–820, 2001.

[4] J. Valle, H. Wasan, D. H. Palmer et al., "Cisplatin plus gemcitabine versus gemcitabine for biliary tract cancer," *The New England Journal of Medicine*, vol. 362, no. 14, pp. 1273–1281, 2010.

[5] K. Ishige, J. Shoda, T. Kawamoto et al., "Potent in vitro and in vivo antitumor activity of interleukin-4-conjugated Pseudomonas exotoxin against human biliary tract carcinoma," *International Journal of Cancer*, vol. 123, no. 12, pp. 2915–2922, 2008.

[6] T. Shimamura, R. E. Royal, M. Kioi, A. Nakajima, S. R. Husain, and R. K. Puri, "Interleukin-4 cytotoxin therapy synergizes with gemcitabine in a mouse model of pancreatic ductal adenocarcinoma," *Cancer Research*, vol. 67, no. 20, pp. 9903–9912, 2007.

[7] R. J. Kreitman, "Immunotoxins in cancer therapy," *Current Opinion in Immunology*, vol. 11, no. 5, pp. 570–578, 1999.

[8] F. Weber, A. Asher, R. Bucholz et al., "Safety, tolerability, and tumor response of IL4-Pseudomonas exotoxin (NBI-3001) in patients with recurrent malignant glioma," *Journal of Neuro-Oncology*, vol. 64, no. 1-2, pp. 125–137, 2003.

[9] P. Attia, D. J. Powell Jr., A. V. Maker, R. J. Kreitman, I. Pastan, and S. A. Rosenberg, "Selective elimination of human regulatory T lymphocytes in vitro with the recombinant immunotoxin LMB-2," *Journal of Immunotherapy*, vol. 29, no. 2, pp. 208–214, 2006.

[10] R. J. Kreitman, "Immunotoxins in cancer therapy," *Current Opinion in Immunology*, vol. 11, no. 5, pp. 570–578, 1999.

[11] S. Choudhary, M. Mathew, and R. S. Verma, "Therapeutic potential of anticancer immunotoxins," *Drug Discovery Today*, vol. 16, no. 11-12, pp. 495–503, 2011.

[12] M. Kohno, T. Horibe, M. Haramoto et al., "A novel hybrid peptide targeting EGFR-expressing cancers," *European Journal of Cancer*, vol. 47, no. 5, pp. 773–783, 2011.

[13] M. Kawamoto, T. Horibe, M. Kohno, and K. Kawakami, "A novel transferrin receptor-targeted hybrid peptide disintegrates cancer cell membrane to induce rapid killing of cancer cells," *BMC Cancer*, vol. 11, article 359, 2011.

[14] T. Horibe, M. Kohno, M. Haramoto, K. Ohara, and K. Kawakami, "Designed hybrid TPR peptide targeting Hsp90 as a novel anticancer agent," *Journal of Translational Medicine*, vol. 9, article 8, 2011.

[15] N. Tada, T. Horibe, M. Haramoto, K. Ohara, M. Kohno, and K. Kawakami, "A single replacement of histidine to arginine in EGFR-lytic hybrid peptide demonstrates the improved anticancer activity," *Biochemical and Biophysical Research Communications*, vol. 407, no. 2, pp. 383–388, 2011.

[16] H. Ueyama, T. Horibe, O. Nakajima, K. Ohara, M. Kohno, and K. Kawakami, "Semaphorin 3A lytic hybrid peptide binding to neuropilin-1 as a novel anti-cancer agent in pancreatic cancer," *Biochemical and Biophysical Research Communications*, vol. 414, no. 1, pp. 60–66, 2011.

[17] L. Yang, T. Horibe, M. Kohno et al., "Targeting interleukin-4 receptor $\alpha$ with hybrid peptide for effective cancer therapy," *Molecular Cancer Therapeutics*, vol. 11, no. 1, pp. 235–243, 2012.

[18] H. Yano, M. Maruiwa, A. Iemura, A. Mizoguchi, and M. Kojiro, "Establishment and characterization of a new human extrahepatic bile duct carcinoma cell line (KMBC)," *Cancer*, vol. 69, no. 7, pp. 1664–1673, 1992.

[19] A. Knuth, H. Gabbert, W. Dippold et al., "Biliary adenocarcinoma. Characterisation of three new human tumor cell lines," *Journal of Hepatology*, vol. 1, no. 6, pp. 579–596, 1985.

[20] K. Saito, H. Minato, N. Kono, Y. Nakanuma, F. Ishida, and M. Kosugi, "Establishment of the human cholangiocellular carcinoma cell line (CCKS1)," *Kanzo*, vol. 34, no. 2, pp. 122–129, 1993 (Japanese).

[21] B. Sripa, S. Leungwattanawanit, T. Nitta et al., "Establishment and characterization of an opisthorchiasis-associated cholangiocarcinoma cell line (KKU-100)," *World Journal of Gastroenterology*, vol. 11, no. 22, pp. 3392–3397, 2005.

[22] N. Tepsiri, L. Chaturat, B. Sripa et al., "Drug sensitivity and drug resistance profiles of human intrahepatic cholangiocarcinoma cell lines," *World Journal of Gastroenterology*, vol. 11, no. 18, pp. 2748–2753, 2005.

[23] N. Koike, T. Todoroki, T. Kawamoto et al., "The invasion potentials of human biliary tract carcinoma cell lines: correlation between invasiveness and morphologic characteristics," *International Journal of Oncology*, vol. 13, no. 6, pp. 1269–1274, 1998.

[24] T. Fujisawa, H. Nakashima, A. Nakajima, B. H. Joshi, and R. K. Puri, "Targeting IL-13R$\alpha$2 in human pancreatic ductal adenocarcinoma with combination therapy of IL-13-PE and gemcitabine," *International Journal of Cancer*, vol. 128, no. 5, pp. 1221–1231, 2011.

[25] K. Seto, J. Shoda, T. Horibe et al., "Interleukin-4 receptor -based hybrid peptide effectively induced antitumor activity in head and neck squamous cell carcinoma," *Oral Oncology*, vol. 29, pp. 2147–2153, 2013.

[26] T. Okusaka, H. Ishii, A. Funakoshi et al., "Phase II study of single-agent gemcitabine in patients with advanced biliary tract cancer," *Cancer Chemotherapy and Pharmacology*, vol. 57, no. 5, pp. 647–653, 2006.

# 5

# Genetic Diseases That Predispose to Early Liver Cirrhosis

**Manuela Scorza,[1,2] Ausilia Elce,[1,2,3] Federica Zarrilli,[1,4] Renato Liguori,[1,2] Felice Amato,[1,2] and Giuseppe Castaldo[1,2]**

[1] *CEINGE—Biotecnologie Avanzate Scarl, Via Gaetano Salvatore 486, 80145 Napoli, Italy*
[2] *Dipartimento di Medicina Molecolare e Biotecnologie Mediche, Università di Napoli Federico II, Via Sergio Pansini 5, 80131 Napoli, Italy*
[3] *Università Telematica Pegaso, Piazza Trieste e Trento 48, 80132 Napoli, Italy*
[4] *Dipartimento di Bioscienze e Territorio, Università del Molise, Contrada Fonte Lappone, Pesche, 86090 Isernia, Italy*

Correspondence should be addressed to Giuseppe Castaldo; giuseppe.castaldo@unina.it

Academic Editor: Mohammad Ahmad al-Shatouri

Inherited liver diseases are a group of metabolic and genetic defects that typically cause early chronic liver involvement. Most are due to a defect of an enzyme/transport protein that alters a metabolic pathway and exerts a pathogenic role mainly in the liver. The prevalence is variable, but most are rare pathologies. We review the pathophysiology of such diseases and the diagnostic contribution of laboratory tests, focusing on the role of molecular genetics. In fact, thanks to recent advances in genetics, molecular analysis permits early and specific diagnosis for most disorders and helps to reduce the invasive approach of liver biopsy.

## 1. Introduction

An early chronic liver involvement may be observed in a number of genetic and metabolic diseases although with different penetrance, age at onset, and outcome. Clinical symptoms and laboratory data are frequently overlapping, thus rendering a differential diagnosis difficult. A great improvement both in imaging [1] and in molecular genetics [2] in the last years helped to discriminate between the different diseases thus reducing the need of pathology (Table 1). On the other hand, liver biopsy is often complex in children, mainly due to the smaller specimen size [3]. For some diseases, prenatal diagnosis is also available [4].

Specific therapies are available for several genetic and metabolic diseases and their effectiveness is strongly related to the precocity of diagnosis. A growing number of children with such diseases now survive well into adulthood [5]. On the other hand, liver transplantation now offers a long-term survival [6].

We will review the genetic and metabolic entities responsible for early chronic liver diseases focusing on the contribution of laboratory and molecular diagnosis (Table 2).

## 2. Alpha-1 Antitrypsin Deficiency

Alpha-1 antitrypsin (AAT) deficiency (OMIM 613490) is an autosomal recessive (codominant) disease due to mutations in the *SERPINA1* gene that encodes the serine protease inhibitor AAT. The protein, mainly synthesized by liver cells, inhibits proinflammatory proteases such as neutrophil elastase, thus, protecting the lung from proteolytic damage. AAT deficiency has an incidence of 1 : 2,000–5,000 but the number of diagnosed patients is underestimated.

AAT deficiency appears with chronic obstructive pulmonary disease, emphysema, and disseminated bronchiectasis usually between the 4th and the 5th decade [7]. The liver involvement is widely heterogeneous according to age at onset (between the 1st year of life up to the 6th decade) and clinical severity that ranges from chronic hepatitis and cirrhosis to fulminant liver failure. The most likely pathogenic mechanism is the accumulation of AAT polymers in hepatocytes. The progression of liver disease is slow, even if few cases develop early cirrhosis with the need for transplantation; furthermore, hepatocellular carcinoma has a very high incidence among AAT deficient subjects [8].

Table 1: Inherited liver diseases that predispose to early cirrhosis.

| Disease | Incidence | Gene |
|---|---|---|
| Disorders of bile acid synthesis | | |
| Wilson disease | 1 : 30,000 | *ATP7B* |
| Progressive familial intrahepatic cholestasis type 3 | 1 : 100,000 | *ABCB4* |
| Disorders of carbohydrate metabolism | | |
| Hereditary fructose intolerance | 1 : 20,000 | *ALDOB* |
| Glycogen storage disease type IV | 1 : 600,000 | *GBE1* |
| Disorders of amino acids metabolism | | |
| Tyrosinemia type I | 1 : 100,000 | *FAH* |
| Urea cycle disorders | | |
| Argininosuccinate lyase deficiency | 1 : 70,000 | *ASL* |
| Citrin deficiency (CTLN2, NICCD) | CTLN2 1 : 100,000<br>NICCD 1 : 19,000 | *SLC25A13* |
| Disorders of lipid metabolism | | |
| Cholesteryl ester storage disease | 1 : 40,000 (Germany)<br>1 : 300,000–1 : 500,000 | *LIPA* |
| Other diseases | | |
| Alpha-1 antitrypsin deficiency | 1 : 2,000–1 : 5,000 | *SERPINA1* |
| Cystic fibrosis | 1 : 2,500 | *CFTR* |
| Hereditary hemochromatosis | 1 : 250 | *HFE* |
| Alström syndrome | 1 : 1.000.000 | *ALMS1* |
| Congenital hepatic fibrosis | 1 : 20,000 | Unknown |

The replacement therapy has no effect because liver damage is due to the accumulation of the AAT mutant polymers and not to the lack of circulating AAT [9].

The indications to laboratory diagnosis include various conditions exhaustively revised [10], but all infants with prolonged jaundice or nonspecific signs of liver disease should be tested for AAT deficiency.

Laboratory diagnosis includes serum AAT measured by nephelometry followed by the qualitative determination of AAT alleles by isoelectric focusing (IEF) and, finally, genotyping [11]. Serum AAT must be performed in subjects free from acute inflammation since AAT is an acute phase protein, and thus inflammation enhances its serum levels [12]. Then, AAT levels should not be considered if serum C-reactive protein levels are increased. The IEF analysis reveals the alleles of each subject. The M alleles (M1 to M6) are the most common and are considered "wild type alleles." Most patients with liver or lung involvement are homozygous for the Z or the S or compound heterozygous for the two alleles. In these patients serum AAT levels are reduced by 40–60%. Heterozygous individuals (MZ or MS) rarely develop clinical signs. However, the IEF analysis may provide false negative results. Also for this reason, molecular analysis is indicated [11]. In the *SERPINA1* disease gene (official name: serpin peptidase inhibitor, clade A), more than 120 allelic variants have been identified so far; thus molecular analysis must be performed by gene sequencing. Gene variants are classified according to their effect on serum levels of alpha-1 antitrypsin [13]. Patients must be counseled before molecular analysis, and when severe mutations are identified the consanguineous should be counseled in turn and analyzed to reveal asymptomatic carriers.

## 3. Cystic Fibrosis

Cystic fibrosis (CF, OMIM 219700) is the most frequent lethal autosomal recessive disease among Caucasians (incidence: 1 : 2,500). CF is a systemic disease that appears mainly with pancreatic insufficiency in more than 90% of cases and pulmonary disease due to inflammation and opportunistic colonization that gradually causes respiratory insufficiency [14]. About 20% of patients experience meconium ileus.

Liver disease in CF appears mainly in the first decade of life and it is observed in up to 30% of patients, but it is still obscure why only some patients develop liver disease. In fact, CF liver disease depends on the altered activity of cystic fibrosis transmembrane regulator (CFTR) chloride channel on the apical membrane of cholangiocytes. It causes an altered bile flow followed by a cholangiocyte-induced inflammatory response with proliferation of stellate cells, which gives rise to cholangitis and progressive periportal fibrosis [15]. CF-associated liver disease is slowly progressive, but in up to 10% of patients it may rapidly evolve to multilobular biliary cirrhosis and portal hypertension.

The possibility to predict CF patients that will develop a severe liver involvement would be useful given the efficacy of ursodeoxycholic acid in the early stages of liver disease [15], but its pathogenesis is poorly known. The scarce correlation between the *CFTR* genotype and liver expression in CF patients is well known [16], as it is the discordant severity

Table 2: Main characteristics of genetic liver disease that predispose to early cirrhosis.

| | Age at onset (ys) | Pathogenic mechanism of liver damage | Laboratory diagnosis | Molecular genetics |
|---|---|---|---|---|
| Alpha-1 antitrypsin deficiency | 40–50 | Accumulation of AAT polymers in hepatocytes | Low serum AAT; AAT alleles by isoelectric focusing | 120 allelic variants in *SERPINA1* gene; *ZZ* genotype associated with liver cirrhosis |
| Cystic fibrosis | 0–12 | Altered activity of CFTR; increased bile flow that causes cholangitis and fibrosis | Sweat test | About 2000 known mutations in *CFTR* gene; no mutation specific for liver disease |
| Wilson disease | 20–22 | Copper hepatocyte increased levels dislocate the ATP7B protein impairing copper excretion through the bile | Low serum ceruloplasmin; high urine copper | About 300 known mutations in *ATP7B* gene; severe mutations (nonsense, frameshift) are associated with liver disease |
| Hereditary hemochromatosis | 30–50 | Iron-induced lipid peroxidation causes hepatocellular injury | Enhanced serum ferritin; high transferrin saturation | p.C282Y in *HFE* gene associated with liver cirrhosis |
| Type I tyrosinemia | Variable | The metabolite succinylacetone accumulates, resulting in toxicity to liver | Enhanced plasma/urine succinylacetone; high plasma tyrosine, methionine, and phenylalanine | Most frequent mutations analysis in *FAH* gene; no mutation specific for liver disease |
| Glycogen storage disease type IV | Variable | The altered stored glycogen impairs the osmotic pressure within the hepatocyte | / | Sequence analysis in *GBE1* gene; no mutation specific for liver disease |
| Argininosuccinate lyase deficiency | 0–15 | Decreased endogenous synthesis of arginine that leads to a decrease in arginine metabolites in various tissues | High serum citrulline; increased argininosuccinic acid in plasma/urine | *ASL* exons 4, 5, and 7 are hotspots of most frequent mutations; no mutation specific for liver disease |
| Citrin deficiency | NICCD: 0-1; CTLN2: 20–40 | Defective aspartate export from the mitochondria to the cytosol and defects in the malate aspartate shuttle | Enhanced plasma ammonia, citrulline, and arginine. NICCD: high plasma threonine, methionine, tyrosine, bilirubin, and bile acids | Sequence analysis in *SLC25A13* gene; no mutation specific for liver disease |
| Cholesteryl ester storage disease | 0–20 | Accumulation of cholesteryl esters and triglycerides in lysosomal hepatocytes | High serum AST, ALT, cholesterol, and low HDL cholesterol | About 40 mutations in *LIPA* gene; (exons 16, 10, and 8 are hotspots of mutations); no mutation specific for liver disease |
| Alström syndrome | Variable | Unclear mechanism | / | About 80 mutations in *ALMS1* gene; no mutation specific for liver disease |
| Congenital hepatic fibrosis | Variable | Immature duct structures stimulate the formation of portal fibrous tissue | / | The disease gene is unknown |
| Hereditary fructose intolerance | Variable | Accumulation of fructose in hepatocytes; fibrosis | Breath test | About 45 known mutations in *ALDOB* gene; no mutation specific for liver disease |
| Progressive familial intrahepatic cholestasis type 3 | 0–20 | The defect of MDR3 results in impaired biliary phospholipid excretion that impairs bile formation | High serum $\gamma$-GT activity, normal serum cholesterol and moderately raised bile salts concentrations | Most of known mutations in *ABCB4* are point mutations |

of liver disease in CF sib pairs [17]. A decade of studies concluded that liver expression in CF patients is influenced by modifier genes like mannose-binding lectin and AAT [18], but such genes modulate the risk for liver disease only in a small percentage of CF patients.

Finally, clinical forms showing pancreatic sufficiency, single organ involvement, and a milder outcome are included under the term of *CFTR*-related disorders (*CFTR*-RD) [19]. These disorders are not associated with liver disease.

The gold standard for CF diagnosis is the sweat test (i.e., sweat chloride levels after pilocarpine stimulation) followed by molecular analysis. Sweat test requires a specific skill and the knowledge of all conditions that may cause false positives, while the rate of false negative results is very low. However, CF diagnosis or exclusion must be based on two concordant sweat tests. The indications to sweat test include a large variety of clinical conditions [14, 15].

The search of *CFTR* mutations is one of the most diffuse molecular analyses worldwide, because it is used to confirm CF diagnosis and prenatal [20] or preimplantation [21] diagnosis. About 2000 mutations have been identified in the *CFTR* gene so far (http://www.genet.sickkids.on.ca/). Guidelines suggest a two-step molecular analysis. In the first step a panel of the most frequent mutations is analyzed, including the mutations peculiar to the geographic area of each patient [22], and commercial kits are used [16, 23]. The first step identifies about 80% alleles from CF patients; the analysis of mutations peculiar to specific ethnic or geographic groups may increase the detection rate [24], and the scanning of *CFTR* coding regions reveals mutations in up to 90% alleles [25]. Large gene rearrangements are present in about 2-3% of CF alleles [16]. Finally, pathogenic mutations in noncoding region of the *CFTR* gene have been described [26, 27], but they are not analyzed for routine purposes. The detection rate of molecular analysis is lower in *CFTR*-RD [28]. No mutations are specifically associated with liver disease [29].

The diagnosis of liver disease in CF patients is difficult, because neither laboratory nor imaging has a great specificity. Liver biopsy contributes to the aim, but the patchy distribution of liver alterations in CF patients reduces its sensitivity [15].

## 4. Wilson Disease

Wilson disease (WD, 277900) is an autosomal recessive disorder with an incidence of about 1:30,000. It typically appears with liver disease in the second decade and neurological disorders in the third decade, even if cases with earlier or later onset have been described [30]. Wilson disease depends on mutations in the gene encoding the ATP7B Cu translocase, a protein mainly expressed by the hepatocyte that regulates the levels of copper in the liver. Furthermore, ATP7B modulates the synthesis of ceruloplasmin [31]. When the activity of ATP7B is reduced, copper accumulates within the hepatocyte. The severity of liver involvement in WD patients is heterogeneous ranging from asymptomatic cases with mild hepatomegaly to cirrhosis with severe liver failure [32]. About two-thirds of patients show haemolytic anemia, coagulopathy, and renal failure. About 6% of WD cases appear with acute liver onset [33]. Kayser-Fleischer rings are present in about 50% of WD cases at diagnosis. About half of patients show psychiatric alterations, up to psychotic symptoms, reverted by adequate therapy [34]. Novel therapies can now effectively treat WD patients and gene therapy is effective in animal models [35].

Low serum ceruloplasmin and high urine copper help to perform the diagnosis in most cases, even if some false negatives are described [35].

Molecular analysis is available [36, 37]. Wilson disease is due to mutations in the *ATP7B* gene: about 300 different mutations are known so far (http://www.wilsondisease.med.ualberta.ca/database.asp); thus gene sequencing is required, reaching a detection rate of about 95%. Severe mutations (i.e., nonsense, frameshift) are associated with the most severe disease, while patients with missense mutations (about 60% of all mutations) show a variable severity and outcome [30]. Liver biopsy is now used in cases with ambiguous biochemical parameters and to evaluate liver copper levels [3].

## 5. Hereditary Hemochromatosis

Hereditary hemochromatosis (HH, OMIM 235200) is an autosomal recessive disease characterized by iron overload that may cause liver cirrhosis, cardiomyopathy, diabetes, arthritis, and skin pigmentation that appear during the third to fifth decade. The incidence is about 1:250. A myriad of diseases cause secondary hemochromatosis. However, while in secondary hemochromatosis the iron overload involves macrophages; in HH iron mainly accumulates in hepatocytes, causing chronic liver damage that ends in cirrhosis [38], with a percentage of cases evolving to hepatocellular carcinoma [39]. The pathogenesis of liver damage in HH is mainly due to the iron-induced lipid peroxidation that occurs in hepatocytes and causes hepatocellular injury or death. Kupffer cells become activated and produce cytokines, which in turn stimulate hepatic stellate cells to synthesize collagen, thereby leading to cirrhosis [38]. Symptoms of hemochromatosis depend on the phase of the disease. When HH is diagnosed by occasional laboratory evaluation, most patients are still asymptomatic; if the diagnosis is performed for symptoms, HH may appear with cirrhosis, bronze-colored skin, diabetes (and other endocrine diseases), joint inflammation, heart disease, arthralgia, and hepatomegaly.

The diagnosis is based on enhanced serum ferritin that correlates with the increased iron content of liver and the high transferrin saturation. Unsaturated iron-binding capacity has been proposed as an alternative to transferrin saturation [40], but it has a higher biological variability [41]. Molecular analysis in *HFE* gene with different protocols [42–47] would confirm hereditary hemochromatosis but surprisingly it has a lower diagnostic sensitivity because the mutations are different in each geographic area. Homozygous patients for p.Cys282Tyr have a higher risk for iron overload.

Liver biopsy is performed in suspected patients with negative molecular analysis and ambiguous laboratory results; in addition, it may be used to assess the degree of liver fibrosis and cirrhosis and the degree of iron liver overload [3, 48]. Laboratory has a role also in the monitoring of patients through biochemical markers of (i) liver fibrosis [49]; (ii) liver protidosynthesis [50]; and (iii) hepatocarcinoma in patients with cirrhosis [51].

## 6. Type I Tyrosinemia

Type I tyrosinemia (TYRSN1, OMIM 276700) is an autosomal recessive disease with an incidence of about 1 : 100,000. It is the most severe form of genetic tyrosinemia and is the only one that causes a severe liver involvement [52, 53].

Type I tyrosinemia is classified in two forms: the first, more frequent, appears with a severe liver expression in the first months of life that may progress to ascites, jaundice, and gastrointestinal bleeding; the second includes cases with acute liver failure at about one year and a chronic evolution with renal-tubular dysfunction [54]. Untreated patients die within the first decade of liver failure or of early hepatocarcinoma. The use of nitisinone and a tyrosine-restricted diet quite completely revert symptoms [55]. Type I tyrosinemia is due to the altered activity of fumarylacetoacetate hydrolase, which causes the elevation of plasma and urine succinylacetone (diagnostic golden standard) and high plasma concentration of tyrosine, methionine, and phenylalanine. Sequence analysis in *FAH* gene may be performed for molecular diagnosis including prenatal [56].

## 7. Glycogen Storage Disease Type IV

Glycogen storage disease (GSD, OMIM 232500) type IV is an autosomal recessive disease with an incidence of about 1 : 600,000. It is due to mutations in the gene encoding the glycogen branching enzyme (GBE1) that catalyzes the alpha 1,6 bond of the first glucose in the side chains of glycogen [57]. The altered glycogen branching reduces its solubility, thus impairing the osmotic pressure within the hepatocyte [58]. Several clinical forms of GSD have been described including (i) a neuromuscular form that appears in the perinatal age or in childhood; most of these cases have an early fatal evolution and are typically due to two null mutations; (ii) a hepatic form that may have a progressive or a nonprogressive evolution; patients are usually compound heterozygous for a severe (null) and a mild (missense) mutation; and (iii) the polyglucosan body disease that appears in adulthood with upper and lower motor neuron involvement and executive dysfunction [59]. The hepatic form is the most frequent phenotype. In the progressive subtype, the clinical expression appears in the first months of life with failure to thrive and hepatomegaly that evolves (in a variable time) to cirrhosis with portal hypertension requiring liver transplantation [60]. In the rare nonprogressive subtype the patients show a variable combination of liver disease (that usually does not evolve to cirrhosis), myopathy, and hypotonia. The diagnosis of GSD is based on biochemical findings from a liver biopsy that reveals an abnormal glycogen content, and on the evidence of enzymatic deficiency in the liver, muscle, or fibroblasts. Now it is based on molecular analysis, that is, the sequence of the *GBE1* gene followed by the search of large gene deletions [61]. In about 10% of patients a negative molecular analysis despite clinical symptoms suggests to perform the enzyme assay on cultured fibroblasts [62]. Prenatal diagnosis is possible if the disease-causing mutations in the family proband are known [63].

## 8. The Urea Cycle

The urea cycle includes a series of reactions that convert nitrogen from ammonia and aspartate into urea [64]. Urea cycle disorders (UCDs) are a group of inborn errors that typically cause a life-threatening hyperammonemia. Among these, argininosuccinate lyase (ASL) and citrin deficiency are usually associated with severe liver disease.

*8.1. Argininosuccinate Lyase Deficiency.* Argininosuccinate lyase deficiency (ASLD, OMIM 207900) is the second most common UCD with an incidence of about 1 : 70,000 and is due to the deficiency of the enzyme that cleaves argininosuccinic acid into arginine and fumarate. The disease includes a severe neonatal onset form and a late onset form: the first appears with hyperammonemia within the first few days of life with vomiting, lethargy, hypothermia, and poor feeding. On the contrary, the late onset form ranges from episodic hyperammonemia triggered by acute infections or stress to cognitive impairment, behavioral abnormalities, and/or learning disabilities in the absence of episodes of hyperammonemia [65]. Symptoms of ASL deficiency are unrelated to the severity or duration of hyperammonemic episodes and include neurocognitive deficiencies with attention deficit hyperactivity disorder and developmental disability [66]. Liver disease ranges from hepatomegaly to severe liver fibrosis and cirrhosis [67]. Systemic hypertension [68] and electrolyte imbalance may be present.

Laboratory diagnosis of ASL deficiency is based on enhanced levels of citrulline and increased argininosuccinic acid in plasma and/or in urine [64]. A newborn screening for ASLD is available in all US citrulline testing. ASLD is due to heterogeneous mutations in the *ASL* gene [69] and sequence analysis detects mutations in about 90% of patients. ASL enzyme activity can be measured in cell homogenates from liver biopsy or from skin fibroblasts or erythrocytes [70]. Prenatal diagnosis is available [71].

*8.2. Citrin Deficiency.* Citrin deficiency is an autosomal recessive disorder and may appear with two phenotypes: neonatal intrahepatic cholestasis caused by citrin deficiency (NICCD, OMIM 605814) and the adult form called citrullinemia type II ($CTLN_2$, OMIM 603471). A form that appears with dyslipidemia (FTTDCD) was described more recently [72]. Typically, citrin deficiency is characterized by food preference (protein-rich/lipid-rich foods) or aversion (carbohydrate-rich foods).

Neonatal intrahepatic cholestasis has an incidence of about 1 : 19,000 and appears with aminoacidemias, galactosemia, hypoproteinemia, cholestasis, and variable hepatic dysfunction [73]. Although such symptoms self-resolve by the first year in most cases, some infants die of infection or of liver cirrhosis [74, 75]. Citrullinemia type II has an incidence of about 1 : 100,000 and appears later between second and fourth decade with recurrent hyperammonemia with neuropsychiatric symptoms; death can be due to brain edema [76]. Symptoms are frequently triggered by alcohol and sugar intake, medication, and/or surgery. Affected patients may or may not have a prior history of NICCD or FTTDCD.

The diagnosis of citrin deficiency is based on clinical and biochemical findings that include enhanced plasma ammonia, citrulline and arginine, and threonine : serine ratio. In neonatal intrahepatic cholestasis plasma threonine, methionine, and tyrosine are elevated as bilirubin, bile acids, and alpha-fetoprotein [73]. Plasma levels of galactose, methionine, and/or phenylalanine are elevated in newborn screening blood spots in about 40% of children.

Citrin deficiency is caused by mutations in *SLC25A13* gene and is characterized by a liver-specific decrease in argininosuccinate synthetase (ASS) [77, 78]. The liver reduction of ASS in CTLN2 patients is secondary to citrin deficiency [79], although its cause still remains to be clarified.

## 9. Cholesteryl Ester Storage Disease

Cholesterol ester storage disease (CESD, OMIM 278000) is an autosomal recessive disorder of lysosomal storage with an incidence ranging between 1 in 40,000 in the Germanic population and 1 : 300,000–1 : 500,000 in the general Caucasian population [80]. It is due to deficiency of lysosomal acid lipase (LAL), which catalyzes the intracellular hydrolysis of triacylglycerols and cholesteryl esters. Its deficiency causes a progressive accumulation of cholesteryl esters (CE), and to a lesser extent, triglycerides, mainly in lysosomal hepatocytes, adrenal glands, and macrophages [81].

Usually patients develop hepatomegaly that leads to fibrosis and micronodular cirrhosis [82] within the first ten years of life. CESD can appear as two forms: Wolman disease, that is, the severe pediatric form, fatal within 1-2 years of life, and the later onset CESD, a more benign disease, associated with some residual LAL activity [80].

Wolman disease is a rare, neonatal onset, lethal disorder that appears in the first months of life with vomiting and diarrhea and severe hepatosplenomegaly. About 50% of patients show adrenal calcifications [83]. In contrast, CESD is often undiagnosed, has a later onset, and may appear in infancy or childhood, depending on the residual levels of LAL activity [83, 84]. CESD should be suspected in children with hepatomegaly and splenomegaly with elevated transaminases, high cholesterol, and low HDL [85].

Liver biopsy helps the diagnosis even if false negatives were reported [86, 87]. To confirm the diagnosis of CESD, LAL activity and molecular analysis of the acid lipase gene (*LIPA*) are available.

To date, over 40 *LIPA* mutations have been identified in patients with CESD [88]. No genotype-phenotype correlation has been established. Prenatal diagnosis is also available [80].

## 10. Alström Syndrome

Alström syndrome (ALMS, OMIM 203800) is a rare autosomal recessive disease with an incidence of 1 : 1,000,000. It appears in infancy with a wide variability in age at onset and severity, and typically leads to organ failure causing a reduced life expectancy, rarely exceeding 50 years. Alström syndrome appears with cone-rod dystrophy, obesity, progressive sensorineural hearing impairment, dilated or restrictive cardiomyopathy, the insulin resistance syndrome, and multiple organ failure [89, 90]. Therapy is complex due to the combination of multiple endocrine disorders, sensorineural deficits, cardiac, renal, and hepatic abnormalities [91]. Fibrosis develops in multiple organs [89]. Liver expression ranges from steatohepatitis to portal hypertension and cirrhosis and can cause hepatic encephalopathy and life-threatening esophageal varices. The diagnosis is based on clinical features [92], and genetic testing is used when major (vision) and minor criteria do not permit a clinical diagnosis. Molecular testing of the disease gene, *ALMS1*, detects mutations in up to 80% of patients of northern European descent, and in about 40% of cases worldwide [93, 94]. Carrier and prenatal diagnosis can be offered if the disease-causing mutations have been identified in a family proband [95].

## 11. Congenital Hepatic Fibrosis

Congenital hepatic fibrosis (CHF) is an autosomal recessive disease characterized by periportal fibrosis and irregularly shaped proliferating bile ducts. The incidence is about 1 : 20,000 [96].

In most patients, the first symptom is portal hypertension (PH) with gastrointestinal bleeding [97]. Pulmonary hypertension and pulmonary vascular shunts are typical complications of PH. Frequently CHF is associated with ciliopathies and renal disease, the so-called hepatorenal fibrocystic disease [98].

Congenital hepatic fibrosis involves various organs (e.g. renal, central nervous system, etc.), but most cases are referred for liver diseases. Four clinical forms have been described [99]: (i) portal hypertension (most common and more severe in the presence of portal vein abnormality); (ii) cholangitis with cholestasis and recurrent cholangitis; (iii) both portal hypertension and cholangitic symptoms; and (iv) latency that appears at a late age with hard hepatomegaly.

Symptoms of CHF are nonspecific, making the diagnosis difficult. The late onset and the clinical evolution suggest that CHF is a dynamic and progressive condition [100, 101].

The diagnosis of CHF can be made by liver biopsy that shows a progressive hepatic fibrosis with nodular formation. Such findings may be mistaken for cirrhosis, but, unlike cirrhosis, hepatic lobules are usually normal with normal hepatocyte morphology, particularly in the early phases [100, 102]. The gene/s causing CHF is/are unknown.

## 12. Hereditary Fructose Intolerance

Hereditary fructose intolerance (HFI, OMIM 229600) is an autosomal recessive disease (incidence 1 : 20,000) due to the deficiency of fructose 1-phosphate aldolase (aldolase B) involved in the metabolism of fructose-1-phosphate (exogenous fructose) into dihydroxyacetone phosphate and D-glyceraldehyde [103].

Onset of symptoms can occur at any age. The persistent intake of fructose, sucrose, or sorbitol in childhood leads to chronic toxicity [104, 105] that causes irreversible damage to the liver (early cirrhosis) and kidney [105]. The strict dietary exclusion leads to normal growth and longevity, but it is difficult to achieve [106].

The early diagnosis of HFI is crucial to start the strict exclusion diet thus avoiding tissue injury and growthretardation. $^{31}P$ nuclear magnetic resonance spectroscopy has been used successfully [107]. The fructose tolerance test (breath test) has a high diagnostic sensitivity [106]. Molecular diagnosis of HFI consists in direct sequencing of the gene encoding aldolase B (*ALDOB*). About 45 different mutations are known so far (http://www.bu.edu/aldolase/HFI/hfidb/hfidb.html) and it is now the diagnostic gold standard [108–111].

## 13. Progressive Familial Intrahepatic Cholestasis Type 3

Progressive familial intrahepatic cholestasis (PFIC) refers to a heterogeneous group of inherited cholestatic disorders that impair bile formation and appear with cholestasis of hepatocellular origin. Three types of PFIC are known. Progressive familial intrahepatic cholestasis type 3 (PFIC3, OMIM 602347) is an autosomal recessive disorder with a prevalence estimated of about 1 : 100,000 [112].

PFIC3 may appear in infancy, in childhood, or during young adulthood. Main symptoms include gastrointestinal bleeding due to portal hypertension, early cirrhosis, and moderate pruritus [113]. The phenotypic expression of PFIC3 ranges from neonatal cholestasis to cirrhosis in young adults [114]. The evolution of the disease is characterized by chronic icteric or anicteric cholestasis, portal hypertension, and liver failure. In about 50% of the patients, liver transplantation is required at a mean age of 7.5 years [115]. Laboratory findings show high serum gamma-glutamyl transferase ($\gamma$-GT) activity (while other two types of PFIC have normal serum $\gamma$-GT activity), normal cholesterol levels, and moderately enhanced bile acid concentrations. Liver histology shows portal fibrosis and true ductular proliferation with mixed inflammatory infiltrate and, in advanced phases, signs of biliary cirrhosis. Interlobular bile ducts are seen in most portal tracts and there is neither periductal fibrosis nor biliary epithelium injury [113].

PFIC3 is caused by mutations in the *ABCB4* gene encoding the multidrug resistance protein 3 (MDR3) protein. This gene is expressed in the canalicular membrane of the hepatocyte and is responsible for phospholipid transport into bile [116]. Reduced or absent activity of the MDR3 transporter causes impaired phospholipid secretion, previously identified as "low phospholipid syndrome" [117]. The diagnosis of PFIC3 is confirmed by molecular genetic analysis of the *ABCB4* gene by sequencing of exons and their splice junctions (http://evs.gs.washington.edu/EVS/) [118]. There are several mutations in *ABCB4* that have a clear effect on the protein and a genotype-phenotype correlation is observed [119–122]. Prenatal diagnosis is available.

## 14. Conclusions and Future Prospects

A chronic liver involvement that can predispose to cirrhosis may be observed in a number of genetic diseases with a different penetrance, age at onset, and outcome. Clinical symptoms and laboratory data are frequently overlapping, thus rendering a differential diagnosis difficult. In the present review we critically discussed the genetic entities responsible for early liver cirrhosis, describing for each disease the laboratory diagnosis and molecular genetics.

In fact, the recent advances made in understanding the genetics and pathophysiology of inherited liver diseases can contribute to the identification of novel strategies for the diagnosis of these conditions. Molecular analysis changed the diagnostic approach in these genetic diseases and led to reduction of invasive and expensive procedures and diagnostic errors.

Disease-genes identification is a step forward in the diagnostic approach to a patient in whom early liver cirrhosisis strongly suspected. However, we have to point out some critical points: (i) molecular analysis would be based on scanning procedures using the gene sequencing; (ii) the negative result of molecular analysis does not exclude the disease, because mutations may involve noncoding, regulatory areas; (iii) some liver diseases are very rare; it is necessary that laboratories also offer molecular diagnosis for such diseases.

However, the availability of new technologies as high throughput sequencing at reasonable costs could help to perform extensive analyses, especially in cases in which more disease genes are involved. No clear genotype-phenotype correlation has been established in most cases, so proteomic and functional studies on the effect of the mutations may guide physicians in the prescription of treatment procedures. In some cases, molecular analysis has been used for prenatal diagnosis to help high risk couples to better plan their reproductive options.

However, given the increased number of genetic liver diseases, the complexity of genotype-phenotype correlations and the need of multidisciplinary counseling to the families, a strict collaboration between physicians and molecular laboratories is mandatory in this field.

## Acknowledgment

Grants from Regione Campania (DGRC 1901/09 and POR, FSE 2007-13, project CREME) are gratefully acknowledged.

## References


[1] T. Taddei, P. Mistry, and M. L. Schilsky, "Inherited metabolic disease of the liver," *Current Opinion in Gastroenterology*, vol. 24, pp. 278–286, 2008.

[2] G. Castaldo, F. Lembo, and R. Tomaiuolo, "Molecular diagnostics: between chips and customized medicine," *Clinical Chemistry and Laboratory Medicine*, vol. 48, pp. 973–982, 2010.

[3] N. Ovchinsky, R. K. Moreira, J. H. Lefkowitch, and J. E. Lavine, "Liver biopsy in modern clinical practice: a pediatric point-of-view," *Advances in Anatomic Pathology*, vol. 19, pp. 250–262, 2012.

[4] G. M. Maruotti, G. Frisso, G. Calcagno et al., "Prenatal diagnosis of inherited diseases: the 20 years experience of an Italian Regional Reference Centre," *Clinical Chemistry and Laboratory Medicine*, vol. 51, pp. 2211–2217, 2013.

[5] M. E. Mailliard and J. L. Gollan, "Metabolic liver disease in the young adult," *Best Practice & Research Clinical Gastroenterology*, vol. 17, pp. 307–322, 2003.

[6] M. Burdelski, B. Rodeck, A. Latta et al., "Treatment of inherited metabolic disorders by liver transplantation," *Journal of Inherited Metabolic Disease*, vol. 14, pp. 604–618, 1991.

[7] S. K. Brode, S. C. Ling, and K. R. Chapman, "Alpha-1 antitrypsin deficiency: a commonly overlooked cause of lung disease," *Canadian Medical Association Journal*, vol. 184, no. 12, pp. 1365–1371, 2012.

[8] K. D. Fairbanks and A. S. Tavill, "Liver disease in alpha 1-antitrypsin deficiency: a review," *The American Journal of Gastroenterology*, vol. 103, pp. 2136–2141, 2008.

[9] A. Kaplan and L. Cosentino, "Alpha1-antitrypsin deficiency: forgotten etiology," *Canadian Family Physician*, vol. 56, pp. 19–24, 2010.

[10] J. K. Stoller, G. L. Snider, M. L. Brantly et al., "American Thoracic Society/European Respiratory Society Statement: standards for the diagnosis and management of individuals with alpha-1 antitrypsin deficiency," *Pneumologie*, vol. 59, pp. 36–68, 2005 (German).

[11] F. Zarrilli, A. Elce, M. Scorza, S. Giordano, F. Amato, and G. Castaldo, "An update on laboratory diagnosis of liver inherited diseases," *BioMed Research International*, vol. 2013, Article ID 697940, 7 pages, 2013.

[12] R. Bals, "Alpha-1-antitrypsin deficiency," *Best Practice & Research Gastroenterology*, vol. 24, pp. 629–633, 2010.

[13] E. K. Silverman and R. A. Sandhaus, "Alpha-1 antitrypsin deficiency," *The New England Journal of Medicine*, vol. 360, pp. 2749–2757, 2009.

[14] B. J. Rosenstein and G. R. Cutting, "The diagnosis of cystic fibrosis: a consensus statement," *The Journal of Pediatrics*, vol. 132, pp. 589–595, 1998.

[15] D. Debray, D. Kelly, R. Houwen, B. Strandvik, and C. Colombo, "Best practice guidelines for the diagnosis and management of cystic fibrosis-associated liver disease," *The Journal of Cystic Fibrosis*, vol. 10, pp. S29–S36, 2011.

[16] R. Tomaiuolo, F. Sangiuolo, C. Bombieri et al., "Epidemiology and a novel procedure for large scale analysis of CFTR rearrangements in classic and atypical CF patients: a multicentric Italian study," *The Journal of Cystic Fibrosis*, vol. 7, no. 5, pp. 347–351, 2008.

[17] G. Castaldo, A. Fuccio, D. Salvatore et al., "Liver expression in cystic fibrosis could be modulated by genetic factors different from the cystic fibrosis transmembrane regulator genotype," *The American Journal of Medical Genetics*, vol. 98, pp. 294–307, 2001.

[18] R. Tomaiuolo, D. Degiorgio, D. A. Coviello et al., "An MBL2 haplotype and ABCB4 variants modulate the risk of liver disease in cystic fibrosis patients: a multicentre study," *Digestive and Liver Disease*, vol. 41, no. 11, pp. 817–822, 2009.

[19] C. Bombieri, M. Claustres, K. de Boeck et al., "Recommendations for the classification of diseases as *CFTR*-related disorders," *The Journal of Fibrosis*, vol. 10, pp. S86–S102, 2011.

[20] R. Tomaiuolo, P. Nardiello, P. Martinelli, L. Sacchetti, F. Salvatore, and G. Castaldo, "Prenatal diagnosis of cystic fibrosis: an experience of 181 cases," *Clinical Chemistry and Laboratory Medicine*, vol. 51, pp. 2227–2232, 2013.

[21] A. Elce, A. Boccia, G. Cardillo et al., "Three novel *CFTR* polymorphic repeats improve segregation analysis for cystic fibrosis," *Clinical Chemistry*, vol. 55, pp. 1372–1379, 2009.

[22] G. Castaldo, E. Rippa, G. Sebastio et al., "Molecular epidemiology of cystic fibrosis mutations and haplotypes in southern Italy evaluated with an improved semiautomated robotic procedure," *Journal of Medical Genetics*, vol. 33, pp. 475–479, 1996.

[23] R. Tomaiuolo, M. Spina, and G. Castaldo, "Molecular diagnosis of cystic fibrosis: comparison of four analytical procedures," *Clinical Chemistry and Laboratory Medicine*, vol. 41, pp. 26–32, 2003.

[24] G. Castaldo, A. Fuccio, C. Cazeneuve et al., "Detection of five rare cystic fibrosis mutations peculiar to Southern Italy: implications in screening for the disease and phenotype characterization for patients with homozygote mutations," *Clinical Chemistry*, vol. 45, pp. 957–962, 1999.

[25] G. Castaldo, A. Polizzi, R. Tomaiuolo et al., "Comprehensive cystic fibrosis mutation epidemiology and haplotype characterization in southern Italy population," *Annals of Human Genetics*, vol. 69, pp. 15–24, 2005.

[26] S. Giordano, F. Amato, A. Elce et al., "Molecular and functional analysis of the large 5' promoter region of *CFTR* gene revealed pathogenic mutations in CF and *CFTR*-related disorders," *The Journal of Molecular Diagnostics*, vol. 15, pp. 331–340, 2013.

[27] F. Amato, M. Seia, S. Giordano et al., "Gene mutation in MicroRNA target sites of *CFTR* gene: a novel pathogenetic mechanism in cystic fibrosis?" *PLoS ONE*, vol. 8, Article ID e60448, 2013.

[28] F. Amato, C. Bellia, G. Cardillo et al., "Extensive molecular analysis of patients bearing *CFTR*-related disorders," *The Journal of Molecular Diagnostics*, vol. 14, pp. 81–89, 2012.

[29] G. Castaldo, E. Rippa, D. Salvatore et al., "Severe liver impairment in a cystic fibrosis-affected child homozygous for the G542X mutation," *American Journal of Medical Genetics*, vol. 69, pp. 155–158, 1997.

[30] T. Okada, Y. Shiono, Y. Kaneko et al., "High prevalence of fulminant hepatic failure among patients with mutant alleles for truncation of ATP7B in Wilsons disease," *Scandinavian Journal of Gastroenterology*, vol. 45, pp. 1232–1237, 2010.

[31] V. Lalioti, I. Sandoval, D. Cassio, and J. C. Duclos-Vallée, "Molecular pathology of Wilson's disease: a brief," *Journal of Hepatology*, vol. 53, no. 6, pp. 1151–1153, 2010.

[32] E. A. Roberts and M. L. Schilsky, "Diagnosis and treatment of Wilson disease: an update," *Hepatology*, vol. 47, no. 6, pp. 2089–2111, 2008.

[33] D. Huster, W. Hermann, and M. Bartels, "Acute Wilson disease," *Der Internist*, vol. 52, pp. 815–822, 2011.

[34] D. Huster, "Wilson disease," *Best Practice Research Clinical Gastroenterology*, vol. 24, no. 5, pp. 531–539, 2010.

[35] K. H. Weiss and W. Stremmel, "Evolving perspectives in Wilson disease: diagnosis, treatment and monitoring," *Current Gastroenterology Reports*, vol. 14, pp. 1–7, 2012.

[36] M. L. Schilsky and A. Ala, "Genetic testing for Wilson disease: availability and utility," *Current Gastroenterology Reports*, vol. 12, pp. 57–61, 2010.

[37] J. Bennett and S. H. Hahn, "Clinical molecular diagnosis of Wilson disease," *Seminars in Liver Disease*, vol. 31, pp. 233–238, 2011.

[38] B. R. Bacon, P. C. Adams, K. V. Kowdley, L. W. Powell, and A. S. Tavill, "Diagnosis and management of hemochromatosis: 2011 practice guideline by the American Association for the Study of Liver Diseases," *Hepatology*, vol. 54, pp. 328–343, 2011.

[39] E. Maillard, "Epidemiology, natural history and pathogenesis of hepatocellular carcinoma," *Cancer/Radiothérapie*, vol. 15, no. 1, pp. 3–6, 2011.

[40] P. C. Adams, D. M. Reboussin, J. C. Barton et al., "Hemochromatosis and iron overload screening in a racially diverse population," *The New England Journal of Medicine*, vol. 352, pp. 1769–1778, 2005.

[41] P. C. Adams, D. M. Reboussin, R. D. Press et al., "Biological variability of transferrin saturation and unsaturated iron-binding capacity," *The American Journal of Medicine*, vol. 120, pp. 999.e1–999.e7, 2007.

[42] A. Piperno, "Molecular diagnosis of hemochromatosis," *Expert Opinion on Medical Diagnostics*, vol. 7, pp. 161–177, 2013.

[43] A. M. Jouanolle, V. Gérolami, C. Ged et al., "Molecular diagnosis of *HFE* mutations in routine laboratories. Results of a survey from reference laboratories in France," *Annales de Biologie Clinique*, vol. 70, pp. 305–313, 2012 (French).

[44] C. J. McDonald, D. F. Wallace, D. H. Crawford, and V. N. Subramaniam, "Iron storage disease in Asia-Pacific populations: the importance of non-*HFE* mutations," *Journal of Gastroenterology and Hepatology*, vol. 28, pp. 1087–1094, 2013.

[45] A. del-Castillo-Rueda, M. I. Moreno-Carralero, N. Cuadrado-Grande et al., "Mutations in the *HFE*, *TFR2*, and *SLC40A1* genes in patients with hemochromatosis," *Gene*, vol. 508, pp. 15–20, 2012.

[46] P. C. Santos, J. E. Krieger, and A. C. Pereira, "Molecular diagnostic and pathogenesis of hereditary hemochromatosis," *International Journal of Molecular Sciences*, vol. 13, pp. 1497–1511, 2012.

[47] I. M. Nadakkavukaran, E. K. Gan, and J. K. Olynyk, "Screening for hereditary haemochromatosis," *Pathology*, vol. 44, pp. 148–152, 2012.

[48] M. L. Bassett, P. E. Hickman, and J. E. Dahlstrom, "The changing role of liver biopsy in diagnosis and management of haemochromatosis," *Pathology*, vol. 43, pp. 433–439, 2011.

[49] G. Fortunato, G. Castaldo, G. Oriani et al., "Multivariate discriminant function based on six biochemical markers in blood can predict the cirrhotic evolution of chronic hepatitis," *Clinical Chemistry*, vol. 47, pp. 1696–1700, 2001.

[50] F. D. Raymond, G. Fortunato, D. W. Moss, G. Castaldo, F. Salvatore, and M. Impallomeni, "Inositol-specific phospholipase D activity in health and disease," *Clinical Science*, vol. 86, pp. 447–451, 1994.

[51] G. Castaldo, G. Oriani, M. M. Lofrano et al., "Differential diagnosis between hepatocellular carcinoma and cirrhosis through a discriminant function based on results from serum analytes," *Clinical Chemistry*, vol. 42, pp. 1263–1269, 1996.

[52] M. De Braekeleer and J. Larochelle, "Genetic epidemiology of hereditary tyrosinemia in Quebec and in Saguenay-Lac-St-Jean," *The American Journal of Human Genetics*, vol. 47, no. 2, pp. 302–307, 1990.

[53] C. J. Ellaway, E. Holme, S. Standing et al., "Outcome of tyrosinaemia type III," *Journal of Inherited Metabolic Disease*, vol. 24, no. 8, pp. 824–832, 2001.

[54] C. de Laet, C. Dionisi-Vici, J. V. Leonard et al., "Recommendations for the management of tyrosinaemia type 1," *Orphanet Journal of Rare Diseases*, vol. 8, article 8, 2013.

[55] P. J. McKiernan, "Nitisinone in the treatment of hereditary tyrosinemia type 1," *Drugs*, vol. 66, pp. 743–750, 2006.

[56] S. I. Demers, P. Russo, F. Lettre, and R. M. Tanguay, "Frequent mutation reversion inversely correlates with clinical severity in a genetic liver disease, hereditary tyrosinemia," *Human Pathology*, vol. 34, pp. 1313–1320, 2003.

[57] C. Lamperti, S. Salani, S. Lucchiari et al., "Neuropathological study of skeletal muscle, heart, liver, and brain in a neonatal form of glycogen storage disease type IV associated with a new mutation in *GBE1* gene," *Journal of Inherited Metabolic Disease*, vol. 32, supplement 1, pp. S161–S168, 2009.

[58] Y. Bao, P. Kishnani, J. Y. Wu, and Y. T. Chen, "Hepatic and neuromuscular forms of glycogen storage disease type IV caused by mutations in the same glycogen-branching enzyme gene," *Journal of Clinical Investigation*, vol. 97, pp. 941–948, 1996.

[59] S. W. Moses and R. Parvari, "The variable presentations of glycogen storage disease type IV: a review of clinical, enzymatic and molecular studies," *Current Molecular Medicine*, vol. 2, pp. 177–188, 2002.

[60] M. K. Davis and D. A. Weinstein, "Liver transplantation in children with glycogen storage disease: controversies and evaluation of the risk/benefit of this procedure," *Pediatric Transplantation*, vol. 12, pp. 137–145, 2008.

[61] P. L. Magoulas, A. W. El-Hattab, A. Roy, D. S. Bali, M. J. Finegold, and W. J. Craigen, "Diffuse reticuloendothelial system involvement in type IV glycogen storage disease with a novel GBE1 mutation: a case report and review," *Human Pathology*, vol. 43, pp. 943–951, 2012.

[62] D. H. Brown and B. I. Brown, "Studies of the residual glycogen branching enzyme activity present in human skin fibroblasts from patients with type IV glycogen storage disease," *Biochemical and Biophysical Research Communications*, vol. 111, pp. 636–643, 1983.

[63] H. O. Akman, C. Karadimas, Y. Gyftodimou et al., "Prenatal diagnosis of glycogen storage disease type IV," *Prenatal Diagnosis*, vol. 26, pp. 951–955, 2006.

[64] S. C. Nagamani, A. Erez, and B. Lee, "Argininosuccinate lyase deficiency," *Genetics in Medicine*, vol. 14, pp. 501–507, 2012.

[65] C. Ficicioglu, R. Mandell, and V. E. Shih, "Argininosuccinate lyase deficiency: longterm outcome of 13 patients detected by newborn screening," *Molecular Genetics and Metabolism*, vol. 98, no. 3, pp. 273–277, 2009.

[66] M. Tuchman, B. Lee, U. Lichter-Konecki et al., "Cross-sectional multicenter study of patients with urea cycle disorders in the United States," *Molecular Genetics and Metabolism*, vol. 94, no. 4, pp. 397–402, 2008.

[67] S. Mercimek-Mahmutoglu, D. Moeslinger, J. Häberle et al., "Long-term outcome of patients with argininosuccinate lyase deficiency diagnosed by newborn screening in Austria," *Molecular Genetics and Metabolism*, vol. 100, pp. 24–28, 2010.

[68] N. Brunetti-Pierri, A. Erez, O. Shchelochkov, W. Craigen, and B. Lee, "Systemic hypertension in two patients with ASL deficiency: a result of nitric oxide deficiency?" *Molecular Genetics and Metabolism*, vol. 98, pp. 195–197, 2009.

[69] M. Linnebank, E. Tschiedel, J. Haberle et al., "Argininosuccinate lyase (ASL) deficiency: mutation analysis in 27 patients and a completed structure of the human *ASL* gene," *Human Genetics*, vol. 111, no. 4-5, pp. 350–359, 2002.

[70] W. J. Kleijer, V. H. Garritsen, M. Linnebank et al., "Clinical, enzymatic, and molecular genetic characterization of a biochemical variant type of argininosuccinic aciduria: prenatal and postnatal diagnosis in five unrelated families," *Journal of Inherited Metabolic Disease*, vol. 25, pp. 399–410, 2002.

[71] J. Häberle and H. G. Koch, "Genetic approach to prenatal diagnosis in urea cycle defects," *Prenatal Diagnosis*, vol. 24, pp. 378–383, 2004.

[72] K. Kobayashi, M. Iijima, M. Ushikai, S. Ikeda, and T. Saheki, "Citrin deficiency," *The Journal of the Pediatric Society*, vol. 110, pp. 1047–1059, 2006.

[73] T. Ohura, K. Kobayashi, Y. Tazawa et al., "Clinical pictures of 75 patients with neonatal intrahepatic cholestasis caused by citrin deficiency," *Journal of Inherited Metabolic Disease*, vol. 30, pp. 139–144, 2007.

[74] A. Tamamori, Y. Okano, H. Ozaki et al., "Neonatal intrahepatic cholestasis caused by citrin deficiency: severe hepatic dysfunction in an infant requiring liver transplantation," *European Journal of Pediatrics*, vol. 161, no. 11, pp. 609–613, 2002.

[75] Y. Z. Song, M. Deng, F. P. Chen et al., "Genotypic and phenotypic features of citrin deficiency: five-year experience in a Chinese pediatric center," *International Journal of Molecular Medicine*, vol. 28, pp. 33–40, 2011.

[76] S. Ikeda, S. Kawa, Y. Takei et al., "Chronic pancreatitis associated with adult-onset type II citrullinemia: clinical and pathological findings," *Annals of Internal Medicine*, vol. 141, pp. W109–W110, 2004.

[77] K. Kobayashi and T. Saheki, "Molecular basis of citrin deficiency," *Seikagaku*, vol. 76, pp. 1543–1559, 2004.

[78] K. Kobayashi, N. Shaheen, R. Kumashiro et al., "A search for the primary abnormality in adult-onset type II citrullinemia," *The American Journal of Human Genetics*, vol. 53, pp. 1024–1030, 1993.

[79] T. Yasuda, N. Yamaguchi, K. Kobayashi et al., "Identification of two novel mutations in the *SLC25A13* gene and detection of seven mutations in 102 patients with adult-onset type II citrullinemia," *Human Genetics*, vol. 107, no. 6, pp. 537–545, 2000.

[80] D. L. Bernstein, H. Hülkova, M. G. Bialer, and R. J. Desnick, "Cholesteryl ester storage disease: review of the findings in 135 reported patients with an underdiagnosed disease," *Journal of Hepatology*, vol. 58, pp. 1230–1243, 2013.

[81] G. A. Grabowski, L. Charnas, and H. Du, "Lysosomal acid lipase deficiencies: the Wolman disease/cholesteryl ester storage disease spectrum," in *Metabolic and Molecular Bases of Inherited Disease—OMMBID*, D. Scriver Valle, A. L. Beaudet, B. Vogelstein, K. W. Kinzler, S. E. Antonarakis, and A. Ballabio, Eds., McGraw-Hill, New York, NY, USA, 2012.

[82] H. Chatrath, S. Keilin, and B. M. Attar, "Cholesterol ester storage disease (CESD) diagnosed in an asymptomatic adult," *Digestive Diseases and Sciences*, vol. 54, no. 1, pp. 168–173, 2009.

[83] G. Assmann and U. Seedorf, "Acid lipase deficiency: Wolman disease and cholesteryl ester storage disease," in *The Metabolic and Molecular Bases of Inherited Disease*, C. R. Scriver, A. L. Beaudet, W. S. Sly, and D. Valle, Eds., pp. 3551–3572, McGraw-Hill, New York, NY, USA, 2001.

[84] L. Pisciotta, R. Fresa, A. Bellocchio et al., "Cholesteryl ester storage disease (CESD) due to novel mutations in the *LIPA* gene," *Molecular Genetics and Metabolism*, vol. 97, pp. 143–148, 2009.

[85] B. Zhang and A. F. Porto, "Cholesteryl ester storage disease: protean presentations of lysosomal acid lipase deficiency," *Journal of Pediatric Gastroenterology and Nutrition*, vol. 56, pp. 682–685, 2003.

[86] H. Hulkova and M. Elleder, "Distinctive histopathological features that support a diagnosis of cholesterol ester storage disease in liver biopsy specimens," *Histopathology*, vol. 60, pp. 1107–1113, 2012.

[87] S. Vom Dahl, K. Harzer, A. Rolfs et al., "Hepatosplenomegalic lipidosis: what unless Gaucher? Adult cholesteryl ester storage disease (CESD) with anemia, mesenteric lipodystrophy, increased plasma chitotriosidase activity and a homozygous lysosomal acid lipase-1 exon 8 splice junction mutation," *Journal of Hepatology*, vol. 31, pp. 741–746, 1999.

[88] H. Klima, K. Ullrich, C. Aslanidis, P. Fehringer, K. J. Lackner, and G. Schmitz, "A splice junction mutation causes deletion of a 72-base exon from the mRNA for lysosomal acid lipase in a patient with cholesteryl ester storage disease," *The Journal of Clinical Investigation*, vol. 92, no. 6, pp. 2713–2718, 1993.

[89] J. D. Marshall, R. T. Bronson, G. B. Collin et al., "New Alström syndrome phenotypes based on the evaluation of 182 cases," *Archives of Internal Medicine*, vol. 165, no. 6, pp. 675–683, 2005.

[90] E. Malm, V. Ponjavic, P. M. Nishina et al., "Full-field electroretinography and marked variability in clinical phenotype of Alström syndrome," *Archives of Ophthalmology*, vol. 126, pp. 51–57, 2008.

[91] J. D. Marshall, P. Maffei, G. B. Collin, and J. K. Naggert, "Alström syndrome: genetics and clinical overview," *Current Genomics*, vol. 12, pp. 225–235, 2011.

[92] J. D. Marshall, S. Beck, P. Maffei, and J. K. Naggert, "Alström syndrome," *European Journal of Human Genetics*, vol. 15, pp. 1193–1202, 2007.

[93] J. D. Marshall, E. G. Hinman, G. B. Collin et al., "Spectrum of *ALMS1* variants and evaluation of genotype-phenotype correlations in Alström syndrome," *Human Mutation*, vol. 28, pp. 1114–1123, 2007.

[94] I. Pereiro, B. E. Hoskins, J. D. Marshall et al., "Arrayed Primer Extension technology simplifies mutation detection in Bardet Biedl and Alström Syndrome," *European Journal of Human Genetics*, vol. 19, pp. 485–488, 2011.

[95] C. J. Bell, D. L. Dinwiddie, N. A. Miller et al., "Carrier testing for severe childhood recessive diseases by next-generation sequencing," *Science Translational Medicine*, vol. 3, p. 65ra4, 2011.

[96] M. De Vos, F. Barbier, and C. Cuvelier, "Congenital hepatic fibrosis," *Journal of Hepatology*, vol. 6, no. 2, pp. 222–228, 1988.

[97] O. Yönem, N. Ozkayar, F. Balkanci et al., "Is congenital hepatic fibrosis a pure liver disease?" *The American Journal of Gastroenterology*, vol. 101, pp. 1253–1259, 2006.

[98] J. A. Summerfield, Y. Nagafuchi, S. Sherlock, J. Canafalch, and P. J. Scheuer, "Hepatobiliary fibropolycystic disease: a clinical and histological review of 51 patients," *Journal of Hepatology*, vol. 2, pp. 141–156, 1986.

[99] A. M. di Bisceglie and A. S. Befeler, "Cystic and nodular diseases on the liver," in *Schiff's Diseases of the Liver*, E. R. Schiff, W. C. Maddrey, and M. Sorrell, Eds., pp. 1231–1251, Lippincott Williams & Wilkins, Philadelphia, Pa, USA, 10th edition, 2007.

[100] A. Shorbagi and Y. Bayraktar, "Experience of a single center with congenital hepaticfibrosis a review of the literature," *The World Journal of Gastroenterology*, vol. 16, pp. 683–690, 2010.

[101] G. Brancatelli, M. P. Federle, V. Vilgrain, M. P. Vullierme, D. Marin, and R. Lagalla, "Fibropolycystic liver disease: CT and MR imaging findings," *Radiographics*, vol. 25, no. 3, pp. 659–670, 2005.

[102] S. K. Sarin and A. Kumar, "Noncirrhotic portal hypertension," *Clinical Liver Disease*, vol. 10, pp. 627–651, 2006.

[103] G. Castaldo, G. Calcagno, R. Sibillo et al., "Quantitative analysis of aldolase A mRNA in liver discriminates between hepatocellular carcinoma and cirrhosis," *Clinical Chemistry*, vol. 46, pp. 901–906, 2000.

[104] G. Esposito, L. Vitagliano, R. Santamaria, A. Viola, A. Zagari, and F. Salvatore, "Structural and functional analysis of aldolase B mutants related to hereditary fructose intolerance," *FEBS Letters*, vol. 531, no. 2, pp. 152–156, 2002.

[105] C. Ciacci, D. Gennarelli, G. Esposito, R. Tortora, F. Salvatore, and L. Sacchetti, "Hereditary fructose intolerance and celiac disease: a novel genetic association," *Clinical Gastroenterology and Hepatology*, vol. 4, pp. 635–638, 2006.

[106] M. I. Yasawy, U. R. Folsch, W. E. Schmidt, and M. Schwend, "Adult hereditary fructose intolerance," *World Journal of Gastroenterology*, vol. 15, pp. 2412–2413, 2009.

[107] R. D. Oberhaensli, B. Rajagopalan, D. J. Taylor et al., "Study of hereditary fructose intolerance by use of $^{31}$P magnetic resonance spectroscopy," *The Lancet*, vol. 2, pp. 931–934, 1987.

[108] G. Esposito, M. R. Imperato, L. Ieno et al., "Hereditary fructose intolerance: functional study of two novel ALDOB natural variants and characterization of a partial gene deletion," *Human Mutation*, vol. 31, no. 12, pp. 1294–1303, 2010.

[109] G. Esposito, R. Santamaria, L. Vitagliano et al., "Six novel alleles identified in Italian fructose intolerance enlarge the mutation spectrum of the *aldolase B* gene," *Human Mutation*, vol. 24, p. 534, 2004.

[110] R. Santamaria, L. Vitagliano, S. Tamasi et al., "Novel six-nucleotide deletion in the hepatic fructose-1,6-bisphosphate aldolase gene in a patient with hereditary fructose intolerance and enzyme structure-function implications," *European Journal of Human Genetics*, vol. 7, pp. 409–414, 1999.

[111] R. Santamaria, S. Tamasi, G. Del Piano et al., "Molecular basis of hereditary fructose intolerance in Italy: identification of two novel mutations in the aldolase B gene," *Journal of Medical Genetics*, vol. 33, pp. 786–788, 1996.

[112] E. Gonzales, A. Spraul, and E. Jacquemin, "Clinical utility gene card for: progressive familial intrahepatic cholestasis type 3," *European Journal of Human Genetics*, vol. 22, 2014.

[113] E. Jacquemin, O. Bernard, M. Hadchouel et al., "The wide spectrum of multidrug resistance 3 deficiency: from neonatal cholestasis to cirrhosis of adulthood," *Gastroenterology*, vol. 120, no. 6, pp. 1448–1458, 2001.

[114] M. Ziol, V. Barbu, O. Rosmorduc et al., "ABCB4 heterozygous gene mutations associated with fibrosing cholestatic liver disease in adults," *Gastroenterology*, vol. 135, pp. 131–141, 2008.

[115] A. Davit-Spraul, E. Gonzales, C. Baussan, and E. Jacquemin, "Progressive familial intrahepatic cholestasis," *Clinical Pediatrics*, vol. 51, pp. 689–691, 2012.

[116] R. Ramraj, M. J. Finegold, and S. J. Karpen, "Progressive familial intrahepatic cholestasis type 3: overlapping presentation with Wilson disease," *Clinical Pediatrics*, vol. 51, pp. 689–691, 2012.

[117] O. Rosmorduc and R. Poupon, "Low phospholipid associated cholelithiasis: association with mutation in the *MDR3/ABCB4* gene," *Orphanet Journal of Rare Diseases*, vol. 2, article 29, 2007.

[118] D. Degiorgio, P. A. Corsetto, A. M. Rizzo et al., "Two ABCB4 point mutations of strategic NBD-motifs do not prevent protein targeting to the plasma membrane but promote MDR3 dysfunction," *European Journal of Human Genetics*, vol. 22, pp. 633–639, 2014.

[119] C. Colombo, P. Vajro, D. Degiorgio et al., "Clinical features and genotype-phenotype correlations in children with progressive familial intrahepatic cholestasis type 3 related to ABCB4 mutations," *Journal of Pediatric Gastroenterology and Nutrition*, vol. 52, pp. 73–83, 2011.

[120] R. Tomaiuolo, D. Degiorgio, D. A. Coviello et al., "An MBL2 haplotype and *ABCB4* variants modulate the risk of liver disease in cystic fibrosis patients: a multicentre study," *Digestive and Liver Disease*, vol. 41, pp. 817–822, 2009.

[121] D. Tavian, D. Degiorgio, N. Roncaglia et al., "A new splicing site mutation of the *ABCB4* gene in intrahepatic cholestasis of pregnancy with raised serum gamma-GT," *Digestive and Liver Disease*, vol. 41, pp. 671–675, 2009.

[122] D. Degiorgio, C. Colombo, M. Seia et al., "Molecular characterization and structural implications of 25 new *ABCB4* mutations in progressive familial intrahepatic cholestasis type 3 (PFIC3)," *European Journal of Human Genetics*, vol. 15, pp. 1230–1238, 2007.

# 6

# Demonstration of Hepatitis C Virus RNA with *In Situ* Hybridization Employing a Locked Nucleic Acid Probe in Humanized Liver of Infected Chimeric Mice and in Needle-Biopsied Human Liver

**Kazuya Shiogama,[1] Ken-ichi Inada,[1] Michinori Kohara,[2] Hidemi Teramoto,[3] Yasuyoshi Mizutani,[1] Takanori Onouchi,[1] and Yutaka Tsutsumi[1]**

[1] *Department of Pathology, Fujita Health University School of Medicine, Toyoake, Aichi 470-1192, Japan*
[2] *Department of Microbiology and Cell Biology, Tokyo Metropolitan Institute of Medical Science, Tokyo 156-8506, Japan*
[3] *Department of Internal Medicine, Kojin Hospital, Nagoya 463-8530, Japan*

Correspondence should be addressed to Yutaka Tsutsumi; tsutsumi@fujita-hu.ac.jp

Academic Editor: Hervé Lerat

*Background. In situ* hybridization (ISH) with high sensitivity has been requested to demonstrate hepatitis C virus (HCV) RNA in formalin-fixed, paraffin-embedded (FFPE) sections of the liver. *Methods.* ISH employing a locked-nucleic-acid- (LNA-)modified oligonucleotide probe and biotin-free catalyzed signal amplification system (CSAII) was applied to HCV-RNA detection in the liver tissue. Nested reverse-transcription polymerase chain reaction (RT-PCR) was performed for HCV genotyping using total RNA extracted from FFPE sections. The target tissues included FFPE tissue sections of humanized livers in HCV-infected chimeric mice (HCV genotypes 1a, 1b, and 2a and noninfected) and of needle-biopsied livers from HCV-infected patients. *Results.* HCV-RNA was demonstrated with the ISH technique in HCV-infected liver tissues from both chimeric mice and 9 (82%) of 11 patients with HCV infection. The HCV signals were sensitive to RNase. Nested RT-PCR confirmed the genotype in 8 (73%) of 11 livers (type 1b: 6 lesions and type 2a: 2 lesions). HCV-RNA was not identified in chronic hepatitis B lesions, fatty liver, autoimmune hepatitis, and hepatocellular carcinoma. *Conclusion.* ISH using the LNA-modified oligonucleotide probe and CSAII was applicable to detecting HCV-RNA in routinely prepared FFPE liver specimens.

## 1. Introduction

Hepatitis C virus (HCV) is a single-stranded RNA virus, a member of the Flaviviridae family. Since the first identification of the HCV genome by Choo et al. [1], HCV study has progressed mainly in the field of HCV functional analysis and therapeutic implications. Because of low viral levels in the serum, the diagnosis of HCV infection has been made with a branched chain DNA signal amplification assay and reverse-transcription polymerase chain reaction (RT-PCR) [2–4]. The sensitivity of HCV detection in the serum thus became reproducible and clinically relevant.

Pathologists are often requested to detect viral pathogens within the routinely prepared biopsy tissue samples, and therefore simple and reliable histochemical techniques are needed. Techniques for visualizing HCV localization within diseased hepatocytes have also been developed. Reports have described the detection of HCV in human liver tissue by using immunohistochemistry and *in situ* hybridization (ISH) [4–14], as well as by *in situ* RT-PCR [4, 6, 15–20]. At the moment, HCV detection with immunohistochemistry and ISH is not yet reproducible enough, we believe. *In situ* RT-PCR may demonstrate highly sensitive signals, but with concomitant increase of false positivity. Reliable histochemical techniques for detecting HCV in formalin-fixed, paraffin-embedded (FFPE) liver tissues are needed, particularly for routine diagnostic purpose.

In the present study, we established an ISH technique using a locked nucleic acid (LNA) probe and biotin-free tyramide amplification system (CSAII) for detecting HCV-RNA in FFPE tissue sections of the liver.

## 2. Materials and Methods

*2.1. Samples.* As positive controls, we sampled the humanized liver of HCV-infected chimeric mice [21, 22], and FFPE tissue sections were prepared. The chimeric mice were maintained by M. Kohara, Department of Microbiology and Cell Biology, Tokyo Metropolitan Institute of Medical Science, Tokyo. A total of 13 humanized liver specimens from HCV-infected chimeric mice were used (noninfected 3, genotype 1a-infected 3, genotype 1b-infected 4, and genotype 2a-infected 3).

A total of 11 needle biopsy liver specimens of chronic hepatitis C were culled from the computer file at the Diagnostic Pathology Division of Fujita Health University Hospital, Toyoake, Japan, and FFPE sections were cut. Needle biopsy specimens of hepatitis-B-virus- (HBV-)infected chronic hepatitis, virus-negative fatty liver and autoimmune hepatitis ($n = 1$, resp.), as well as two surgically removed HCC lesions caused by HCV or HBV infection, were also examined. The nonneoplastic part of the liver tissue (chronic hepatitis B) in the HBV-related HCC case was also evaluated. Nonneoplastic liver tissue was scarcely included in the HCV-related HCC case. Hematoxylin and eosin (HE) staining was performed for demonstrating histological features. The activity of inflammation and the degree of fibrosis were evaluated according to the New Inuyama Classification (1996) [23]. Serum HCV-RNA levels in the patients were measured using an RT-PCR assay, the Amplicor HCV Monitor Assay (Roche Diagnostics), and serum HCV subtypes were determined with nested RT-PCR (Roche Diagnostics).

*2.2. LNA-Modified Oligonucleotide Probe.* The sequence of an HCV-common probe was designed according to the previous description [15]. The target was within the HCV 5′-untranslated region (HCV-5′UTR), which is a highly conserved portion in the HCV genome. An LNA-modified oligonucleotide probe labeled with digoxygenin at the 3′-end was prepared in Gene Design Inc., Ibaraki, Osaka, Japan. The nucleotide sequence of the 45-mer probe was 5′-ALtTTLgGGLcGTLgCCLcCCLgCGLaGALcTGLcTALg-CCLgAGLtAGLtGTLtGGLgT-3′, in which La, Lt, Lc, and Lg represent LNA monomers corresponding to the bases A, T, C, and G, respectively.

*2.3. ISH.* FFPE sections were dewaxed in xylene and rehydrated in graded ethanol. Endogenous peroxidase activity was quenched with 0.3% hydrogen peroxide in methanol for 60 minutes at room temperature (RT). After rinsing thrice in diethyl-pyrocarbonate- (DEPC-)treated water, sections were digested with 40 $\mu$g/mL proteinase K (Roche Diagnostics, Tokyo, Japan) at 37°C for 15 minutes, washed thrice in DEPC-treated water, submerged in 95% ethanol for 1 minute, and air-dried completely. Then, sections were heat-treated for 5 minutes at 95°C on a hot plate and hybridized with 0.01 $\mu$mol/L LNA-modified oligonucleotide probe diluted with *in situ* Hybridization Buffer (Enzo Life Science, Bulter Pike, PA, USA) in an incubation chamber overnight at 37°C. After rinsing in 1x saline sodium citrate (SSC) for 30 minutes at 50°C, sections were rinsed twice in 50 mM Tris-HCl-buffered saline (TBS), pH 7.6, at RT. A horseradish-peroxidase-labeled antidigoxygenin antibody (Roche Diagnostics) diluted at 1 : 100 with 1% bovine serum albumin in TBS was applied for 60 minutes at RT. For amplifying signals, fluorescein-isothiocyanate- (FITC-)conjugated tyramide enclosed in CSAII (Dako, Glostrup, Denmark) was applied to the sections for 15 minutes at RT. Finally, a horseradish-peroxidase-labeled anti-FITC antibody equipped in the CSAII kit was reacted for 30 minutes at RT. Reaction products were visualized in 50 mM Tris-HCl buffer, pH 7.6, containing 20 mg/dL diaminobenzidine tetrahydrochloride and 0.006% hydrogen peroxidase. The nuclei were lightly counterstained with Mayer's hematoxylin.

In order to verify the specificity of the ISH technique for HCV-RNA detection, we carried out the treatment with DNase and RNase before the hybridization with the LNA probe on consecutive sections. Namely, either 10 IU/mL DNase I (Wako, Osaka, Japan) or 100 $\mu$g/mL RNase (Sigma-Aldrich, St. Louis, MO, USA) was incubated for 30 minutes at 37°C.

*2.4. Immunostaining Using a Human Specific Cytokeratin 8/18 (CK8/18) Antibody.* In order to distinguish mouse hepatocytes from chimeric human hepatocytes in HCV-infected chimeric mice, we utilized a human-specific CK8/18 monoclonal antibody (clone: NCL 5D3, MP Biochemicals, Santa Ana, CA, USA). After blocking endogenous peroxidase activity, hydrated heat-assisted epitope retrieval was employed using a pressure pan cooker (Delicio 6L, T-FAL, Clichy, France) for 10 minutes. Preliminary study revealed that as a soaking solution, 1 mM ethylenediamine tetraacetic acid solution, pH 8.0, was optimal to retrieve the antigenicity. After pressure cooking, sections were left for 30 minutes at RT for cooling. In order for avoiding nonspecific signals in mouse hepatocytes, a Mouse Stain kit (Nichirei Bioscience, Tokyo) was applied before and after the primary antibody incubation. The human-specific CK8/18 monoclonal antibody at a 1 : 100 dilution was incubated overnight at RT. After rinsing in 10 mM phosphate-buffered saline (PBS), pH 7.2, the sections were reacted with a secondary polymer reagent, Novolink (Novocastra, Newcastle, UK). Reaction products were visualized in the diaminobenzidine-hydrogen peroxide solution. Nuclear counterstaining with hematoxylin followed.

*2.5. HCV Genotyping by Nested RT-PCR.* Five slices of 5 $\mu$m thickness sections were collected in Eppendorf tubes. Total RNA was extracted from dewaxed sections using RecoverAll Total Nucleic Acid Isolation kit (Applied Biosytems, Austin, TX, USA), according to the manufacturer's protocol, and stored at −80°C until use. Nested RT-PCR for HCV genotyping was performed, as described previously [24].

Table 1: HCV-RNA demonstration with LNA-based ISH and nested RT-PCR in FFPE human liver tissues.

| Patient | Biopsy or surgery | Diagnosis New Inuyama Classification | Serum | | FFPE liver tissue | | |
|---|---|---|---|---|---|---|---|
| | | | HCV-RNA (KIU/mL) | Nested RT-PCR | Nested RT-PCR | ISH | |
| Case 1 | B | Chronic hepatitis C, A2F2 | $5{,}1 \times 10^2 \leqq$ | 1b | 1b | + | Focal/partial |
| Case 2 | B | Chronic hepatitis C, A1F1 | $2{,}8 \times 10^2$ | 1b | 1b | + | Focal/partial |
| Case 3 | B | Chronic hepatitis C, A2,F1 | $2{,}4 \times 10^2$ | 2a | 2a | + | Diffuse |
| Case 4 | B | Chronic hepatitis C, A1F0 | $1{,}9 \times 10^2$ | 2a | 2a | – | |
| Case 5 | B | Chronic hepatitis C, A1F1 | $2{,}5 \times 10^2$ | 1b | 1b | + | Focal/partial |
| Case 6 | B | Chronic hepatitis C, A2F3 | $2{,}7 \times 10^2$ | 1b | – | – | |
| Case 7 | B | Chronic hepatitis C, A2F1 | $2{,}2 \times 10^2$ | 2a | – | + | Focal/partial |
| Case 8 | B | Chronic hepatitis C, A3F3 | $5{,}1 \times 10^2$ | 1b | 1b | + | Focal/partial |
| Case 9 | B | Chronic hepatitis C, A2F1 | $2{,}9 \times 10^2$ | 1b | 1b | + | Diffuse |
| Case 10 | B | Chronic hepatitis C, A2F2 | $3{,}1 \times 10^2$ | 2a | – | + | Focal/partial |
| Case 11 | B | Chronic hepatitis C, A2F3 | $3{,}3 \times 10^2$ | 1b | 1b | + | Diffuse |
| Case 12 | B | Chronic hepatitis B, A3F3 | Not detected | Not done | – | – | |
| Case 13 | B | Fatty liver, A0F0 | Not detected | Not done | – | – | |
| Case 14 | B | Autoimmune hepatitis, A3F3 | Not detected | Not done | – | – | |
| Case 15 | S | Hepatitis-B-related HCC<br>Chronic hepatitis B, A2F2 | Not detected | Not done | – | –<br>– | |
| Case 16 | S | Hepatitis-C-related HCC | 84 | Not done | – | – | |

New Inuyama Classification (1996).
Activity of inflammation: A1: mild, A2: moderate, and A3: severe.
Fibrosis: F0: none, F1: portal widening, F2: bridging fibrosis, and F3: bridging fibrosis with lobular distortion.

*2.6. Ethical Issue.* The present study was approved by the institutional ethical review board for clinical and epidemiological investigations at Fujita Health University, Toyoake. The approval number is 12-193. Written informed consent was obtained from each patient.

## 3. Results

*3.1. HCV-RNA Localization in Humanized Liver of HCV-Infected Chimeric Mice.* In HE-stained sections, mouse hepatocytes showed densely eosinophilic cytoplasm, while chimeric human hepatocytes were weakly eosinophilic with frequent deposition of fat droplets. Immunoreactivity of human CK8/18 was seen only in human hepatocytes. In all the 10 HCV-infected livers but not the livers of three HCV noninfected mice, ISH demonstrated diffuse cytoplasmic signals in the human hepatocytes. In Figure 1 employing consecutive sections, HCV-RNA was visualized with the ISH technique in human CK8/18-positive chimeric hepatocytes from chimeric mice infected HCV genotypes 1a, 1b, and 2a (in Figure 1, dotted lines encircle the mouse hepatocyte area). No signals were detected in the noninfected chimeric liver tissue. It is of note that HCV-RNA was demonstrated in the cytoplasm of almost all chimeric human hepatocytes. The positive signals remained after DNase treatment but were completely abolished after RNase treatment. Figure 2 illustrates HCV genotype 1b-infected chimeric mouse liver, showing HE histology and positive cytoplasmic signals, which were resistant to DNase but sensitive to RNase.

*3.2. HCV-RNA Localization in Needle-Biopsied or Surgically Removed Human Liver Tissues.* Results of the human material are summarized in Table 1. Most of the HCV-positive patients showed high levels of HCV-RNA in the serum. Exceptionally, a surgical case of HCV-related HCC showed a low level of HCV-RNA in the serum. Nested RT-PCR genotyping for HCV using total RNA extracted from FFPE sections was successful in 8 (73%) of 11 biopsied chronic hepatitis C lesions, and in all the 8 cases, the genotypes were comparable with the serum analysis. LNA-based ISH detected signals in 9 (82%) of 11 chronic hepatitis C lesions, including three showing diffuse cytoplasmic positivity, and six showing focal or partial positivity. In three nested RT-PCR negative lesions, ISH revealed negativity (1 lesion) or focal/partial positivity (2 lesions). One lesion was nested RT-PCR-positive and ISH-negative. No HCV-RNA was detected in HBV-related lesions, fatty liver, autoimmune hepatitis, and in HCC lesions. Figure 3 demonstrates representative histochemical findings. Nonspecific binding of the CSAII reagent to Kupffer cells or lymphoid cells was occasionally observed in both the HCV-infected and HCV-unrelated lesions, as arrows indicate.

## 4. Discussion

We showed herein that LNA-based ISH for HCV-RNA yielded clear cytoplasmic reactivity in infected hepatocytes in FFPE sections. The LNA-modified oligonucleotide probe we employed represents one of the most sensitive probes for

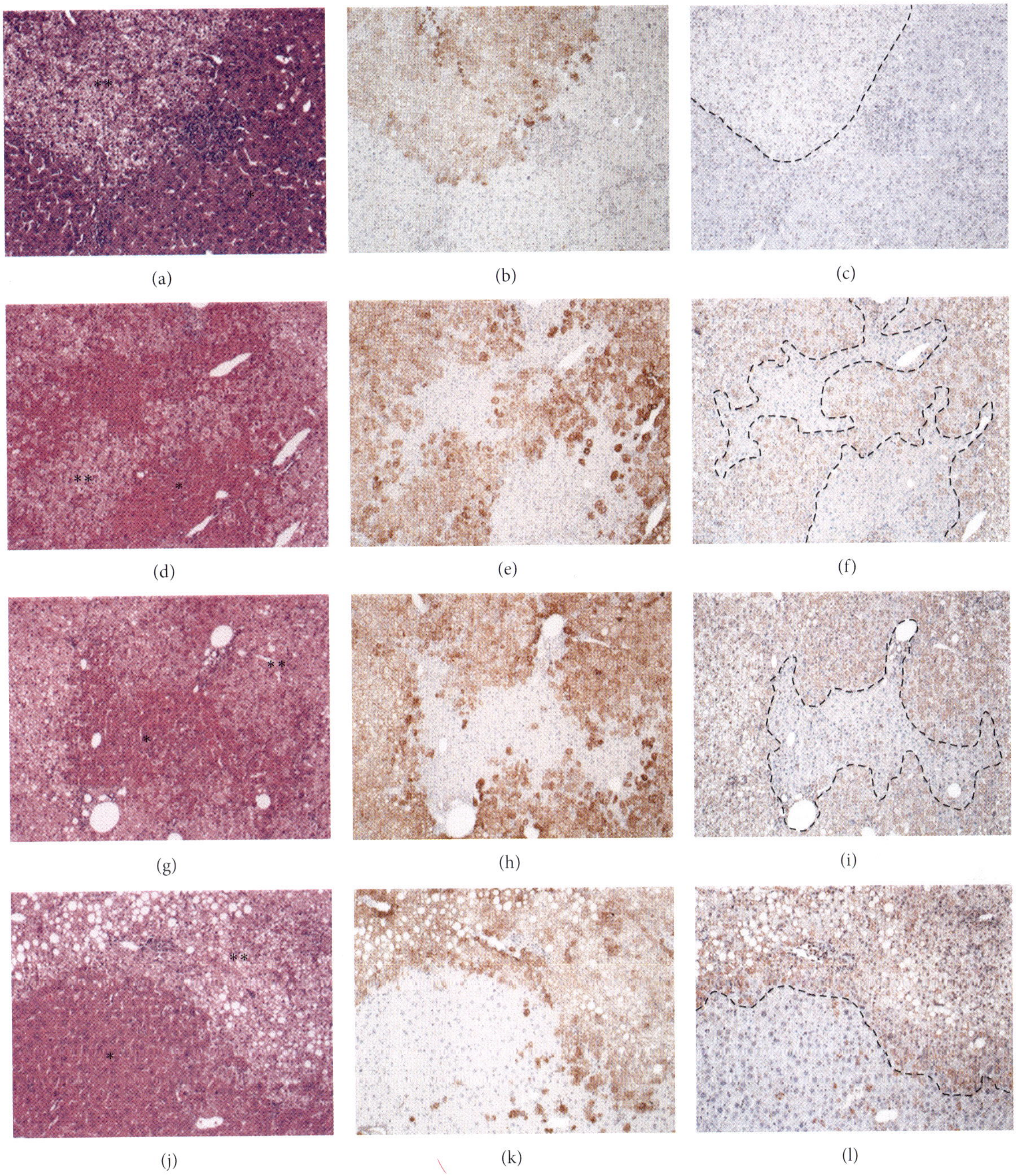


FIGURE 1: HCV-RNA localization with LNA-based ISH in the liver of chimeric mice infected with HCV of different genotypes. (a)–(c) HCV noninfected, (d)–(f) HCV genotype 1a-infected, (g)–(i) HCV genotype 1b-infected, (j)–(l) HCV genotype 2a-infected, ((a), (d), (g), (j)) HE stain, ((b), (e), (h), (k)) immunostaining for human-specific CK8/18, ((c), (f), (i), (l)) LNA-based ISH, (∗) mouse hepatocytes, and (∗∗) human hepatocytes. HCV-RNA is demonstrated diffusely in the cytoplasm of human hepatocytes in the chimeric livers. No signals are seen in the noninfected liver.

ISH [25–29]. LNA-based ISH has been applied to detecting cellular microRNA in FFPE tumor tissues [30–32]. The 45-mer LNA probe was targeted at the HCV-5′UTR containing a sequence common to the HCV subtypes. Positive signals for HCV-RNA were clearly demonstrated in HCV 1a-, 1b-, and 2a-infected humanized livers of chimeric mice. HCV-infected chimeric mice with humanized liver thus functioned as a useful model for histochemically demonstrating the HCV genome, particularly when immunostaining for human-specific CK8/18 was combined.

In needle-biopsied human liver specimens, HCV-RNA was detected in 8 of 11 HCV-infected samples with the nested RT-PCR analysis and in 9 of 11 with the ISH technique. In nested RT-PCR negative cases, ISH was negative or partially

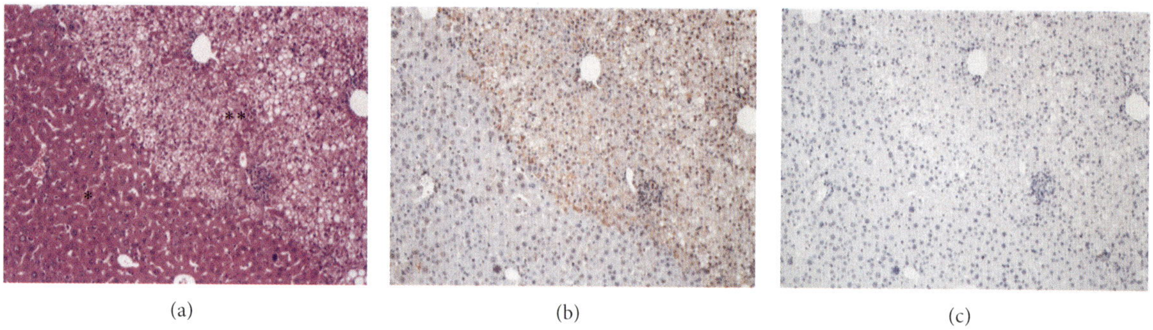


Figure 2: Confirmation of the specificity of LNA-based ISH. (a) HE stain, (b) ISH after DNase treatment, (c) ISH after RNase treatment, (∗) mouse hepatocytes, and (∗∗) human hepatocytes. The mouse hepatocytes are densely eosinophilic, while the human hepatocytes appear pale with deposition of fat droplets. HCV-RNA is observed only in the human hepatocytes in the chimeric liver infected with HCV genotype 1b. The HCV-RNA signals are resistant to DNase treatment but disappear after RNase treatment.

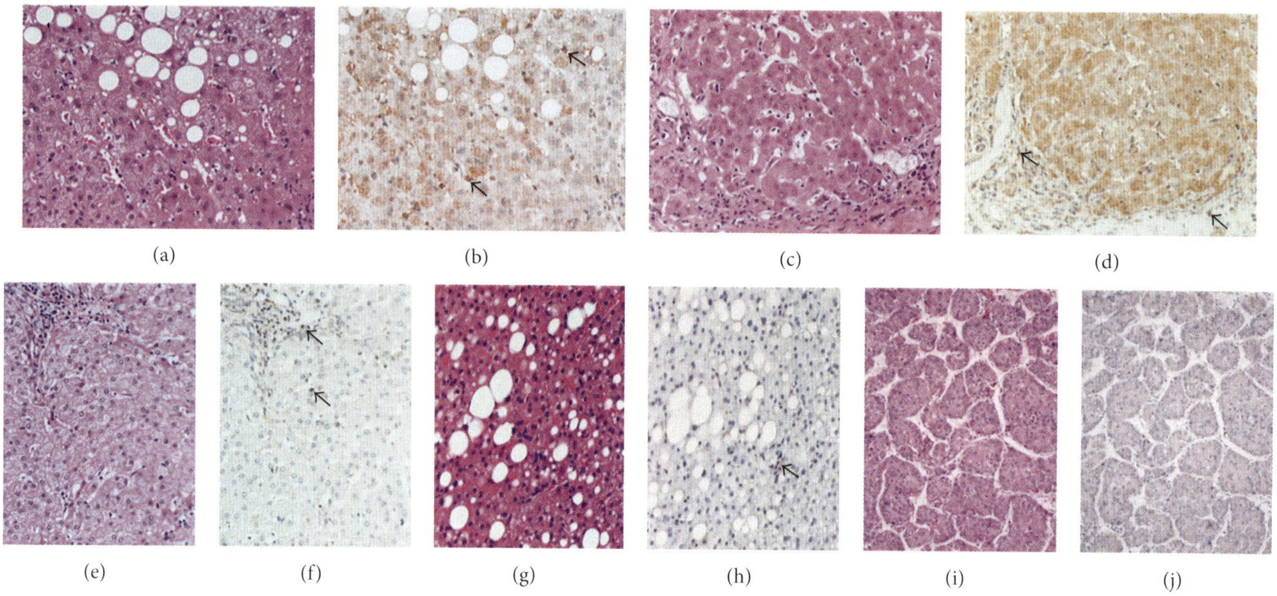


Figure 3: HCV-RNA localization with LNA-based ISH in FFPE biopsy or surgical specimens of the liver. ((a), (b)) Case 10 with chronic hepatitis C, ((c), (d)) case 11 with chronic hepatitis C, ((e), (f)) case 15 with chronic hepatitis B (noncancerous portion of a surgical case for HCC), ((g), (h)) case 13 with fatty liver, ((i), (j)) case 16 with surgically removed hepatitis-C-related HCC, ((a), (c), (e), (g), (i)) HE stain, and ((b), (d), (f), (h), (j)) LNA-based ISH. In HCV-infected human livers, the HCV-RNA signals are demonstrated in a focal/partial pattern (b) or in a diffuse pattern (d). Signals are not demonstrated in the hepatocytes of HBV-infected liver (f), fatty liver (h), and hepatitis-C-related HCC (j). Nonspecific binding of the reagent to Kupffer cells and lymphoid cells is occasionally observed (arrows in the panels (b), (d), (f), and (h)).

positive, suggesting that the detection threshold may depend on the virus load. Diffuse HCV expression pattern in the hepatocytes was already reported by Nuriya et al. [15], Liang et al. [33], and Li et al. [34].

In the present ISH study, HCV-RNA was undetectable in the hepatocytes in HBV-infected livers, nonviral liver disorders (fatty liver and autoimmune hepatitis), and in HCV-related HCC. With ISH using a digoxygenin-labeled cDNA probe, Tang et al. reported positivity in 8 (67%) of 12 HCV-related HCC [12]. It has been documented with an *in situ* RT-PCR technique that HCV-RNA decreases along with the progression from liver cirrhosis to HCC [35]. More cases of HCC need to be analyzed, in relation to the distribution of the HCV genome in cancerous lesions.

Revie and Salahuddin reviewed that HCV replicated in macrophages, B and T lymphocytes, and other nonhepatocellular components [36]. However, we judged the nonhepatocellular bindings as nonspecific reactions, primarily because of the staining in non-HCV cases. Under our present condition, nonspecific binding of the reagents, particularly CSAII, to Kupffer cells and lymphoid cells was observed. Further technical improvement is requested for reliable and reproducible HCV-RNA detection in FFPE specimens.

In conclusion, the ISH technique using the LNA-modified oligonucleotide probe and CSAII can be applied to detecting

HCV-RNA in liver biopsy specimens, the sensitivity probably being comparable to *in situ* RT-PCR. For detecting the HCV genome in routinely prepared liver biopsy specimens, our ISH sequence is relatively simple and requires no special equipment to perform. At the moment, this method seems to be suitable for demonstrating HCV genome in FFPE sections and will become a valuable tool for routine histopathological diagnosis of HCV infection using FFPE liver biopsy specimens.

## Acknowledgments

The authors thank Mr. Yutaka Hirasawa and Ms. Satomi Ito, Division of Diagnostic Pathology, Fujita Health University Hospital, for their cooperation in culling the specimens. Professor Kentaro Yoshioka, Department of Liver, Biliary Tract and Pancreas Diseases, and Professor Atsushi Sugioka, Department of Surgery, Fujita Health University School of Medicine, Toyoake, kindly allowed the authors to use the biopsy specimens. The skillful technical assistance by Ms. Mika Maeshima and Ms. Sayaka Takeuchi, Department of Pathology, Fujita Health University School of Medicine, is also cordially acknowledged. This work was in part supported by the Research Grant-in-Aid from the Japanese Ministry of Education, Culture, Sports, Science and Technology (no. 24790367).

## References

[1] Q.-L. Choo, G. Kuo, A. J. Weiner, L. R. Overby, D. W. Bradley, and M. Houghton, "Isolation of a cDNA clone derived from a blood-borne non A, non-B viral hepatitis genome," *Science*, vol. 244, no. 4902, pp. 359–362, 1989.

[2] A. M. Majid and D. R. Gretch, "Current and future hepatitis C virus diagnostic testing: problems and advancements," *Microbes and Infection*, vol. 4, no. 12, pp. 1227–1236, 2002.

[3] L. Muratori, "*In situ* reverse transcriptase-polymerase chain reaction: an innovative tool for hepatitis C virus RNA detection and localisation, and for quantification of infected cells," *European Journal of Histochemistry*, vol. 42, no. 2, pp. 133–136, 1998.

[4] P. Komminoth, V. Adams, A. A. Long et al., "Evaluation of methods for hepatitis C virus detection in archival liver biopsies. Comparison of histology, immunohistochemistry, *in-situ* hybridization, reverse transcriptase polymerase chain reaction (RT-PCR) and *in-situ* RT-PCR," *Pathology Research and Practice*, vol. 190, no. 11, pp. 1017–1025, 1994.

[5] H. S. Carvalho, M. L. Baptista, M. A. Pinto et al., "Detection of hepatitis C virus RNA by *in situ* hybridization in paraformaldehyde fixed biopsies," *Memorias do Instituto Oswaldo Cruz*, vol. 100, no. 3, pp. 269–272, 2005.

[6] X. Qian, R. B. Guerrero, T. B. Plummer, V. F. Alves, and R. V. Lloyd, "Detection of hepatitis C virus RNA in formalin-fixed paraffin-embedded sections with digoxigenin-labeled cRNA probes," *Diagnostic Molecular Pathology*, vol. 13, no. 1, pp. 9–14, 2004.

[7] S. de Lucas, J. Bartolomé, E. Rodríguez-Iñigo et al., "Distribution of hepatitis C virus infection in liver biopsies from children and adults with chronic hepatitis C," *Journal of Medical Virology*, vol. 64, no. 1, pp. 1–5, 2001.

[8] M. Chang, A. P. Marquardt, B. L. Wood et al., "*in situ* distribution of hepatitis C virus replicative-intermediate RNA in hepatic tissue and its correlation with liver disease," *Journal of Virology*, vol. 74, no. 2, pp. 944–955, 2000.

[9] V. Agnello, G. Ábel, G. B. Knight, and E. Muchmore, "Detection of widespread hepatocyte infection in chronic hepatitis C," *Hepatology*, vol. 28, no. 2, pp. 573–584, 1998.

[10] D. Sansonno, V. Cornacchiulo, V. Racanelli, and F. Dammacco, "*In situ* simultaneous detection of hepatitis C virus RNA and hepatitis C virus-related antigens in hepatocellular carcinoma," *Cancer*, vol. 80, no. 1, pp. 22–33, 1997.

[11] S. W. Cho, S. G. Hwang, D. C. Han et al., "*In situ* detection of hepatitis C virus RNA in liver tissue using a digoxigenin-labeled probe created during a polymerase chain reaction," *Journal of Medical Virology*, vol. 48, no. 3, pp. 227–233, 1996.

[12] L. Tang, Y. Tanaka, N. Enomoto, F. Marumo, and C. Sato, "Detection of hepatitis C virus RNA in hepatocellular carcinoma by *in situ* hybridization," *Cancer*, vol. 76, no. 11, pp. 2211–2216, 1995.

[13] M. Gastaldi, A. Massacrier, R. Planells et al., "Detection by *in situ* hybridization of hepatitis C virus positive and negative RNA strands using digoxigenin-labeled cRNA probes in human liver cells," *Journal of Hepatology*, vol. 23, no. 5, pp. 509–518, 1995.

[14] Y. Tanaka, N. Enomoto, S. Kojima et al., "Detection of hepatitis C virus RNA in the liver by *in situ* hybridization," *Liver*, vol. 13, no. 4, pp. 203–208, 1993.

[15] H. Nuriya, K. Inoue, T. Tanaka et al., "Detection of hepatitis B and C viruses in almost all hepatocytes by modified PCR-based *in situ* hybridization," *Journal of Clinical Microbiology*, vol. 48, no. 11, pp. 3843–3851, 2010.

[16] A. J. Alzahrani, P. J. Vallely, and R. F. T. McMahon, "Development of a novel nested *in situ* PCR-ISH method for detection of hepatitis C virus RNA in liver tissue," *Journal of Virological Methods*, vol. 99, no. 1-2, pp. 53–61, 2002.

[17] P. Biagini, L. Benkoel, F. Dodero et al., "Hepatitis C virus RNA detection by *in situ* RT-PCR in formalin-fixed paraffin-embedded liver tissue. Comparison with serum and tissue results," *Cellular and Molecular Biology*, vol. 47, pp. OL167–OL171, 2001.

[18] D. Bettinger, C. Mougin, B. Fouqué, B. Kantelip, J. P. Miguet, and M. Lab, "Direct *in situ* reverse transcriptase-linked polymerase chain reaction with biotinylated primers for the detection of hepatitis C virus RNA in liver biopsies," *Journal of Clinical Virology*, vol. 12, no. 3, pp. 233–241, 1999.

[19] F. M. Walker, M. Dazza, M. Dauge et al., "Detection and localization by *in situ* molecular biology techniques and immunohistochemistry of hepatitis C virus in livers of chronically infected patients," *Journal of Histochemistry and Cytochemistry*, vol. 46, no. 5, pp. 653–660, 1998.

[20] G. K. K. Lau, J. W. S. Fang, P. C. Wu, G. L. Davis, and J. Y. N. Lau, "Detection of hepatitis C virus genome in formalin-fixed paraffin-embedded liver tissue by *in situ* reverse transcription polymerase chain reaction," *Journal of Medical Virology*, vol. 44, no. 4, pp. 406–409, 1994.

[21] C. Tateno, Y. Yoshizane, N. Saito et al., "Near completely humanized liver in mice shows human-type metabolic responses to drugs," *American Journal of Pathology*, vol. 165, no. 3, pp. 901–912, 2004.

[22] D. F. Mercer, D. E. Schiller, J. F. Elliott et al., "Hepatitis C virus replication in mice with chimeric human livers," *Nature Medicine*, vol. 7, no. 8, pp. 927–933, 2001.

[23] F. Ichida, "Histological grading criteria of chronic hepatitis: new Inuyama classification," in *Proceedings of the 19th Inuyama Symposium*, pp. 183–188, Chugai Igaku, 1996.

[24] K. Shiogama, H. Teramoto, Y. Morita et al., "Hepatitis C virus infection in a Japanese leprosy sanatorium for the past 67 years," *Journal of Medical Virology*, vol. 82, no. 4, pp. 556–561, 2010.

[25] L. A. Neely, S. Patel, J. Garver et al., "A single-molecule method for the quantitation of microRNA gene expression," *Nature Methods*, vol. 3, no. 1, pp. 41–46, 2006.

[26] W. P. Kloosterman, E. Wienholds, E. de Bruijn, S. Kauppinen, and R. H. A. Plasterk, "*In situ* detection of miRNAs in animal embryos using LNA-modified oligonucleotide probes," *Nature Methods*, vol. 3, no. 1, pp. 27–29, 2006.

[27] K. Kubota, A. Ohashi, H. Imachi, and H. Harada, "Improved *in situ* hybridization efficiency with locked-nucleic-acid- incorporated DNA probes," *Applied and Environmental Microbiology*, vol. 72, no. 8, pp. 5311–5317, 2006.

[28] R. Thomsen, P. S. Nielsen, and T. H. Jensen, "Dramatically improved RNA *in situ* hybridization signals using LNA-modified probes," *RNA*, vol. 11, no. 11, pp. 1745–1748, 2005.

[29] A. Válóczi, C. Hornyik, N. Varga, J. Burgyán, S. Kauppinen, and Z. Havelda, "Sensitive and specific detection of microRNAs by northern blot analysis using LNA-modified oligonucleotide probes," *Nucleic Acids Research*, vol. 32, no. 22, article e175, 2004.

[30] K. Sakurai, C. Furukawa, T. Haraguchi et al., "MicroRNAs miR-199a-5p and -3p target the Brm subunit of SWI/SNF to generate a double-negative feedback loop in a variety of human cancers," *Cancer Research*, vol. 71, no. 5, pp. 1680–1689, 2011.

[31] N. Yamamichi, R. Shimomura, K. Inada et al., "Locked nucleic acid *in situ* hybridization analysis of miR-21 expression during colorectal cancer development," *Clinical Cancer Research*, vol. 15, no. 12, pp. 4009–4016, 2009.

[32] P. T. Nelson, D. A. Baldwin, W. P. Kloosterman, S. Kauppinen, R. H. A. Plasterk, and Z. Mourelatos, "RAKE and LNA-ISH reveal microRNA expression and localization in archival human brain," *RNA*, vol. 12, no. 2, pp. 187–191, 2006.

[33] Y. Liang, T. Shilagard, S. Xiao et al., "Visualizing hepatitis C virus infections in human liver by two-photon microscopy," *Gastroenterology*, vol. 137, no. 4, pp. 1448–1458, 2009.

[34] G. Li, K. Li, A. S. Lea et al., "*In situ* hybridization for the detection of hepatitis C virus RNA in human liver tissue," *Journal of Viral Hepatitis*, vol. 20, no. 3, pp. 183–192, 2013.

[35] T. Tanaka, K. Inoue, Y. Hayashi et al., "Virological significance of low-level hepatitis B virus infection in patients with hepatitis C virus associated liver disease," *Journal of Medical Virology*, vol. 72, no. 2, pp. 223–229, 2004.

[36] D. Revie and S. Z. Salahuddin, "Human cell types important for Hepatitis C Virus replication *in vivo* and *in vitro*. Old assertions and current evidence," *Virology Journal*, vol. 8, pp. 346–370, 2011.

7

# Circulating MicroRNAs in Plasma of Hepatitis B e Antigen Positive Children Reveal Liver-Specific Target Genes

**Thilde Nordmann Winther,[1,2] Kari Stougaard Jacobsen,[1,2] Aashiq Hussain Mirza,[2] Ida Louise Heiberg,[1] Claus Heiner Bang-Berthelsen,[2] Flemming Pociot,[2] and Birthe Hogh[1]**

[1]*Department of Paediatrics, Hvidovre Hospital, University of Copenhagen, Kettegaard Allé 30, 2650 Hvidovre, Denmark*
[2]*Department of Paediatrics and Center for Non-Coding RNA in Technology and Health, Herlev Hospital, University of Copenhagen, Arkaden, 2730 Herlev, Denmark*

Correspondence should be addressed to Thilde Nordmann Winther; thildewinther@gmail.com

Academic Editor: Daisuke Morioka

*Background and Aim.* Hepatitis B e antigen positive (HBeAg-positive) children are at high risk of severe complications such as hepatocellular carcinoma and cirrhosis. Liver damage is caused by the host immune response to infected hepatocytes, and we hypothesise that specific microRNAs play a role in this complex interaction between virus and host. The study aimed to identify microRNAs with aberrant plasma expressions in HBeAg-positive children and with liver-specific target genes. *Methods.* By revisiting our previous screen of microRNA plasma levels in HBeAg-positive and HBeAg-negative children with chronic hepatitis B (CHB) and in healthy controls, candidate microRNAs with aberrant plasma expressions in HBeAg-positive children were identified. MicroRNAs targeting liver-specific genes were selected based on bioinformatics analysis and validated by qRT-PCR using plasma samples from 34 HBeAg-positive, 26 HBeAg-negative, and 60 healthy control children. *Results.* Thirteen microRNAs showed aberrant plasma expressions in HBeAg-positive children and targeted liver-specific genes. In particular, three microRNAs were upregulated and one was downregulated in HBeAg-positive children compared to HBeAg-negative and healthy control children, which showed equal levels. *Conclusion.* The identified microRNAs might impact the progression of CHB in children. Functional studies are warranted, however, to elucidate the microRNAs' role in the immunopathogenesis of childhood CHB.

## 1. Introduction

Children with chronic hepatitis B (CHB) have a lifetime risk of developing hepatocellular carcinoma (HCC) up to 25% and an incidence of cirrhosis of 2-3% per year [1, 2]. It is widely accepted that the natural course of CHB is determined by the host-virus interaction; however, the exact mechanisms responsible for disease progression in children are not fully understood.

Evidence suggests that microRNAs play a role in the complex interaction between the hepatitis B virus and host [3]. Our group recently identified a panel of 16 microRNAs aberrantly expressed in plasma of children with CHB and suggested a potential role of these microRNAs in the pathogenesis of childhood CHB [4].

Risk of progressive liver disease primarily applies to hepatitis B e antigen positive (HBeAg-positive) children and seroclearance of HBeAg is a key event in the natural course of disease [5]. Most children who undergo HBeAg seroconversion are defined inactive carriers, with absent or low viral replication, and usually inactive liver histology [5]. Inactive carriers with no signs of cirrhosis at seroconversion do not show disease progression over long-term follow-up (24–29 years) [6–8]. In the present study we hypothesise that microRNAs aberrantly expressed in plasma of HBeAg-positive children might be involved in the development of progressive liver disease.

It is well known that specific host factors in the liver tissue are tightly regulated in patients with CHB [9]. MicroRNAs may regulate specific individual targets or function as master regulators of cellular processes, and many microRNAs regulate their targets cooperatively [10, 11]. Identifying liver-specific target genes for aberrantly expressed microRNAs in HBeAg-positive children may provide better insight in understanding the role of microRNAs in the pathogenesis of childhood CHB.

The present study aimed to identify circulating microRNAs targeting liver-specific genes—specifically in HBeAg-positive children. Our data provide an important resource for future investigations aiming at deciphering the role of specific microRNAs in the pathogenesis of childhood CHB.

## 2. Patients and Methods

*2.1. Patients and Healthy Controls.* CHB is a notifiable disease in Denmark [12] and the definition of CHB is hepatitis B surface antigen (HBsAg) seropositivity for more than six months [13]. Danish children with CHB are mainly adoptees and immigrants from highly endemic countries. During the period from July 2005 to April 2011, all children aged 0–18 years with CHB who were reported to Statens Serum Institut, Copenhagen, Denmark ($n = 202$), were invited to participate in the study. Parents of 60 children volunteered, and these children were included in the study. The cohort of children with CHB was previously described [4].

Characteristics of the chronically HBV infected children in brief included mean age: 10.1 years (SD ± 3.9 years, range 0.9–17.3 years); gender: 26 males and 34 females; racial origin: 62% ($n = 37$) were Asian, 17% ($n = 10$) were African, and 22% ($n = 13$) were Caucasian.

Of the 60 children studied, 34 were HBeAg-positive and 26 were HBeAg-negative (and anti-HBe positive). Mean alanine aminotransferase (ALT) and HBV DNA (± SD) were as follows: HBeAg-positive: ALT 47 ± 28 U/L and HBV DNA $5E + 08 \pm 1E + 09$ IU/mL, and HBeAg-negative: ALT 26 ± 13 U/L and HBV DNA $9E + 02 \pm 2E + 03$ IU/mL. Among HBeAg-positive children, genotypes A, B, C, D, E, and F were identified, and among HBeAg-negative children, genotypes A, B, C, D, and E were identified. Eleven out of 26 HBeAg-negative patients were not successfully genotyped due to low HBV DNA levels (Table 1) [4]. None of the children showed symptoms of their HBV infection, and none of them had received antiviral treatment. The children were followed in accordance with international guidelines [13–15]. All patients were negative for HIV, hepatitis A virus, and hepatitis C virus.

Furthermore, 60 healthy control children (previously described [4]) were included between August 2010 and August 2011. These children were recruited prior to elective surgery for a hernia or prior to minor orthopaedic surgery at Hvidovre Hospital, University of Copenhagen, Denmark.

Characteristics of the healthy controls in brief are mean age: 7.1 years (SD ± 3.7, range 0.7–15.7); gender: 33 males and 27 females; racial origin: 15% ($n = 9$) were Asian, 2% ($n = 1$) were African, and 83% ($n = 50$) were Caucasian (Table 1) [4]. The children were tested HBsAg-negative and none of the children had received vaccination against HBV. The children were free from known medical conditions. Blood samples were obtained prior to anaesthesia.

Table 1: Characteristics of children with chronic hepatitis B and of healthy controls [4].

| | Chronic hepatitis B | | Healthy controls |
|---|---|---|---|
| | HBeAg pos. | HBeAg neg. | |
| Number of patients | **34** | **26** | **60** |
| Male | 14 (41%) | 12 (46%) | 33 (55%) |
| Female | 20 (59%) | 14 (54%) | 27 (45%) |
| Age (years) | | | |
| Mean | **8.8** | **12.0** | **7.1** |
| SD | 3.7 | 3.4 | 3.7 |
| Race | | | |
| African | 4 | 6 | 1 |
| Asian | 22 | 15 | 9 |
| Caucasian | 8 | 5 | 50 |
| ALT (U/L ref. value 5–45) | | | |
| Mean | **46.5** | **25.6** | **14.3** |
| SD | 27.6 | 12.6 | 5.3 |
| HBV DNA (IU/mL) | | | |
| Mean | **5.1*E* + 08** | **8.5*E* + 02** | **NA** |
| SD | 1.2*E* + 09 | 2.0*E* + 03 | |
| Genotypes | | | |
| A | **2** (6%) | **2** (8%) | |
| B | **11** (32%) | **2** (8%) | |
| C | **5** (15%) | **2** (8%) | |
| D | **12** (35%) | **7** (27%) | |
| E | **3** (9%) | **2** (8%) | |
| F | **1** (3%) | **0** (0%) | |
| N/A | **0** (0%) | **11** (42%) | **60** (100%) |

ALT: alanine aminotransferase.
N/A: not analysed.

*2.2. Ethical Considerations.* The study was performed in accordance with the criteria of the Helsinki II Declaration and was approved by the Ethics Committee, Capital Region of Denmark, Reference number H-KF-255584, and the Danish Data Protection Agency, Journal number 2009-41-4193. Parents of all participants provided informed written consent prior to any study procedure.

*2.3. Blood Samples.* Blood samples were processed as previously described [4]. Briefly, blood samples were collected in EDTA tubes, centrifuged at 2,500 g for 10 minutes at room temperature, separated, aliquoted, and stored at −80°C until further use.

*2.4. HBsAg Quantification.* HBsAg was quantified as previously described [4], using ARCHITECT HBsAg assay (Abbott, Chicago, IL, USA) according to manufacturer's instructions.

*2.5. Screen of Plasma MicroRNA Levels in Children with CHB and in Healthy Controls.* Recently, our group published an initial screen of plasma microRNA levels in HBeAg-positive, HBeAg-negative, and healthy children [4]. Briefly, microRNA polymerase-chain-reaction (PCR) panels (human panel I and II V2.M/R), miRCURY LNA Universal RT PCR system (Exiqon, Vedbaek, Denmark) were employed to measure plasma levels of 739 human microRNAs in a total of three samples: one sample contained plasma from 10 HBeAg-positive children, one sample contained plasma from 10 HBeAg-negative children, and one sample contained plasma from 10 healthy controls. Analyses were performed per Exiqon's instructions. According to the manufacturer, the microRNAs covered in the microRNA PCR panels are generally higher expressed and more likely differentially expressed in disease, or more often cited in the literature.

*2.6. Selection of Candidate MicroRNAs.* For selection of candidate microRNAs we followed stringent criteria and included only data from HBeAg-positive and HBeAg-negative children. Firstly, based on raw data, microRNAs with $C_T$ values above 35 in HBeAg-positive and/or HBeAg-negative children were excluded. Secondly, raw data were normalised using three differentapproaches: global mean, U6, and geometric mean of miR-22-5p, -26a-5p, and 221-3p as previously described [4]. By using the comparative $C_T$ method, the relative expression of each microRNA between the groups was calculated [16]. We focused on microRNAs aberrantly expressed in HBeAg-positive children and identified the top up- and downregulated microRNAs for further analyses.

*2.7. Bioinformatics Analysis.* Bioinformatics analysis was performed on all candidate microRNAs identified by revisiting our previous screen. Our analysis included retrieval of microRNA target genes with CLIP-Seq (cross-linking immunoprecipitation-high-throughput sequencing) overlap from starBase (sRNA target Base, release 2.1) and subsequently liver-specificity filters were applied on the retrieved microRNA target genes with CLIP-Seq overlap.

*2.8. Retrieval of MicroRNA Target Genes with CLIP-Seq Overlap.* MicroRNA target genes were retrieved using the starBase, a database that allows a comprehensive exploration of microRNA-target gene interaction maps from CLIP-Seq and Degradome-Seq data [17]. The predicted microRNA-target gene interactions in starBase are processed from five target prediction tools (TargetScan, PicTar, PITA, miRanda, and RNA22) overlapping with the CLIP-Seq data. Only those target genes that intersected the CLIP-Seq data sets with a biological complexity ≥2 (a measure of reproducibility between biological replicates or experiments to further reduce false positives) were retrieved.

*2.9. Liver-Specificity Filter for MicroRNA Target Genes.* Human liver-specific genes were retrieved from the TiGER (Tissue Specific-Gene-Expression and Regulation, version 1.0) [18] and TiSGeD (Tissue-Specific Genes Database) [19] databases. The TiGER database encompasses human tissue-specific gene expression profiles or expressed sequence tag (EST) data, cis-regulatory module (CRM) data, and combinatorial gene regulation data for interacting transcription factor (TF) pairs.

TiGER data is based on analyses of 30 human tissues identifying tissue-specific genes (specificity is determined by expression enrichment scores and associated −log10 ($P$ value)), TFs and CRMs. A gene is defined as tissue-specific if it satisfies the following two conditions: enrichment score >5 and $P$ value $< 10^{-3.5}$. In case of the TiSGeD, tissue-specific genes are based on biomedical literature and data mining of gene expression profiles for over 100 human tissues. In TiSGeD, relative tissue-specificity of a gene is based on a statistical parameter, SPM, to quantitatively measure the specificity of a gene over tissues. An SPM parameter is a sensitive indicator in quantitative estimation of gene expression patterns. SPM ranges from 0 to 1.0. A value close to 1.0 indicates high tissue specificity of a gene.

From the TiGER database, liver-specific genes were retrieved: 383 genes based on ESTs (309 nonredundant genes); 300 CRM detections (105 nonredundant genes); and 160 TF pairs coregulating in liver (96 nonredundant genes). Two-hundred-and-fifty liver-specific genes were retrieved from the TiSGeD database that included human liver, fetal liver, hepatoma, and HepG2 specific genes. In total, 542 liver-specific genes were retrieved from these resources.

Liver-specific target genes were identified for the microRNAs of interest by comparing all the target genes with four liver-specific gene lists based on TiGER (EST, CRM, TF) and TiSGeD. A target gene was deemed to be liver-specific if it was present in any of the four liver-specific gene lists.

*2.10. Validation of Candidate MicroRNAs.* Candidate microRNAs targeting liver-specific genes were selected for further validation by quantitative real-time PCR (qRT-PCR). Candidate microRNAs were individually quantified by standard qRT-PCR using total RNA extracted from plasma of 34 HBeAg-positive, 26 HBeAg-negative, and 60 healthy controls.

*2.11. RNA Extraction.* Total RNA was extracted from plasma using the miRNeasy mini kit (Qiagen, Hilden, Germany) as previously described [4]. RNA was stored at −80°C until further use.

*2.12. cDNA Synthesis.* cDNA synthesis was performed using the Universal cDNA Synthesis kit (Exiqon, Vedbaek, Denmark) as previously described [4] and cDNA was stored at −20°C.

*2.13. qRT-PCR.* qRT-PCRs were performed on Pick & Mix microRNA PCR panels including predesigned primers for 23 microRNAs: mir-16-2-3p, -28-5p, -30a-5p, -30b-5p, -30c-5p, -30e-3p, -144-5p, -148a-3p, -224-3p, -378a-3p, -548c-5p, -574-3p, -589-3p, -605, -636, -639, -654-3p, -let-7c, -23a-3p, -451a, 22-5p, -26a-5p, 221-3p (Exiqon, Vedbaek, Denmark).

Resultant cDNA was diluted ×50 and assayed in 10 $\mu$L PCR reactions according to the protocol for miRCURY LNA Universal RT microRNA PCR (Exiqon, Vedbaek, Denmark). Negative controls with no template from the reverse transcription reaction were included and profiled like the samples. Thermal cycling was performed on a CFX384 Real-Time thermal cycler (Biorad, Hercules, California, USA) in 384 well plates as per Exiqon's instruction. $C_T$ (max) was set to 40 amplification cycles. Analyses were run in triplicate.

*2.14. Analysis of qRT-PCR Data.* Quality control of the qRT-PCR was performed as previously described [4, 20]. Raw data were normalised using the geometric mean of miR-22-3p, -26a-5p, and -221-3p [4, 21, 22] and the comparative $C_T$ method was used to analyse the data [16]. Statistical analyses were performed as previously described [4], by using SAS software, version 9.2 (SAS Institute, Cary, NC, USA). Briefly, statistical significances were determined using Mann-Whitney test and correlation analyses were performed in two steps, both of which used analysis of variance on ranks ($P$ values from Chi-Squared tests). Due to multiple testing only $P < 0.0028$ was regarded as significant (Bonferroni correction).

## 3. Results

*3.1. Clinical Parameters.* HBsAg was quantified in plasma from 48 out of 60 (80%) children with CHB. Plasma levels of HBsAg were significantly higher in HBeAg-positive children ($1.1E + 08 \pm$ SD $9.3E + 07$) compared to HBeAg-negative children ($1.4E + 07 \pm$ SD $1.2E + 07$), $P < 0.001$. It was not possible to measure HBsAg in plasma from 12 chronically infected children due to lack of sample material (7 HBeAg-positive and 5 HBeAg-negative).

*3.2. Selection of Candidate MicroRNAs.* We revisited our previous screen on plasma levels of 739 microRNAs in HBeAg-positive, HBeAg-negative, and healthy children [4]. Only data from children with CHB were included in the present study. Firstly, we included only microRNAs with raw $C_T$-values at or below 35 for further downstream analyses. Based on this cut-off, 227 candidate microRNAs were taken for subsequent analysis. Secondly, raw data of the 227 candidate microRNAs were normalised against the global mean; U6; and geometric mean of miR-22-5p, -26a-5p, and -221-3p. The plasma microRNAs levels in HBeAg-positive and HBeAg-negative children were compared and the top up- and downregulated microRNAs were selected. A total of 32 microRNAs were selected as candidate microRNAs. The candidate microRNAs included 14 microRNAs that were previously identified (miR-99a-5p, -100-5p, -122-5p, -122-3p, -125b-5p, -192-5p, -192-3p, -193b-3p, -194-5p, -215, -365a-3p, -455-5p, -455-3p, and -855-5p) [4] and 18 "new" candidate microRNAs of which 9 showed higher levels in plasma from HBeAg-positive children compared to HBeAg-negative children (miR-28-5p, -30a-5p, -30b-5p, -30c-5p, -30e-3p, -148a-3p, -378a-3p, -574-3p, and -let-7c) and nine showed lower levels (miR-16-2-3p, -144-5p, -224-3p, -548c-5p, -589-3p, -605, -636, -639, and 654-3p).

*3.3. Identification of Liver-Specific MicroRNA Target Genes.* All 32-candidate microRNAs were included in bioinformatics analysis. MicroRNA target genes with CLIP-seq overlap were retrieved from the starBase, 26 microRNAs (miR-28-5p, -30a-5p, -30b-5p, -30c-5p, -30e-3p, -99a-5p, -100-5p, -122-5p, -125b-5p, -148a-3p, -192-5p, -193b-3p, -194-5p, -215, -365a-3p, -378a-3p, -455-5p, -455-3p, -548c-5p, -574-3p, -605, -636, -639, -654-3p, -855-5p, and -let-7c) had target genes with CLIP-seq overlap, and a total of 1822 target genes with CLIP-seq overlap were retrieved from the starBase.

A liver-specificity filter was applied on the retrieved microRNA target genes with CLIP-seq-overlap. Sixteen out of 26 microRNAs had liver-specific target genes with CLIP-seq overlap (miR-28-5p, -30a-5p, -30e-3p, -125b-5p, -148a-3p, -193b-3p, -215, -365a-3p, -378a-3p, -455-5p, -455-3p, -548c-5p, -574-3p, -639, -654-3p, and -let-7c), and in total 28 (16 non-redundant) target genes were retrieved. The 16 non-redundant target genes were *ACADSB, ARIDIA, BTG3, CEBPG, CPOX, E2F1, FRAT2, GABBR1, GATA6, HOXA9, LEF1, MAZ, PAPD5, SF1, SMAD4*, and *ZXDB* (Table 2).

Furthermore, the remaining ten microRNAs had no liver-specific target genes and did not pass the liver-specificity filter. For these microRNAs, the total numbers of non-liver-specific target genes with CLIP-seq overlap retrieved from the starBase were 1378 (833 nonredundant). Only those target genes predicted by two or more target prediction tools are presented: in total 522 target genes of which 299 are nonredundant (Table S1 in Supplementary Material, available online at http://dx.doi.org/10.1155/2014/791045).

*3.4. Validation of Candidate MicroRNAs.* Of the 16 candidate microRNAs targeting liver-specific genes, six microRNAs (miR-125b-5p, -193b-3p, -215, -365a-3p, -455-5p, and -455-3p) were validated in our previous study. Interestingly, all these microRNAs were significantly expressed at higher levels in plasma from HBeAg-positive children than in the HBeAg-negative children [4]. The remaining 10 microRNAs were selected for validation in the present study (miR-28-5p, -30a-5p, -30e-3p, -148a-3p, -378a-3p, -548c-5p, -574-3p, -639, -654-3p, and -let-7c). Individual qRT-PCR analyses of these microRNAs were performed on plasma samples from 34 HBeAg-positive, 26 HBeAg-negative, and 60 healthy children. Quality control led to the exclusion of samples from four children (one sample from a HBeAg-negative child and three samples from healthy controls) and the exclusion of two microRNAs (miR-148a-3p and -639).

*3.5. MicroRNAs Showing Aberrant Plasma Levels in HBeAg-Positive Children.* We measured the quantity of the eight microRNAs in plasma from 34 HBeAg-positive and 25 HBeAg-negative children. Six microRNAs (miR-28-5p, -30a-5p, -30e-3p, -378a-3p, -574-3p, and -let-7c) were significantly expressed ($P < 0.001$) at higher levels in plasma from HBeAg-positive children than in the HBeAg-negative children. One microRNA (miR-654-3p) was expressed at a lower

TABLE 2: Liver-specific target genes with CLIP-seq overlap for 16 microRNAs.

| MicroRNA (hsa) | Target gene | Gene description |
|---|---|---|
| 28-5p | MAZ | MYC-associated zinc finger protein (purine-binding transcription factor) |
| 30a-5p | ARID1A | AT rich interactive domain 1A (SWI-like) |
| 30e-3p | CEBPG | CCAAT/enhancer binding protein (C/EBP), gamma |
| 125b-5p | FRAT2 | Frequently rearranged in advanced T-cell lymphomas 2 |
| | MAZ | MYC-associated zinc finger protein (purine-binding transcription factor) |
| 148a-3p | ZXDB | Zinc finger, X-linked, duplicated B |
| | ARID1A | AT rich interactive domain 1A (SWI-like) |
| | CEBPG | CCAAT/enhancer binding protein (C/EBP), gamma |
| 193b-3p | MAZ | MYC-associated zinc finger protein (purine-binding transcription factor) |
| 215 | ACADSB | Acyl-CoA dehydrogenase, short/branched chain |
| 365a-3p | HOXA9 | Homeobox A9 |
| | MAZ | MYC-associated zinc finger protein (purine-binding transcription factor) |
| 378a-3p | ARID1A | AT rich interactive domain 1A (SWI-like) |
| 455-5p | SMAD4 | SMAD family member 4 |
| 455-3p | PAPD5 | PAP associated domain containing 5 |
| | MAZ | MYC-associated zinc finger protein (purine-binding transcription factor) |
| 548c-5p | BTG3 | B-cell translocation gene 3 |
| | SF1 | Splicing factor 1 |
| | GATA6 | GATA binding protein 6 |
| 574-3p | GABBR1 | Gamma-aminobutyric acid (GABA) B receptor, 1 |
| | E2F1 | E2F transcription factor 1 |
| 639 | LEF1 | Lymphoid enhancer-binding factor 1 |
| 654-3p | CPOX | Coproporphyrinogen oxidase |
| | SF1 | Splicing factor 1 |
| let-7c | HOXA9 | Homeobox A9 |
| | GATA6 | GATA binding protein 6 |
| | CEBPG | CCAAT/enhancer binding protein (C/EBP), gamma |
| | SF1 | Splicing factor 1 |

level ($P = 0.012$) (Figure 1). Due to multiple testing, however, only $P < 0.0028$ was regarded as significant. miR-548c-5p was expressed at the same level in plasma from HBeAg positive and HBeAg-negative children, $P = 0.542$ (Figure 1).

To further investigate the microRNA expression patterns of children with CHB we included data from 57 healthy controls in the statistical analyses. Of the six microRNAs with significantly higher plasma levels in HBeAg-positive children than in HBeAg-negative children, two microRNAs (miR-28-5p and miR-30a-5p) showed similar expression levels in plasma from HBeAg-negative and healthy children, $P > 0.004$, whereas four microRNAs (miR-30e-3p, 378a-3p, 574-3p, and let-7c) showed lowest expression in plasma from healthy controls, $P < 0.001$ (Figure 1).

miR-654-3p that showed lower expression in HBeAg-positive children compared to HBeAg-negative children was expressed at same levels in plasma from HBeAg-negative and healthy control children, $P = 0.52$ (Figure 1).

Levels (fold changes) of the eight microRNAs in plasma from HBeAg-positive and HBeAg-negative children were calculated relative to the plasma levels in healthy controls (Table 3).

*3.6. MicroRNA Plasma Levels and Virological Parameters.* We examined the correlations between plasma microRNA levels and the virological parameters: viral load and HBsAg quantity. Only children with CHB were included in these analyses. Firstly, focusing on univariate analyses, we observed strong positive correlations between plasma levels of six microRNAs (miR-28-5p, -30a-5p, -30e-3p, -378a-3p, -574-3p, and -let-7c) and with both viral load and HBsAg quantity, $P < 0.001$. All six of these microRNAs showed significantly higher plasma levels in HBeAg-positive children when compared to HBeAg-negative children.

Secondly, multivariate analyses were performed taking into account the effect on plasma microRNA levels of the different virological parameters: HBeAg-status, viral load, and HBsAg quantity. Interestingly, the strongest correlations were observed between plasma microRNA levels and HBsAg quantity. The correlations were significant for four microRNAs (miR-28-5p, -30e-3p, -574-3p, and -let-7c), $P < 0.001$, all of which showed significantly higher levels in HBeAg-positive children when compared to HBeAg-negative children (Figure 2).

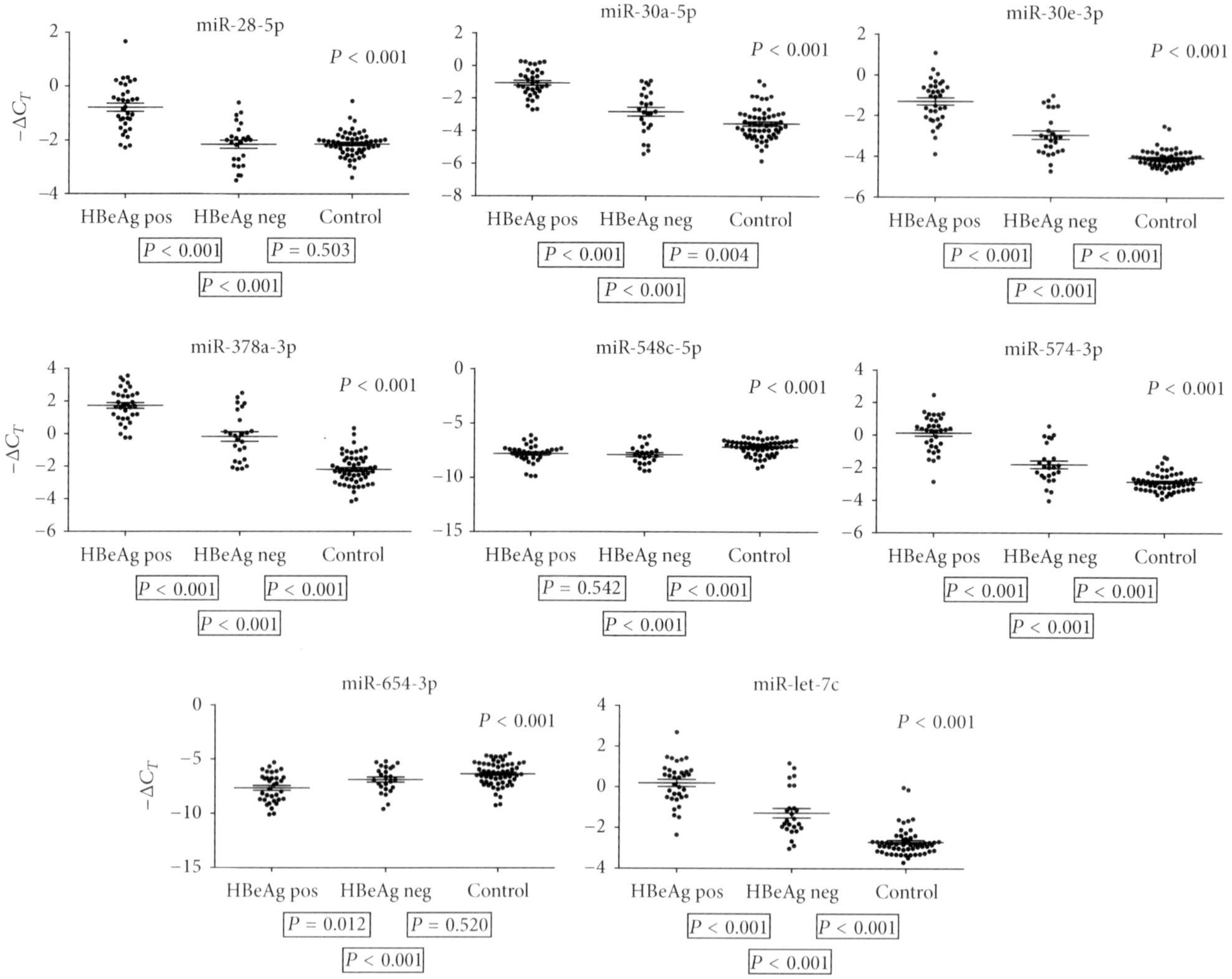


FIGURE 1: MicroRNA plasma levels in HBeAg-positive, HBeAg-negative, and healthy children. qRT-PCR-data on 34 HBeAg-positive, 25 HBeAg-negative, and 57 healthy control children. The $P$ values shown above the individual figures are results of statistical analyses on HBeAg-positive, HBeAg-negative, and healthy children, and $P$ values shown below left are results on HBeAg-positive versus HBeAg-negative, below centred HBeAg-positive versus healthy controls, and below right HBeAg-negative versus healthy controls. The bars represent geometric means $-\Delta C_T \pm$ SEM. Due to multiple testing only $P < 0.0028$ was considered significant.

## 4. Discussion

HBeAg-positive children are especially vulnerable to developing HCC and cirrhosis, and we hypothesise that specific microRNAs impact the progression of CHB. This study is the first to identify microRNAs with aberrant plasma expressions specifically in HBeAg-positive children and with liver-specific target genes.

A total of 13 microRNAs showed aberrant plasma expressions in HBeAg-positive children and revealed liver-specific target genes (miR-28-5p, -30a-5p, -30e-3p, -125b-5p, -193b-3p, -215, -365a-3p, -378a-3p, -455-5p, -455-3p, -574-3p, -654-3p, and -let-7c). Our bioinformatics approach led to the identification of 21 liver-specific target genes for the 13 microRNAs. Of these, 13 were nonredundant. All target genes retrieved for two or more microRNAs (*ARIDIA, CEBPG, HOXA9*, and *MAZ*), and the majority of the remaining target genes (*CPOX, E2F1, FRAT2, GATA6, SF1*, and *SMAD4*) are regulators of carcinogenesis, functioning both as promoters and as suppressors, and/or are implicated in the replication of HBV [23–34]. However, three of the target genes, to our knowledge, are not described in relation to cancer or HBV infection (*ACADSB, GABBR1*, and *PAPD5*).

For miR-122, known to be highly expressed in liver tissue [35], we could not identify liver-specific target genes due to nonavailability of CLIP-seq data for a number of microRNAs, including mir-122-3p. Additionally, the application of a liver-specificity filter excluded candidate microRNAs with substantial functions in tissues other than the liver.

Of the 13 microRNAs targeting liver-specific genes, seven microRNAs (validated in the present study) were aberrantly expressed in HBeAg-positive children when compared to HBeAg-negative children. Six microRNAs (miR-28-5p, -30a-5p, -30e-3p, -378a-3p, -574-3p, and -let-7c) showed significantly higher levels in HBeAg-positive children when compared to HBeAg-negative children, and one microRNA

TABLE 3: MicroRNA plasma levels in children with CHB relative to healthy controls.

| MicroRNA (hsa) | Sample | Mean Ct | SD | Fold change | SE | *P* value |
|---|---|---|---|---|---|---|
| 28-5p | HBeAg pos. | 28.21 | 1.35 | 3.1 | 2.8–3.5 | <0.001 |
| | HBeAg neg. | 29.89 | 1.80 | 1.0 | 0.9–1.1 | |
| | Control | 29.39 | 1.34 | 1 | | |
| 30a-5p | HBeAg pos. | 28.50 | 1.22 | 5.6 | 4.9–6.4 | <0.001 |
| | HBeAg neg. | 30.55 | 1.07 | 1.6 | 1.3–2.0 | |
| | Control | 30.80 | 0.65 | 1 | | |
| 30e-3p | HBeAg pos. | 28.72 | 1.60 | 6.8 | 6.0–7.8 | <0.001 |
| | HBeAg neg. | 30.77 | 1.36 | 2.9 | 2.5–3.3 | |
| | Control | 31.34 | 1.25 | 1 | | |
| 378a-3p | HBeAg pos. | 25.69 | 1.39 | 15.1 | 13.0–17.5 | <0.001 |
| | HBeAg neg. | 27.88 | 0.93 | 4.0 | 3.3–5.0 | |
| | Control | 29.43 | 0.71 | 1 | | |
| 548c-5p | HBeAg pos. | 35.17 | 1.57 | 0.7 | 0.6-0.7 | <0.001 |
| | HBeAg neg. | 35.43 | 1.94 | 0.9 | 0.8–1.0 | |
| | Control | 34.40 | 1.46 | 1 | | |
| 574-3p | HBeAg pos. | 27.30 | 1.48 | 7.8 | 6.8–9.0 | <0.001 |
| | HBeAg neg. | 29.51 | 1.22 | 2.1 | 1.7–2.4 | |
| | Control | 30.07 | 0.98 | 1 | | |
| 654-3p | HBeAg pos. | 35.11 | 1.82 | 0.4 | 0.3–0.5 | <0.001 |
| | HBeAg neg. | 34.68 | 2.16 | 0.7 | 0.6–0.8 | |
| | Control | 33.62 | 1.94 | 1 | | |
| let-7c | HBeAg pos. | 27.24 | 1.53 | 7.4 | 6.5–8.5 | <0.001 |
| | HBeAg neg. | 29.02 | 1.36 | 2.7 | 2.3–3.2 | |
| | Control | 29.94 | 1.15 | 1 | | |

(miR-654-3p) showed lower levels ($P = 0.012$). Additionally, six out of the 13 microRNAs with liver-specific target genes were validated in our previous study. All six microRNAs (miR-125b-5p, -193b-3p, -215, -365a-3p, -455-5p, and -455-3p) [4] showed significantly higher levels in HBeAg-positive children when compared to HBeAg-negative children. Interestingly, all 12 microRNAs upregulated in HBeAg-positive children are previously reported aberrantly expressed in adults with different types of cancer [36–44]. Indeed, seven microRNAs (miR-30a-5p, -125b-5p, -193b-3p, -215, -378a-3p, -574-3p, and -let-7c) have previously been associated with HCC [39–43, 45, 46].

By including data on healthy controls in the analyses we identified two interesting microRNA expression profiles. Firstly, three microRNAs (miR-28-5p, -30a-5p, and -125b-5p) were significantly upregulated in HBeAg-positive children when compared to HBeAg-negative and healthy control children, which showed equal levels. The liver-specific target genes identified for these three microRNAs were *ARID1A*, *FRAT2*, and *MAZ*. *ARID1A* encodes an AT-rich interactive domain-containing protein 1A (SWI-like). *ARID1A* is a tumour suppressor and has been found mutated in HBV associated HCC [24, 47]. *FRAT2* encodes a GSK-3-binding protein, and the expression of *FRAT2* may be upregulated in tumour progression [25]. *MAZ* gene encodes a MYC-associated zinc finger protein and the expression of MAZ is significantly increased in HCC [26]. Interestingly, the signalling pathways regulated by *ARID1A, FRAT2*, and *MAZ* have at least one target in common, namely, c-*MYC* [48–50], which is known to be overexpressed in mouse HCC [51].

The other interesting microRNA expression profile observed in the present study was for miR-654-3p. miR-654-3p was downregulated in HBeAg-positive children when compared to HBeAg-negative and healthy control children, which showed equal levels. In line with our finding, miR-654-3p has an inhibitory role in the H1N1 Influenza A virus [52] and acts as a tumor suppressor in prostate cancer [53]. Two liver-specific target genes, *CPOX* and *SF1*, are targeted by miR-654-3p. *CPOX* encodes the enzyme Coproporphyrinogen-III oxidase that has a role in the haem and chlorophyll biosynthetic pathways [54] whereas *SF1* encodes Splicing Factor 1 that is involved in the formation of the spliceosome complex [55].

We propose that these microRNAs identified with aberrant plasma expressions specifically in HBeAg-positive children and with liver-specific target genes are biomarkers for disease progression and might impact the development of HCC, and perhaps also cirrhosis, in children with CHB. Functional studies are warranted, however, to further elucidate these microRNAs' role in the immunopathogenesis of childhood CHB.

To date few therapies have been licensed to treat CHB in children, and most are only partially effective [5]. Interestingly, the potential of microRNAs as targets for therapeutic

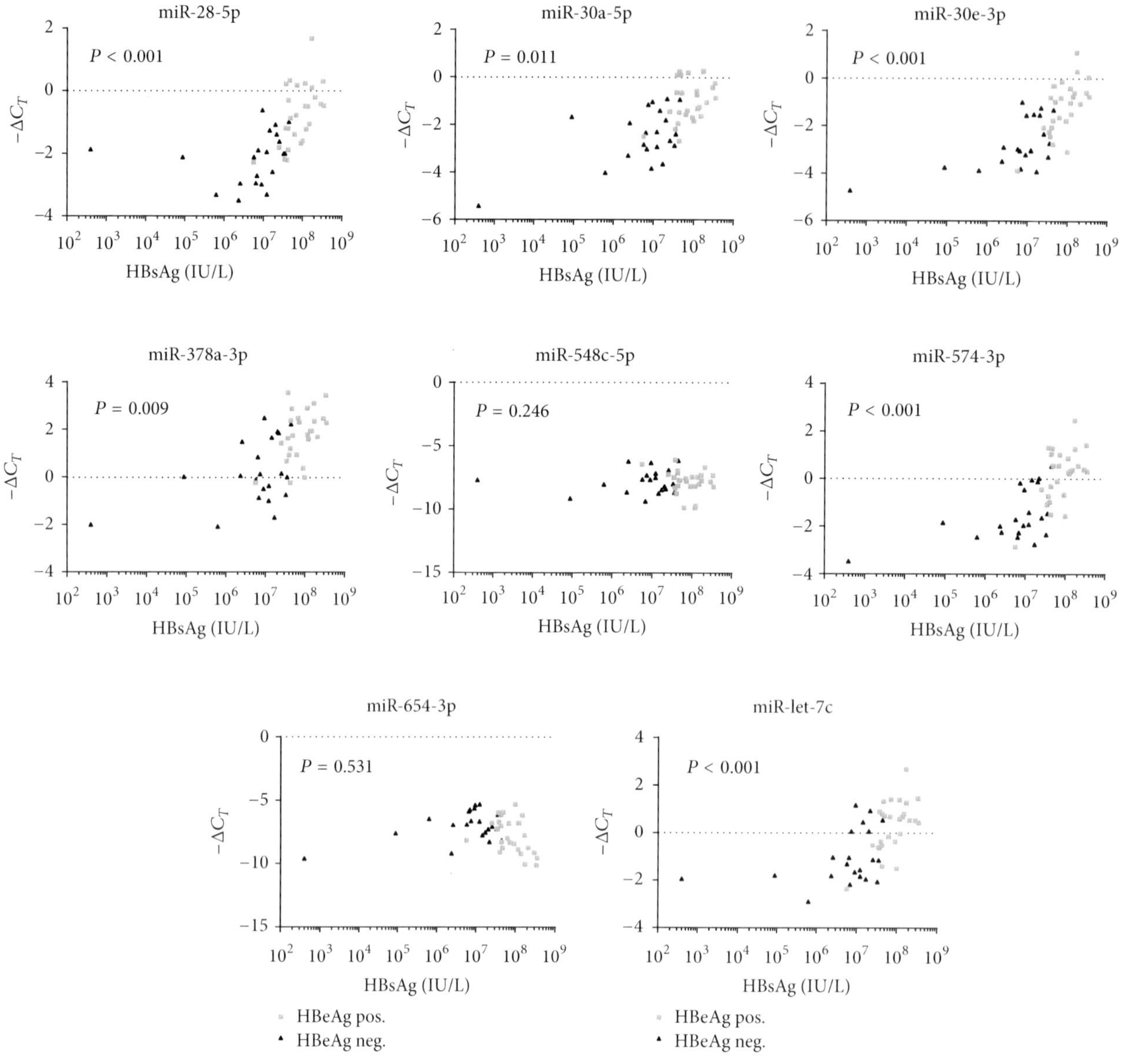


FIGURE 2: MicroRNA plasma levels and HBsAg quantity. qRT-PCR and HBsAg data on 34 HBeAg-positive and 25 HBeAg-negative children. $P$ values are based on multivariate analyses. Due to multiple testing only $P < 0.0028$ was considered significant.

interventions has shown great promise [11], and the first artificial microRNA antagonist is already in clinical trial [56]. MicroRNAs with a biological function in the immunopathogenesis of childhood CHB might serve as targets for the development of new antiviral treatment strategies. Whether the microRNAs identified in the present study would have the potential to serve as targets in future therapeutics needs to be investigated.

In conclusion, we identified 13 microRNAs with aberrant plasma expressions of HBeAg-positive children and with liver-specific target genes. In particular, we observed two distinct microRNA expression patterns: three microRNAs were upregulated and one was downregulated in HBeAg-positive children compared to HBeAg-negative and healthy control children, which showed equal levels. Five liver-specific target genes were identified for the four microRNAs. The microRNAs might be biomarkers for disease progression in children with CHB. Further studies are needed to elucidate the microRNAs' role in childhood CHB, hopefully leading to the identification of future therapeutic targets and to enhanced management of childhood CHB.

## Acknowledgments

The authors would like to thank all of the participating children and their parents. They are grateful for the collaboration with the participating hospitals and the staff. A special thanks goes to Dr. Thomas Hoffmann, Nina Lambertus, and Lena Vang, Department of Paediatrics, Hvidovre Hospital, University of Copenhagen, Copenhagen, Denmark.

## References

[1] M.-W. Yu, H.-C. Chang, Y.-F. Liaw et al., "Familial risk of hepatocellular carcinoma among chronic hepatitis B carriers and their relatives," *Journal of the National Cancer Institute*, vol. 92, no. 14, pp. 1159–1164, 2000.

[2] Z. Luo, L. Li, and B. Ruan, "Impact of the implementation of a vaccination strategy on hepatitis B virus infections in China over a 20-year period," *International Journal of Infectious Diseases*, vol. 16, no. 2, pp. e82–e88, 2012.

[3] Y.-F. Wei, G.-Y. Cui, P. Ye, J.-N. Chen, and H.-Y. Diao, "MicroRNAs may solve the mystery of chronic hepatitis B virus infection," *World Journal of Gastroenterology*, vol. 19, no. 30, pp. 4867–4876, 2013.

[4] T. N. Winther, C. H. Bang-Berthelsen, I. L. Heiberg, F. Pociot, and B. Hogh, "Differential plasma microRNA profiles in HBeAg positive and HBeAg negative children with chronic hepatitis B," *PLoS ONE*, vol. 8, no. 3, Article ID e58236, 2013.

[5] E. M. Sokal, M. Paganelli, S. Wirth et al., "Management of chronic hepatitis B in childhood: ESPGHAN clinical practice guidelines: consensus of an expert panel on behalf of the European Society of Pediatric Gastroenterology, Hepatology and Nutrition," *Journal of Hepatology*, vol. 59, no. 4, pp. 814–829, 2013.

[6] F. Bortolotti, M. Guido, S. Bartolacci et al., "Chronic hepatitis B in children after e antigen seroclearance: final report of a 29-year longitudinal study," *Hepatology*, vol. 43, no. 3, pp. 556–562, 2006.

[7] R. Iorio, A. Giannattasio, F. Cirillo, L. D'Alessandro, and A. Vegnente, "Long-term outcome in children with chronic hepatitis B: a 24-year observation period," *Clinical Infectious Diseases*, vol. 45, no. 8, pp. 943–949, 2007.

[8] Y.-H. Ni, M.-H. Chang, P.-J. Chen et al., "Viremia profiles in children with chronic hepatitis B virus infection and spontaneous e antigen seroconversion," *Gastroenterology*, vol. 132, no. 7, pp. 2340–2345, 2007.

[9] Y. Chen, A. Shen, P. J. Rider et al., "A liver-specific microRNA binds to a highly conserved RNA sequence of hepatitis B virus and negatively regulates viral gene expression and replication," *The FASEB Journal*, vol. 25, no. 12, pp. 4511–4521, 2011.

[10] R. M. O'Connell, D. S. Rao, A. A. Chaudhuri, and D. Baltimore, "Physiological and pathological roles for microRNAs in the immune system," *Nature Reviews Immunology*, vol. 10, no. 2, pp. 111–122, 2010.

[11] M. Esteller, "Non-coding RNAs in human disease," *Nature Reviews Genetics*, vol. 12, no. 12, pp. 861–874, 2011.

[12] Statens Serum Institut (SSI), *Mandatory Notification Systems*, SSI, Copenhagen, Denmark, 2013, http://www.ssi.dk/English/HealthdataandICT/Surveillance%20in%20Denmark/Mandatory%20notification%20systems.aspx.

[13] "EASL clinical practice guidelines: management of chronic hepatitis B virus infection," *Journal of Hepatology*, vol. 57, no. 1, pp. 167–185, 2012.

[14] B. A. Haber, J. M. Block, M. M. Jonas et al., "Recommendations for screening, monitoring, and referral of pediatric chronic hepatitis B," *Pediatrics*, vol. 124, no. 5, pp. e1007–e1013, 2009.

[15] A. S. F. Lok and B. J. McMahon, "Chronic hepatitis B: update of recommendations," *Hepatology*, vol. 39, no. 3, pp. 857–861, 2004.

[16] K. J. Livak and T. D. Schmittgen, "Analysis of relative gene expression data using real-time quantitative PCR and the 2-ΔΔCT method," *Methods*, vol. 25, no. 4, pp. 402–408, 2001.

[17] J.-H. Yang, J.-H. Li, P. Shao, H. Zhou, Y.-Q. Chen, and L.-H. Qu, "StarBase: a database for exploring microRNA-mRNA interaction maps from Argonaute CLIP-Seq and Degradome-Seq data," *Nucleic Acids Research*, vol. 39, no. 1, pp. D202–D209, 2011.

[18] X. Liu, X. Yu, D. J. Zack, H. Zhu, and J. Qian, "TiGER: a database for tissue-specific gene expression and regulation," *BMC Bioinformatics*, vol. 9, article 271, 2008.

[19] S.-J. Xiao, C. Zhang, Q. Zou, and Z.-L. Ji, "TiSGeD: a database for tissue-specific genes," *Bioinformatics*, vol. 26, no. 9, Article ID btq109, pp. 1273–1275, 2010.

[20] T. N. Winther, I. L. Heiberg, C. H. Bang-Berthelsen, F. Pociot, and B. Hogh, "Hepatitis B surface antigen quantity positively correlates with plasma levels of microRNAs differentially expressed in immunological phases of chronic hepatitis B in children," *PLoS ONE*, vol. 8, no. 11, Article ID e80384, 2013.

[21] H.-T. Zhu, Q.-Z. Dong, G. Wang et al., "Identification of suitable reference genes for qRT-PCR analysis of circulating microRNAs in hepatitis B virus-infected patients," *Molecular Biotechnology*, vol. 50, no. 1, pp. 49–56, 2012.

[22] J. Vandesompele, K. De Preter, F. Pattyn et al., "Accurate normalization of real-time quantitative RT-PCR data by geometric averaging of multiple internal control genes," *Genome Biology*, vol. 3, no. 7, 2002.

[23] G. Amaddeo, C. Guichard, S. Imbeaud, and J. Zucman-Rossi, "Next-generation sequencing identified new oncogenes and tumor suppressor genes in human hepatic tumors," *OncoImmunology*, vol. 1, no. 9, pp. 1612–1613, 2012.

[24] J. Huang, Q. Deng, Q. Wang et al., "Exome sequencing of hepatitis B virus-associated hepatocellular carcinoma," *Nature Genetics*, vol. 44, no. 10, pp. 1117–1121, 2012.

[25] T. Saitoh, J. Moriwaki, J. Koike et al., "Molecular cloning and characterization of FRAT2, encoding a positive regulator of the WNT signaling pathway," *Biochemical and Biophysical Research Communications*, vol. 281, no. 3, pp. 815–820, 2001.

[26] J. Dudas, T. Mansuroglu, F. Moriconi et al., "Altered regulation of Prox1-gene-expression in liver tumors," *BMC Cancer*, vol. 8, article 92, 2008.

[27] Q. Feng, J. E. Stern, S. E. Hawes, H. Lu, M. Jiang, and N. B. Kiviat, "DNA methylation changes in normal liver tissues and hepatocellular carcinoma with different viral infection," *Experimental and Molecular Pathology*, vol. 88, no. 2, pp. 287–292, 2010.

[28] N. Trehanpati, S. Shrivastav, B. Shivakumar et al., "Analysis of Notch and TGF-$\beta$ signaling expression in different stages of disease progression during hepatitis B virus infection," *Clinical and Translational Gastroenterology*, vol. 3, article e23, 2012.

[29] L. Yao, F.-J. Li, Z.-Q. Tang, S. Gao, and D.-Q. Wu, "Smad4 expression in hepatocellular carcinoma differs by hepatitis status," *Asian Pacific Journal of Cancer Prevention*, vol. 13, no. 4, pp. 1297–1303, 2012.

[30] E. A. Conner, E. R. Lemmer, M. Omori, P. J. Wirth, V. M. Factor, and S. S. Thorgeirsson, "Dual functions of E2F-1 in a transgenic mouse model of liver carcinogenesis," *Oncogene*, vol. 19, no. 44, pp. 5054–5062, 2000.

[31] K. Takahashi, N. Ikeda, N. Nonoguchi et al., "Enhanced expression of coproporphyrinogen oxidase in malignant brain tumors: CPOX expression and 5-ALA-induced fluorescence," *Neuro-Oncology*, vol. 13, no. 11, pp. 1234–1243, 2011.

[32] F. Shen, J. Li, W. Cai et al., "GATA6 predicts prognosis and hepatic metastasis of colorectal cancer," *Oncology Reports*, vol. 30, no. 3, pp. 1355–1361, 2013.

[33] T. Heise, G. Sommer, K. Reumann, I. Meyer, H. Will, and H. Schaal, "The hepatitis B virus PRE contains a splicing regulatory element," *Nucleic Acids Research*, vol. 34, no. 1, pp. 353–363, 2006.

[34] Y.-H. Ou, P.-H. Chung, F.-F. Hsu, T.-P. Sun, W.-Y. Chang, and S.-Y. Shieh, "The candidate tumor suppressor BTG3 is a transcriptional target of p53 that inhibits E2F1," *The EMBO Journal*, vol. 26, no. 17, pp. 3968–3980, 2007.

[35] P. Landgraf, M. Rusu, R. Sheridan et al., "A mammalian microRNA expression atlas based on small RNA library sequencing," *Cell*, vol. 129, no. 7, pp. 1401–1414, 2007.

[36] Z. Li, X. Gu, Y. Fang, J. Xiang, and Z. Chen, "microRNA expression profiles in human colorectal cancers with brain metastases," *Oncology Letters*, vol. 3, no. 2, pp. 346–350, 2012.

[37] H. Xie, L. Lee, S. Caramuta et al., "MicroRNA expression patterns related to merkel cell polyomavirus infection in human Merkel cell carcinoma," *The Journal of Investigative Dermatology*, vol. 134, no. 2, pp. 507–517, 2014.

[38] A. Markou, I. Sourvinou, P. A. Vorkas, G. M. Yousef, and E. Lianidou, "Clinical evaluation of microRNA expression profiling in non small cell lung cancer," *Lung Cancer*, vol. 81, no. 3, pp. 388–396, 2013.

[39] L. Li, Z. Guo, J. Wang, Y. Mao, and Q. Gao, "Serum miR-18a: a potential marker for hepatitis B virus-related hepatocellular carcinoma screening," *Digestive Diseases and Sciences*, vol. 57, no. 11, pp. 2910–2916, 2012.

[40] J. Gui, Y. Tian, X. Wen et al., "Serum microRNA characterization identifies miR-885-5p as a potential marker for detecting liver pathologies," *Clinical Science*, vol. 120, no. 5, pp. 183–193, 2011.

[41] X.-M. Zhu, L.-J. Wu, J. Xu, R. Yang, and F.-S. Wu, "Let-7c MicroRNA expression and clinical significance in hepatocellular carcinoma," *Journal of International Medical Research*, vol. 39, no. 6, pp. 2323–2329, 2011.

[42] H.-Y. Jia, Y.-X. Wang, W.-T. Yan et al., "MicroRNA-125b functions as a tumor suppressor in hepatocellular carcinoma cells," *International Journal of Molecular Sciences*, vol. 13, no. 7, pp. 8762–8774, 2012.

[43] C. Xu, S. Liu, H. Fu et al., "MicroRNA-193b regulates proliferation, migration and invasion in human hepatocellular carcinoma cells," *European Journal of Cancer*, vol. 46, no. 15, pp. 2828–2836, 2010.

[44] S.-M. Kang, H.-J. Lee, and J.-Y. Cho, "MicroRNA-365 regulates NKX2-1, a key mediator of lung cancer," *Cancer Letters*, vol. 335, no. 2, pp. 487–494, 2013.

[45] S. Shimizu, T. Takehara, H. Hikita et al., "The let-7 family of microRNAs inhibits Bcl-xL expression and potentiates sorafenib-induced apoptosis in human hepatocellular carcinoma," *Journal of Hepatology*, vol. 52, no. 5, pp. 698–704, 2010.

[46] L. Zeng, J. Yu, T. Huang et al., "Differential combinatorial regulatory network analysis related to venous metastasis of hepatocellular carcinoma," *BMC Genomics*, vol. 13, supplement 8, article S14, 2012.

[47] A. Fujimoto, Y. Totoki, T. Abe et al., "Whole-genome sequencing of liver cancers identifies etiological influences on mutation patterns and recurrent mutations in chromatin regulators," *Nature Genetics*, vol. 44, no. 7, pp. 760–764, 2012.

[48] S. A. Bossone, C. Asselin, A. J. Patel, and K. B. Marcu, "MAZ, a zinc finger protein, binds to c-MYC and C2 gene sequences regulating transcriptional initiation and termination," *Proceedings of the National Academy of Sciences of the United States of America*, vol. 89, no. 16, pp. 7452–7456, 1992.

[49] N. G. Nagl Jr., D. R. Zweitzig, B. Thimmapaya, G. R. Beck Jr., and E. Moran, "The *c-myc* gene is a direct target of mammalian SWI/SNF-related complexes during differentiation-associated cell cycle arrest," *Cancer Research*, vol. 66, no. 3, pp. 1289–1293, 2006.

[50] M. Bechard, R. Trost, A. M. Singh, and S. Dalton, "Frat is a phosphatidylinositol 3-kinase/akt-regulated determinant of glycogen synthase kinase 3$\beta$ subcellular localization in pluripotent cells," *Molecular and Cellular Biology*, vol. 32, no. 2, pp. 288–296, 2012.

[51] C. Coulouarn, L. E. Gomez-Quiroz, J.-S. Lee et al., "Oncogene-specific gene expression signatures at preneoplastic stage in mice define distinct mechanisms of hepatocarcinogenesis," *Hepatology*, vol. 44, no. 4, pp. 1003–1011, 2006.

[52] L. Song, H. Liu, S. Gao, W. Jiang, and W. Huang, "Cellular microRNAs inhibit replication of the H1N1 influenza A virus in infected cells," *Journal of Virology*, vol. 84, no. 17, pp. 8849–8860, 2010.

[53] A. Formosa, E. K. Markert, A. M. Lena et al., "MicroRNAs, miR-154, miR-299-5p, miR-376a, miR-376c, miR-377, miR-381, miR-487b, miR-485-3p, miR-495 and miR-654-3p, mapped to the 14q32.31 locus, regulate proliferation, apoptosis, migration and invasion in metastatic prostate cancer cells," *Oncogene*, vol. 33, pp. 5173–5182, 2014.

[54] S. Taketani, T. Furukawa, and K. Furuyama, "Expression of coproporphyrinogen oxidase and synthesis of hemoglobin in human erythroleukemia K562 cells," *European Journal of Biochemistry/FEBS*, vol. 268, no. 6, pp. 1705–1711, 2001.

[55] M. Corioni, N. Antih, G. Tanackovic, M. Zavolan, and A. Krämer, "Analysis of in situ pre-mRNA targets of human splicing factor SF1 reveals a function in alternative splicing," *Nucleic Acids Research*, vol. 39, no. 5, pp. 1868–1879, 2011.

[56] H. L. Janssen, H. W. Reesink, E. J. Lawitz et al., "Treatment of HCV infection by targeting microRNA," *The New England Journal of Medicine*, vol. 368, no. 18, pp. 1685–1694, 2013.

# 8

# Diagnosis of Spontaneous Bacterial Peritonitis and an *In Situ* Hybridization Approach to Detect an "Unidentified" Pathogen

**Hirayuki Enomoto,[1] Shin-ichi Inoue,[2] Akio Matsuhisa,[2] and Shuhei Nishiguchi[1]**

[1] *Division of Hepatobiliary and Pancreatic Disease, Department of Internal Medicine, Hyogo College of Medicine, Mukogawacho 1-1, Nishinomiya, Hyogo 663-8501, Japan*
[2] *Research & Development Center, Fuso Pharmaceutical Industries, Ltd., Morinomiya 2-3-30, Joto-ku, Osaka 536-8523, Japan*

Correspondence should be addressed to Hirayuki Enomoto; enomoto@hyo-med.ac.jp

Academic Editor: Yong-Song Guan

Spontaneous bacterial peritonitis (SBP) is a frequent and severe complication in cirrhotic patients with ascites. Although identifying the pathogen(s) plays a major role in the management of infectious diseases, ascitic fluid cultures often show negative results in patients with clinical signs and symptoms of SBP, and ascitic fluid cell analyses are the gold standard method for diagnosing SBP. SBP is generally diagnosed based on an increased number of polymorphonuclear neutrophils in the ascitic fluid (>250/mm$^3$), and the identification of the causal pathogen may not be given consideration. We newly developed an *in situ* hybridization (ISH) method to provide early and direct evidence of bacterial infection in ascites in patients with SBP. This paper will review the diagnosis of SBP, including our novel approach with ISH method to detect bacterial DNA in SBP ascitic fluid.

## 1. Introduction

Spontaneous bacterial peritonitis (SBP) is a frequent and severe complication in patients with cirrhosis and ascites. SBP is a bacterial infection that occurs in the absence of an evident intra-abdominal and surgically treatable source of infection, such as the perforation or inflammation of intra-abdominal organs [1–4]. Although the precise mechanism(s) underlying the development of SBP have not been fully clarified, bacterial translocation (BT) is believed to be the most important causative factor. Mild BT to the mesenteric lymph nodes is a documented physiological event; however, only a few intestinal bacteria, including *Escherichia coli*, *Klebsiella pneumoniae*, and other Enterobacteriaceae, are able to efficiently translocate from the lumen of the gut to the mesenteric lymph nodes [5, 6]. Since the bacterial species with a capacity for BT are also major pathogens of SBP, unphysiological disease-related BT is thought to be significantly associated with the development of SBP. In addition, several conditions frequently noted in cirrhotic patients, including alterations in gut flora, increased intestinal permeability, and a compromised immune system, have been reported to be involved in disease-related BT and the subsequent onset of SBP [6].

The prevalence of SBP in cirrhotic hospitalized patients with ascites ranges from 10% to 30% [1, 2, 7]. Although the mortality rate was initially reported to exceed 90%, the prognosis has improved with early diagnosis and treatment [8]. The diagnosis of SBP is established based on positive ascitic fluid bacterial cultures and the detection of an elevated absolute fluid polymorphonuclear neutrophil (PMN) count in the ascites (>250/mm$^3$) without an evident intra-abdominal surgically treatable source of infection [1, 9]. Although identifying the pathogen(s) plays a major role in the management of infectious diseases, it takes several days to identify the casual bacteria. In addition, ascitic fluid cultures are negative in approximately 10–60% of patients with clinical manifestations of SBP [3, 9, 10]. Therefore, SBP is usually diagnosed based only on an increased (>250/mm$^3$) PMN count in the ascitic fluid in cases in which there is no obvious source of bacteria spreading to the ascites, regardless of whether ascitic fluid cultures are positive [6, 11–13].

This paper reviews the diagnosis of SBP, focusing on a novel *in situ* hybridization (ISH) method for detecting bacterial DNA in the ascites of patients with SBP.

## 2. Standard Approach to Diagnosing SBP

*2.1. Diagnostic Paracentesis.* Paracentesis is extremely important, as the PMN count in the ascitic fluid plays an essential role in obtaining a diagnosis of SBP. Diagnostic paracentesis should be performed in all patients who present with (1) compatible signs or symptoms (abdominal pain and/or tenderness on palpation, fever, and chills); (2) impairment of the hepatic or renal function; (3) unexplained hepatic encephalopathy; (4) gastrointestinal bleeding [6, 9, 11–13]. However, clinical signs and symptoms are occasionally absent in patients with SBP [11–16]. Although all cirrhotic patients with ascites are at risk of SBP, the prevalence of SBP among hospitalized patients (10%) is higher than that observed in outpatients (1.5–3.5%) [14, 15]. It is therefore recommended that diagnostic paracentesis be performed in all cirrhotic patients with ascites who require hospital admission, regardless of whether they exhibit clinical symptom(s) of SBP [1, 6, 9, 11–13].

*2.2. Ascitic Fluid Cell Analysis.* Despite the use of a sensitive method (the culture-bottle method; please refer to the Ascitic Fluid Culture section), ascites cultures often show negative results, even in patients with an increased ascitic PMN count and clinical symptoms suggestive of SBP [3, 9, 10, 18]. Therefore, the diagnosis of SBP is confirmed based on a PMN count in the ascites of >250 cells/mm$^3$ in the absence of an intra-abdominal and surgically treatable source of infection. The cutoff value of 250 PMN cells/mm$^3$ has the greatest sensitivity, whereas 500 PMN cells/mm$^3$ exhibits the greatest specificity [19–21]. However, the most sensitive cutoff value should be used for diagnosis, as it is important not to miss cases of SBP. Physicians should subtract one PMN for every 250 red blood cells in patients with hemorrhagic ascites with a fluid red blood cell count of >10,000/mm$^3$ (due to the effects of concomitant malignancy or traumatic tap) in order to adjust for the presence of blood in the ascites [9, 11–13].

The PMN count in the ascitic fluid may be determined according to a hematological method using either a light microscope and manual counting chamber or an automated cell counter [22–24]. The ascitic fluid is centrifuged in order to manual count the number of ascitic cells, after which a smear of the collected cells is stained with Giemsa and the total and differential cell counts are determined using a light microscope [1, 4, 25]. The microscopic cell counting method requires several hours and carries a risk at inter- and/or intraobserver discrepancy. On the other hand, automated cell counters provide reproducible results within a few minutes; however, coulter counter findings of the neutrophil count have been shown to be inaccurate for relatively low levels of neutrophils in the ascitic fluid. Therefore, the manual PMN counting method is conventionally preferred [1, 6]. However, a recent study demonstrated that automated cell counts have sufficient sensitivity for diagnosing SBP [22], thus suggesting that this simple method may be used in place of traditional manual counting.

*2.3. Ascitic Fluid Culture.* Conventional bacterial culture methods, such as laboratory analyses of fluid collected in syringes or tubes, effectively detect bacteria in less than 50% of ascites samples with an elevated PMN count (>250/mm$^3$). Therefore, it is recommended to inoculate the ascitic fluid into blood culture bottles at the patient's bedside in order to increase the sensitivity of the bacterial culture [10, 26–29]. The culture-positive rate of SBP ascites is approximately 80%, namely, between 72% and 90% of cases assessed using the culture-bottle method [9, 11]. However, several recent studies have reported lower culture-positive rates for SBP ascites, ranging from approximately 40% to 60% [3, 30–32]. In addition, even with the sensitive culture-bottle method, positive results for ascitic cultures are estimated to be approximately 40–70%, according to various recent guidelines [6, 11–13]. Since patients with an increased PMN count in the ascitic fluid (>250 cells/mm$^3$) and negative cultures exhibit a clinical presentation similar to that of bacteriologically confirmed SBP [1, 33], these patients are categorized as having "culture-negative SBP" and should be treated in the same manner as those with culture-positive SBP.

*2.4. Differentiation from Secondary Bacterial Peritonitis.* Differentiating SBP from secondary peritonitis due to perforation or inflammation of intra-abdominal organs is clinically very important. Secondary bacterial peritonitis should be suspected in patients with relevant abdominal signs or symptoms, multiple organisms in ascitic cultures, and a very high PMN count and/or high protein concentration in the ascites, as well as those who display an inadequate response to therapy [25]. However, accurately diagnosing secondary peritonitis based on these criteria generally takes a long time, and patients with perforated secondary peritonitis require surgical treatment in a timely fashion [34]. Therefore, performing abdominal CT to detect perforation is recommended in patients with suspected secondary bacterial peritonitis [6, 9, 11–13].

Various parameters available at the time of paracentesis have been proposed to assist in rapidly detecting secondary peritonitis. Parameters in the ascitic fluid in patients with secondary peritonitis, as proposed by Runyon and Hoefs [35], are as follows: (1) an elevated PMN count in the ascitic fluid (>250/mm$^3$: usually many thousands) and (2) at least two of the following: a total protein level of >1 g/dL, a serum lactate dehydrogenase level above the upper limit of normal, and a glucose level of <50 mg/dL. In addition, both an alkaline phosphatase level of >240 U/l and carcinoembryonic antigen level of >5 ng/mL in the ascitic fluid have been reported to exhibit good diagnostic performance for detecting gut perforation into the ascitic fluid, with a sensitivity of 92% and specificity of 88% [30]. However, it is not easy to differentiate SBP from secondary peritonitis based only on biochemical parameters of ascitic samples, and abdominal CT is essential in the clinical setting [6, 11–13, 34, 35].

## 3. Potential Diagnostic Methods for SBP

*3.1. Leukocyte Esterase Reagent Strips (LERS).* It takes several hours to obtain the results of an ascitic fluid cell count. Therefore, the use of leukocyte reagent strips (LERS) has been proposed as a fast and inexpensive method for diagnosing SBP. These reagent strips, which were originally developed to diagnose urinary tract infections, detect leukocytes based on their esterase activity according to a colorimetric method [36]. However, a large, multicenter prospective study recently showed that the Multistix 8 SG has a low level of diagnostic accuracy for diagnosing SBP, with a high false-negative rate (55%) [14]. In addition, a systemic review of 19 studies of several strips (including Multistix, Aution, Combur, Nephur, and UriScan) demonstrated that these LERS have both low sensitivity and a high risk of false-negative results [36]. According to a recent review of 26 studies regarding the validity of LERS for SBP diagnosis [37], LERS display low sensitivity for diagnosing SBP, with significant interstudy variability among brands of LERS. However, LERS have consistently shown high negative predictive value (>95% in the majority of studies) and may therefore be used as a preliminary screening tool to diagnose SBP. However, the utility of LERS for diagnosing SBP has not been confirmed.

Most of the above strips were developed for use in urine with a threshold of >50 PMN cells/mm$^3$; however, the diagnostic performance of a reagent strip test calibrated for ascitic fluid with a cutoff of 250 PMN cells/mm$^3$ has recently been reported [38]. That study showed excellent results, with a sensitivity of 100% and a negative predictive value of 100%. Although these conclusions have yet to be confirmed in large multicenter trials, this method may provide a new and useful diagnostic tool for detecting SBP.

*3.2. Measurement of Leukocyte-Derived Proteins.* The levels of proteins, such as granulocyte elastase [39] and lactoferrin [40], released by activated PMNs are elevated in patients with SBP. Lactoferrin shows notable sensitivity (95.5%) and specificity (97%) for diagnosing SBP, with a cutoff value of 242 ng/mL [40]. Nevertheless, the diagnostic performance of this parameter must be further evaluated in other studies with a larger number of patients due to the small number of SBP cases in that study. In addition to the proteins described above, the levels of several inflammatory cytokines and chemokines in the ascitic fluid are reported to be associated with the severity of SBP [41, 42]. However, these potential diagnostic biomarkers are generated by host reactions against inflammatory stimulation and fail to provide any direct evidence of bacterial infection in SBP ascites.

*3.3. Detection of Bacterial DNA Using Polymerase Chain Reaction (PCR).* Bacterial cultures require several days to obtain results. Hence, bacterial DNA detection and sequencing is increasingly being used to diagnose various infectious diseases [43–45]. Some PCR-based methods for detecting bacterial DNA have also been applied to the microbiological diagnosis of SBP [46–49]. However, these methods have received several major criticisms regarding the detection of bacterial DNA. First, most previous studies enrolled a limited number of patients, and a recent report including a large number of patients showed poor results for diagnosis. Furthermore, previous studies have revealed serious concerns regarding contamination of bacterial DNA in the PCR system [50–53]. Commercially available Taq-polymerases may be contaminated with bacterial DNA [50, 51]. Moreover, the reagents used for DNA extraction procedures carry a risk of exposing the clinical samples to exogenous bacterial DNA [52, 53]. Although PCR is a very sensitive method for detecting DNA, PCR-based methods display discrepant and controversial findings with respect to diagnostic performance in detecting the causative pathogen(s) in SBP patients with ascites [46–49], perhaps, or at least in part, due to the problems described above. Therefore, no definitive PCR-based method for providing an accurate diagnosis of SBP has been established.

## 4. A Novel Approach for Detecting Bacterial DNA in SBP Ascites Using *In Situ* Hybridization

A new strategy using an ISH method for detecting the genomic DNA of bacteria phagocytized in neutrophils and macrophages was recently developed to identify causal bacteria in cases of sepsis [54–56]. The utility of this ISH method for detecting bacterial genomic DNA phagocytized in the leukocytes of patients with sepsis has been demonstrated, providing evidence for the presence of bacterial infection in such cases. Notably, the ISH method is almost four times more sensitive than blood cultures in detecting the causal bacteria of sepsis [55]. In addition, the results of ISH tests can be acquired within one day, whereas it takes several days, at least, to obtain the results of cultures. Based on the rapid and sensitive detection of bacterial DNA provided by the ISH method, we investigated whether this method can be used to obtain direct evidence of bacterial infection in SBP patients with ascites [17].

The concept of the ISH method for detecting bacterial DNA in SBP patients with ascites is shown in Figure 1. In addition to the low amount of bacteria present in the ascitic fluid of SBP patients, phagocytosis and the digestion of bacteria by leukocytes may reduce the amount of proliferative, suspended bacteria in the ascitic fluid, thus making it difficult to identify the pathogen using standard methods. Phagocytosis is thought be responsible for the low rate of detectable causative bacteria [17]. Therefore, we attempted to detect ingested bacterial DNA using the ISH method. Since all bacteria have the 23S ribosomal RNA gene, a novel cDNA probe for this gene was generated to detect the genomic DNA of the causative bacteria.

Several cDNA fragments corresponding to the 23S rRNA genes of various bacteria were obtained using PCR. Since we found no single cDNA probe able to detect all types of bacteria universally, we mixed plural cDNA fragments to create a new probe cocktail. This cocktail was able to detect the genomic DNA of all 59 bacterial strains examined, including the leading species accounting for SBP (Table 1). The new probe was designated the "global bacteria (GB)

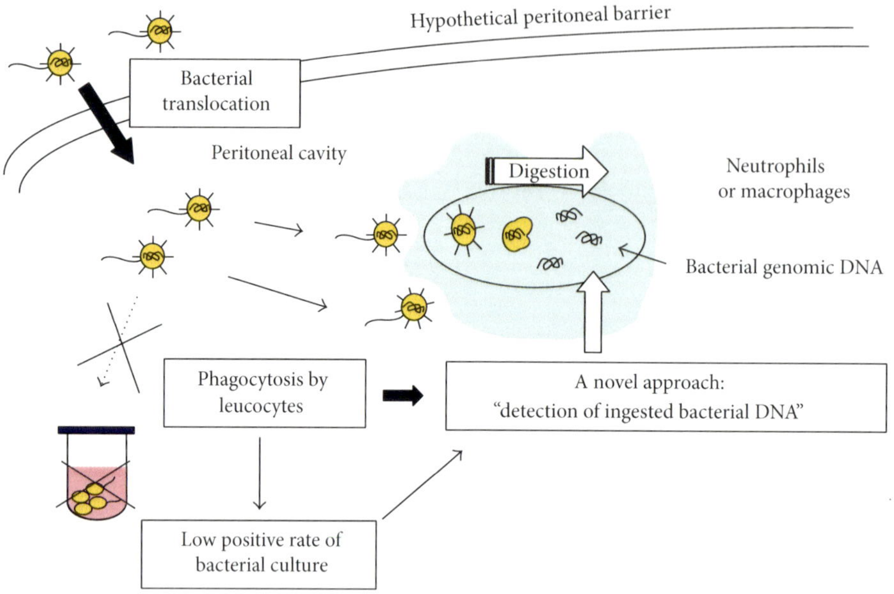


FIGURE 1: The concept of the ISH method for detecting bacterial DNA in SBP ascites.

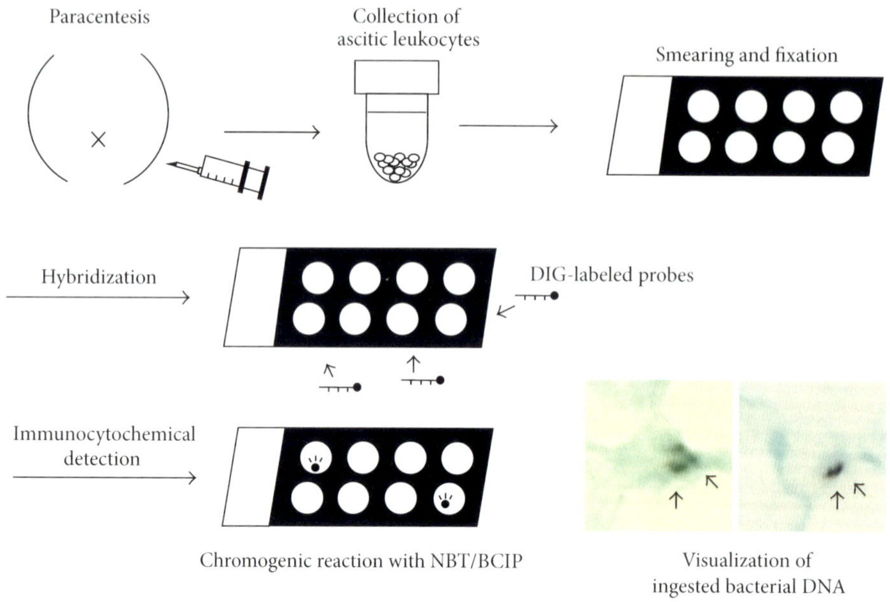


FIGURE 2: Schematic representation of the *in situ* hybridization (ISH) method used to assess the ascitic samples. Floating leukocytes in the ascitic fluid were collected via centrifugation and used for the ISH tests. DIG- (digoxigenin-) labeled probes were used for hybridization, and positive signals were detected with NBT (nitro-blue tetrazolium chloride) and BCIP (5-bromo-4-chloro-3′-indolyphosphate p-toluidine salt). Positive (purple brown) signals were observed in the leukocytes with intracellular bacterial DNA (arrows).

probe," and its utility for detecting phagocytized bacterial DNA in SBP ascites was evaluated. An outline of the ISH method for assessing leukocytes in the ascitic fluid is shown in Figure 2. Floating leukocytes in the ascites were collected via centrifugation and prepared for the ISH tests. Intracellular bacterial DNA was detected as positive (purple brown) signals of leukocytes in the SBP samples.

The ISH tests showed positive results in 10 of 11 SBP ascites samples, whereas negative results were obtained in all remaining 40 non-SBP ascites samples. These findings suggest that the ISH test yields high sensitivity (91%) and specificity (100%) for detecting phagocytized bacterial DNA in leukocytes the ascites of SBP patients. Importantly, the ISH tests showed positive findings in seven cases with negative culture results, thus suggesting that the ISH method can be used to identify bacterial infections that are not detected using the bacterial culture method [17]. Furthermore, the ISH test results were obtained within one day, consistent with that observed for septic blood samples. Therefore, this newly established ISH method resulted in the rapid and sensitive

Table 1: Bacterial strains detected by the *in situ* hybridization method [17]. ISH test was able to detect the genomic DNA of all bacterial strains tested.

| Genus | Species |
|---|---|
| *Eggerthella* | *lenta* |
| *Corynebacterium* | *diphtheriae* |
| | *pseudodiphteriticum* |
| | *jeikeium* |
| *Propionibacterium* | *acnes* |
| *Micrococcus* | *luteus* |
| *Lactobacillus* | *fermentum* |
| | *acidophilus* |
| *Bacillus* | *cereus* |
| *Staphylococcus* | *aureus* |
| | *epidermidis* |
| *Enterococcus* | *faecalis* |
| | *faecium* |
| | *avium* |
| *Streptococcus* | *pneumoniae* |
| | *sanguinis* |
| | *pyogenes* |
| | *agalactiae* |
| | *salivarius* |
| *Clostridium* | *perfringens* |
| *Peptoniphilus* | *asaccharolyticus* |
| *Bacteroides* | *fragilis* |
| | *ovatus* |
| *Porphyromonas* | *asaccharolytica* |
| *Fusobacterium* | *nucleatum* |
| | *necrophorum* |
| *Brevundimonas* | *diminuta* |
| *Burkholderia* | *cepacia* |
| *Achromobacter* | *xylosoxidans* |
| *Pseudomonas* | *aeruginosa* |
| | *fluorescens* |
| | *putida* |
| *Acinetobacter* | *calcoaceticus* |
| *Escherichia* | *coli* |
| *Enterobacter* | *cloacae* |
| | *sakazakii* |
| | *aerogenes* |
| | *gergoviae* |
| *Klebsiella* | *pneumoniae* |
| | *aerogenes* |
| | *oxytoca* |
| *Raoultella* | *terrigena* |
| *Haemophilus* | *influenzae* |
| *Serratia* | *marcescens* |
| | *liquefaciens* |
| *Citrobacter* | *koseri* |
| *Hafnia* | *alvei* |

Table 1: Continued.

| Genus | Species |
|---|---|
| *Edwardsiella* | *tarda* |
| *Proteus* | *vulgaris* |
| | *mirabilis* |
| *Providencia* | *rettgeri* |
| | *alcalifaciens* |
| | *stuartii* |
| *Morganella* | *morganii* |
| *Salmonella* | *enterica* |
| *Pantoea* | *agglomerans* |
| *Kluyvera* | *intermedia* |
| *Raoultella* | *planticola* |
| *Stenotrophomonas* | *maltophilia* |

detection of bacterial DNA in SBP ascites, thereby implying its utility for providing early and direct evidence of bacterial infection. Although additional large-scale clinical trials are required to evaluate the ISH method in detail, this new test may offer a novel and effective approach for the management of SBP.

## 5. Conclusion

Rapid diagnosis and treatment play a key role in the management of SBP. In general, potentially fatal cirrhosis-related infectious disease is diagnosed based only on an increased PMN count in the ascitic fluid, and the identification of the causal pathogen is sometimes not taken into consideration. Although no ideal method for detecting causal bacteria has been established, our novel ISH test may be used to provide early and direct evidence of bacterial infection in SBP patients with ascites. The current findings therefore shed new light on the management of SBP.

## Abbreviations

SBP: Spontaneous bacterial peritonitis
BT: Bacterial translocation
PMN: Polymorphonuclear neutrophil
ISH: *In situ* hybridization
PCR: Polymerase chain reaction.

## Acknowledgment

This study was supported by a Grant-in-Aid for Health and Labour Sciences Research from the Ministry of Health, Labour and Welfare of Japan.

## References


[1] A. Rimola, G. García-Tsao, M. Navasa et al., "Diagnosis, treatment and prophylaxis of spontaneous bacterial peritonitis: a consensus document," *Journal of Hepatology*, vol. 32, no. 1, pp. 142–153, 2000.

[2] W. R. Caly and E. Strauss, "A prospective study of bacterial infections in patients with cirrhosis," *Journal of Hepatology*, vol. 18, no. 3, pp. 353–358, 1993.

[3] J. Fernández, M. Navasa, J. Gómez et al., "Bacterial infections in cirrhosis: epidemiological changes with invasive procedures and norfloxacin prophylaxis," *Hepatology*, vol. 35, no. 1, pp. 140–148, 2002.

[4] F. Wong, M. Bernardi, R. Balk et al., "Sepsis in cirrhosis: report on the 7th meeting of the International Ascites Club," *Gut*, vol. 54, no. 5, pp. 718–725, 2005.

[5] C. L. Wells, "Relationship between intestinal microecology and the translocation of intestinal bacteria," *Antonie van Leeuwenhoek, International Journal of General and Molecular Microbiology*, vol. 58, no. 2, pp. 87–93, 1990.

[6] R. Wiest, A. Krag, and A. Gerbes, "Spontaneous bacterial peritonitis: recent guidelines and beyond," *Gut*, vol. 61, no. 2, pp. 297–310, 2012.

[7] G. Garcia-Tsao, "Spontaneous bacterial peritonitis," *Gastroenterology Clinics of North America*, vol. 21, no. 1, pp. 257–275, 1992.

[8] G. Garcia-Tsao, "Spontaneous bacterial peritonitis: a historical perspective," *Journal of Hepatology*, vol. 41, no. 4, pp. 522–527, 2004.

[9] B. A. Runyon, "Management of adult patients with ascites due to cirrhosis: an update," *Hepatology*, vol. 49, no. 6, pp. 2087–2107, 2009.

[10] B. A. Runyon, H. N. Canawati, and E. A. Akriviadis, "Optimization of ascitic fluid culture technique," *Gastroenterology*, vol. 95, no. 5, pp. 1351–1355, 1988.

[11] K. P. Moore and G. P. Aithal, "Guidelines on the management of ascites in cirrhosis," *Gut*, vol. 55, no. S6, pp. vi1–vi12, 2006.

[12] G. Garcia-Tsao, J. Lim, and Members of Veterans Affairs Hepatitis C Resource Center Program, "Management and treatment of patients with cirrhosis and portal hypertension: recommendations from the department of veterans affairs hepatitis C resource center program and the national hepatitis C program," *The American Journal of Gastroenterology*, vol. 104, no. 7, pp. 1802–1829, 2009.

[13] European Association for the Study of the Liver, "EASL clinical practice guidelines on the management of ascites, spontaneous bacterial peritonitis, and hepatorenal syndrome in cirrhosis," *Journal of Hepatology*, vol. 53, no. 3, pp. 397–417, 2010.

[14] J. B. Nousbaum, J. F. Cadranel, P. Nahon et al., "Diagnostic accuracy of the Multistix 8 SG reagent strip in diagnosis of spontaneous bacterial peritonitis," *Hepatology*, vol. 45, no. 5, pp. 1275–1281, 2007.

[15] L. T. Evans, W. R. Kim, J. J. Poterucha, and P. S. Kamath, "Spontaneous bacterial peritonitis in asymptomatic outpatients with cirrhotic ascites," *Hepatology*, vol. 37, no. 4, pp. 897–901, 2003.

[16] B. Chinnock, H. Afarian, H. Minnigan, J. Butler, and G. W. Hendey, "Physician clinical impression does not rule out spontaneous bacterial peritonitis in patients undergoing emergency department paracentesis," *Annals of Emergency Medicine*, vol. 52, no. 3, pp. 268–273, 2008.

[17] H. Enomoto, S. Inoue, A. Matsuhisa et al., "Development of a new *in situ* hybridization method for the detection of global bacterial DNA to provide early evidence of a bacterial infection in spontaneous bacterial peritonitis," *Journal of Hepatology*, vol. 56, no. 1, pp. 85–94, 2012.

[18] G. Garcia-Tsao, "Current management of the complications of cirrhosis and portal hypertension: variceal hemorrhage, ascites, and spontaneous bacterial peritonitis," *Gastroenterology*, vol. 120, no. 3, pp. 726–748, 2001.

[19] G. Garcia-Tsao, H. O. Conn, and E. Lerner, "The diagnosis of bacterial peritonitis: comparison of pH, lactate concentration and leukocyte count," *Hepatology*, vol. 5, no. 1, pp. 91–96, 1985.

[20] C.-Y. Yang, Y.-F. Liaw, C.-M. Chu, and I.-S. Sheen, "White count, pH and lactate in ascites in the diagnosis of spontaneous bacterial peritonitis," *Hepatology*, vol. 5, no. 1, pp. 85–90, 1985.

[21] W. N. Stassen, A. J. McCullough, B. R. Bacon et al., "Immediate diagnostic criteria for bacterial infection of ascitic fluid: evaluation of ascitic fluid polymorphonuclear leukocyte count, pH, and lactate concentration, alone and in combination," *Gastroenterology*, vol. 90, no. 5, part 1, pp. 1247–1254, 1986.

[22] S. Angeloni, G. Nicolini, M. Merli et al., "Validation of automated blood cell counter for the determination of polymorphonuclear cell count in the ascitic fluid of cirrhotic patients with or without spontaneous bacterial peritonitis," *The American Journal of Gastroenterology*, vol. 98, no. 8, pp. 1844–1848, 2003.

[23] O. Riggio, S. Angeloni, A. Parente et al., "Accuracy of the automated cell counters for management of spontaneous bacterial peritonitis," *World Journal of Gastroenterology*, vol. 14, no. 37, pp. 5689–5694, 2008.

[24] F. Cereto, J. Genescà, and R. Segura, "Validation of automated blood cell counters for the diagnosis of spontaneous bacterial peritonitis," *The American Journal of Gastroenterology*, vol. 99, no. 7, article 1400, 2004.

[25] C. Guarner and G. Soriano, "Spontaneous bacterial peritonitis," *Seminars in Liver Disease*, vol. 17, no. 3, pp. 203–217, 1997.

[26] M. Bobadilla, J. Sifuentes, and G. Garcia-Tsao, "Improved method for bacteriological diagnosis of spontaneous bacterial peritonitis," *Journal of Clinical Microbiology*, vol. 27, no. 10, pp. 2145–2147, 1989.

[27] B. A. Runyon, M. R. Antillon, E. A. Akriviadis, and J. G. McHutchison, "Bedside inoculation of blood culture bottles with ascitic fluid is superior to delayed inoculation in the detection of spontaneous bacterial peritonitis," *Journal of Clinical Microbiology*, vol. 28, no. 12, pp. 2811–2812, 1990.

[28] P. D. Siersema, S. de Marie, J. H. van Zeijl, D.-J. Bac, and J. H. P. Wilson, "Blood culture bottles are superior to lysis-centrifugation tubes for bacteriological diagnosis of spontaneous bacterial peritonitis," *Journal of Clinical Microbiology*, vol. 30, no. 3, pp. 667–669, 1992.

[29] J. Castellote, X. Xiol, R. Verdaguer et al., "Comparison of two ascitic fluid culture methods in cirrhotic patients with spontaneous bacterial peritonitis," *The American Journal of Gastroenterology*, vol. 85, no. 12, pp. 1605–1608, 1990.

[30] S. S. Wu, O. S. Lin, Y. Y. Chen, K. L. Hwang, M. S. Soon, and E. B. Keeffe, "Ascitic fluid carcinoembryonic antigen and alkaline phosphatase levels for the differentiation of primary from secondary bacterial peritonitis with intestinal perforation," *Journal of Hepatology*, vol. 34, no. 2, pp. 215–221, 2001.

[31] M. Navasa, A. Follo, J. M. Llovet et al., "Randomized, comparative study of oral ofloxacin versus intravenous cefotaxime in spontaneous bacterial peritonitis," *Gastroenterology*, vol. 111, no. 4, pp. 1011–1017, 1996.

[32] A. Rimola, J. M. Salmerón, G. Clemente et al., "Two different dosages of cefotaxime in the treatment of spontaneous bacterial peritonitis in cirrhosis: results of a prospective, randomized, multicenter study," *Hepatology*, vol. 21, no. 3, pp. 674–679, 1995.

[33] R. Terg, D. Levi, P. Lopez et al., "Analysis of clinical course and prognosis of culture-positive spontaneous bacterial peritonitis and neutrocytic ascites. Evidence of the same disease," *Digestive Diseases and Sciences*, vol. 37, no. 10, pp. 1499–1504, 1992.

[34] G. Soriano, J. Castellote, C. Álvarez et al., "Secondary bacterial peritonitis in cirrhosis: a retrospective study of clinical and analytical characteristics, diagnosis and management," *Journal of Hepatology*, vol. 52, no. 1, pp. 39–44, 2010.

[35] B. A. Runyon and J. C. Hoefs, "Ascitic fluid analysis in the differentiation of spontaneous bacterial peritonitis from gastrointestinal tract perforation into ascitic fluid," *Hepatology*, vol. 4, no. 3, pp. 447–450, 1984.

[36] E. Nguyen-Khac, J.-F. Cadranel, T. Theveno, and J.-B. Nousbaum, "Review article: the utility of reagent strips in the diagnosis of infected ascites in cirrhotic patients," *Alimentary Pharmacology and Therapeutics*, vol. 28, no. 3, pp. 282–288, 2008.

[37] A. Koulaouzidis, "Diagnosis of spontaneous bacterial peritonitis: an update on leucocyte esterase reagent strips," *World Journal of Gastroenterology*, vol. 17, no. 9, pp. 1091–1094, 2011.

[38] M. H. Mendler, A. Agarwal, M. Trimzi et al., "A new highly sensitive point of care screen for spontaneous bacterial peritonitis using the leukocyte esterase method," *Journal of Hepatology*, vol. 53, no. 3, pp. 477–483, 2010.

[39] F. Casafont, M. Rivero, M. D. Fernandez et al., "Granulocyte elastase in cirrhotic patients with spontaneous bacterial peritonitis," *Digestive Diseases and Sciences*, vol. 44, no. 10, pp. 1985–1989, 1999.

[40] M. A. Parsi, S. N. Saadeh, N. N. Zein et al., "Ascitic fluid lactoferrin for diagnosis of spontaneous bacterial peritonitis," *Gastroenterology*, vol. 135, no. 3, pp. 803–807, 2008.

[41] M. Navasa, A. Follo, X. Filella et al., "Tumor necrosis factor and interleukin-6 in spontaneous bacterial peritonitis in cirrhosis: relationship with the development of renal impairment and mortality," *Hepatology*, vol. 27, no. 5, pp. 1227–1232, 1998.

[42] J. A. Giròn-González, C. Rodríguez-Ramos, J. Elvira et al., "Serial analysis of serum and ascitic fluid levels of soluble adhesion molecules and chemokines in patients with spontaneous bacterial peritonitis," *Clinical and Experimental Immunology*, vol. 123, no. 1, pp. 56–61, 2001.

[43] E. J. Baron, "Implications of new technology for infectious diseases practice," *Clinical Infectious Diseases*, vol. 43, no. 10, pp. 1318–1323, 2006.

[44] P. C. Y. Woo, S. K. P. Lau, J. L. L. Teng, H. Tse, and K. Y. Yuen, "Then and now: use of 16S rDNA gene sequencing for bacterial identification and discovery of novel bacteria in clinical microbiology laboratories," *Clinical Microbiology and Infection*, vol. 14, no. 10, pp. 908–934, 2008.

[45] S. Sontakke, M. B. Cadenas, R. G. Maggi, P. P. V. P. Diniz, and E. B. Breitschwerdt, "Use of broad range16S rDNA PCR in clinical microbiology," *Journal of Microbiological Methods*, vol. 76, no. 3, pp. 217–225, 2009.

[46] R. Francés, P. Zapater, J. M. González-Navajas et al., "Bacterial DNA in patients with cirrhosis and noninfected ascites mimics the soluble immune response established in patients with spontaneous bacterial peritonitis," *Hepatology*, vol. 47, no. 3, pp. 978–985, 2008.

[47] T. Sugihara, M. Koda, Y. Maeda et al., "Rapid identification of bacterial species with bacterial DNA microarray in cirrhotic patients with spontaneous bacterial peritonitis," *Internal Medicine*, vol. 48, no. 1, pp. 3–10, 2009.

[48] T. Bruns, S. Sachse, E. Straube et al., "Identification of bacterial DNA in neutrocytic and non-neutrocytic cirrhotic ascites by means of a multiplex polymerase chain reaction," *Liver International*, vol. 29, no. 8, pp. 1206–1214, 2009.

[49] G. Soriano, Ó. Esparcia, M. Montemayor et al., "Bacterial DNA in the diagnosis of spontaneous bacterial peritonitis," *Alimentary Pharmacology and Therapeutics*, vol. 33, no. 2, pp. 275–284, 2011.

[50] C. E. Corless, M. Guiver, R. Borrow, V. Edwards-Jones, E. B. Kaczmarski, and A. J. Fox, "Contamination and sensitivity issues with a real-time universal 16s rRNA PCR," *Journal of Clinical Microbiology*, vol. 38, no. 5, pp. 1747–1752, 2000.

[51] S. Philipp, H. P. Huemer, E. U. Irschick, and C. Gassner, "Obstacles of multiplex real-time PCR for bacterial 16S rDNA: primer specifity and DNA decontamination of Taq polymerase," *Transfusion Medicine and Hemotherapy*, vol. 37, no. 1, pp. 21–28, 2010.

[52] G. E. Evans, D. R. Murdoch, T. P. Anderson, H. C. Potter, P. M. George, and S. T. Chambers, "Contamination of Qiagen DNA extraction kits with Legionella DNA," *Journal of Clinical Microbiology*, vol. 41, no. 7, pp. 3452–3453, 2003.

[53] J. J. H. C. Tilburg, M. H. Nabuurs-Franssen, E. J. van Hannen, A. M. Horrevorts, W. J. G. Melchers, and C. H. W. Klaassen, "Contamination of commercial PCR master mix with DNA from Coxiella burnetii," *Journal of Clinical Microbiology*, vol. 48, no. 12, pp. 4634–4635, 2010.

[54] A. Matsuhisa, Y. Saito, Y. Sakamoto et al., "Detection of bacteria in phagocyte-smears from septicemia-suspected blood by in situ hybridization using biotinylated probes," *Microbiology and Immunology*, vol. 38, no. 7, pp. 511–517, 1994.

[55] J. Shimada, I. Hayashi, T. Inamatsu et al., "Clinical trial of in-situ hybridization method for the rapid diagnosis of sepsis," *Journal of Infection and Chemotherapy*, vol. 5, no. 1, pp. 21–31, 1999.

[56] M. Kudo, Y. Matsuo, A. Nakasendo et al., "Potential clinical benefit of the in situ hybridization method for the diagnosis of sepsis," *Journal of Infection and Chemotherapy*, vol. 15, no. 1, pp. 23–26, 2009.

9

# Diagnosis and Management of Giant Hepatic Hemangioma: The Usefulness of Contrast-Enhanced Ultrasonography

**Masaki Maruyama,[1] Osamu Isokawa,[2] Koki Hoshiyama,[3] Ayako Hoshiyama,[4] Mari Hoshiyama,[4] and Yoshihiro Hoshiyama[5]**

[1] *Division of Gastroenterology and Hepatology, Department of Internal Medicine, Kashiwazaki Central Hospital, 2-1-25 Ekimae, Niigata, Kashiwazaki 9450055, Japan*
[2] *Division of Gastroenterology and Hepatology, Kashiwazaki General Hospital and Medical Center, 2-11-3 Kitahanda, Kashiwazaki, Niigata, 9458535, Japan*
[3] *Division of Cardiology, Department of Internal Medicine, Kashiwazaki Central Hospital, 2-1-25 Ekimae, Niigata, Kashiwazaki 9450055, Japan*
[4] *Division of Endocrinology and Metabolism, Department of Internal Medicine, Kashiwazaki Central Hospital, 2-1-25 Ekimae, Niigata, Kashiwazaki 9450055, Japan*
[5] *Department of Surgery, Kashiwazaki Central Hospital, 2-1-25 Ekimae, Niigata, Kashiwazaki 9450055, Japan*

Correspondence should be addressed to Masaki Maruyama; gontax@nifty.com

Academic Editor: Kenya Kamimura

Giant hepatic hemangiomas, though often asymptomatic, may require intervention if rapid growth occurs. The imaging studies including the computed tomography, magnetic resonance imaging, and ultrasonography, and so on are effective for the diagnosis and the management of this tumor; however, due to its size and various patterns of these studies, we need to carefully consider the therapeutic methods. Compared to the cost needed for these modalities, recently developed and approved Perflubutane- (Sonazoid-) based contrast agent enhanced ultrasonography is reasonable and safe. The major advantage is the real-time observation of the vascular structure and function of the Kupffer cells. By this procedure, we can carefully follow the tumor growth or character change in a hemangioma and decide the timing of therapeutic intervention, since abdominal pain, abdominal mass, consumptive coagulopathy, and hemangioma growth are the signs for the therapeutic intervention. We reviewed recent reports about Sonazoid-based enhancement and also showed the representative images collected in our department. This is the first review showing the detailed findings of the giant hemangiomas using Perflubutane (Sonazoid). This review will help the physician in making the decision, and we hope that Sonazoid will gain widespread acceptance in the near future.

## 1. Introduction

Hepatic hemangiomas are the most common benign tumors of the liver and usually do not grow [1]. In cases with giant hepatic hemangiomas, intervention is necessary since clinical symptoms due to rapid growth are present [2, 3]. Detailed follow-up imaging examinations of giant hepatic hemangiomas are essential for relevant medical treatment or surgical intervention. Although computed tomography (CT) or magnetic resonance imaging (MRI) is useful for diagnosing hepatic hemangioma, these modalities are expensive and there are several risks associated with the contrast agents used as well as radiation exposure. There are many recent reports describing contrast-enhanced ultrasonography (US) as being safe, inexpensive, and useful for the diagnosis of focal liver lesions [4, 5]. Perflubutane (Sonazoid) is a new contrast agent for contrast-enhanced US approved only Japan. The only contraindication to its use is an allergy to eggs. Sonazoid contrast-enhanced US is very useful for the diagnosis of hemangioma of the liver, since real-time images can be shown that is unable to be obtained by CT or MRI, and yielding information about Kupffer cell function [6, 7]. However, there have been few reports describing Sonazoid contrast-enhanced US for the diagnosis and followup of "giant hepatic hemangioma." For the followup of huge hemangiomas to decide the timing of therapeutic intervention, the use of Sonazoid is easy, cost effective, and detailed real-time information can be obtained. For the understanding of the procedure and images, we have shown the representative 2 giant hepatic hemangiomas, with maximum diameters of 17 cm and 6 cm, respectively, observed with Sonazoid contrast-enhanced US. Both tumors showed typical imaging patterns using Sonazoid and its reinjection procedure. We herein review the diagnosis and management of giant hepatic hemangiomas and discuss the usefulness of Sonazoid contrast-enhanced US for the diagnosis, observation, and management of giant hepatic hemangiomas.

## 2. Diagnosis and Management of Giant Hepatic Hemangioma

Hepatic hemangioma is the most common benign liver tumor and typically remains stable in size [1]. Hepatic hemangioma is diagnosed in most patients using noninvasive studies such as CT, MRI, and US. A hepatic hemangioma shows hypodensity at unenhanced CT. At the enhanced CT, a hepatic hemangioma shows the characteristic pattern, and the tumor existence is represented clearly and shows "nodular peripheral puddling" pattern in early phase and subsequently "fill-in" pattern. In cases where a central scar exists, this portion is not enhanced on delayed phase of dynamic CT. MRI imaging features of hepatic hemangioma are usually low signal intensity and well defined on T1-weighted images and very high intensity on T2-weighted images [8, 9]. Hepatic hemangiomas larger than 4-5 cm demonstrate a nonhomogeneously hypoechoic area on B-mode US. At contrast-enhanced US, hepatic hemangiomas show the characteristic puddling and peripheral-nodular enhancement in the early vascular phase followed by a progressive and centripetal fill-in during the late vascular phase. The real-time images like those of dynamic CT and dynamic MRI can be obtained by contrast-enhanced US. It is the same as that of the enhanced CT; the centripetal fill-in may be incomplete on a central scar [5]. CT angiography can be a particularly valuable preoperative study in patients with large tumors [10]. Hemangiomas in the liver greater than 4-5 cm in diameter are usually defined as giant hepatic hemangiomas, according to several reports. Observation is justified in patients with minimal or no symptoms, even those with giant hepatic hemangiomas. The decision to perform surgical resection or another invasive intervention should not be made based solely on size [11–13]. Indications for surgical interventions are abdominal pain, an abdominal mass, a consumptive coagulopathy (Kasabach-Merritt syndrome), and hemangioma growth. Since the safety of hepatectomy and enucleation with normal liver function is improving, it is essential that radical surgery should be appropriately timed [14–16]. Jiang et al. advocated that liver resection is indicated for giant hepatic hemangiomas causing abdominal discomfort, especially for lesions greater than 20 cm [17]. It is possible for consumptive coagulopathy (Kasabach-Merritt syndrome), spontaneous tumor rupture, and tumor hemorrhage to occur in patients with giant hepatic hemangiomas [18–20]. Therefore, it is important to confirm tumor growth or a change in the character of a hemangioma by performing detailed follow-up imaging examinations. On the other hand, large unresectable hemangiomas have been treated with transcatheter arterial embolization (TAE) [21] and liver transplantation [22, 23]. TAE is reportedly useful for reducing the tumor volume, which could potentially facilitate radical resection [24, 25]. A case of hepatic hemangioma with consumptive coagulopathy was also reported, and TAE appeared to ameliorate the coagulopathy and increase the safety of surgery [26]. As mentioned above, in order to treat giant hepatic hemangioma with optimal timing, close observation is required.

## 3. The Usefulness of Contrast-Enhanced Ultrasonography

Sonazoid is the recently developed and approved phase contrast agent for the contrast-enhanced US. It is a powerful modality for the various liver tumors.

Since the US is safe, inexpensive, has few side effects, and can obtain real-time images comparable to those of dynamic CT, it is useful for achieving meticulous follow-up care of various liver tumors, including giant hepatic hemangioma patients. This agent also provides the function of Kupffer's cells inside of the tumors; therefore, we can determine the possible malignancy. In this section, we show the representative images obtained from 2 tumors in our department.

Representative images from tumor 1: multidetector CT (MDCT) revealed a giant hepatic hemangioma, 17 cm in maximum diameter, replacing the right lobe of the liver (Figures 1(a), 1(b), and 2(a)). The hemangioma was near the middle hepatic vein. A small tumor (2 cm) suggestive of hemangioma was also seen in the left hepatic lobe on MDCT. These two tumors showed no changes in either size or character as compared to the MDCT findings obtained 2 years previously. For Sonazoid contrast-enhanced US examination, Sonazoid, injected intravenously as a 0.5 mL bolus followed by 10 mL of normal saline flush using a 22-gauge peripheral intravenous cannula, was used as the US contrast agent. The images showed intratumoral perfusion with "cotton wool-like pooling" in the early vascular phase (Figure 2(b)) and "gradual fill-in" persisting through the late vascular phase (Figure 2(c)). This main tumor showed a slightly inhomogeneous positive uptake in the Kupffer phase (Figure 2(d)). A small tumor, only 2 cm in diameter, suggestive of hemangioma, was also seen in the left lobe in the Kupffer phase (Figure 3(a)). This lesion displayed a slightly negative uptake rather than normal liver parenchymal enhancement. After Sonazoid reinjection according to the US technique reported by Kudo et al., termed as "defect reperfusion ultrasound imaging" [27], we observed slight "peripheral-nodular enhancement" (Figure 3(b)).

Representative images from tumor 2: MDCT showed a huge hypodense mass in the right lobe of the liver measuring approximately 6 cm. In Sonazoid contrast-enhanced US

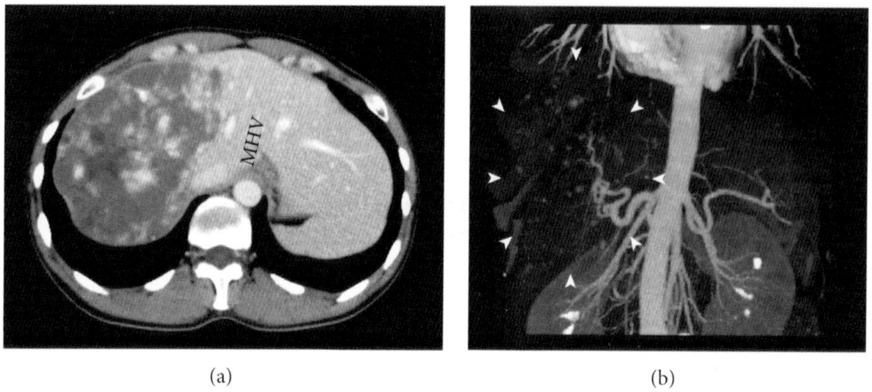


FIGURE 1: Multidetector computed tomography (MDCT) images. (a) Axial MDCT image shows a huge hypodense mass in the right lobe of the liver measuring about 17 cm, extending to the middle hepatic vein (MHV). (b) Vascular reconstruction image shows "cotton wool-like pooling" (arrowhead).

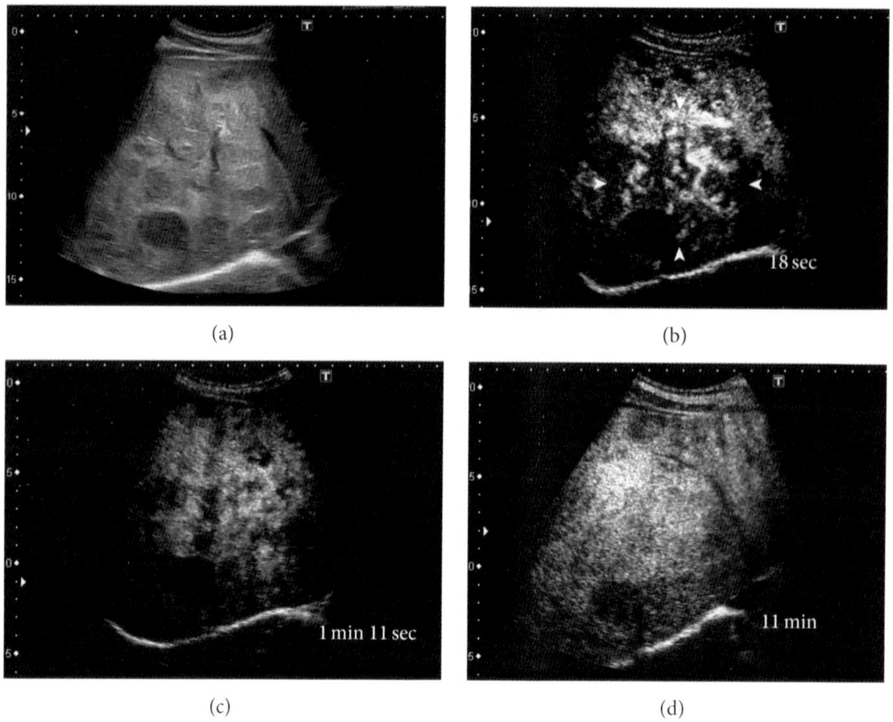


FIGURE 2: Ultrasonography (US) scan. (a) B-mode US scan shows a huge nonhomogeneously hypoechoic lesion in the right lobe of the liver. (b) Sonazoid contrast-enhanced US in the early vascular phase reveals "cotton wool-like pooling" (arrowhead). (c) Gradual fill-in through the late vascular phase. (d) The fill-in was completed in the Kupffer phase.

examination (Figure 4(a)), the images showed intratumoral perfusion with "peripheral-nodular enhancement" in the early vascular phase (Figure 4(b)) and "partial centripetal filling" in the late vascular phase (Figure 4(c)). The tumor showed slightly negative uptake in the Kupffer phase with a partial defect (Figure 4(d)). After Sonazoid reinjection in this tumor, according to the "defect reperfusion ultrasound imaging" technique, we observed typical "peripheral-nodular enhancement" and typical Kupffer images 13 min after reinjection (Figures 4(e) and 4(f)).

## 4. Discussion

Contrast-enhanced US with Sonazoid is a useful modality for differentially diagnosing hepatic tumors [6, 7]. Giant hepatic hemangiomas greater than 20 cm in maximum diameter are often reported [24]. In a case with a giant hepatic hemangioma, since the image pick-up range of an ultrasonic probe is narrow, it is difficult to obtain an overall picture of the tumor. However, as Sonazoid contrast-enhanced US is low cost and minimally invasive, it is much easier to scan

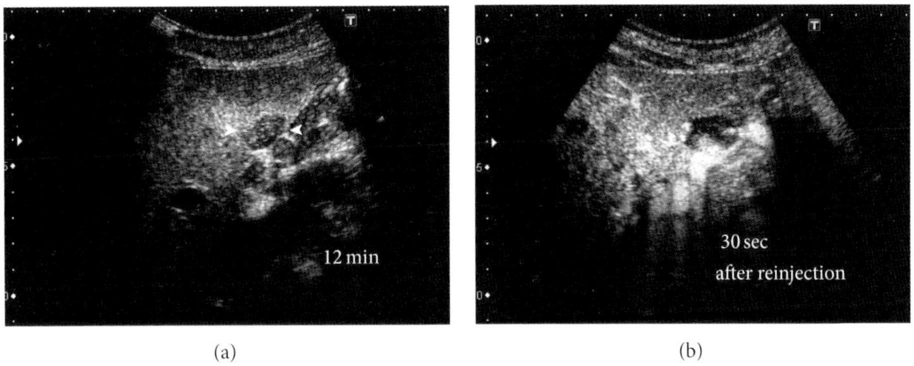


Figure 3: US, employing the "defect reperfusion US imaging" technique with Sonazoid, was performed on another hepatic hemangioma, in the left lobe of the liver, in tumor 1. (a) Preinjection image shows a hypoechoic mass measuring about 2 cm (arrowhead). (b) The lesion shows "peripheral-nodular enhancement" 30 s after reinjection of Sonazoid.

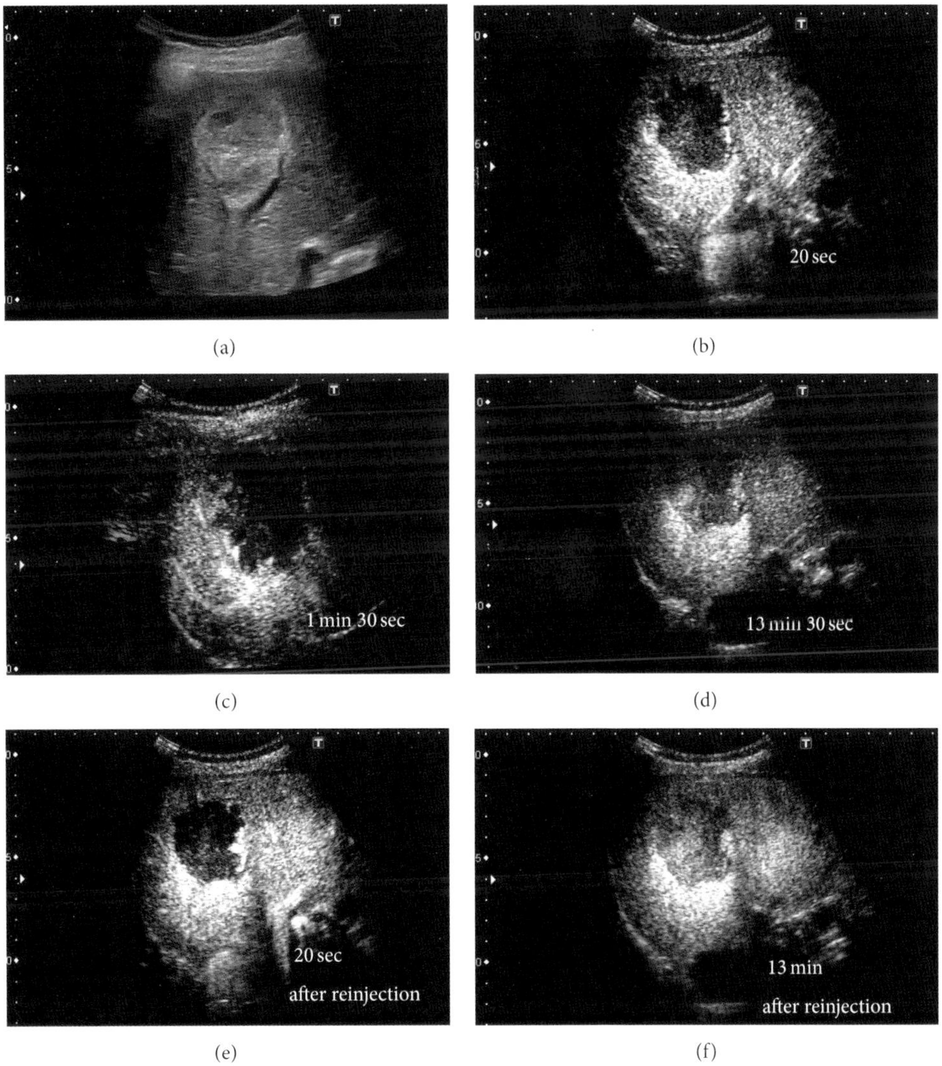


Figure 4: Intranodular dynamic image of the hepatic hemangioma in tumor 2. (a) B-mode US shows a nonhomogeneously hyperechoic lesion approximately 6 cm in size in the right lobe of the liver. (b) Sonazoid contrast-enhanced US in the early vascular phase reveals typical "peripheral globular enhancement" of the lesion. (c) The lesion shows progressive "partial centripetal filling-in" during the late vascular phase. (d) The tumor is visualized as a hypoperfusion image in the Kupffer phase. (e) The same pattern is apparent 20 s after reinjection of Sonazoid: typical "peripheral globular enhancement" of the lesion in the early vascular phase 20 s after the first injection of Sonazoid. (f) Parenchymal perfusion 13 min after reinjection results in a hypoperfusion image similar to that in the Kupffer phase after the first injection of Sonazoid.

the hepatic tumor repeatedly. There are few reports describing the observation of giant hepatic hemangiomas with Sonazoid contrast-enhanced US.

We are performing Sonazoid contrast-enhanced US on giant hepatic hemangiomas for the effective followup of the tumors. The giant hepatic hemangioma in representative tumor 1, when observed with Sonazoid contrast-enhanced US (Figure 2(b)), showed intratumoral vessels in the early vascular phase image that has been only obtained by angiography. The findings appeared to represent a general view of both arterial vascularity and portal flow, in practice, despite being in the early vascular phase. In huge hemangiomas, the enhancement pattern is in proportion to the annular form or has a form, in many cases, in which the central portion is a defect due to a central scar. Thus, tumor vessels exist in the periphery of the hepatic hemangioma [28]. Therefore, since an image similar to the projection image of a tumor vessel on angiography will be obtained if the periphery of a giant hepatic hemangioma is scanned on US with tangential adjustment, the typical pattern of a hemangioma on angiography is the so-called "cotton wool-like pooling" which can more easily be represented than "globular pooling." In our tumor 1, the spatial relationship of a vessel and the corresponding stain portioned was clearly shown. This was considered to be an important finding, greatly facilitating our understanding that the image reflected the blood supply from the hepatic artery to many vascular spaces and thereby clarifying the pathological structure of the hemangioma [8, 9]. If, however, the hemangioma in representative tumor 2, which had a smaller diameter than that in tumor 1, was observed by crossing the image of the tumor at the equatorial plane, rather than calling it "cotton wool-like pooling", the features known as "puddling" and "centripetal filling" were present (Figures 4(b) and 4(c)). In tumor 1, we recognized the coexistence of a low echoic lesion, which was faint in the Kupffer phase. We examined this low echoic lesion employing the reinjection method known as "defect reperfusion ultrasound imaging" [27] and obtained an image showing "peripheral-nodular enhancement" in the vascular phase (Figures 3(a) and 3(b)). The coexisting lesion was also considered to be a hemangioma, based on these findings. In tumor 2, because there were no other lesions, we performed secondary imaging examinations in the main tumor with Sonazoid contrast-enhanced US according to the "defect reperfusion ultrasound imaging" technique but acquired essentially the same image as the first time (Figures 4(e) and 4(f)). When a coexisting lesion is present, this raises the question of whether blood-flow evaluation is also possible, if Sonazoid contrast-enhanced US is also used to examine another tumor. Moreover, it seems that a second examination is possible, if the first observation of the same lesion was unsuccessful. In this way, if the "reperfusion imaging" is used, Sonazoid contrast-enhanced US may be useful for diagnosis and observation in cases with multiple hemangiomas. Hamaloglu et al. reported that the size average in their series of giant hepatic hemangiomas was 90 mm [29]. Many giant liver hemangiomas with a diameter of 10 cm or less, as on our tumor 2, may also be accurately examined and tested only with Sonazoid contrast-enhanced US and B-mode US with neither CT nor MRI. Furthermore, the Sonazoid contrast agent has a high probability of being useful even in cases with CT contrast media contraindications or relative contraindications such as renal insufficiency, Graves' disease, contrast media allergy, and bronchial asthma. These findings suggest observation of giant hepatic hemangiomas with Sonazoid contrast-enhanced US to be useful, safe, and cost effective.

In conclusion, even giant hepatic hemangiomas usually have nearly the same Sonazoid contrast-enhanced US findings as hepatic hemangiomas with smaller diameters. We observed the "cotton wool-like pooling" finding on Sonazoid contrast-enhanced US of giant hepatic hemangioma to be similar to the image obtained by angiography. This appears to be a very important image for understanding the histological structure of hemangioma. Moreover, Sonazoid contrast-enhanced US is also expected to be useful for the identification and examination of multiple liver hemangiomas. Although the ultrasonic contrast agent Sonazoid is currently a powerful and easy-to-use tool for diagnosis and meticulous follow-up observation of giant hepatic hemangioma, it is, unfortunately, only available in Japan. It is hoped that Sonazoid will gain widespread acceptance in the future.

## References

[1] J. A. Mungovan, J. J. Cronan, and J. Vacarro, "Hepatic cavernous hemangiomas: lack of enlargement over time," *Radiology*, vol. 191, no. 1, pp. 111–113, 1994.

[2] M. N. Sinanan and T. Marchioro, "Management of cavernous hemangioma of the liver," *American Journal of Surgery*, vol. 157, no. 5, pp. 519–522, 1989.

[3] L. Belli, L. De Carlis, C. Beati, G. Rondinara, V. Sansalone, and G. Brambilla, "Surgical treatment of symptomatic giant hemangiomas of the liver," *Surgery Gynecology and Obstetrics*, vol. 174, no. 6, pp. 474–478, 1992.

[4] C. F. Dietrich, J. C. Mertens, B. Braden, G. Schuessler, M. Ott, and A. Ignee, "Contrast-enhanced ultrasound of histologically proven liver hemangiomas," *Hepatology*, vol. 45, no. 5, pp. 1139–1145, 2007.

[5] T. V. Bartolotta, A. Taibbi, M. Midiri, and R. Lagalla, "Focal liver lesions: contrast-enhanced ultrasound," *Abdominal Imaging*, vol. 34, no. 2, pp. 193–209, 2009.

[6] V. Salvatore, A. Borghi, and F. Piscaglia, "Contrast-enhanced ultrasound for liver imaging: recent advances," *Current Pharmaceutical Design*, vol. 18, no. 15, pp. 2236–2252, 2012.

[7] K. Hatanaka, M. Kudo, Y. Minami et al., "Differential diagnosis of hepatic tumors: value of contrast-enhanced harmonic sonography using the newly developed contrast agent, Sonazoid," *Intervirology*, vol. 51, no. 1, pp. 61–69, 2008.

[8] K. M. Horton, D. A. Bluemke, R. H. Hruban, P. Soyer, and E. K. Fishman, "CT and MR imaging of benign hepatic and biliary tumors," *Radiographics*, vol. 19, no. 2, pp. 431–451, 1999.

[9] F. Caseiro-Alves, J. Brito, A. E. Araujo et al., "Liver haemangioma: common and uncommon findings and how to improve the differential diagnosis," *European Radiology*, vol. 17, no. 6, pp. 1544–1554, 2007.

[10] S. S. Yoon, C. K. Charny, Y. Fong et al., "Diagnosis, management, and outcomes of 115 patients with hepatic hemangioma," *Journal of the American College of Surgeons*, vol. 197, no. 3, pp. 392–402, 2003.

[11] D. Erdogan, O. R. C. Busch, O. M. Van Delden et al., "Management of liver hemangiomas according to size and symptoms," *Journal of Gastroenterology and Hepatology*, vol. 22, no. 11, pp. 1953–1958, 2007.

[12] M. S. Duxbury and O. J. Garden, "Giant haemangioma of the liver: observation or resection," *Digestive Surgery*, vol. 27, no. 1, pp. 7–11, 2010.

[13] T. Schnelldorfer, A. L. Ware, R. Smoot, C. D. Schleck, W. S. Harmsen, and D. M. Nagorney, "Management of giant hemangioma of the liver: resection versus observation," *Journal of the American College of Surgeons*, vol. 211, no. 6, pp. 724–730, 2010.

[14] J. Choi, Y. J. Lee, D. W. Hwang, S. H. Chon, A. Nagpal, and K. M. Park, "Surgical treatment of giant hepatic hemangiomas: technical point of view," *American Surgeon*, vol. 77, no. 1, pp. 48–54, 2011.

[15] T. Uetama, H. Yoshida, A. Hirakata et al., "A symptomatic giant hepatic hemangioma treated with hepatectomy," *Journal of Nippon Medical School*, vol. 78, no. 1, pp. 34–39, 2011.

[16] H. Y. Ho, T. H. Wu, M. C. Yu, W. C. Lee, T. C. Chao, and M. F. Chen, "Surgical management of giant hepatic hemangiomas: complications and review of the literature," *Chang Gung Medical Journal*, vol. 35, no. 1, pp. 70–78, 2012.

[17] H. Jiang, Z. Chen, P. Prasoon, H. Wu, and Y. Zeng, "Surgical management for giant liver hemangiomas greater than 20 cm in size," *Gut and Liver*, vol. 5, no. 2, pp. 228–233, 2011.

[18] H. H. Watzke, W. Linkesch, and U. Hay, "Giant hemangioma of the liver (Kasabach-Merritt syndrome): successful suppression of intravascular coagulation permitting surgical removal," *Journal of Clinical Gastroenterology*, vol. 11, no. 3, pp. 347–350, 1989.

[19] J. H. Sewell and K. Weiss, "Spontaneous rupture of hemangioma of the liver. A review of the literature and presentation of illustrative case," *Archives of Surgery*, vol. 83, pp. 729–733, 1961.

[20] H. Papafragkakis, M. Moehlen, M. T. Garcia-Buitrago, B. Madrazo, E. Island, and P. Martin, "A case of a ruptured sclerosing liver hemangioma," *International Journal of Hepatology*, vol. 2011, Article ID 942360, 5 pages, 2011.

[21] Q. Zeng, Y. Li, Y. Chen, Y. Ouyang, X. He, and H. Zhang, "Gigantic cavernous hemangioma of the liver treated by intra-arterial embolization with pingyangmycin-lipiodol emulsion: a multi-center study," *CardioVascular and Interventional Radiology*, vol. 27, no. 5, pp. 481–485, 2004.

[22] A. A. Bandeira Ferraz, M. J. Antunes Sette, M. Maia et al., "Liver transplant for the treatment of giant hepatic hemangioma," *Liver Transplantation*, vol. 10, no. 11, pp. 1436–1437, 2004.

[23] M. Meguro, Y. Soejima, A. Taketomi et al., "Living donor liver transplantation in a patient with giant hepatic hemangioma complicated by Kasabach-Merritt syndrome: report of a case," *Surgery Today*, vol. 38, no. 5, pp. 463–468, 2008.

[24] N. Akamasu, Y. Sugawara, M. Komagome et al., "Giant liver hemangioma resected by trisectorectomy after efficient volume reduction by transcatheter arterial embolization: a case report," *Journal of Medical Case Reports*, vol. 4, article 283, 2010.

[25] K. Vassiou, H. Rountas, P. Liakou, D. Arvanitis, I. Fezoulidis, and K. Tepetes, "Embolization of a giant hepatic hemangioma prior to urgent liver resection. Case report and review of the literature," *CardioVascular and Interventional Radiology*, vol. 30, no. 4, pp. 800–802, 2007.

[26] H. Suzuki, Y. Nimura, J. Kamiya et al., "Preoperative transcatheter arterial embolization for giant cavernous hemangioma of the liver with consumption coagulopathy," *American Journal of Gastroenterology*, vol. 92, no. 4, pp. 688–691, 1997.

[27] M. Kudo, K. Hatanaka, and K. Maekawa, "Newly developed novel ultrasound technique, defect reperfusion ultrasound imaging, using Sonazoid in the management of hepatocellular carcinoma," *Oncology*, vol. 78, no. 1, pp. 40–45, 2010.

[28] M. J. McLoughlin, "Angiography in cavernous hemangioma of the liver," *The American Journal of Roentgenology, Radium Therapy, and Nuclear Medicine*, vol. 113, no. 1, pp. 50–55, 1971.

[29] E. Hamaloglu, H. Altun, A. Ozdemir, and A. Ozenc, "Giant liver hemangioma: therapy by enucleation or liver resection," *World Journal of Surgery*, vol. 29, no. 7, pp. 890–893, 2005.

# 10

# The Role of Bridging Therapy in Hepatocellular Carcinoma

**Roberto Galuppo, Angie McCall, and Roberto Gedaly**

*Department of Surgery, College of Medicine, University of Kentucky, Lexington, KY 40536-0293, USA*

Correspondence should be addressed to Roberto Gedaly; rgeda2@uky.edu

Academic Editor: Daisuke Morioka

Hepatocellular carcinoma (HCC) is the most common primary malignancy of the liver accounting for 7% of all cancers worldwide. Most cases of HCC develop within an established background of chronic liver disease. For that reason, liver resection is only possible in selected patients. Liver transplantation has become the treatment of choice in patients with HCC, end-stage liver disease, and significant portal hypertension. Shortage of organ donors has resulted in overall increase of waiting list time with increased risk of dropout due to tumor progression. Neoadjuvant therapies have emerged as an alternative to control tumor growth in patients while waiting. The aim of this study is to review the literature on the role of bridging therapy and downstaging prior to liver transplantation in patients with HCC. We are also presenting our single-center experience of 96 patients undergoing transplantation for HCC with and without bridging therapy.

## 1. Introduction

Hepatocellular carcinoma (HCC) is the most common primary malignancy of the liver, the sixth most common cancer (749,000 new cases each year), and the third cause of cancer-related death worldwide [1].

In the western world, most cases of HCC develop within an established background of chronic liver disease and portal hypertension (70%–90% of all patients). Liver resection is only possible in selected cases due to the high incidence of morbidity and mortality in patients with cirrhosis and elevated portal pressures. Liver transplantation (LT) has become the treatment of choice for patients with HCC and end-stage liver disease, as it has the advantage of eradicating the tumor and the premalignant cirrhotic liver. Recurrence after LT ranges from 8% to 15% when a specific criterion for selection of patients is used. Surgical resection and ablation therapies have been associated with much higher rates of recurrence [2].

After Milan criteria were established (single nodule less than 5 cm or 3 nodules less than 3 cm), excellent results have been reported with survival in the range of 60%–70% at 5 years [3, 4]. Nonetheless, shortage of organ donors is increasing the waiting time and consequently leading to 30%–40% dropout per year because of tumor progression [5].

Therefore, the practice of treating HCC patients with locoregional therapies before LT, as they are waiting to be transplanted, has become standard in most centers [6].

We reviewed the literature on the use of locoregional therapies prior to liver transplantation and analyzed patients undergoing transplantation for HCC in our institution with emphasis on bridging therapy.

## 2. Locoregional Therapies as a Bridge to Liver Transplantation

Locoregional therapies play a major role in the current therapeutic management of HCC. They encompass a broad range of modalities including radiofrequency ablation (RFA), percutaneous ethanol injection (PEI), transarterial chemoembolization (TACE), liver resection, and microwave ablation [7, 8].

The most significant problem in patients with HCC on the waiting list is the possibility of tumor progression. For this reason, most centers started to use locoregional or neoadjuvant therapies to control tumor growth in patients while waiting. Although bridging therapies using ablation, TACE, resection, or combination treatments have been used by different transplant centers worldwide, the real impact and indication of any type of neoadjuvant treatments are still in debate. Some authors propose that patients with HCC waiting for more than 3 to 6 months should be treated [9, 10]. Various studies have suggested that treatment of HCC prior to LT in patients with a waiting time less than 6 months is not associated with an impact in patient survival or tumor recurrence and raises the question of cost effectiveness of treatment [11]. The overall risk of dropout in patients with diagnosis of HCC waiting for liver transplantation has been reported in the range of 15% to 30% at one year. New studies have reported that a lower incidence of dropout in the range of 0% to 25% may be related to the use of neoadjuvant therapies.

However, locoregional or neoadjuvant treatments prior to liver transplantation have been used to reduce tumor burden if patients are considered to be outside criteria for transplantation in a strategy called downstaging. The group from Paris, France, at L'Hopital Paul Brousse, initially recommended this strategy in 1997. They observed higher rates of survival in TACE responders than in nonresponders in an analysis of patients with more than three nodules or nodules greater than 3 cm [12]. LT was then performed only in patients that fulfilled Milan criteria after treatment. Furthermore, several prospective studies have reported good patient survival compared to patients undergoing LT without prior intervention.

*2.1. Ablation.* The use of radiofrequency ablation (RFA) for the treatment of liver tumors started in the early 1990s both in Europe and in the USA [13]. Radiofrequency ablation (RFA) is a form of locoregional therapy that utilizes a high-frequency alternating current using a probe inserted into the tumor.

The radiofrequency waves are converted into thermal energy within the conducting tissue, destroying the tumor [14]. Early experiences reported high risk of seeding, making RFA not an appealing treatment in patients while waiting to be transplanted. However, in the last few years, a well-conducted cohort study demonstrated that seeding is a rare event [7].

Percutaneous ethanol injection was used for several years in Asia and then in Europe and the USA to treat HCC with excellent results in patients with small tumors and was usually limited to less than 3-4 lesions. PEI was used for many years as treatment and more recently as bridging therapy in patients waiting for liver transplantation.

Other authors previously published that PEI can produce similar amounts of tumor necrosis although it requires a significant additional number of sessions compared to RFA. For that reason, most centers in the USA use RFA as the preferred method of ablative therapy to treat or as neoadjuvant treatment in patients with HCC. Llovet et al. demonstrated in a Markov model that ablation in patients awaiting liver transplantation had a possible gain in life expectancy and cost per year of life saved.

Several studies [7, 15–19] validated the efficacy of RFA as the most promising therapy for bridging patients to transplantation. Patients with single nodules treated with RFA showed drop-out rates ranging from 0% to 21%, while historical nontreated controls showed drop-out rates at 1 year of 30% [20].

RFA has few theoretical advantages over TACE. It has less posttreatment discomfort and simple percutaneous access, and it can be applied in patients with mild-moderate to severe liver dysfunction [21].

Ethanol injection could still be recommended in cases where radiofrequency ablation is not technically feasible such as lesions located close to large vascular structures where heat sinking effect can be observed (around 10%–15%) [22].

Other therapies such as microwave ablation have been used in some centers, but they are still under investigation. Irreversible electroporation is another ablation technique that has been used in patients with tumors abutting major vascular structures where heat sink and collateral damage must be avoided. The role of this technique as neoadjuvant treatment in HCC patients awaiting transplantation is still to be determined [23].

*2.2. Transarterial Chemoembolization.* TACE combines two different therapeutic approaches. First, application of chemotherapeutic agents is usually mixed with lipiodol as a vehicle into the feeding vessels of the tumor. Lipiodol is an oily contrast used for lymphographic studies and is selectively retained within the tumor, raising the exposure of neoplastic cells to chemotherapy. Second, the feeding artery is occluded by microparticles inducing ischemia and a prolonged exposure to the chemotherapeutic agent. Hepatic artery obstruction is usually achieved by Gelfoam particles, but not polyvinyl alcohol (PVA), starch microspheres, metallic coils, and autologous blood clots [24]. Drug-eluting beads (DEB) are a novel system consisting of PVA beads (500–700 $\mu$m) that are specifically designed to release chemotherapy at a slow rate.

Survival of patients with advanced HCC not suitable for radical therapies treated with TACE is improved compared with best supportive care [25]. Side effects range from the postembolization syndrome up to hepatic insufficiency, which is very rare. The main purpose of TACE as a bridge to transplantation is to reach local tumor control until a donor organ becomes available [26].

TACE is the preferred single-treatment modality in downstaging protocols, especially for multifocal tumors [10]. But combined modalities of TACE, RFA, PEI, and resection seem to downstage patients more effectively than TACE alone [27].

TACE is the most commonly used form of neoadjuvant therapy, alone or in combination with ablation/resection, in patients listed for LT or included in a program of downstaging [6].

The use of external beam radiation therapy in HCC treatment has been limited by the low radiation tolerance of the nontumoral cirrhotic liver. Transarterial radioembolization (TARE) instead has been recently used in the management of HCC not suitable for curative treatment with similar indications as those of TACE. Radioembolization consists of infusion of radioactive substances including microspheres containing yttrium-90 (Y90), iodine-131-iodized oil, or similar agents into the hepatic artery [9]. It represents an interesting alternative, as it appears to induce a more efficient decrease in tumor size, with a shorter time to response (4.2 versus 10.9 months) [28]. In addition, TARE could be performed in cases of portal vein thrombosis, a relative contraindication to TACE [29].

There are no randomized control trials available to assess the real place of this treatment modality in HCC patients or as a bridge to transplantation.

*2.3. Resection.* Surgery is the mainstay of HCC treatment. Resection and transplantation achieve the best overall outcomes in well-selected candidates (5-year survival of 60%–80%) and compete as the first options in patients with early tumors.

Resection is the first-line treatment option for patients with solitary tumors and very well-preserved liver function, defined as normal bilirubin with either hepatic venous pressure gradient ≤10 mmH or platelet count ≥100,000. While selected patients with cirrhosis are best treated with resection, patients with ESLD and portal hypertension are at increased risk of morbidity and mortality compared to noncirrhotic counterparts. For these reasons, only 20%–30% of patients with cirrhosis, portal hypertension, and HCC are candidates for resection. Selection of the ideal candidate requires an adequate assessment of the liver functional reserve, tumor extension, and risk of postoperative complications and mortality.

Several different systems have been used to try to address risk of morbidity and mortality after resection in patients with portal hypertension and cirrhosis. The Child-Pugh classification system initially permitted assessment of liver function. Nowadays, more sophisticated measurements such as indocyanine green retention rate at 15 min (ICG15) [30] and hepatic venous pressure gradient (HVPG) as direct measurements of relevant portal hypertension are utilized [31, 32]. Low platelet count has been confirmed as a strong independent predictor of mortality in patients with HCC and cirrhosis [22, 33].

Resection can be used as a therapy for HCC prior to LT in different settings. Initially, resection can be used as a first-line treatment for patients with small HCC and preserved liver function. Also resection could help refine the selection process for LT according to detailed pathological examination of the tumor and the surrounding liver parenchyma. It could help in selection of candidates for LT in patients with tumors slightly outside the Milan criteria but with histological features of good prognosis or in denying LT in patients within the Milan criteria but with histological features of poor prognosis such as undetected macrovascular invasion.

Several groups considered surgical resection as one of the bridging treatment modalities prior to LT. Other groups consider liver resection as one of the options for downstaging patients with tumors outside the transplantation criteria [34].

Tumor recurrence represents one of the major difficulties after resection. The pattern of recurrence influences subsequent treatment allocation and outcomes. In these instances, the patients could be reassessed, staged, and retreated accordingly.

## 3. Downstaging

The role of downstaging HCC patients prior to LT is not very clear. There are several centers in the USA and Europe trying to use different types of neoadjuvant therapy to treat HCC to decrease tumor burden to fulfill usually Milan criteria and then perform liver transplantation. The type of therapy that should be used and the upper limit of tumor size that should be downstaged are not clear. Some authors have recommended putting the candidate on hold until downstaging by local ablation and/or chemoembolization is achieved and maintained (disease stability) for a period of at least three months [22]. However, the real waiting time after successful downstaging is not clear.

There is not a single randomized control trial or a large cohort study available on patients consistently treated and properly followed. Various prospective small studies suggested that downstaging tumors to reach Milan criteria using RFA and/or TACE achieves 5-year survival rates similar to those within the conventional criteria after LT.

Ravaioli et al. presented a prospective study providing validation of a downstaging protocol, in which patients, initially excluded by the conventional transplant criteria, undergoing successful downstaging obtained satisfactory survival after LT [35]. Still efficacy of downstaging in patients exceeding conventional criteria is strictly related to tumor size and number at presentation. The bigger the tumor bulk, the lower the efficacy of downstaging in terms of tumor response [10].

Considering the existing information, downstaging of patients beyond Milan criteria still remains controversial, and criteria for selecting candidates are not well established. Chapman et al. considered most patients beyond Milan criteria and did not exclude a priori any patients. This group reported that 17 out of 76 patients were transplanted after successful downstaging. They reported comparable outcomes in these 17 patients to those in patients within Milan criteria [36]. Yao et al. restricted downstaging eligibility criteria to one lesion >5 cm and up to 8 cm; 2 to 3 tumors with at least one lesion >3 cm but not exceeding 5 cm, with total tumor diameter up to 8 cm; or 4 to 5 lesions with none >3 cm with total tumor diameter less than 8 cm. Using these criteria as an upper limit for downstaging, 57.4% (35/61) of their patients were successfully downstaged and transplanted [37]. Ravaioli et al. prospectively analyzed patients with a single HCC 5 cm to 6 cm, 2 lesions ≤5 cm, or less than 6 HCC lesions ≤4 cm and sum diameter ≤12 cm, and they achieved a 67% transplantation rate (32/48 patients). They achieved similar outcomes in patients treated versus those within conventional Milan criteria [35].

## 4. Our Experience

In the Transplant Center at the University of Kentucky, the strategy for management of HCC has evolved with a multimodality algorithm approach similar to that adopted in other centers [38].

We retrospectively analyzed our experience of 96 consecutive patients undergoing transplantation for HCC from September 1999 to September 2011. Of the 96 patients, 78 were

Table 1: Patient demographics.

| Patient demographics | | |
|---|---|---|
| Age | 56 | (36–72) |
| Sex | | |
| Male | 78 | 81.30% |
| Female | 18 | 18.70% |
| Incidental | 31 | 32.30% |
| ALD | 40 | 41.70% |
| HCV | 48 | 50% |
| BT | 19 | 29.20% |
| Size of greater lesion (mean) | 2.3 | (0.7–7.6 cm) |
| Single | 51 | 54.40% |
| Vascular invasion | 22 | 22.90% |

Alcoholic liver disease (ALD); hepatitis C cirrhosis (HCV); bridging therapy (BT).

males (81.3%). As expected, hepatitis C (HCV) was the most common indication in this group (48 patients, 50%), followed by alcoholic liver disease (40 patients, 41.7%). Among the 96 patients who underwent LT, 31 patients were identified as having incidental HCC on the explanted livers, undetected on preoperative imaging (Table 1).

A total of 49 patients (54.4%) had single lesions. The mean diameter of the greatest lesion was 2.3 cm, ranging from 0.7 to 7.6 cm. Vascular invasion was found in 22 patients (22.9%).

Analysis of survival was performed using the Kaplan-Meier method. For intention-to-treat survival, all 96 patients were followed up from the time of listing to death or last followup. Overall survival rates of 89.2%, 74.1%, and 62.1% at one, three, and five years were observed, respectively. As expected, patients with vascular invasion had significantly worse survival compared to those patients with tumors without vascular invasion ($P < 0.005$). Rates at one, three, and five years for patients without vascular invasion were 90.9%, 77.6%, and 66.1%, respectively, while for patients with vascular invasion survival was considerably lower; 71.6%, 61.7%, and 46.3% (Figures 1 and 2).

We compared patient characteristics in individuals undergoing bridging therapy with those without preoperative treatment (Table 2). Patients characteristics were similar in both groups other than tumor size greater than 3 cm that was more common in patients in the BT group ($P < 0.005$).

Nineteen liver transplant candidates representing 29.2% of known HCC cases were treated with locoregional therapies (Table 2). Of those patients undergoing neoadjuvant treatments, 10 were treated with RFA (15.4%), 8 with TACE (12.3%), 1 with resection (1.5%), and 1 with RFA/TACE combination (1.5%).

Recurrence was seen in 13 patients representing 13.2% or our cases transplanted for HCC. Survival and recurrence rates were similar in treated patients versus nontreated individuals ($P$ = ns).

## 5. Discussion

Liver transplantation represents the best curative option for HCC and cirrhosis as it has the advantage of removing the tumor and treating the underlying disease. Despite that, HCC can progress significantly in patients awaiting LT. It has been reported an approximate doubling time for these cancers of around 6 months [39]. As a consequence, tumors can grow beyond conventional criteria, increasing the possibility of microvascular invasion and occult metastasis and further worsening the patient condition.

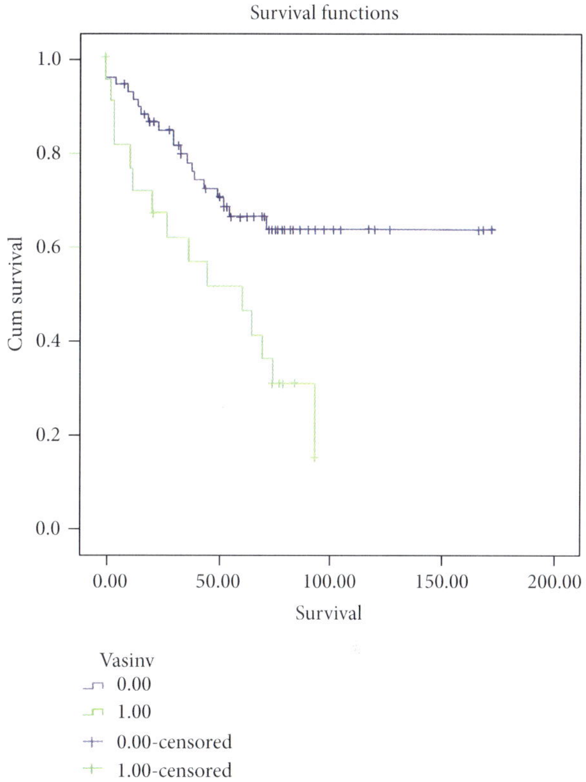


Figure 1: This graphic shows survival among patients undergoing LT with and without vascular invasion. Survival is significantly better in those patients transplanted without vascular invasion ($P < 0.05$).

Recent advances in imaging techniques, especially with the use of liver-specific contrast MRI, are making diagnosis of HCC and quantification of the amount of disease more accurate. Gadolinium-ethoxybenzyl-diethylenetriamine pentaacetic acid (Gd-EOB-DTPA) is a liver-specific magnetic resonance imaging contrast agent that has up to 50% hepatobiliary excretion in the normal liver. After intravenous injection, Gd-EOB-DTPA distributes into the vascular and extravascular spaces during the arterial, portal venous and late dynamic phases and then progressively into the hepatocytes and bile ducts during the hepatobiliary phase. The role of gadolinium-ethoxybenzyl-diethylenetriamine pentaacetic acid-enhanced magnetic resonance imaging (EOB-MRI) in the management of HCC is still to be determined. However, most centers are now using EOVIST when regular dynamic CT/MRI images do not show conclusive findings.

Selection criteria for liver transplantation in HCC patients are still controversial [22, 40–43]. Although initial

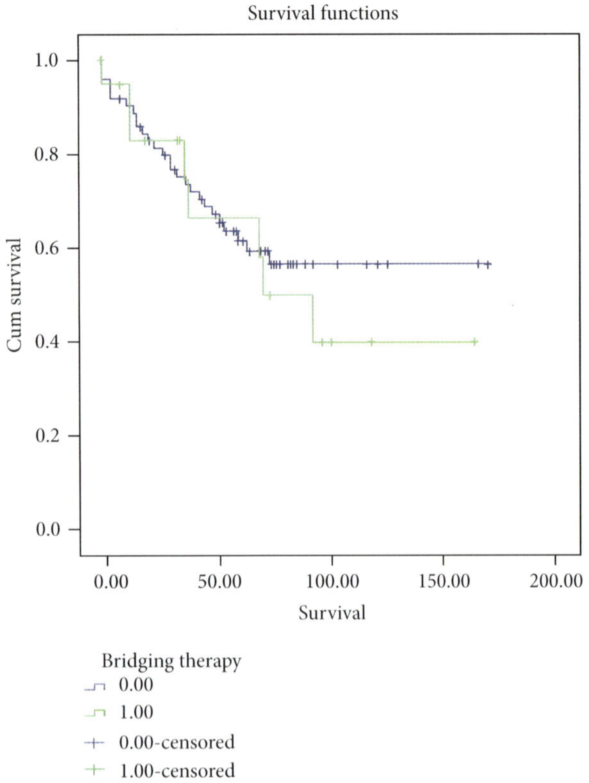


FIGURE 2: This graphic demonstrates survival among patients undergoing LT with and without bridging treatment. Similar survival rates were observed in patients transplanted with and without BT ($P$ = ns).

TABLE 2: Comparison of patients, characteristics.

| Comparison of patients' characteristics<br>Bridging therapy versus nonbridging therapy | | | |
|---|---|---|---|
| | BT | Non-BT | Sig |
| Age | 59.4 | 55.9 | 0.47 |
| Sex (male) | 16 | 58 | 0.46 |
| AFP | 168 | 160 | 0.98 |
| MELD | 13 | 16 | 0.86 |
| Waiting time | 59.5 | 152.1 | 0.09 |
| Vascular invasion | 5 | 15 | 0.45 |
| Multiple | 7 | 33 | 0.32 |
| Size > 3 cm | 7 | 11 | 0.04* |
| HCV | 11 | 36 | 0.26 |

*Statistically significant ($P < 0.05$).
Bridging therapy (BT); alpha-fetoprotein (AFP); hepatitis C cirrhosis (HCV).

LT results in nonselected patients with HCC were discouraging, subsequent series proved that better results could be achieved by employing defined selection criteria [44]. The criteria proposed by Mazzaferro et al. in 1996 are used as a basic stratification tool by numerous transplantation centers worldwide [2]. Using these criteria, a patient with a single tumor measuring 5 cm or less, or three or fewer nodules each smaller than 3 cm, would be a candidate for LT. Excellent 5-year survival rates in the range of 60%–70% or higher have been reported when these criteria are followed. Subsequently, the University of California at San Francisco reported 57% survival for patients with HCC who exceeded Milan criteria but were within the limits of their expanded criteria, including patients with solitary lesions less than 6.5 cm in size or up to three tumors with the largest not more than 4.5 cm and a combined tumor diameter of not more than 8 cm [45]. The TNM criteria by Marsh et al. at the University of Pittsburgh are based on HCC characteristics including microvascular or macrovascular invasion, lobar distribution, tumor size, and lymph node involvement, and they seemed to provide a more clear-cut discrimination with respect to post-OLT survival for each TNM tumor stage (I to IV) [46].

Yao et al. compared the previous three proposed criteria and supported a modest expansion of the tumor size limits of the Milan criteria (the UCSF criteria) while still preserving acceptable survival after OLT. The expanded criteria offered the benefits of OLT to about 20% of our patients who would have otherwise been excluded from OLT under the more restrictive Milan criteria. The UCSF criteria also confer an advantage over the Pittsburgh criteria, which require information on microvascular invasion that is difficult to ascertain preoperatively without the attendant risks of biopsy [47].

Candidacy is now decided based on size and number of lesions (Milan, UCSF criteria, etc.). However, there are other important predictors of recurrence and patient survival that have not been included in the current selection system such as AFP/AFPL3% levels, tumor differentiation, and microvascular invasion. AFP is the most widely tested biomarker in HCC [22]. Lens culinaris agglutinin-reactive AFP (AFP-L3) is an isoform of AFP that is very specific for screening and diagnosis of HCC in the background of cirrhosis or hepatitis. However, the clinical usefulness of AFP-L3 in HCC has been inconsistent. Unfortunately, there has been large heterogeneity on the results of multiple studies when assessing AFP-L3% and AFP in the same population [48].

The relationship between AFP levels and tumor burden has been determined in HCC patients. Our group reported that tumor size and AFP were strongly related to the presence of microvascular invasion (MVI) on the explanted liver. AFP in conjunction with other markers such as des-gamma-carboxyprothrombin and AFP-L3 has been associated with tumor burden as well [49]. Because of the relationship with tumor burden and outcomes, several centers are now using highly elevated levels of AFP to rule out patients for liver transplantation. In 2012, Duvoux et al. published that levels of AFP greater than 1000 U/dL are associated with high risk of recurrence and suggested that AFP should be incorporated to the Milan criteria in order to select patients for liver transplantation [50].

Based on UNOS data, the 3 most common indications for liver transplantation in the USA are hepatitis C, alcoholic liver disease, and hepatocellular carcinoma. Interestingly, in 2010, HCC is already the second most common indication for transplantation, second only to hepatitis C. A significant amount of patients with HCC have concomitant HCV infection which could compromise outcomes in this subgroup of patients.

Reinfection of the liver graft by HCV is constant, and the natural history of HCV recurrence is accelerated compared with nontransplanted patients when serum HCV RNA remains detectable at LT. Approximately 20% to 30% of patients will develop cirrhosis within 5 years after LT.

The best strategy to prevent recurrence of HCV is to eradicate HCV infection prior to LT. Treatment before the development of injury to the graft in the early phase is currently not recommended because studies have shown that it is difficult to initiate antiviral therapy with IFN during the postoperative period and that it has a poor efficacy with remarkable side effects such as bacterial infections, hematological toxicity, and rejections, which lead to dose reduction or discontinuation of treatment.

HCV therapy should be initiated in the presence of severe and rapid progression of fibrosis with a higher risk of graft loss, especially in the setting of cholestatic hepatitis. Current regimens included antiviral therapy with PEG-IFN/RBV, and several studies have shown that a sustained virological response is achieved in 8%–45%. Three different systematic reviews of PEG-IFN/RBV after LT showed that the SVR rate is around 30% [51–53]. The duration of therapy is usually 48 weeks, and therapy is influence by several factors which influences the prognosis before and during therapy such as viral genotype, donor age, baseline viral load, IL28B donor and recipient, absence of prior antiviral therapy, severity of baseline fibrosis, adherence to therapy, duration of therapy, rapid virological response, and early virological response.

Due to the development of new drugs for the treatment of HCV infection, most experts believe that treatment of HCV recurrence after LT will change in the next few years. The role of triple therapy using PEG-IFN/RBV plus protease inhibitors is not clear. Verna EC et al. recently published the results of a multicenter study using triple therapy with Telaprevir in HCV recurrence after LT reporting increased sustained viral response rates exceeding those with standard treatment with PEG-IFN/RBV alone [54]. These results must be balanced with high rates of adverse events including increased risk of readmissions, kidney dysfunction, and death. There are now other protocols under investigation in patients with cirrhosis including noninterferon regimens. The role of these treatment combinations in the LT setting is still to be determined.

The timing and adequacy of HCC treatment before liver transplantation to control the disease are unclear. New minimally invasive strategies are being implemented to decrease tumor progression in patients with diagnosis of HCC while waiting to be transplanted.

The appropriate treatment alternative that should be used as neoadjuvant therapy prior to LT such as liver resection, radiofrequency ablation (RFA), transarterial chemoembolization (TACE), or combination remains under debate.

Considering the strength and existing evidence, it is recommended to treat patients waiting for transplant with local ablation and/or chemoembolization when waiting time is estimated to exceed 6 months. Furthermore, several cohort studies and a preliminary analysis of large registries suggest that bridging strategies with locoregional therapy are likely to be beneficial for patients waiting for 6 months or longer. The recommendation of bridging therapy is more important in UNOS T2 HCC patients to decrease dropout rates and achieve good posttransplant outcomes [55, 56]. A Markov-based cost-effectiveness analysis by Llovet et al. pointed out the benefits of neoadjuvant therapies when waiting time exceeded 6 months [5]. In our center, the decision to use bridging therapy is done on an individual basis by a multidisciplinary team integrated by hepatologist, radiologist, interventional radiologists, oncologist, radiation oncologists, and transplant surgeons. We usually recommend TACE and/or RFA in patients with UNOS stage 2 HCC prior to LT if 6 months or longer waiting time is expected in rapidly growing tumors or in large lesions close to the upper size limits of the Milan criteria.

Based on the International Consensus Conference held in December 2010 in Zurich, Switzerland, specific recommendations regarding downstaging cannot be properly made due to the lack of evidence, and further research is needed [22].

Although adjuvant therapy is currently used in most centers in the USA and Europe, further investigation is needed to determine the efficacy and timing of neoadjuvant treatment modalities for HCC in patients awaiting liver transplantation.

## References


[1] http://www-dep.iarc.fr/, http://globocan.iarc.fr/factsheet.asp.

[2] V. Mazzaferro, E. Regalia, R. Doci et al., "Liver transplantation for the treatment of small hepatocellular carcinomas in patients with cirrhosis," *The New England Journal of Medicine*, vol. 334, no. 11, pp. 693–699, 1996.

[3] V. Mazzaferro, Y. S. Chun, R. T. P. Poon et al., "Liver transplantation for hepatocellular carcinoma," *Annals of Surgical Oncology*, vol. 15, no. 4, pp. 1001–1007, 2008.

[4] P. P. McHugh, J. Gilbert, S. Vera, A. Koch, D. Ranjan, and R. Gedaly, "Alpha-fetoprotein and tumour size are associated with microvascular invasion in explanted livers of patients undergoing transplantation with hepatocellular carcinoma," *HPB*, vol. 12, no. 1, pp. 56–61, 2010.

[5] J. M. Llovet, X. Mas, J. J. Aponte et al., "Cost effectivenessof adjuvant therapy for hepatocellular carcinoma during the waiting list for liver transplantation," *Gut*, vol. 50, no. 1, pp. 123–128, 2002.

[6] M. Cescon, A. Cucchetti, M. Ravaioli, and A. D. Pinna, "Hepatocellular carcinoma locoregional therapies for patients in the waiting list. Impact on transplantability and recurrence rate," *Journal of Hepatology*, vol. 58, no. 3, pp. 609–618, 2013.

[7] V. Mazzaferro, C. Battiston, S. Perrone et al., "Radiofrequency ablation of small hepatocellular carcinoma in cirrhotic patients awaiting liver transplantation: a prospective study," *Annals of Surgery*, vol. 240, no. 5, pp. 900–909, 2004.

[8] D. Ansari and R. Andersson, "Radiofrequency ablation or percutaneous ethanol injection for the treatment of liver tumors," *World Journal of Gastroenterology*, vol. 18, no. 10, pp. 1003–1008, 2012.

[9] R. Lencioni, L. Crocetti, P. De Simone, and F. Filipponi, "Locoregional interventional treatment of hepatocellular carcinoma:

techniques, outcomes, and future prospects," *Transplant International*, vol. 23, no. 7, pp. 698–703, 2010.

[10] S. Bhoori, C. Sposito, A. Germini, J. Coppa, and V. Mazzaferro, "The challenges of liver transplantation for hepatocellular carcinoma on cirrhosis," *Transplant International*, vol. 23, no. 7, pp. 712–722, 2010.

[11] A. Díaz-Sánchez, A. Matilla, O. Núñez et al., "Influence of treatment of hepatocellular carcinoma before liver transplantation on post transplant tumor recurrence and survival," *Journal of Gastroenterology and Hepatology*, vol. 33, no. 3, pp. 155–164, 2010.

[12] P. E. Majno, R. Adam, H. Bismuth et al., "Influence of preoperative transarterial lipiodol chemoembolization on resection and transplantation for hepatocellular carcinoma in patients with cirrhosis," *Annals of Surgery*, vol. 226, no. 6, pp. 688–703, 1997.

[13] J. P. McGahan, P. D. Browning, J. M. Brock, and H. Tesluk, "Hepatic ablation using radiofrequency electrocautery," *Investigative Radiology*, vol. 25, no. 3, pp. 267–270, 1990.

[14] S.-F. Li, A. M. Hawxby, R. Kanagala, H. Wright, and A. Sebastian, "Liver transplantation for hepatocellular carcinoma: indications, bridge therapy and adjuvant therapy," *The Journal of the Oklahoma State Medical Association*, vol. 105, no. 1, pp. 12–16, 2012.

[15] R. J. Fontana, H. Hamidullah, H. Nghiem et al., "Percutaneous radiofrequency thermal ablation of hepatocellular carcinoma: a safe and effective bridge to liver transplantation," *Liver Transplantation*, vol. 8, no. 12, pp. 1165–1174, 2002.

[16] P.-Y. Brillet, V. Paradis, G. Brancatelli et al., "Percutaneous radiofrequency ablation for hepatocellular carcinoma before liver transplantation: a prospective study with histopathologic comparison," *American Journal of Roentgenology*, vol. 186, no. 5, pp. S296–S305, 2006.

[17] D. S. K. Lu, N. C. Yu, S. S. Raman et al., "Percutaneous radiofrequency ablation of hepatocellular carcinoma as a bridge to liver transplantation," *Hepatology*, vol. 41, no. 5, pp. 1130–1137, 2005.

[18] F. Y. Yao, M. Kinkhabwala, J. M. LaBerge et al., "The impact of pre-operative loco-regional therapy on outcome after liver transplantation for hepatocellular carcinoma," *American Journal of Transplantation*, vol. 5, no. 4, pp. 795–804, 2005.

[19] A. Bharat, D. B. Brown, J. S. Crippin et al., "Pre-liver transplantation locoregional adjuvant therapy for hepatocellular carcinoma as a strategy to improve longterm survival," *Journal of the American College of Surgeons*, vol. 203, no. 4, pp. 411–420, 2006.

[20] J. M. Llovet, M. Schwartz, and V. Mazzaferro, "Resection and liver transplantation for hepatocellular carcinoma," *Seminars in Liver Disease*, vol. 25, no. 2, pp. 181–200, 2005.

[21] D. S. Lu, N. C. Yu, S. S. Raman et al., "Percutaneous radiofrequency ablation of hepatocellular carcinoma as a bridge to liver transplantation," *Hepatology*, vol. 41, no. 5, pp. 1130–1137, 2005.

[22] European Association for the Study of the Liver and European Organisation for Research and Treatment of Cancer, "EASL—EORTC clinical practice guidelines: management of hepatocellular carcinoma," *Journal of Hepatology*, vol. 56, no. 4, pp. 908–943, 2012.

[23] K. P. Charpentier, "Irreversible electroporation for the ablation of liver tumors: are we there yet?" *Archives of Surgery*, vol. 147, no. 11, pp. 1053–1061, 2012.

[24] L. Marelli, R. Stigliano, C. Triantos et al., "Transarterial therapy for hepatocellular carcinoma: which technique is more effective? a systematic review of cohort and randomized studies," *CardioVascular and Interventional Radiology*, vol. 30, no. 1, pp. 6–25, 2007.

[25] J. M. Llovet and J. Bruix, "Systematic review of randomized trials for unresectable hepatocellular carcinoma: chemoembolization improves survival," *Hepatology*, vol. 37, no. 2, pp. 429–442, 2003.

[26] J. Petersen, B. Henninger, B. Glodny, and W. Jaschke, "Transarterial chemoembolisation in hepatocellular carcinoma," *Wiener Medizinische Wochenschrift*, vol. 163, no. 5–6, pp. 123–127, 2013.

[27] Z. W. Peng, Y. J. Zhang, M. S. Chen et al., "Radiofrequency ablation with or without transcatheter arterial chemoembolization in the treatment of hepatocellular carcinoma: a prospective randomized trial," *Journal of Clinical Oncology*, vol. 31, no. 4, pp. 426–432, 2013.

[28] R. J. Lewandowski, L. M. Kulik, A. Riaz et al., "A comparative analysis of transarterial downstaging for hepatocellular carcinoma: chemoembolization versus radioembolization," *American Journal of Transplantation*, vol. 9, no. 8, pp. 1920–1928, 2009.

[29] C. Toso, G. Mentha, N. M. Kneteman, and P. Majno, "The place of downstaging for hepatocellular carcinoma," *Journal of Hepatology*, vol. 52, no. 6, pp. 930–936, 2010.

[30] M. Makuuchi, T. Kosuge, T. Takayama et al., "Surgery for small liver cancers," *Seminars in Surgical Oncology*, vol. 9, no. 4, pp. 298–304, 1993.

[31] J. Bruix, A. Castells, J. Bosch et al., "Surgical resection of hepatocellular carcinoma in cirrhotic patients: prognostic value of preoperative portal pressure," *Gastroenterology*, vol. 111, no. 4, pp. 1018–1022, 1996.

[32] T. Ishizawa, K. Hasegawa, T. Aoki et al., "Neither multiple tumors nor portal hypertension are surgical contraindications for hepatocellular carcinoma," *Gastroenterology*, vol. 134, no. 7, pp. 1908–1916, 2008.

[33] W. Bleibel, S. H. Caldwell, M. P. Curry, and P. G. Northup, "Peripheral platelet count correlates with liver atrophy and predicts long-term mortality on the liver transplant waiting list," *Transplant International*, vol. 26, no. 4, pp. 435–442, 2013.

[34] J. Belghiti, "Resection and liver transplantation for HCC," *Journal of Gastroenterology*, vol. 44, supplement 19, pp. 132–135, 2009.

[35] M. Ravaioli, G. L. Grazi, F. Piscaglia et al., "Liver transplantation for hepatocellular carcinoma: results of down-staging in patients initially outside the Milan selection criteria," *American Journal of Transplantation*, vol. 8, no. 12, pp. 2547–2557, 2008.

[36] W. C. Chapman, M. B. Majella Doyle, J. E. Stuart et al., "Outcomes of neoadjuvant transarterial chemoembolization to downstage hepatocellular carcinoma before liver transplantation," *Annals of Surgery*, vol. 248, no. 4, pp. 617–624, 2008.

[37] F. Y. Yao, R. K. Kerlan Jr., R. Hirose et al., "Excellent outcome following down-staging of hepatocellular carcinoma prior to liver transplantation: an intention-to-treat analysis," *Hepatology*, vol. 48, no. 3, pp. 819–827, 2008.

[38] J. M. Llovet, J. Fuster, and J. Bruix, "The Barcelona approach: diagnosis, staging, and treatment of hepatocellular carcinoma," *Liver Transplantation*, vol. 10, no. 2, pp. S115–S120, 2004.

[39] L. Barbara, G. Benzi, S. Gaiani et al., "Natural history of small untreated hepatocellular carcinoma in cirrhosis: a multivariate analysis of prognostic factors of tumor growth rate and patient survival," *Hepatology*, vol. 16, no. 1, pp. 132–137, 1992.

[40] J. Bruix, M. Sherman, J. M. Llovet et al., "Clinical management of hepatocellular carcinoma. Conclusions of the Barcelona-2000 EASL conference," *Journal of Hepatology*, vol. 35, no. 3, pp. 421–430, 2001.

[41] J. Bruix and M. Sherman, "Management of hepatocellular carcinoma," *Hepatology*, vol. 42, no. 5, pp. 1208–1236, 2005.

[42] B. E. Van Beers, C. M. Pastor, and H. K. Hussain, "Primovist, Eovist: what to expect?" *Journal of Hepatology*, vol. 57, no. 2, pp. 421–429, 2012.

[43] T. Inoue, M. Kudo, M. Komuta et al., "Assessment of Gd-EOB-DTPA-enhanced MRI for HCC and dysplastic nodules and comparison of detection sensitivity versus MDCT," *Journal of Gastroenterology*, vol. 47, no. 9, pp. 1036–1047, 2012.

[44] J. M. Llovet, M. Schwartz, and V. Mazzaferro, "Resection and liver transplantation for hepatocellular carcinoma," *Seminars in Liver Disease*, vol. 25, no. 2, pp. 181–200, 2005.

[45] J. P. Duffy, A. Vardanian, E. Benjamin et al., "Liver transplantation criteria for hepatocellular carcinoma should be expanded: a 22-year experience with 467 patients at UCLA," *Annals of Surgery*, vol. 246, no. 3, pp. 502–509, 2007.

[46] J. W. Marsh, I. Dvorchik, C. A. Bonham, and S. Iwatsuki, "Is the pathologic TNM staging system for patients with hepatoma predictive of outcome?" *Cancer*, vol. 88, no. 3, pp. 538–543, 2000.

[47] F. Y. Yao, N. M. Bass, B. Nikolai et al., "Liver transplantation for hepatocellular carcinoma: analysis of survival according to the intention-to-treat principle and dropout from the waiting list," *Liver Transplantation*, vol. 8, no. 10, pp. 873–883, 2002.

[48] X. Yi, S. Yu, and Y. Bao, "Alpha-fetoprotein-L3 in hepatocellular carcinoma: a meta-analysis," *Clinica Chimica Acta*, vol. 425, pp. 212–220, 2013.

[49] F. A. Durazo, L. M. Blatt, W. G. Corey et al., "Des-$\gamma$-carboxyprothrombin, $\alpha$-fetoprotein and AFP-L3 in patients with chronic hepatitis, cirrhosis and hepatocellular carcinoma," *Journal of Gastroenterology and Hepatology*, vol. 23, no. 10, pp. 1541–1548, 2008.

[50] C. Duvoux, F. Roudot-Thoraval, T. Decaens et al., "Liver transplantation for hepatocellular carcinoma: a model including $\alpha$-fetoprotein improves the performance of Milan criteria," *Gastroenterology*, vol. 143, no. 4, pp. 986–994, 2012.

[51] M. Berenguer, "Systematic review of the treatment of established recurrent hepatitis C with pegylated interferon in combination with ribavirin," *Journal of Hepatology*, vol. 49, no. 2, pp. 274–287, 2008.

[52] C. S. Wang, H. H. Ko, E. M. Yoshida, C. A. Marra, and K. Richardson, "Interferon-based combination anti-viral therapy for hepatitis C virus after liver transplantation: a review and quantitative analysis," *American Journal of Transplantation*, vol. 6, no. 7, pp. 1586–1599, 2006.

[53] E. Xirouchakis, C. Triantos, P. Manousou et al., "Pegylated-interferon and ribavirin in liver transplant candidates and recipients with HCV cirrhosis: systematic review and meta-analysis of prospective controlled studies," *Journal of Viral Hepatitis*, vol. 15, no. 10, pp. 699–709, 2008.

[54] E. C. Verna, J. R. Burton, J. G. O'Leary et al., "Multicenter study of protease inhibitor-triple therapy in HCV-infected liver transplant recipients: report from the crush-C group," *Journal of Hepatology*, vol. 58, supplement 1, pp. S10–S11, 2013.

[55] P. Majno, R. Lencioni, F. Mornex, N. Girard, R. T. Poon, and D. Cherqui, "Is the treatment of hepatocellular carcinoma on the waiting list necessary?" *Liver Transplantation*, vol. 17, no. S2, pp. S98–S108, 2011.

[56] O. B. Lao, J. Weissman, and J. D. Perkins, "Pre-transplant therapy for hepatocellular carcinoma is associated with a lower recurrence after liver transplantation," *Clinical Transplantation*, vol. 23, no. 6, pp. 874–881, 2009.

# 11

# Pretreatment of Small-for-Size Grafts *In Vivo* by $\gamma$-Aminobutyric Acid Receptor Regulation against Oxidative Stress-Induced Injury in Rat Split Orthotopic Liver Transplantation

**Tomohide Hori,[1,2] Shinji Uemoto,[2] Lindsay B. Walden,[1,3] Feng Chen,[1] Ann-Marie T. Baine,[1] Toshiyuki Hata,[1,2] and Justin H. Nguyen[3]**

[1] *Department of Neuroscience, Mayo Clinic, Jacksonville, FL 32224, USA*
[2] *Division of Hepato-Biliary-Pancreatic and Transplant Surgery, Department of Surgery, Kyoto University Graduate School of Medicine, 54 Shogoinkawara-cho, Sakyo-ku, Kyoto 606-8507, Japan*
[3] *Division of Transplant Surgery, Department of Transplantation, Mayo Clinic, Jacksonville, FL 32224, USA*

Correspondence should be addressed to Tomohide Hori; horit@kuhp.kyoto-u.ac.jp

Academic Editor: Matthias Bahr

*Background.* Graft pretreatment to limit postoperative damage has the advantage of overcoming a current issue in liver transplantation (LT). The strategic potential of graft pretreatment *in vivo* by a specific agonist for $\gamma$-aminobutyric acid receptor (GABAR) was investigated in the rat LT model with a small-for-size graft (SFSG). *Methods.* Recipient rats were divided into three groups according to donor treatments and recipient surgeries: (i) saline and laparotomy, (ii) saline and split orthotopic liver transplantation (SOLT) with 40%-SFSG, and (iii) GABAR agonist and SOLT with 40%-SFSG. Survival was evaluated. Blood and liver samples were collected 6 h after surgery. Immunohistological assessment for apoptotic induction and western blotting for 4-hydroxynonenal, ataxia-telangiectasia mutated kinase (ATM), histone H2AX, phosphatidylinositol-3 kinase (PI3K), Akt, and free radical scavenging enzymes were performed. *Results.* Pretreatment by GABAR showed improvement in survival, histopathological assessment, and biochemical tests. Apoptotic induction and oxidative stress were observed after SOLT with an SFSG, and this damage was limited by GABAR regulation. GABAR regulation appeared to reduce DNA damage via the ATM/H2AX pathway and to promote cell survival via the PI3K/Akt pathway. *Conclusions.* Pretreatment *in vivo* by GABAR regulation improves graft damage after SOLT with an SFSG. This strategy may be advantageous in LT.

## 1. Introduction

Oxygen is required for cell survival. However, oxygen also poses a potential hazard via reactive oxygen species (ROS) and reactive nitrogen species (RNS), with biological and functional alterations of lipids, proteins, and deoxyribonucleic acid (DNA) [1–3]. Therefore, ROS/RNS have been initially considered as harmful products of the normal aerobic metabolism. The control of ROS/RNS production plays physiological roles, especially, in regulating cell signaling to involve cell proliferation, differentiation, and apoptosis [1–3]. Oxidative stress (OS) mediated by free radicals is defined as an imbalance between the production of ROS/RNS and the antioxidant capacity of the cell [1–3]. These antioxidants ensure a defense against ROS/RNS-induced OS [2].

The predominant inhibitory neurotransmitter in the brain is $\gamma$-aminobutyric acid (GABA), and almost all researchers have focused on GABA or the regulation of GABA receptor (GABAR) in the brain [4–8]. Currently, GABA is considered to be a multifunctional molecule with various physiological effects throughout the body [9, 10]. In the brain, many researchers have found that the regulation of GABAR has preventive effects against OS-induced damage [5, 7, 8]. These results in the brain were mainly explained via specific pathways against OS (i.e., inhibition of the response to DNA damage [5, 11, 12] and promotion of cell survival [13, 14] or the free radical scavenging system [15, 16]). Liver contains GABA and its transporter [10], and hepatic GABAR has been also detected [17]. However, in the liver, the effects of GABAR regulation have not been reported.

Orthotopic liver transplantation (OLT) is an accepted therapy for children and adults with end-stage liver disease, and it currently provides long-term survival and quality lifestyle. However, cold ischemia during organ storage and subsequent reperfusion severely damage the transplanted liver [18]. During cold ischemic preservation, parenchymal cells swell and bleb [18], and then Kupffer and endothelial cells trigger ROS/RNS production after warm reperfusion [18]. This cold ischemia/warm reperfusion (CIWR) injury is still a major cause of morbidity and mortality after OLT due to primary graft dysfunction or a nonfunctioning graft [18]. Reperfusion not only triggers the liver regeneration cascade but also causes fatal damage in the liver graft due to OS [18, 19]. Currently, strategic procedures are required to improve liver tolerance against CIWR injury. Proactive strategies through pharmacological pretreatment to limit graft damage from CIWR injury have the advantage of excellent graft function after OLT.

A small-for-size graft (SFSG) is also an issue in deceased-donor liver transplantation (DDLT) and living-donor liver transplantation (LDLT). An SFSG is defined as a ratio of graft weight against standard liver volume <40% [20, 21]. An inevitable insufficiency of graft size cannot be avoided in LDLT or split orthotopic liver transplantation (SOLT) for DDLT. Shear stress not only triggers the liver regeneration cascade but also causes fatal damage in the SFSG by OS [22, 23]. An SFSG in LDLT or SOLT is accompanied by CIWR injury, as well as shear stress with portal hypertension. Therefore, SFSGs result in a higher mortality and morbidity after LDLT or SOLT. The choice of a left-side graft is preferred from the viewpoint of greater donor safety and expanded donor candidates in LDLT [20, 24]. Guaranteed SOLT with successful outcomes resolves a donor shortage in DDLT [24, 25]. Currently, the 40%-SFSG is a critical issue [24].

Our laboratory has focused on the effect of GABAR regulation on liver damage by using rodent models [26–28]. We failed to show beneficial effects in GABAR regulation *ex vivo* and in GABAR regulation by a specific antagonist [27, 28]. However, GABAR regulation *in vivo* by a specific agonist showed a subtle reduction in liver damage in a murine hepatectomy model involving shear stress with portal hypertension [27] and in a rat orthotopic liver transplantation model with a whole-liver graft involving CIWR injury [26]. Proactive strategies through pharmacological pretreatment to limit graft damage from CIWR injury and shear stress with portal hypertension have advantages for overcoming a current issue.

As a final goal of GABAR regulation in the liver, we investigated the strategic potential of graft pretreatment *in vivo* by a GABAR agonist in the rat SOLT model with a 40%-SFSG, and we examined the possible pathways involved.

## 2. Materials and Methods

*2.1. Animals.* Lewis rats (RT-$1^l$) were purchased from Harlan Laboratories, Inc. (Indianapolis, IN, USA). Graft donors and recipients were 8–12-week-old rats (approximately 250 g). The experimental protocols were approved by the Ethical Committee of our institution (Mayo Clinic, Institutional Animal Care and Use Committee, no. A19609). Rats were cared for in accordance with the institutional guidelines for Animal Welfare based on The National Institutes of Health Guide for the Care and Use of Laboratory Animals.

*2.2. Intravenous Injection of a GABAR Agonist.* A dose of 43.56 nmol/g body weight of GABAR agonist ($GABA_A$ receptor agonist, muscimol, 114.10 g/mol; 70015, Fluka, Sigma-Aldrich Co., St. Louis, MO, USA) was used [5]. Four hours before graft harvest, the donor rat intravenously received 1.0 mL of GABAR agonist into the penile vein.

*2.3. SOLT with 40%-SFSG and Postoperative Care.* Comprehensive details of the surgical procedures for rat SOLT and postoperative care in our institution have been previously described [29, 30]. Briefly, the syngeneic graft had a cold ischemic time of 2 h at 4°C in normal Ringer's solution. The liver graft was washed twice by 10 mL of normal Ringer's solution, immediately after the graft harvest and before graft implantation. The 40%-SFSG was made by the left median and lateral segments at the back table [29, 30]. To avoid any irrelevant signaling, the hepatic artery was reconstructed by ultramicrosurgery in this study [29, 30]. Each rat was housed separately after surgery, and body temperature was maintained by a heating pad. Postoperative observation was performed every 30 min until 6 h after SOLT, and 1.0 mL of warm lactate Ringer's solution was routinely administered every 1 h until 6 h after SOLT. In this model, we previously demonstrated the importance of a shortened anhepatic phase and exclusion of unreliable samples based on autopsy findings [29, 30]. In this study, the anhepatic phase was maintained within 20 min in each SOLT, and no surgical complications were observed in each case at autopsy.

*2.4. Study Design.* Recipient rats were divided into three groups according to donor treatments and the recipient's surgery as follows: (i) saline (normal saline, 1.0 mL, i.v.) and laparotomy, (ii) saline (normal saline, 1.0 mL, i.v.) and SOLT with 40%-SFSG, and (iii) GABAR agonist (muscimol, 43.56 nmol (4.98 $\mu$g)/g body weight, 1.0 mL, i.v.) and SOLT with 40%-SFSG.

First, a survival study was performed ($n = 10$ in each group). Cell signalings involving cell proliferation, differentiation, and apoptosis were investigated from the early postoperative period [18, 31–33], and subsequently, progressive necrosis was observed [18, 31–33]. Serum, plasma, and liver samples for histopathological/immunohistological assessment and western blotting analyses were then collected 6 h after SOLT ($n = 5$ in each group).

*2.5. Biochemical Assay and Coagulation Profile.* Aspartate aminotransferase (AST), alanine aminotransferase (ALT), and total bilirubin (T-Bil) levels, and the international normalized ratio of prothrombin time (PT-INR) were measured. Serum AST, ALT, and T-Bil levels were assessed (SGOT, SGPT, and total bilirubin reagent, respectively, Biotron, Hemet, CA, USA). The PT-INR in plasma was measured by the i-STAT System (Abbott, Princeton, NJ, USA).

*2.6. Histopathological and Immunohistological Assessments.* Liver tissue was fixed in 10% neutral-buffered formalin, embedded in paraffin, and sliced into 4 $\mu$m sections. Morphological characteristics and graft injury scores were assessed after hematoxylin-eosin (HE) staining. The graft damage score (points) has previously been described elsewhere [30, 34, 35]. Scores were counted in 10 fields (×100) in each slide, and then these scores were averaged.

Induction of apoptosis was assessed by immunostaining of terminal deoxynucleotidyl transferase-mediated deoxyuridine triphosphate nick-end labeling (TUNEL) (ApopTag Peroxidase *in situ* Apoptosis Detection Kit, S7100, Chemicon International, Inc., Billerica, MA, USA) and cysteine aspartic acid protease (caspase) 3 (cleaved caspase-3 (Asp175) antibody, 9661S, Cell Signaling Technology, Inc., Danvers, MA, USA). TUNEL-positive nuclei were stained brown, and negative nuclei were counterstained light blue. Caspase-3-positive nuclei were stained brown, and negative nuclei were counterstained blue. Slides were scanned with an automated high-throughput scanning system (Scanscope XT, Aperio Technologies, Inc., Vista, CA, USA). To quantify the immunohistological findings, positively stained nuclei were counted by Aperio Imagescope software (Aperio Technologies, Inc.). All nuclei were classified into four color intensity levels, and the higher two levels were considered as positive. The ratio of positively stained nuclei to all nuclei was calculated, and the mean ratio per $mm^2$ was determined.

*2.7. Western Blotting Analysis.* The primary antibodies for 4-hydroxynonenal (4-HNE) (4 hydroxynonenal antibody, ab46545, Abcam, Cambridge, MA, USA), ataxia-telangiectasia mutated kinase (ATM) (phospho-ATM/ATR substrate rabbit mAb, Cell Signaling Technology), phosphorylated histone H2AX (phospho-histone H2AX antibody, 2577, Cell Signaling Technology), phosphatidylinositol-3 kinase (PI3K) (phospho-PI3K p85/p55 antibody, 4228, Cell Signaling Technology), Akt (phospho-Akt rabbit mAb, 4058, Cell Signaling Technology), superoxide dismutase (SOD) 1 (Cu/Zn superoxide dismutase, LS-B2907, LifeSpan BioSciences, Seattle, WA, USA), SOD 2 (Mn superoxide dismutase, LS-C62194, LifeSpan BioSciences), and catalase (catalase, LS-B2554, LifeSpan BioSciences) were used. Liver samples were collected, homogenized, and centrifuged at high speed for 10 min at 4°C. The supernatant was then collected and used for bicinchoninic acid protein determination (BCA Protein Assay Reagent, Thermo Fisher Scientific, Rockford, IL, USA) and western blot analysis. Forty micrograms of protein were run on 4–20% Tris-glycine gels and transferred onto 0.45 $\mu$m nitrocellulose membranes. The membranes were then blocked with 5% nonfat milk made up in a Tris-buffered saline solution. After blocking, the membranes were incubated at 4°C overnight with the primary antibody. The next day, the membranes were washed three times for 10 min with Tris-buffered saline solution and then incubated with the peroxidase-conjugated secondary antibody for 1 h, with shaking at room temperature. After incubation, the membranes were once again washed three times for 10 min with Tris-buffered saline solution and then developed using chemiluminescence. Glyceraldehyde-3-phosphate dehydrogenase (GAPDH) served as a control. Signals were quantified by using ImageQuant 5.0 software (Molecular Dynamics, Sunnyvale, CA, USA).

*2.8. Statistical Analysis.* The results are presented as mean ± standard deviation. The Student's $t$-test was used for the comparison of unpaired continuous variables between groups. Survival curves were constructed by the Kaplan-Meier method (log-rank test). Statistical calculations were performed using SPSS Software Version 16.0 (SPSS Inc., Chicago, IL, USA). A $P$ value <0.05 was considered statistically significant.

## 3. Results

*3.1. Survival Curves.* Survival curves in each group are shown in Figure 1(a). SOLT with a 40%-SFSG clearly showed poorer survival than laparotomy ($P < 0.0001$), and graft pretreatment by GABAR agonist prolonged survival after SOLT ($P = 0.0369$).

*3.2. Parenchymal Damage in Grafts.* Inflammatory cell infiltration, vacuolization, hepatocyte ballooning, and necrosis were confirmed after SOLT with a 40%-SFSG. Actual histopathological findings in H-E staining are shown in each group in Figures 1(b)–1(d).

There were significant differences between laparotomy and SOLT with saline (0.0 ± 0.0 versus 5.8 ± 1.1 points, $P < 0.0001$) and between SOLT with saline and SOLT with GABAR agonist (5.8 ± 1.1 versus 4.1 ± 1.0 points; $P = 0.0280$) (Figure 1(e)).

*3.3. Biochemical and Coagulation Profiles.* There were significant differences in serum AST levels between laparotomy and SOLT with saline (45.4 ± 10.3 versus 387.4 ± 36.8 U/L; $P < 0.0001$) and between SOLT with saline and SOLT with GABAR agonist (387.4 ± 36.8 versus 296.0 ± 32.3 U/L; $P = 0.0031$) (Figure 2(a)).

There were significant differences in serum ALT levels between laparotomy and SOLT with saline (54.2 ± 9.2 versus 354.2 ± 32.1 U/L; $P < 0.0001$) and between SOLT with saline and SOLT with GABAR agonist (354.2 ± 32.1 versus 272.4 ± 31.3 U/L; $P = 0.0035$) (Figure 2(b)).

There were significant differences in serum T-Bil levels between laparotomy and SOLT with saline (0.28 ± 0.04 versus 1.37 ± 0.29 mg/dL; $P < 0.0001$) and between SOLT with saline and SOLT with GABAR agonist (1.37 ± 0.29 versus 1.02 ± 0.15 mg/dL; $P = 0.0453$) (Figure 2(c)).

There were significant differences in PT-INR between laparotomy and SOLT with saline (0.99 ± 0.04 versus

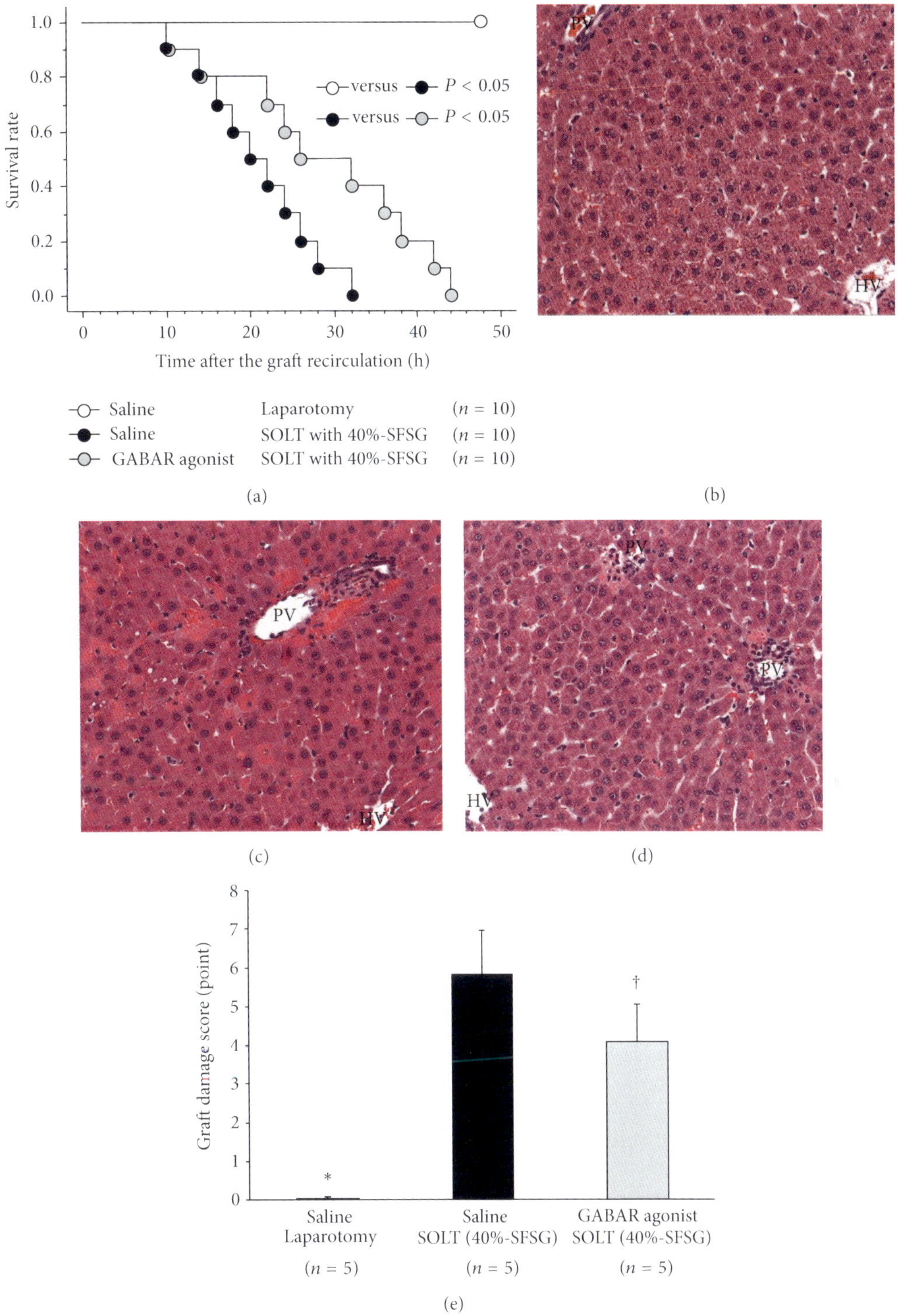


FIGURE 1: Survival curves, histopathological findings from HE staining, and graft damage scores. (a) Survival curves after SOLT with a 40%-SFSG. There were significant differences between laparotomy and SOLT with saline ($P < 0.05^{*}$) and between SOLT with saline and SOLT with GABAR agonist ($P < 0.05^{\dagger}$). (b) Laparotomy with saline: H-E, ×100. (c) SOLT with saline: H-E, ×100. (d) SOLT with GABAR agonist: H-E, ×100. (e) Graft damage score: There were significant differences between laparotomy and SOLT with saline ($P < 0.05^{*}$) and between SOLT with saline and SOLT with GABAR agonist ($P < 0.05^{\dagger}$). GABAR, γ-aminobutyric acid receptor; HE, hematoxylin-eosin; HV, hepatic vein; PV, portal vein; SFSG, small-for-size graft; and SOLT, split orthotopic liver transplantation.

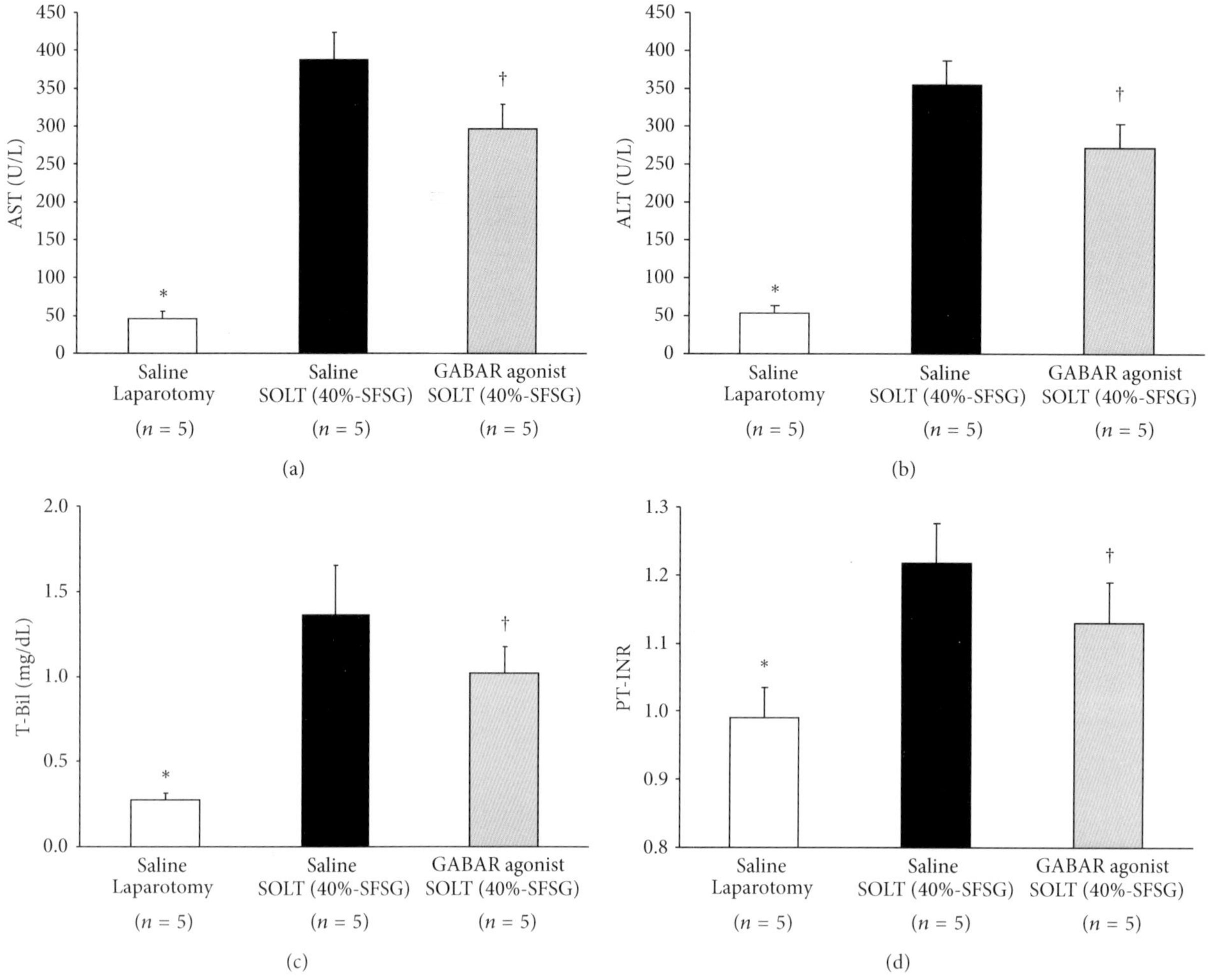


Figure 2: Biochemical and coagulation profiles. (a) AST levels. There were significant differences between laparotomy and SOLT with saline ($P < 0.05^*$) and between SOLT with saline and SOLT with GABAR agonist ($P < 0.05^\dagger$). (b) ALT levels. There were significant differences between laparotomy and SOLT with saline ($P < 0.05^*$) and between SOLT with saline and SOLT with GABAR agonist ($P < 0.05^\dagger$). (c) T-Bil levels. There were significant differences between laparotomy and SOLT with saline ($P < 0.05^*$) and between SOLT with saline and SOLT with GABAR agonist ($P < 0.05^\dagger$). (d) PT-INR. There were significant differences between laparotomy and SOLT with saline ($P < 0.05^*$) and between SOLT with saline and SOLT with GABAR agonist ($P < 0.05\dagger$). AST, aspartate aminotransferase; ALT, alanine aminotransferase; GABAR, $\gamma$-aminobutyric acid receptor; SFSG, small-for-size graft; SOLT, split orthotopic liver transplantation; PT-INR, international normalized ratio of prothrombin time; and T-Bil, total bilirubin.

$1.22 \pm 0.06$; $P = 0.0001$) and between SOLT with saline and SOLT with GABAR agonist ($1.22 \pm 0.06$ versus $1.13 \pm 0.06$; $P = 0.0456$) (Figure 2(d)).

*3.4. Apoptotic Induction.* TUNEL immunostaining in each group is shown in Figures 3(a)–3(c). The ratio of TUNEL-positive nuclei was significantly different between laparotomy and SOLT with saline ($0.001 \pm 0.002$ versus $0.166 \pm 0.052$; $P < 0.0001$) and between SOLT with saline and SOLT with GABAR agonist ($0.166 \pm 0.052$ versus $0.092 \pm 0.038$; $P = 0.0324$) (Figure 3(d)).

Caspase 3 immunostaining in each group is shown in Figures 4(a)–4(c). The ratio of caspase 3-positive nuclei was significantly different between laparotomy and SOLT with saline ($0.0001 \pm 0.0001$ versus $0.115 \pm 0.019$; $P < 0.0001$) and between SOLT with saline and SOLT with GABAR agonist ($0.115 \pm 0.019$ versus $0.080 \pm 0.024$; $P = 0.0347$) (Figure 4(d)).

*3.5. Lipoperoxidation.* Actual intensities of 4-HNE are shown in Figure 5(a). Normalized 4-HNE showed significant differences between laparotomy and SOLT with saline ($1.00 \pm 0.06$ versus $1.38 \pm 0.22$; $P = 0.0068$) and between SOLT with saline and SOLT with GABAR agonist ($1.38 \pm 0.22$ versus $1.05 \pm 0.15$; $P = 0.0276$) (Figure 5(b)).

*3.6. Response to and Repair of DNA Damage.* Actual intensities of ATM and H2AX in each group are shown in Figure 6(a).

Normalized ATM showed significant differences between laparotomy and SOLT with saline ($1.00 \pm 0.11$ versus $1.21 \pm 0.11$; $P = 0.0131$) and between SOLT with saline and SOLT with GABAR agonist ($1.21 \pm 0.11$ versus $0.90 \pm 0.28$; $P = 0.0477$) (Figure 6(b)).

Normalized H2AX showed significant differences between laparotomy and SOLT with saline ($1.00 \pm 0.10$ versus

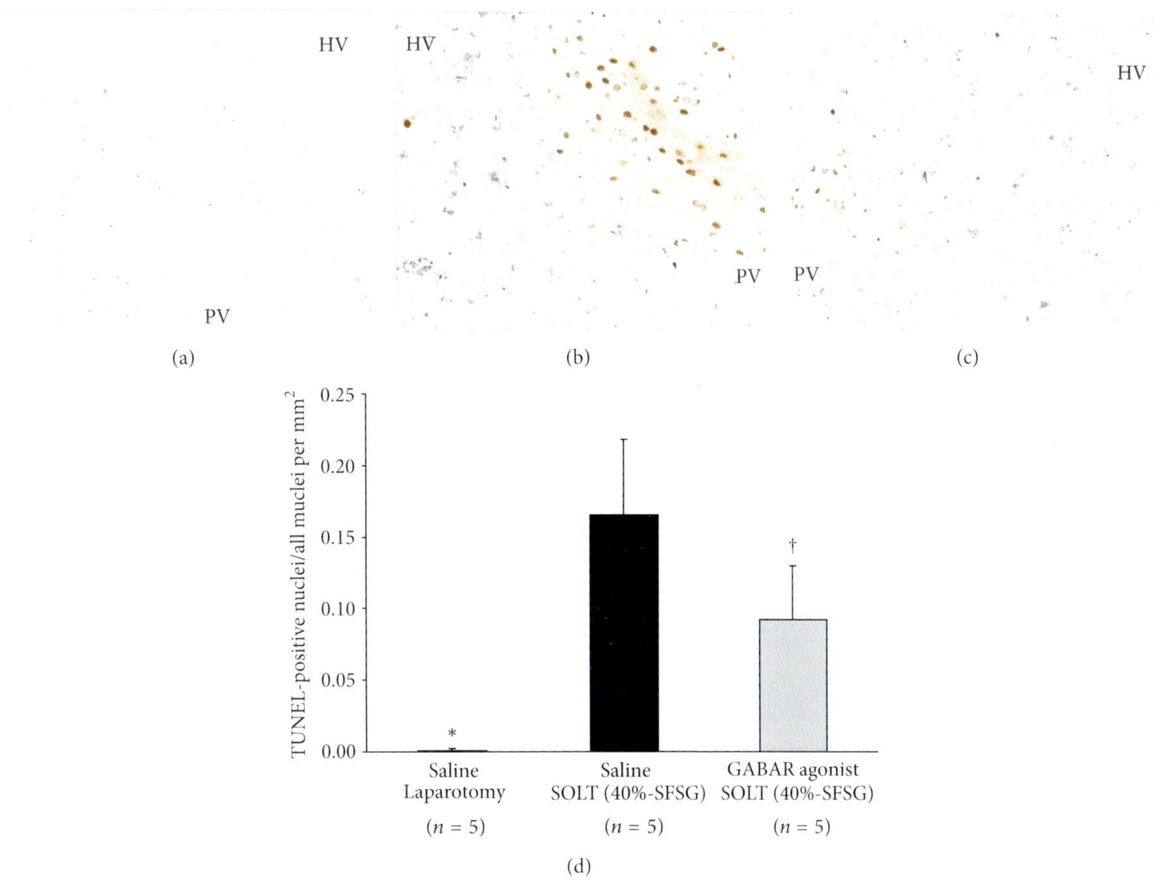


FIGURE 3: Immunohistological assessment by TUNEL. (a) Laparotomy with saline: TUNEL, ×100. (b) SOLT with saline: TUNEL, ×100. (c) SOLT with GABAR agonist: TUNEL, ×100. (d) Ratio of TUNEL-positive nuclei. There were significant differences between laparotomy and SOLT with saline ($P < 0.05^*$) and between SOLT with saline and SOLT with GABAR agonist ($P < 0.05^\dagger$). GABAR, γ-aminobutyric acid receptor; HV, hepatic vein; SFSG, small-for-size graft; SOLT, split orthotopic liver transplantation; PV, portal vein; and TUNEL, terminal deoxynucleotidyl transferase-mediated deoxyuridine triphosphate nick-end labeling.

2.59 ± 0.66; $P = 0.0007$) and between SOLT with saline and SOLT with GABAR agonist (2.59 ± 0.66 versus 0.83 ± 0.25; $P = 0.0005$) (Figure 6(c)).

*3.7. Promotion of Cell Survival.* Actual intensities of PI3K and Akt in each group are shown in Figure 7(a).

Normalized PI3K showed significant differences between laparotomy and SOLT with saline (1.00 ± 0.11 versus 0.59 ± 0.27; $P = 0.0139$) and between SOLT with saline and SOLT with GABAR agonist (0.59 ± 0.27 versus 0.92 ± 0.13; $P = 0.0443$) (Figure 7(b)).

Normalized Akt showed significant differences between laparotomy and SOLT with saline (1.00 ± 0.12 versus 0.34 ± 0.24; $P = 0.0006$) and between SOLT with saline and SOLT with GABAR agonist (0.34 ± 0.24 versus 1.11 ± 0.22; $P = 0.0007$) (Figure 7(c)).

*3.8. Activities of Antioxidant Enzymes.* Actual intensities of SOD 1, SOD 2, and catalase in each group are shown in Figure 8(a).

Normalized SOD 1 showed significant differences between laparotomy and SOLT with saline (1.00 ± 0.10 versus 0.81 ± 0.16; $P = 0.0445$) but not between SOLT with saline and SOLT with GABAR agonist (0.81 ± 0.16 versus 0.82 ± 0.12; $P = 0.8248$) (Figure 8(b)).

Normalized SOD 2 showed significant differences between laparotomy and SOLT with saline (1.00 ± 0.13 versus 0.79 ± 0.14; $P = 0.0361$) but not between SOLT with saline and SOLT with GABAR agonist (0.79 ± 0.14 versus 0.84 ± 0.15; $P = 0.5765$) (Figure 8(c)).

Normalized catalase showed no significant differences between laparotomy and SOLT with saline (1.00 ± 0.14 versus 0.95 ± 0.14; $P = 0.6904$) and between SOLT with saline and SOLT with GABAR agonist (0.95 ± 0.14 versus 0.96 ± 0.26; $P = 0.9764$) (Figure 8(d)).

## 4. Discussion

Based on the current situation in the clinical field, the 40%-SFSG needs to be investigated in detail because successful SOLT overcomes a donor shortage in DDLT, and the shift to a left-lobe graft provides donor safety in LDLT [20, 24, 30]. However, the 40%-SFSG is prone to ischemia/reperfusion injury and shear stress with portal hypertension, and therefore, the OS-induced damage after SOLT is more fatal [18, 36–38]. In our study, a survival study, biochemical assays,

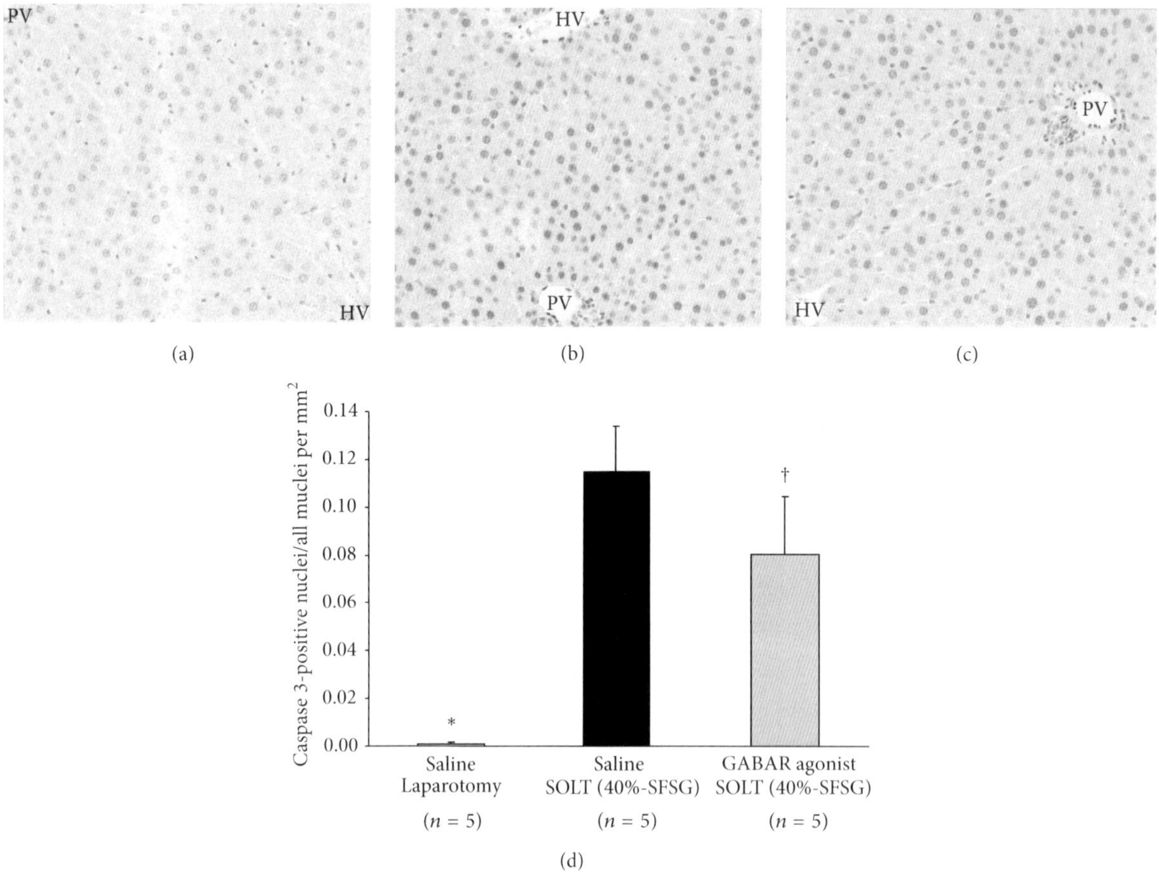


Figure 4: Immunohistological assessment by caspase 3. (a) Laparotomy with saline: caspase 3, ×100. (b) SOLT with saline: caspase 3, ×100. (c) SOLT with GABAR agonist: caspase 3, ×100. (d) The ratio of caspase 3-positive nuclei. There were significant differences between laparotomy and SOLT with saline ($P < 0.05^*$) and between SOLT with saline and SOLT with GABAR agonist ($P < 0.05^\dagger$). Caspase, cysteine aspartic acid protease; GABAR, $\gamma$-aminobutyric acid receptor; HV, hepatic vein; SFSG, small-for-size graft; SOLT, split orthotopic liver transplantation; and PV, portal vein.

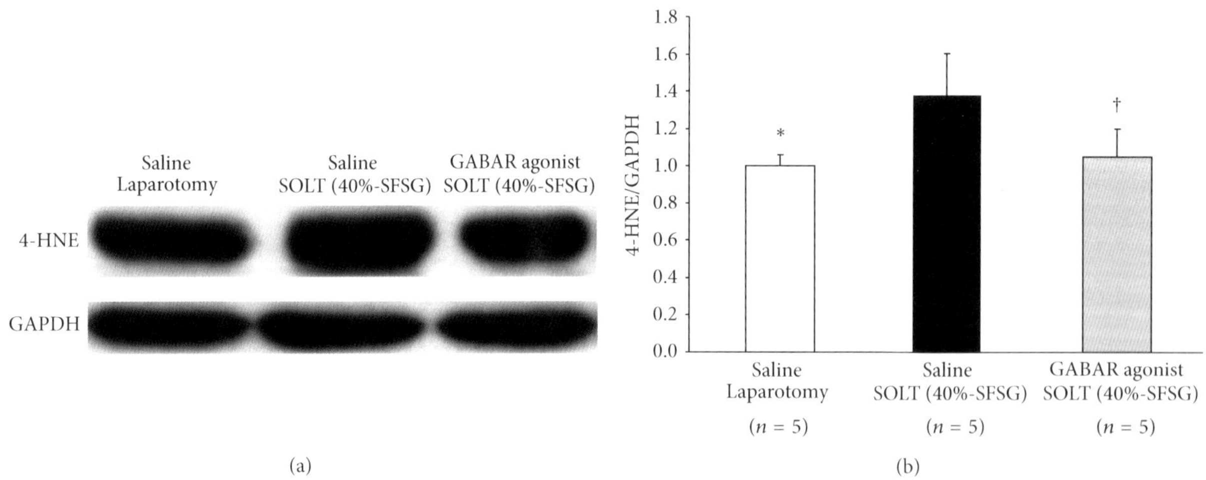


Figure 5: Western blot analysis of 4-HNE. (a) Intensities of 4-HNE and GAPDH. (b) Normalized 4-HNE. There were significant differences between laparotomy and SOLT with saline ($P < 0.05^*$) and between SOLT with saline and SOLT with GABAR agonist ($P < 0.05^\dagger$). 4-HNE, 4-hydroxynonenal; GABAR, $\gamma$-aminobutyric acid receptor; GAPDH, glyceraldehyde-3-phosphate dehydrogenase; SFSG, small-for-size graft; and SOLT, split orthotopic liver transplantation.

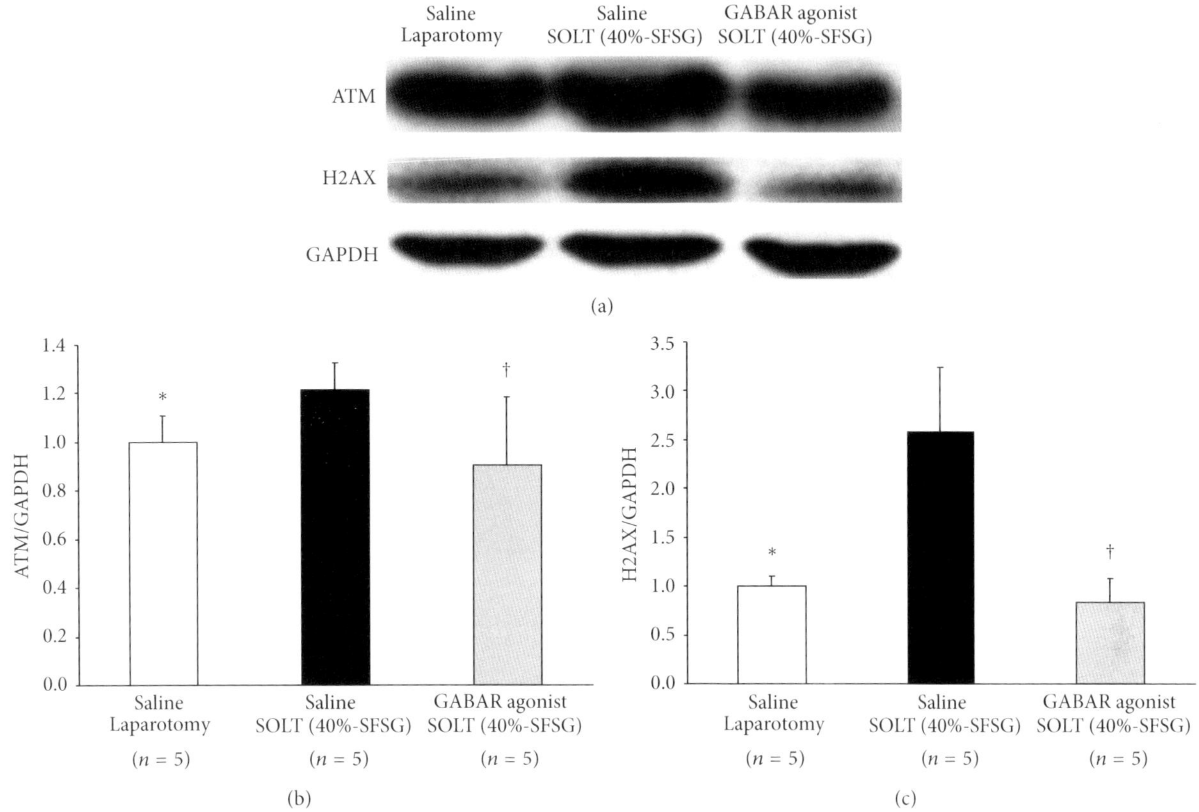


FIGURE 6: Western blot analyses of ATM and H2AX. (a) Intensities of ATM, H2AX, and GAPDH. (b) Normalized ATM. There were significant differences between laparotomy and SOLT with saline ($P < 0.05^*$) and between SOLT with saline and SOLT with GABAR agonist ($P < 0.05^\dagger$). (c) Normalized H2AX. There were significant differences between laparotomy and SOLT with saline ($P < 0.05^*$) and between SOLT with saline and SOLT with GABAR agonist ($P < 0.05^\dagger$). ATM, ataxia-telangiectasia mutated kinase; GABAR, γ-aminobutyric acid receptor; GAPDH, glyceraldehyde-3-phosphate dehydrogenase; SFSG, small-for-size graft; and SOLT, split orthotopic liver transplantation.

and histopathological assessment showed that the 40%-SFSG received the liver injury enough. OS causes DNA damage and subsequent apoptosis [1–3], and in our study, immunohistochemistry showed that SOLT induced apoptosis in the 40%-SFSG. ROS/RNS can attack and damage a variety of critical biological molecules [1–3], and the products of lipid peroxidation reliably and rapidly reflect sensitive and specific signals due to OS occurring *in vivo* [39, 40]. The fatty aldehyde 4-HNE is an end product of lipoperoxidation [39, 40]. Our results of 4-HNE showed that OS occurred after SOLT. Therefore, OS after SOLT with a 40%-SFSG resulted in apoptotic induction and subsequent necrosis.

OS mediated by free radicals is defined as an imbalance between the production of ROS/RNS and antioxidant capacity [1–3]. ROS/RNS have been suggested as a major contributing factor for DNA damage in the progression of OS. As a sensor of DNA damage responses, the protein kinase ATM can be initiated through rapid intermolecular autophosphorylation induced by DNA damage [12, 41]; it phosphorylates various proteins, and subsequently amplifies the responses to DNA damage [12]. This DNA damage-inducible kinase activates histone H2AX [5]. H2AX is required for cell cycle arrest and DNA repair following double-stranded DNA breaks [5, 42]. DNA damage results in the rapid phosphorylation of H2AX by ATM at sites of DNA damage [5, 43 45]. Our study showed that this response to and repair of DNA damage via ATM/H2AX was clearly triggered after SOLT with a 40%-SFSG and that this cascade is a possible pathway in the process of OS-induced injury after SOLT with SFSG. Our preliminary data in the rat OLT model with whole-liver grafts (i.e., a model for only CIWR injury) suggested that GABAR regulation by a specific agonist showed differences in ATM/H2AX [26]. We consider that GABAR regulation may have a beneficial effect against CIWR injury via the ATM/H2AX pathway in the liver.

From the viewpoint of the production of ROS/RNS in the process of OS, Akt also plays a critical role in controlling apoptosis [41, 46, 47] and promotes cell survival [47–50]. Apoptotic machinery is inhibited by the activation of Akt [46, 51, 52]. Akt is a component of the antiapoptotic process related to the activation of PI3K [14], and PI3K is upstream from Akt [47, 53]. The cell survival pathway via PI3K/Akt is also considered as an important signaling pathway to control apoptotic induction in the liver [54, 55]. Our study showed that this promotion of cell survival via PI3K/Akt was disturbed after SOLT with a 40%-SFSG and that this cascade could be one of the possible pathways in the process of OS-induced injury after SOLT with SFSG. Our preliminary

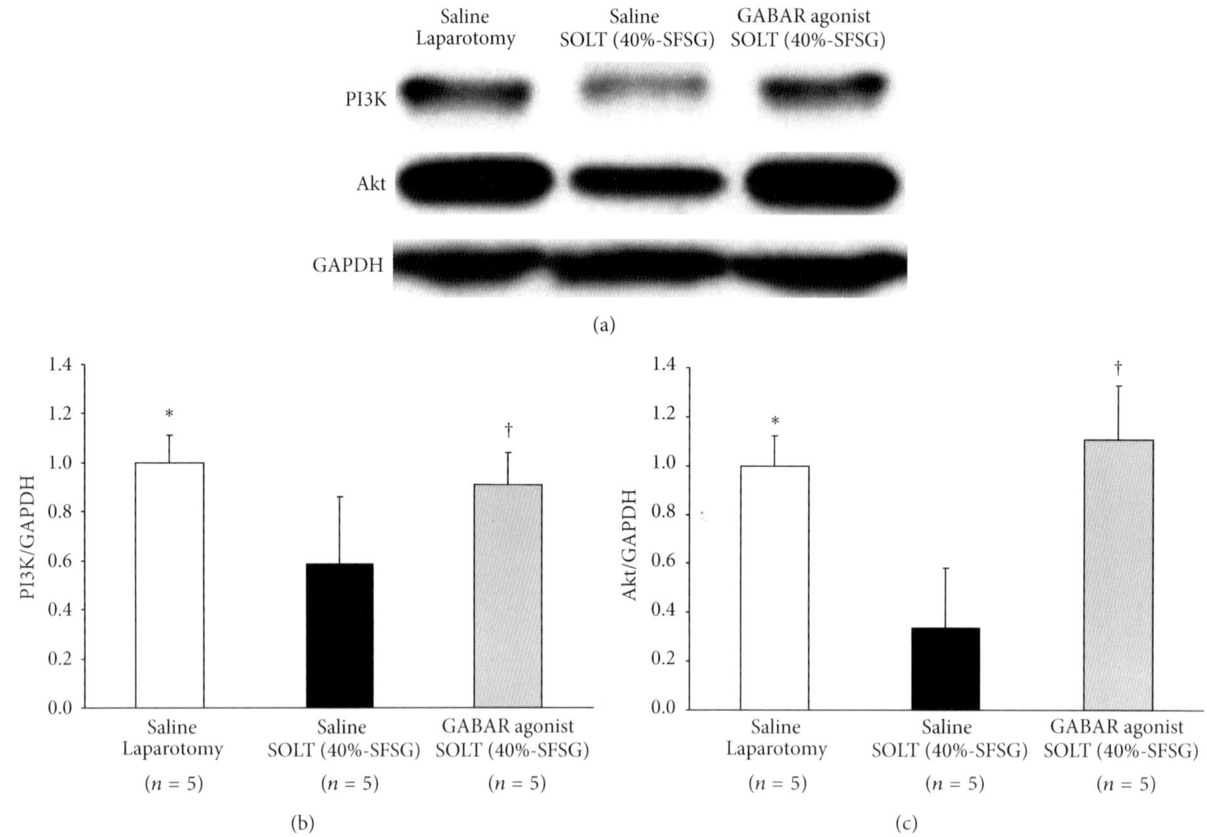


Figure 7: Western blot analyses of PI3K and Akt. (a) Intensities of PI3K. Akt, and GAPDH. (b) Normalized PI3K: There were significant differences between laparotomy and SOLT with saline ($P < 0.05^*$) and between SOLT with saline and SOLT with GABAR agonist ($P < 0.05^\dagger$). (c) Normalized Akt. There were significant differences between laparotomy and SOLT with saline ($P < 0.05^*$) and between SOLT with saline and SOLT with GABAR agonist ($P < 0.05^\dagger$). GABAR, $\gamma$-aminobutyric acid receptor; GAPDH, glyceraldehyde-3-phosphate dehydrogenase; PI3K, phosphatidylinositol-3 kinase; SFSG, small-for-size graft; and SOLT, split orthotopic liver transplantation.

data in the murine hepatectomy model (i.e., a model for only shear stress with portal hypertension) suggested that GABAR regulation by a specific agonist showed differences in PI3K/Akt [27]. Therefore, we consider that GABAR regulation may have a beneficial effect against shear stress with portal hypertension via the PI3K/Akt pathway in the liver.

From the viewpoint of antioxidant defenses, free radical scavenging enzymes, such as SOD and catalase, also play an important role in reducing DNA damage and subsequent apoptosis [2, 3, 56]. Normal cells are able to defend themselves against OS through this scavenging system [3, 56]. Our study showed a decrease in SOD 1 and SOD 2 levels after SOLT with a 40%-SFSG, although we initially expected that antioxidant enzymes would increase. Our results appear to be consistent with a previous opinion that OS impairs mitochondrial importing and processing of SOD [57]. However, another possible explanation for our results may be that this scavenging system failed, and some reactive molecules evaded the detoxification process and damaged potential targets because of drastic damage after SOLT with a 40%-SFSG, even though these scavenging enzymes can handle large amounts of ROS/RNS [58].

Our results of the survival study, histopathological assessment, and biochemical assays showed that pretreatment for SFSG by GABAR regulation *in vivo* affected graft damage after SOLT. Moreover, immunohistochemistry showed that this pretreatment reduced apoptotic induction after SOLT. In the field of brain research, the effect of GABAR regulation on the prevention of OS has been reported [5–7]. Although GABA was initially thought to be confined to the central nervous system, GABA is currently considered to be a multifunctional molecule with various physiological effects throughout the body [9, 10]. Although the liver contains GABA and hepatic GABAR [10, 17], the effects of GABAR regulation in the liver are unknown. Our study suggests that GABAR regulation may have a strategic potential for 40%-SFSGs as a pharmacological pretreatment for reducing OS-induced damage after SOLT, although SOLT with a 40%-SFSG involves fatal OS due to dual damage (i.e., CIWR injury and shear stress with portal hypertension).

Any pretreatment in a living donor violates ethical policy and spoils donor regulations. Whether GABAR regulation *ex vivo* (i.e., a procedure during organ storage) is more suitable for LDLT is unknown. Although our results showed the strategic potential of GABAR regulation *in vivo* as a pretreatment for liver grafts, we failed to confirm a positive effect of GABAR regulation *ex vivo* [28]. Therefore, some innovations are still required for clinical application.

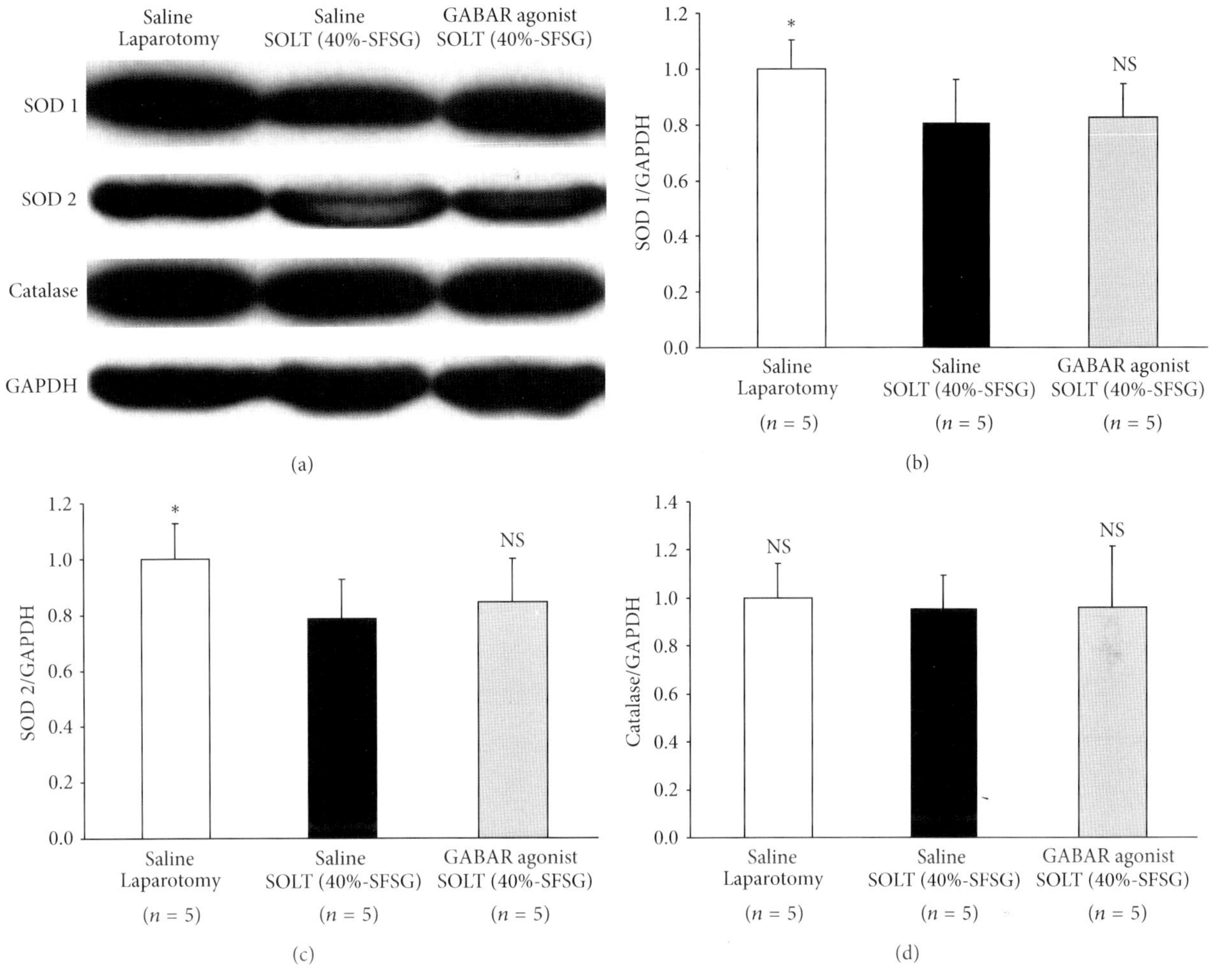


FIGURE 8: Western blot analyses of SOD 1, SOD 2, and catalase. (a) Intensities of SOD 1, SOD 2, catalase, and GAPDH. (b) Normalized SOD 1. There were significant differences between laparotomy and SOLT with saline ($P < 0.05^*$) but no differences between SOLT with saline and SOLT with GABAR agonist. (c) Normalized SOD 2. There were significant differences between laparotomy and SOLT with saline ($P < 0.05^*$) but no differences between SOLT with saline and SOLT with GABAR agonist. (d) Normalized catalase. There were no significant differences between laparotomy and SOLT with saline and between SOLT with saline and SOLT with GABAR agonist. GABAR, γ-aminobutyric acid receptor; GAPDH, glyceraldehyde-3-phosphate dehydrogenase; NS, not significant ($P \geq 0.05$); SFSG, small-for-size graft; SOD, superoxide dismutase; SOLT, split orthotopic liver transplantation.

In previous reports on the brain, many investigators have suggested that GABAR regulation by a specific agonist or antagonist affects the response to reduce OS-induced injury [5, 7, 8]. Their preventive effects in the brain have been mainly explained via specific pathways against OS (i.e., inhibition of the response to DNA damage [5, 11, 12] and promotion of cell survival [13, 14] or the free radical scavenging system [15, 16]). Many previous investigators have suggested that GABAR regulation in the brain has certain effects on the response to and repair of DNA damage via the ATM/H2AX pathway *in vivo* and *in vitro* in the process of OS [5, 11, 12]. Our study showed that the regulation of hepatic GABAR also appeared to reduce OS-induced DNA damage via the ATM/H2AX pathway as well as to have effects in the brain. With regard to the effects of GABAR regulation on OS in the brain, the PI3K/Akt pathway promotes cell survival against DNA damage [5, 13, 14, 46, 59]. Our study showed that regulation of hepatic GABAR appeared to promote cell survival via the PI3K/Akt pathway against OS-induced DNA damage as well as to have effects in the brain. However, antioxidant enzymes reduce OS-induced damage. From the viewpoint of this scavenging system, some researchers have shown that GABAR regulation in the brain has preventive effects against OS-induced damage via antioxidant enzymes [15, 16]. Although SOD 2 plays an important role in preventing DNA damage in the SFSG [36], our results suggested that the effects of the regulation of hepatic GABAR against OS did not depend on this scavenging system. Overall, we speculate that the regulation of hepatic GABAR has a preventive effect against OS, by reducing DNA damage via the ATM/H2AX pathway and by promoting cell survival via the PI3K/Akt pathway. However, antioxidant enzymes might be important for GABAR regulation in the brain [15, 16].

## 5. Conclusion

In conclusion, regulation of GABAR by a specific agonist *in vivo* works well in the liver, as well as the brain. Even though CIWR injury and shear stress with portal hypertension affect 40%-SFSGs after SOLT and results in fatal OS, graft pretreatment *in vivo* by GABAR regulation clearly improves graft damage after SOLT. This strategy may be advantageous for overcoming current issues in the DDLT and LDLT fields. The effects of GABAR regulation on graft damage after SOLT with a 40%-SFSG appear to prevent OS by reducing DNA damage via the ATM/H2AX pathway and by promoting cell survival via the PI3K/Akt pathway.

## Acknowledgments

This work was partially supported by Grants to J. H. Nguyen from the Deason Foundation, Sandra and Eugene Davenport, Mayo Clinic CD CRT-II, and from the National Institutes of Health (R01NS051646-01A2) and a Grant to T. Hori from the Uehara Memorial Foundation (no. 200940051, Tokyo, Japan). The authors are grateful to Dickson W. Dennis, Monica Castanedes-Casey, Virginia R. Phillips, Linda G. Rousseau, and Melissa E. Murray (Department of Neuroscience, Mayo Clinic Florida, Jacksonville, FL, USA) for their diagnostic and technical support in the histopathological and immunohistological assessments.

## References

[1] D. A. Castroviejo, L. C. Lopez, G. Escames, A. Lopez, J. A. Garcia, and R. J. Reiter, "Melatonin-mitochondria interplay in health and disease," *Current Topics in Medicinal Chemistry*, vol. 11, pp. 221–240, 2011.

[2] N. Ghosh, R. Ghosh, and S. C. Mandal, "Antioxidant protection: a promising therapeutic intervention in neurodegenerative disease," *Free Radical Research*, vol. 45, no. 8, pp. 888–905, 2011.

[3] B. Turan, "Role of antioxidants in redox regulation of diabetic cardiovascular complications," *Current Pharmaceutical Biotechnology*, vol. 11, no. 8, pp. 819–836, 2010.

[4] M. E. Pamenter, D. W. Hogg, J. Ormond, D. S. Shin, M. A. Woodin, and L. T. Buck, "Endogenous $GABA_A$ and $GABA_B$ receptor-mediated electrical suppression is critical to neuronal anoxia tolerance," *Proceedings of the National Academy of Sciences of the United States of America*, vol. 108, no. 27, pp. 11274–11279, 2011.

[5] M. Andäng, J. Hjerling-Leffler, A. Moliner et al., "Histone H2AX-dependent $GABA_A$ receptor regulation of stem cell proliferation," *Nature*, vol. 451, no. 7177, pp. 460–464, 2008.

[6] J. M. Ferreira, A. L. Burnett, and G. A. Rameau, "Activity-dependent regulation of surface glucose transporter-3," *The Journal of Neuroscience*, vol. 31, no. 6, pp. 1991–1999, 2011.

[7] Y. Hirooka, T. Kishi, K. Sakai, A. Takeshita, and K. Sunagawa, "Imbalance of central nitric oxide and reactive oxygen species in the regulation of sympathetic activity and neural mechanisms of hypertension," *American Journal of Physiology—Regulatory Integrative and Comparative Physiology*, vol. 300, no. 4, pp. R818–R826, 2011.

[8] S. Kurt, J. M. Crook, F. W. Ohl, H. Scheich, and H. Schulze, "Differential effects of iontophoretic *in vivo* application of the GABA A-antagonists bicuculline and gabazine in sensory cortex," *Hearing Research*, vol. 212, no. 1-2, pp. 224–235, 2006.

[9] Y. Gong, M. Zhang, L. Cui, and G. Y. Minuk, "Sequence and chromosomal assignment of a human novel cDNA: similarity to gamma-aminobutyric acid transporter," *Canadian Journal of Physiology and Pharmacology*, vol. 79, no. 12, pp. 977–984, 2001.

[10] T. Norikura, A. Kojima-Yuasa, D. O. Kennedy, and I. Matsui-Yuasa, "Protective effect of gamma-aminobutyric acid (GABA) against cytotoxicity of ethanol in isolated rat hepatocytes involves modulations in cellular polyamine levels," *Amino Acids*, vol. 32, no. 3, pp. 419–423, 2007.

[11] R. N. Fernando, B. Eleuteri, S. Abdelhady, A. Nussenzweig, M. Andäng, and P. Ernfors, "Cell cycle restriction by histone H2AX limits proliferation of adult neural stem cells," *Proceedings of the National Academy of Sciences of the United States of America*, vol. 108, no. 14, pp. 5837–5842, 2011.

[12] C. E. Irarrazabal, J. C. Liu, M. S. Burg, and J. D. Ferraris, "ATM, a DNA damage-inducible kinase, contributes to activation by high NaCl of the transcription factor TonEBP/OREBP," *Proceedings of the National Academy of Sciences of the United States of America*, vol. 101, no. 23, pp. 8809–8814, 2004.

[13] J. Xu, C. Li, X. Yin, and G. Zhang, "Additive neuroprotection of GABA A and GABA B receptor agonists in cerebral ischemic injury via PI-3K/Akt pathway inhibiting the ASK1-JNK cascade," *Neuropharmacology*, vol. 54, no. 7, pp. 1029–1040, 2008.

[14] J. E. Lee, J. S. Kang, Y. Ki et al., "Akt/GSK3$\beta$ signaling is involved in fipronil-induced apoptotic cell death of human neuroblastoma SH-SY5Y cells," *Toxicology Letters*, vol. 202, no. 2, pp. 133–141, 2011.

[15] S. Tejada, C. Roca, A. Sureda, R. V. Rial, A. Gamundí, and S. Esteban, "Antioxidant response analysis in the brain after pilocarpine treatments," *Brain Research Bulletin*, vol. 69, no. 5, pp. 587–592, 2006.

[16] J. Zhou, Y. Li, G. Yan et al., "Protective role of taurine against morphine-induced neurotoxicity in C6 cells via inhibition of oxidative stress," *Neurotoxicity Research*, vol. 20, no. 4, pp. 334–342, 2011.

[17] M. P. Biju, S. Pyroja, N. V. Rajeshkumar, and C. S. Paulose, "Hepatic $GABA_A$ receptor functional regulation during rat liver cell proliferation," *Hepatology Research*, vol. 21, no. 2, pp. 136–146, 2001.

[18] J. Lemasters, H. Bunzendahl, and R. Thurman, "Preservation of the liver," in *Transplantation of the Liver*, W. Maddrey and M. Sorrell, Eds., pp. 297–321, Appleton & Lange, East Norwalk, Conn, USA, 2nd edition, 1995.

[19] H. B. Abdennebi, M. A. Zaoualí, I. Alfany-Fernandez, D. Tabka, and J. Roselló-Catafau, "How to protect liver graft with nitric oxide," *World Journal of Gastroenterology*, vol. 17, no. 24, pp. 2879–2889, 2011.

[20] Y. Ogura, T. Hori, W. M. El Moghazy et al., "Portal pressure <15 mm Hg is a key for successful adult living donor liver transplantation utilizing smaller grafts than before," *Liver Transplantation*, vol. 16, no. 6, pp. 718–728, 2010.

[21] F. Wang, K. Pan, S. Chu et al., "Preoperative estimation of the liver graft weight in adult right lobe living donor liver transplantation using maximal portal vein diameters," *Liver Transplantation*, vol. 17, no. 4, pp. 373–380, 2011.

[22] S. He, C. Atkinson, F. Qiao, K. Cianflone, X. Chen, and S. Tomlinson, "A complement-dependent balance between hepatic ischemia/reperfusion injury and liver regeneration in mice," *Journal of Clinical Investigation*, vol. 119, no. 8, pp. 2304–2316, 2009.

[23] J. Wu, Q. Tang, J. Shen et al., "Comparative proteome profile during the early period of small-for-size liver transplantation in rats revealed the protective role of Prdx5," *Journal of Hepatology*, vol. 53, no. 1, pp. 73–83, 2010.

[24] T. Hori, S. Uemoto, L. B. Gardner, L. Sibulesky, Y. Ogura, and J. H. Nguyen, "Left-sided grafts for living-donor liver transplantation and split grafts for deceased-donor liver transplantation: their impact on long-term survival," *Clinics and Research in Hepatology and Gastroenterology*, vol. 36, no. 1, pp. 47–52, 2012.

[25] R. W. Busuttil and J. A. Goss, "Split liver transplantation," *Annals of Surgery*, vol. 229, no. 3, pp. 313–321, 1999.

[26] T. Hori, L. B. Gardner, T. Hata et al., "Pretreatment of liver grafts *in vivo* by γ-aminobutyric acid receptor regulation reduces cold ischemia/warm reperfusion injury in rat," *Annals of Transplantation*, vol. 18, pp. 299–313, 2013.

[27] L. B. Gardner, T. Hori, F. Chen et al., "Effect of specific activation of γ-aminobutyric acid receptor *in vivo* on oxidative stress-induced damage after extended hepatectomy," *Hepatology Research*, vol. 42, pp. 1131–1140, 2012.

[28] T. Hori, L. B. Gardner, F. Chen et al., "Liver graft pretreated *in vivo* or *ex vivo* by γ-aminobutyric acid receptor regulation," *Journal of Surgical Research*, vol. 182, pp. 166–175, 2013.

[29] T. Hori, J. H. Nguyen, X. Zhao et al., "Comprehensive and innovative techniques for liver transplantation in rats: a surgical guide," *World Journal of Gastroenterology*, vol. 16, no. 25, pp. 3120–3132, 2010.

[30] T. Hori, S. Uemoto, X. Zhao et al., "Surgical guide including innovative techniques for orthotopic liver transplantation in the rat: key techniques and pitfalls in whole and split liver grafts," *Annals of Gastroenterology*, vol. 23, no. 4, pp. 270–295, 2010.

[31] S. Padrissa-Altés, M. A. Zaouali, R. Franco-Gou et al., "Matrix metalloproteinase 2 in reduced-size liver transplantation: beyond the matrix," *American Journal of Transplantation*, vol. 10, no. 5, pp. 1167–1177, 2010.

[32] Z. Y. Ma, J. M. Qian, X. H. Rui et al., "Inhibition of matrix metalloproteinase-9 attenuates acute small-for-size liver graft injury in rats," *American Journal of Transplantation*, vol. 10, no. 4, pp. 784–795, 2010.

[33] V. Defamie, M. Laurens, D. Patrono et al., "Matrix metalloproteinase inhibition protects rat livers from prolonged cold ischemia-warm reperfusion injury," *Hepatology*, vol. 47, no. 1, pp. 177–185, 2008.

[34] T. Iida, S. Yagi, K. Taniguchi et al., "Significance of CT attenuation value in liver grafts following right lobe living-donor liver transplantation," *American Journal of Transplantation*, vol. 5, no. 5, pp. 1076–1084, 2005.

[35] T. Hori, T. Iida, S. Yagi et al., "KICGvalue, a reliable real-time estimator of graft function, accurately predicts outcomes in adult living-donor liver transplantation," *Liver Transplantation*, vol. 12, no. 4, pp. 605–613, 2006.

[36] H. Rehman, H. D. Connor, V. K. Ramshesh et al., "Ischemic preconditioning prevents free radical production and mitochondrial depolarization in small-for-size rat liver grafts," *Transplantation*, vol. 85, no. 9, pp. 1322–1331, 2008.

[37] Z. Zhong, H. D. Connor, M. Froh et al., "Free radical-dependent dysfunction of small-for-size rat liver grafts: prevention by plant polyphenols," *Gastroenterology*, vol. 129, no. 2, pp. 652–664, 2005.

[38] K. Man, S. Fan, C. Lo et al., "Graft injury in relation to graft size in right lobe live donor liver transplantation: a study of hepatic sinusoidal injury in correlation with portal hemodynamics and intragraft gene expression," *Annals of Surgery*, vol. 237, no. 2, pp. 256–264, 2003.

[39] Y. C. Awasthi, R. Sharma, A. Sharma et al., "Self-regulatory role of 4-hydroxynonenal in signaling for stress-induced programmed cell death," *Free Radical Biology and Medicine*, vol. 45, no. 2, pp. 111–118, 2008.

[40] G. Voulgaridou, I. Anestopoulos, R. Franco, M. I. Panayiotidis, and A. Pappa, "DNA damage induced by endogenous aldehydes: current state of knowledge," *Mutation Research*, vol. 711, no. 1-2, pp. 13–27, 2011.

[41] J. Kim and P. K. Y. Wong, "Loss of ATM impairs proliferation of neural stem cells through oxidative stress-mediated p38 MAPK signaling," *Stem Cells*, vol. 27, no. 8, pp. 1987–1998, 2009.

[42] J. Yuan, R. Adamski, and J. Chen, "Focus on histone variant H2AX: to be or not to be," *FEBS Letters*, vol. 584, no. 17, pp. 3717–3724, 2010.

[43] E. P. Rogakou, D. R. Pilch, A. H. Orr, V. S. Ivanova, and W. M. Bonner, "DNA double-stranded breaks induce histone H2AX phosphorylation on serine 139," *The Journal of Biological Chemistry*, vol. 273, no. 10, pp. 5858–5868, 1998.

[44] S. Burma, B. P. Chen, M. Murphy, A. Kurimasa, and D. J. Chen, "ATM phosphorylates histone H2AX in response to DNA Double-strand breaks," *The Journal of Biological Chemistry*, vol. 276, no. 45, pp. 42462–42467, 2001.

[45] E. P. Rogakou, C. Boon, C. Redon, and W. M. Bonner, "Megabase chromatin domains involved in DNA double-strand breaks *in vivo*," *Journal of Cell Biology*, vol. 146, no. 5, pp. 905–916, 1999.

[46] S. Maruyama, R. Shibata, K. Ohashi et al., "Adiponectin ameliorates doxorubicin-induced cardiotoxicity through Akt protein-dependent mechanism," *The Journal of Biological Chemistry*, vol. 286, no. 37, pp. 32790–32800, 2011.

[47] Y. Sánchez, D. Amrán, E. de Blas, and P. Aller, "Regulation of genistein induced differentiation in human acute myeloid leukaemia cells (HL60, NB4). Protein kinase modulation and reactive oxygen species generation," *Biochemical Pharmacology*, vol. 77, no. 3, pp. 384–396, 2009.

[48] T. F. Franke, D. R. Kaplan, and L. C. Cantley, "PI3K: downstream AKTion blocks apoptosis," *Cell*, vol. 88, no. 4, pp. 435–437, 1997.

[49] B. M. Burgering and P. J. Coffer, "Protein kinase B (c-Akt) in phosphatidylinositol-3-OH kinase signal transduction," *Nature*, vol. 376, no. 6541, pp. 599–602, 1995.

[50] T. F. Franke, S.-I. Yang, T. O. Chan et al., "The protein kinase encoded by the Akt proto-oncogene is a target of the PDGF-activated phosphatidylinositol 3-kinase," *Cell*, vol. 81, no. 5, pp. 727–736, 1995.

[51] D. Kim and J. Chung, "Akt: versatile mediator of cell survival and beyond," *Journal of Biochemistry and Molecular Biology*, vol. 35, no. 1, pp. 106–115, 2002.

[52] S. R. Datta, H. Dudek, T. Xu et al., "Akt phosphorylation of BAD couples survival signals to the cell-intrinsic death machinery," *Cell*, vol. 91, no. 2, pp. 231–241, 1997.

[53] A. Khalil, R. N. Morgan, B. R. Adams et al., "ATM-dependent ERK signaling via AKT in response to DNA double-strand breaks," *Cell Cycle*, vol. 10, no. 3, pp. 481–491, 2011.

[54] C. Dal Ponte, E. Alchera, A. Follenzi et al., "Pharmacological postconditioning protects against hepatic ischemia/reperfusion injury," *Liver Transplantation*, vol. 17, no. 4, pp. 474–482, 2011.

[55] S. Haga, M. Ozaki, H. Inoue et al., "The survival pathways phosphatidylinositol-3 kinase (PI3-K)/phosphoinositide-dependent protein kinase 1 (PDK1)/Akt modulate liver regeneration through hepatocyte size rather than proliferation," *Hepatology*, vol. 49, no. 1, pp. 204–214, 2009.

[56] D. S. A. Majid and L. Kopkan, "Nitric oxide and superoxide interactions in the kidney and their implication in the development of salt-sensitive hypertension," *Clinical and Experimental Pharmacology and Physiology*, vol. 34, no. 9, pp. 946–952, 2007.

[57] G. Wright, V. Reichenbecher, T. Green, G. L. Wright, and S. Wang, "Paraquat inhibits the processing of human manganese-dependent superoxide dismutase by Sf-9 insect cell mitochondria," *Experimental Cell Research*, vol. 234, no. 1, pp. 78–84, 1997.

[58] N. Maulik and D. K. Das, "Emerging potential of thioredoxin and thioredoxin interacting proteins in various disease conditions," *Biochimica et Biophysica Acta*, vol. 1780, pp. 1368–1382, 2008.

[59] T. Cesetti, T. Fila, K. Obernier et al., "$GABA_A$ receptor signaling induces osmotic swelling and cell cycle activation of neonatal prominin+precursors," *Stem Cells*, vol. 29, no. 2, pp. 307–319, 2011.

# 12

# *E. coli* Induced Experimental Model of Primary Biliary Cirrhosis

**Andreas L. Koutsoumpas,[1] Daniel S. Smyk,[2] and Dimitrios P. Bogdanos[1,2,3]**

[1]*Division of Medicine, School of Health Sciences, University of Thessaly, Thessaly, Viopolis, 40500 Larissa, Greece*
[2]*Institute of Liver Studies, King's College London School of Medicine at King's College Hospital, Denmark Hill Campus, London SE5 9RS, UK*
[3]*Cellular Immunotherapy and Molecular Immunodiagnostics, Biomedical Section, Institute of Research and Technology-Thessaly (IRETETH), 41222 Larissa, Greece*

Correspondence should be addressed to Dimitrios P. Bogdanos; dimitrios.bogdanos@yahoo.com

Academic Editor: Pierluigi Toniutto

Recurrent urinary tract infections (UTI) have been considered potential triggers of primary biliary cirrhosis (PBC), an autoimmune cholestatic liver disease characterised by progressive destruction of intrahepatic bile ducts. Additional support for the link made between PBC and UTI was based on early observations of recurrent episodes of bacteriuria in female patients with PBC. A series of large epidemiological studies demonstrated a strong correlation between recurrent UTI and PBC, initiating a series of studies investigating the role of *Escherichia coli* (*E. coli*, the most prevalent organism isolated in women with UTI) as a trigger of PBC. Immunological evidence of B- and T-cell cross-reactive responses implicating PBC-specific autoantigens and *E. coli* mimics have been clearly demonstrated, adding support to the notion that *E. coli* is a potential infectious inducer of PBC in susceptible individuals. One of the major limitations in proving the *E. coli*/PBC association was the lack of reliable *E. coli*-infected animal models of PBC. This review provides an overview of the evidence linking this infectious agent with PBC and discusses the pros and cons of a recently developed *E. coli*-infected animal model of PBC.

## 1. Introduction

Primary biliary cirrhosis (PBC) is an autoimmune cholestatic liver disease characterized by high-titre antimitochondrial antibodies (AMA), as well as disease-specific antinuclear antibodies (ANA) [1, 2]. The presence of AMA is considered pathognomonic for PBC, as serum AMA positivity predicts disease development in asymptomatic individuals [3]. The natural course of PBC is generally slow, although the disease course is unpredictable. Over the years, the progression of the disease leads to the inflammatory destruction of small intrahepatic bile ducts, which progresses to fibrosis, cirrhosis, and eventual liver failure [1].

As the disease overwhelmingly affects middle-aged females frequently complaining from recurrent urinary tract infections (UTI), *Escherichia coli* (*E. coli*) has been postulated as a potential trigger for the development of the disease [4, 5]. Epidemiological, immunological, and microbiological data have provided strong evidence in support of the pathogenic link between this bacterium and the disease [6–18]. These data are comprehensively discussed elsewhere and will not be mentioned in the present report.

AMA are directed against components of the 2-oxoacid dehydrogenase complexes, which mainly recognise the E2 subunit of the pyruvate dehydrogenase complex (PDC) in 90% of cases [2, 19]. In 20–70% of cases, the E2 subunits of branched-chain 2-oxoacid dehydrogenase complex (BCOADC) and 2-oxoglutarate dehydrogenase complex (OGDC) are also targeted, while the E1$\alpha$ and E1$\beta$ subunits of PDC have been identified as subdominant autoantigenic targets [2, 19]. Anti-PDC-E2 antibodies cross-reactively recognize PDC-E3 binding protein (PDC-E3BP), formerly known as PDC-X [2, 19].

The exact mechanisms that lead to the loss of immunological tolerance to mitochondrial autoantigens (such as PDC-E2) are unclear [20–22]. Nevertheless, specific infectious agents including *E. coli* (the most frequent pathogen

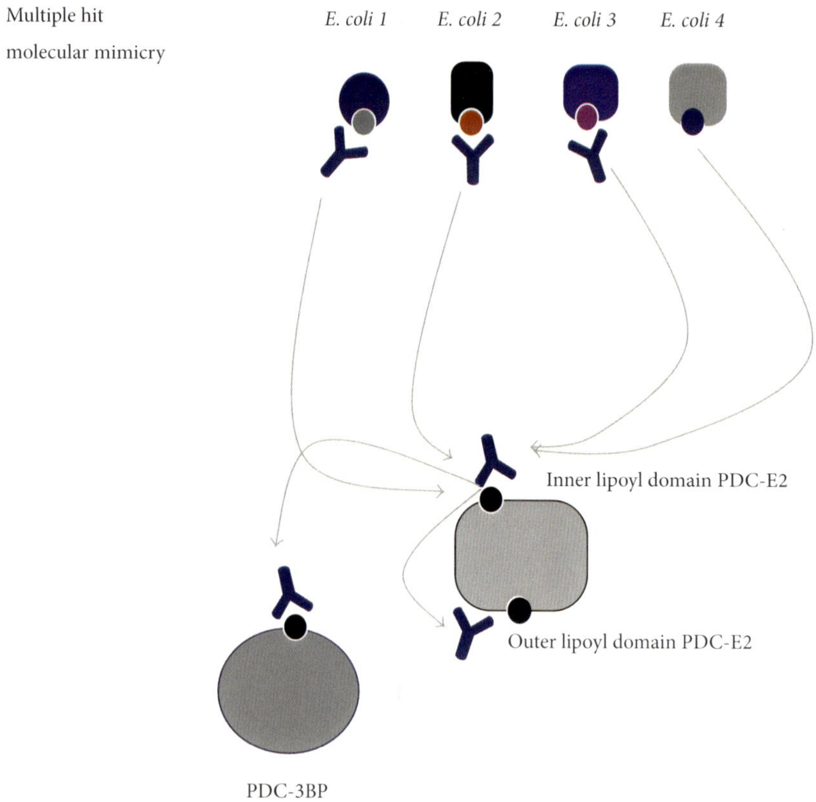


FIGURE 1: A microbial/self-multiple hit mechanism of molecular mimicry including several primary biliary cirrhosis- (PBC-) specific autoepitopes and their *E. coli* mimics (numbered 1–4 corresponding to those with reactivity depicted in Table 2) is likely involved in the induction of antimitochondrial antibody (AMA) responses in PBC. We propose that a multiple hit mechanism of intra- and intermolecular mimicry is operated at the B-cell level. This mechanism involves several mimics from various *E. coli* proteins which share a high degree of homology with the major mitochondrial autoepitope located at the inner lipoyl domain of the pyruvate dehydrogenase complex E2 subunit (PDC-E2). Urinary tract infections initiate an immune response against the *E. coli* mimics which in turn cross-react with the human mitochondrial autoantigens (arrows). Autoantibody responses against the human ILD PDC-E2 autoepitope initiate cross-reactive response to the mimicking sequences of the outer lipoyl domain of PDC-E2 and its mimic on the E3 binding protein (E3BP) of PDC (arrows). This multiple hit intra- (between the inner and the outer lipoyl domain of the same protein) and inter- (between different self-proteins and microbial proteins) mechanism of molecular mimicry may explain several specificities of the multiantigen specificities seen in PBC, as well as in other autoimmune diseases.

for recurrent urinary tract infection in women), as well as *Novosphingobium aromaticivorans* [23] and *Lactobacillus delbrueckii*, have been considered the most significant infectious triggers, but these have been studied more extensively. The mechanism of molecular mimicry and cross-reactivity involving *E. coli* and human PDC-E2 epitopes (or other mitochondrial antigens) has been considered the most likely trigger of the initiation of *E. coli*-associated antimitochondrial immune responses (Figure 1) [24, 25]. In fact, strong evidence regarding CD4 T-cell cross-recognition of *E. coli* and human mitochondrial autoantigens has been obtained over the years, further supporting the concept of molecular mimicry as the driving force of the immunological breakdown characteristic of PBC. An overview of the evidence provided thus far on immunological studies investigating the role of molecular mimicry is given below.

As for other diseases, external support of the pathogenic association between *E. coli* and PBC could stem from studies on animal models of PBC based on *E. coli*-infected mice (Table 1). These long awaited animal models of PBC have now been developed, and the present review discusses the major features of these mice and their relevance to the human disease [26].

## 2. *E. coli*, Molecular Mimicry, and PBC

Anti-PDC-E2 antibody positive PBC cases recognise *E. coli* PDC-E2, but this reactivity is 100-fold lower compared to that against mammalian PDC-E2 [27]. This is also the case for cross-recognition of OGDC-E2, another OADC-E2 subunit [28]. At the B-cell epitope level, antibodies against PDC-$E2_{212-226}$, which is the core antibody autoepitopic region of human PDC-E2, do not appear to cross-react with the corresponding PDC-E2 sequences of *E. coli*. Our group has proposed that the lack of humoral cross-reactivity may be due to differences between human and *E. coli* PDC-E2 on the structural level, which make antigenic cross-recognition impossible. Our hypothesis was a valid one, as

Table 1: Immunological and histological features of patients with primary biliary cirrhosis (PBC) and PBC-resembling experimental *E. coli*-infected NOD.B6 Idd10/Idd18 mice.

| | PBC | *E. coli*-infected NOD.B6 Idd10/Idd18 mice |
|---|---|---|
| Immunological features | | |
| **AMA** | Yes | Yes |
| Anti-PDC-E2 | Yes | Yes |
| Anti-OGDC-E2 | Yes | Yes |
| Anti-BCOADC-E2 | Yes | No |
| **ANA** | Yes | Not tested |
| Histology | | |
| Portal infiltration | Yes | Yes |
| Granuloma formation | Yes | Yes |
| Bile-duct destruction | Yes | Yes |

PDC: pyruvate dehydrogenase complex; OGDC: 2-oxoglutarate dehydrogenase complex; BCOADC: branched-chain 2-oxoacid dehydrogenase complex.

epitope prediction analysis has shown that the extent of 3D mimicry between *E. coli* and human PDC-E2 is not sufficient enough to initiate cross-reactive immune responses [29]. Nevertheless, the core epitopic region of the B-cell PDC-E2 epitope overlaps with the immunodominant CD4 and CD8 T-cell epitope, and HLA class II restricted motifs shared by the human and *E. coli* PDC-E2 do exist [25]. Experimental findings support the presence of cross-reactive CD4 and CD8 T-cell responses between human and *E. coli* PDC-E2 [10, 11, 25, 30]. Shimoda and colleagues have developed CD4 T-cell lines with specificity for the disease-specific human PDC E2 autoepitope (GDLLAEIETDKATI) and its *E. coli* homologue PDC-E2 (EQSLITVEGDKASM). That group also demonstrated that these two cross-react at the CD4 T-cell level. Shimoda and colleagues have delineated the fine specificity of these T-cell lines and demonstrated that the ExDK motif shared by human and *E. coli* PDC-E2 is of paramount importance for epitope recognition [10, 11]. These reports also demonstrated that T-cell lines specific to the human PDC-E2 autoepitope developed from PBC patients peripheral blood mononuclear cells, or liver infiltrating cells, can proliferate in the presence of an *E. coli* OGDC-E2 peptide containing the ExDK motif [10, 11]. Amongst 16 T-cell clones specific for *E. coli* OGDC-E2 peptide, 13 could respond to human OADC-E2 autoepitopes from PDC-E2, OGDC-E2, and BCOADC-E2 [12].

Several investigators have pointed out that motifs shared by *E. coli* and human OADC proteins are to be expected in view of the highly conserved nature of OADC (Table 2). However, previous studies have also shown that *E. coli* sequences not related to PDC-E2, BCOADC-E2, or OGDC-E2 are highly homologous to PDC-E2$_{212-226}$ and some are also cross-reactive targets of antibodies specifically present in patients with PBC, particularly those with recurrent episodes of UTI [10, 15]. Among the six *E. coli* mimics, only 2 originating from the ATP-dependant helicase hrpA, and the periplasmic binding protein cross-recognised, and their respective peptides were able to absorb out reactivity to human PDC-E2$_{212-226}$ [15]. As four other mimicking sequences were totally unreactive, we speculated that reactivity to ATP-dependant helicase hrpA is not epiphenomenal and has potential significance for the pathogenesis of PBC [15, 22, 29].

Two independent studies in PBC cohorts from Spain and the UK have demonstrated a disease-specific presence of antibodies against a short 18-meric sequence from the ATP-dependant Clp protease (ClpP$_{177-194}$). Antibody reactivity against this peptide was found in one-third of the cases with PBC but in less than 4% of the controls tested [8, 16]. This finding was of potential interest for several reasons. First, a three-dimensional model of the *E. coli* ClpP clearly demonstrates that this region of ClpP$_{177-194}$ is exposed on the surface of the molecule and as such could be an easy target for antibody binding, further explaining its high affinity for the respective antibodies [29]. Peculiarly enough, ClpP is in a complex with the regulatory ATP-binding subunit X of the *E. coli* Clp complex ClpX, and a peptide of ClpX shares a striking homology with the dominant human PDC-E2$_{212-226}$ epitope [15]. However, antibody testing of the ClpX mimic did not reveal any evidence of significant humoral response in patients with PBC [15]. Thus, despite being a mimic, *E. coli* ClpX is not an antibody target. This is in contrast to ClpP that is not homologous but is targeted by antibodies. We provided an explanation for this paradoxical finding and suggested that recognition of ClpP/ClpX by PBC-specific antibodies leads to internalization of the ClpP and subsequent B-cell presentation of the Clp X peptide to CD4 helper T-cells [15, 29]. To this end, we have provided preliminary data demonstrating the presence of strong CD4 T-cell responses to *E. coli* ClpX. ClpP was not a T-cell target [29]. The biological significance of these findings requires external validation and further investigation as the ClpP epitope is highly conserved amongst bacteria and the respective ClpP homologue from other bacteria is also a target of cross-reactive responses in PBC women with recurrent UTI [16].

According to these scenarios, recurrent UTI leads to an initiation of anti-*E. coli* and cross-reactive PBC-specific AMA responses and subsequently to liver disease. As PBC is also characterized by disease-specific ANA, evidence must be sought in search for molecular mimics between *E. coli* proteins and human nuclear autoantigens of PBC-specific ANA [14]. It is of interest that the great majority of women with recurrent UTI but no liver disease, who are AMA positive, also react with sp100. None of the AMA negative women in this group showed anti-sp100 antibody reactivity [14]. These data show that antibody reactivity to sp100 correlates with AMA positivity and a history of recurrent UTI. The fact that women without PBC but with a history of recurrent UTI also have anti-sp100 but not anti-gp210 antibodies led us to speculate that *E. coli* is linked to PBC and that this infectious agent is most likely a trigger of AMA and sp100-specific ANA (rather than gp210) production. This scenario would fit with the finding that gp210 and sp100 autoantibodies rarely coexist in the same patient, which suggests that different triggers may account for their initiation during the development of the disease.

Table 2: Amino acid similarities between *E. coli* and self-proteins in patients with primary biliary cirrhosis (PBC). There are three major targets of cross-reactive autoantibodies directed against an epitope located at the inner lipoyl domain (ILD) of human pyruvate dehydrogenase E2 complex (PDC-E2), a cross-reactive one at the outer lipoyl domain (OLD), and one mimic on the PDC E3-binding protein (E3BP). Amongst six PDC-E2 mimics originated from various *E. coli* proteins, four are targets of cross-reactive responses while three are unreactive, including the *E. coli* PDC-E2 mimic which is a weak target. Amino acids appear in standard single letter code. Sequence alignment has been performed using the BLAST2p protein-protein comparison programmes. + indicates conserved or semiconserved substitutions.

| | Protein | Identity | Similarity | Reactivity |
|---|---|---|---|---|
| G Q A M V D L L A E Y E K V G | *E. coli* nitrate reductase 2 | 6 | 53% (8/15) | No |
| K A S E G E L L A Q V E P E D | *E. coli* ATP-dependent Clp-X | 8 | 93% (14/15) | No |
| K V A A E Q S L I T V E G D K | *E. coli* PDC-E2 | 5 | 73% (11/15) | Weak |
| **K L S E G D L L A E I E T D K** | **Human PDC-E2 ILD** | | | |
| L M T D G I L L A E I Q Q D R | *E. coli* ATP-dependent helicase | 7 | 80% (12/15) | Yes |
| G Y A Q S G L L A E I T P D K | *E. coli* periplasmic maltose-binding | 7 | 73% (11/15) | Yes |
| D A A V E D L L A E V S Q P K | *E. coli* fatty acid oxidation-$\alpha$ | 6 | 60% (9/15) | Yes |
| L A T L D D L L A E I G L G N | *E. coli* (P) ppGpp synthetase II | 6 | 60% (9/15) | Yes |
| A V S A G D A L C E I E T D K | **Human PDC-3BP** | **10** | 80% (12/15) | Yes (strong) |

## 3. *E. coli*-Based Animal Models of PBC

There is no doubt that any attempt to consider *E. coli* as a pathogen of PBC has to find experimental support on the basis of a reliable animal model of the disease. This model would have to be induced after exposure of the animals to uropathogenic strains of *E. coli*. As for any other experimental model of a given disease, the animal model would have to be characterized by high reproducibility in terms of disease frequency and prolonged disease maintenance [26]. The immunological and histopathological features of the affected animals would have to show high resemblance with that of the human disease (Table 1). The animal would have to be presented with AMA targeting epitopic regions corresponding to those of the human mitochondrial autoantigens, as well as PBC-specific ANA against nuclear body and nuclear envelope antigens that is similar to those noted in a significant proportion (25–50%) of PBC women. In addition, AMA and ANA seen in sera from affected animals would need to show fine specificity comparable to that noted in women with PBC. Ideally, the fine specificity of cellular immune responses against mitochondrial autoantigens noted in mice would match those noted in humans. In terms of clinical relevance, nonspecific symptoms like those of pruritus and fatigue observed in a considerable proportion of women with PBC could also be seen in experimentally induced PBC. PBC is characterized by the cocurrent presence of other autoimmune diseases (mainly sicca symptomatology and autoimmune thyroiditis); thus, an ideal experimental model would be that showing extrahepatic features similar to those of women affected with PBC.

Practically speaking, all animal models of diseases including those developed for autoimmune diseases such as PBC lack some of the key features of the disease under investigation. Nevertheless, work performed over the years in the field of experimental PBC has led to the development of animal models closely resembling the human condition, including most if not all of the typical features of the disease (reviewed in [26]).

In 2008, Palermo published in the form of an abstract a monography reporting the development of an *E. coli*-based experimental model of PBC [9]. According to the author, the animals used were seven-week-old female C57Bl/6 mice receiving transurethral inoculations with uropathogenic *E. coli*. Four months after the original inoculation, the mice developed histological and immunological features of PBC. The histological features included intrahepatic bile-duct destruction, granuloma formation, and lymphocyte infiltration [9]. AMA were induced at early time points following inoculation. This model, which resembles early PBC, has never been published in a form of a full-length paper, and a detailed analysis of the features of the affected animals has not been performed.

A recent study from the Gershwin's group has described a novel model of *E. coli* induced PBC [31]. NOD.B6 Idd10/Idd18 mice were infected with *E. coli* [31]. These mice were followed up for several weeks following infection and histological as well as immunological features were assessed in great detail.

## 4. AMA Responses in *E. coli*-Infected PBC Animals

In the study by Gershwin's group, the animals developed AMA reaching their peak four weeks after the infection, and subsequently their concentration diminished to levels comparable to those noted in mice infected with *Novosphingobium aromaticivorans* [31]. While AMA reactivity in the *E. coli*-infected mice is stronger than that noted in *N. aromaticivorans*, this reactivity is weaker than that seen in serum samples from women with PBC or in other animal models of PBC. These include the dominant negative transforming growth factor- (dnTGF-) $\beta$RII mice and xenobiotic 2-octynoic acid bovine serum albumin (BSA) conjugate-immunized mice [13, 32].

Antibody measurements showed reactivity against PDC-E2 and OGDC-E2 but not against BCOADC-E2 [31]. The *E. coli*-infected mice developed histological features such as portal inflammation and granuloma formation long after the induction of AMA responses. Thus, while AMA reached their peak at 4 weeks after infection, histological features presented at 26 weeks [31]. This finding is of interest, as several investigators believe that AMA directly or indirectly participate in the destruction of small bile ducts. These findings do not support the notion believed by many investigators that AMA (and in general autoantibodies) are secondary phenomena following the destruction of biliary epithelial destruction and the release of cryptic mitochondrial autoantigens. PBC-specific ANA were not tested in these mice.

## 5. Histological Features of the *E. coli*-Based PBC Animal Model

Histological assessment of the mice showed portal inflammation, granuloma formation, and biliary cell damage in the livers of both *N. aromaticivorans* and *E. coli*-infected mice. Immunohistochemical staining for CK19 showed biliary epithelial cells among lymphoid aggregates and a diverse degree of biliary cell damage [31]. The heterogeneous form of cell destruction involved biliary epithelial cells with moderate to severe inflammatory cell infiltration and cell destruction in some portal tracts, while neighboring tracts were almost undamaged showing only a mild lymphoid aggregation [31].

The results of this study show that *E. coli* infection can inflict PBC-mimicking biliary epithelial cell damage in the biliary disease-prone NOD.B6-Idd10/Idd18 mice.

This model may shed light on the understanding of the long-presumed association of recurrent UTI with the development of primary biliary cirrhosis.

## Abbreviations

AMA: Antimitochondrial antibody
ANA: Antinuclear antibody
BEC: Biliary epithelial cell
*E. coli*: *Escherichia coli*
OADC: Oxoacid dehydrogenase complex
OGDC: 2-Oxoglutarate dehydrogenase complex
PBC: Primary biliary cirrhosis
PDC: Pyruvate dehydrogenase complex
UTI: Urinary tract infection.

## References


[1] M. M. Kaplan and M. E. Gershwin, "Primary biliary cirrhosis," *The New England Journal of Medicine*, vol. 353, no. 12, pp. 1261–1273, 2005.

[2] D.-P. Bogdanos, H. Baum, and D. Vergani, "Antimitochondrial and other autoantibodies," *Clinics in Liver Disease*, vol. 7, no. 4, pp. 759–777, 2003.

[3] J. V. Metcalf, H. C. Mitchison, J. M. Palmer, D. E. Jones, M. F. Bassendine, and O. F. W. James, "Natural history of early primary biliary cirrhosis," *The Lancet*, vol. 348, no. 9039, pp. 1399–1402, 1996.

[4] A. K. Burroughs, I. J. Rosenstein, O. Epstein, J. M. Hamilton-Miller, W. Brumfitt, and S. Sherlock, "Bacteriuria and primary biliary cirrhosis," *Gut*, vol. 25, no. 2, pp. 133–137, 1984.

[5] P. Butler, J. M. T. Hamilton-Miller, N. McIntyre, and A. K. Burroughs, "Natural history of bacteriuria in women with primary biliary cirrhosis and the effect of antimicrobial therapy in symptomatic and asymptomatic groups," *Gut*, vol. 36, no. 6, pp. 931–934, 1995.

[6] D. S. Smyk, D. P. Bogdanos, S. Kriese, C. Billinis, A. K. Burroughs, and E. I. Rigopoulou, "Urinary tract infection as a risk factor for autoimmune liver disease: from bench to bedside," *Clinics and Research in Hepatology and Gastroenterology*, vol. 36, no. 2, pp. 110–121, 2012.

[7] P. Butler, F. Valle, J. M. T. Hamilton-Miller, W. Brumfitt, H. Baum, and A. K. Burroughs, "M2 mitochondrial antibodies and urinary rough mutant bacteria in patients with primary biliary cirrhosis and in patients with recurrent bacteriuria," *Journal of Hepatology*, vol. 17, no. 3, pp. 408–414, 1993.

[8] I. Mayo, P. Arizti, A. Pares et al., "Antibodies against the COOH-terminal region of E. coli ClpP protease in patients with primary biliary cirrhosis," *Journal of Hepatology*, vol. 33, no. 4, pp. 528–536, 2000.

[9] J. J. Palermo, "W1846 recurrent urinary tract infection in mice results in immune-mediated cholangiopathy similar to human primary biliary cirrhosis," *Gastroenterology*, vol. 134, supplement 1, no. 4, p. A837, 2008.

[10] S. Shimoda, M. Nakamura, H. Shigematsu et al., "Mimicry peptides of human PDC-E2 163-176 peptide, the immunodominant T- cell epitope of primary biliary cirrhosis," *Hepatology*, vol. 31, no. 6, pp. 1212–1216, 2000.

[11] S. Shimoda, J. van de Water, A. Ansari et al., "Identification and precursor frequency analysis of a common T cell epitope motif in mitochondrial autoantigens in primary biliary cirrhosis," *The Journal of Clinical Investigation*, vol. 102, no. 10, pp. 1831–1840, 1998.

[12] H. Tanimoto, S. Shimoda, M. Nakamura et al., "Promiscuous T cells selected by Escherichia coli: OGDC-E2 in primary biliary cirrhosis," *Journal of Autoimmunity*, vol. 20, no. 3, pp. 255–263, 2003.

[13] K. Wakabayashi, K. Yoshida, P. S. C. Leung et al., "Induction of autoimmune cholangitis in non-obese diabetic (NOD).1101 mice following a chemical xenobiotic immunization," *Clinical and Experimental Immunology*, vol. 155, no. 3, pp. 577–586, 2009.

[14] D.-P. Bogdanos, H. Baum, P. Butler et al., "Association between the primary biliary cirrhosis specific anti-sp100 antibodies and recurrent urinary tract infection," *Digestive and Liver Disease*, vol. 35, no. 11, pp. 801–805, 2003.

[15] D.-P. Bogdanos, H. Baum, A. Grasso et al., "Microbial mimics are major targets of crossreactivity with human pyruvate dehydrogenase in primary biliary cirrhosis," *Journal of Hepatology*, vol. 40, no. 1, pp. 31–39, 2004.

[16] D.-P. Bogdanos, H. Baum, U. C. Sharma et al., "Antibodies against homologous microbial caseinolytic proteases P characterise primary biliary cirrhosis," *Journal of Hepatology*, vol. 36, no. 1, pp. 14–21, 2002.

[17] A. Parikh-Patel, E. B. Gold, H. Worman, K. E. Krivy, and M. E. Gershwin, "Risk factors for primary biliary cirrhosis in a cohort of patients from the United States," *Hepatology*, vol. 33, no. 1, pp. 16–21, 2001.

[18] M. E. Gershwin, C. Selmi, H. J. Worman et al., "Risk factors and comorbidities in primary biliary cirrhosis: a controlled interview-based study of 1032 patients," *Hepatology*, vol. 42, no. 5, pp. 1194–1202, 2005.

[19] P. S. C. Leung, R. L. Coppel, A. Ansari, S. Munoz, and M. E. Gershwin, "Antimitochondrial antibodies in primary biliary cirrhosis," *Seminars in Liver Disease*, vol. 17, no. 1, pp. 61–69, 1997.

[20] M. E. Gershwin and I. R. Mackay, "Primary biliary cirrhosis: paradigm or paradox for autoimmunity," *Gastroenterology*, vol. 100, no. 3, pp. 822–833, 1991.

[21] M. E. Gershwin and I. R. Mackay, "The causes of primary biliary cirrhosis: convenient and inconvenient truths," *Hepatology*, vol. 47, no. 2, pp. 737–745, 2008.

[22] D. P. Bogdanos and D. Vergani, "Bacteria and primary biliary cirrhosis," *Clinical Reviews in Allergy and Immunology*, vol. 36, no. 1, pp. 30–39, 2009.

[23] C. Selmi, D. L. Balkwill, P. Invernizzi et al., "Patients with primary biliary cirrhosis react against a ubiquitous xenobiotic-metabolizing bacterium," *Hepatology*, vol. 38, no. 5, pp. 1250–1257, 2003.

[24] A. K. Burroughs, P. Butler, M. J. E. Sternberg, and H. Baum, "Molecular mimicry in liver disease," *Nature*, vol. 358, no. 6385, pp. 377–378, 1992.

[25] J. van de Water, H. Ishibashi, R. L. Coppel, and M. E. Gershwin, "Molecular mimicry and primary biliary cirrhosis: premises not promises," *Hepatology*, vol. 33, no. 4, pp. 771–775, 2001.

[26] J. Wang, G. X. Yang, K. Tsuneyama, M. E. Gershwin, W. M. Ridgway, and P. S. Leung, "Animal models of primary biliary cirrhosis," *Seminars in Liver Disease*, vol. 34, pp. 285–296, 2014.

[27] S. P. M. Fussey, S. T. Ali, J. R. Guest, O. F. W. James, M. F. Bassendine, and S. J. Yeaman, "Reactivity of primary biliary cirrhosis sera *Escherichia coli* dihydrolipoamide acetyltransferase (E2p): characterization of the main immunogenic region," *Proceedings of the National Academy of Sciences of the United States of America*, vol. 87, no. 10, pp. 3987–3991, 1990.

[28] S. P. Fussey, M. F. Bassendine, O. F. James, and S. J. Yeaman, "Characterisation of the reactivity of autoantibodies in primary biliary cirrhosis," *FEBS Letters*, vol. 246, no. 1-2, pp. 49–53, 1989.

[29] D. P. Bogdanos, H. Baum, D. Vergani, and A. K. Burroughs, "The role of *E. coli* infection in the pathogenesis of primary biliary cirrhosis," *Disease Markers*, vol. 29, no. 6, pp. 301–311, 2010.

[30] H. Shigematsu, S. Shimoda, M. Nakamura et al., "Fine specificity of T cells reactive to human PDC-E2 163-176 peptide, the immunodominant autoantigen in primary biliary cirrhosis: implications for molecular mimicry and cross-recognition among mitochondrial autoantigens," *Hepatology*, vol. 32, no. 5, pp. 901–909, 2000.

[31] J. J. Wang, G.-X. Yang, W. C. Zhang et al., "*Escherichia coli* infection induces autoimmune cholangitis and anti-mitochondrial antibodies in non-obese diabetic (NOD).B6 (Idd10/Idd18) mice," *Clinical and Experimental Immunology*, vol. 175, no. 2, pp. 192–201, 2014.

[32] S. Oertelt, Z. X. Lian, C. M. Cheng et al., "Anti-mitochondrial antibodies and primary biliary cirrhosis in TGF-$\beta$receptor II dominant-negative mice," *Journal of Immunology*, vol. 177, no. 3, pp. 1655–1660, 2006.

# 13

# The Mind and Liver Test: A New Approach to the Diagnosis of Minimal Hepatic Encephalopathy in Resource-Poor Settings

**Saurav Das,[1] Sajjadh M. J. Ali,[1] James Seward,[2] and Jayanthi Venkataraman[3]**

[1] *Department of Medical Gastroenterology, Stanley Medical College and Hospital, Chennai 600001, India*
[2] *Banner Alzheimer's Institute, E Willetta Street, Phoenix, AZ 85006, USA*
[3] *Global Health City, Perumbakkam, Chennai, Tamil Nadu 600100, India*

Correspondence should be addressed to Saurav Das; sauravmed@gmail.com

Academic Editor: Daisuke Morioka

*Background and Aims.* Minimal hepatic encephalopathy (MHE) is diagnosed using neuropsychometric tests or neurophysiological tests that are either inapplicable to illiterate patient population in resource-poor settings or require sophisticated and expensive equipment. The available tests assess discrete domains of mental impairment. Our aim was (a) to design a neuropsychometric test that measures all domains of mental impairment in MHE using one metric; (b) to evaluate its sensitivity, specificity, and reproducibility. *Methods.* The mind and liver test (MALT), a psychometric test assessing cognition, memory, and psychometric impairment, each on a scale of 20, was designed keeping in mind the requirements of a universal test. 40 cirrhotics and 36 controls were subjected to critical flicker frequency (CFF) and MALT in same sitting. ROC curve was plotted for MALT using CFF as gold standard. Bland-Altman plot was used to find test-retest agreement. *Results.* CFF values and MALT scores varied significantly between the cases and the controls ($P < 0.05$). MALT was 94% sensitive and 83% specific. Using ROC with CFF as gold standard, the AUC for diagnosis of MHE using MALT score was 0.89. Test-retest agreement was high (ICC = 0.89). *Conclusion.* In this pilot study, MALT proved to be highly sensitive, specific, inexpensive, and reproducible.

## 1. Introduction

Hepatic encephalopathy is a major complication of cirrhosis. It is characterized by neuropsychiatric manifestations. In minimal hepatic encephalopathy (MHE), patients have alterations in sleep pattern, and there is difficulty in performing even day-to-day routine activities like driving a vehicle, doing simple calculations, and so forth [1–3]. This is often due to an impairment in multiple faculties of the mind. Initially there is a mild impairment in cognition and psychomotor skills which then progress to a gross impairment in orientation and general consciousness. These manifestations are potentially reversible, especially, if the diagnosis is made early in the course of the disease [4, 5].

The diagnosis of minimal hepatic encephalopathy (MHE) is made using a battery of neuropsychometric or neurophysiological tests [2]. The existing neuropsychometric tests include paper-pencil tests like the number connection tests A and B, the figure connection test (FCT), trail tracing test, block design test, digit symbol test, and the comparatively recent inhibitory control test [6]. Inaccuracies in the paper-pencil tests have been widely reported [7, 8]. Also, there is a lack of consensus on the diagnostic criteria and a limited correction for educational level and age in these studies [4]. The FCT was designed for the Indian population and has been widely accepted as a sensitive test to detect MHE in illiterate individuals [9]. However, this test assesses only a few discrete domains of impairment (attention and psychomotor skills). Similarly the inhibitory control test primarily assesses attention deficit [10]. As a result, much of the tests hitherto mentioned are seldom used in day-to-day clinical practice [11]. More recent objective neurophysiological tests include critical flicker frequency (CFF) and, auditory and visual evoked potentials. All these tests involve expensive specialized equipment and trained experienced personnel [7, 11]. There is therefore a need to design an inexpensive test which would measure all the impaired domains of the mind using the same metric [12].

We designed a test that would examine the three important domains—cognition, memory, and psychomotor skills—and used this test in patients with chronic liver disease to detect MHE.

## 2. Materials and Methods

*2.1. Design of the Mind and Liver Test (MALT).* The impaired domains of mental function in MHE have an impact on the quality of daily life [13]. The mind and liver test (MALT) was conceptualized on a scientific basis and was designed to measure the daily mental needs of an individual as a whole, and not for just one specific domain. MALT was designed such that it served as a single metric measure for all impaired domains like cognition, memory, and psychometric skills.

In order to design the specific tasks which make up the MALT, a questionnaire investigating the specific daily mental demands encountered by the target population was administered to 100 individuals attending the out-patient liver clinic of Institute of Gastroenterology and Hepatology, Stanley Hospital, Chennai, India. Except for 5 patients who were either professionals or businessmen, the rest belonged to lower socioeconomic status and were laborers, unskilled workers, or farmers (Kuppuswamy's socioeconomic status scale) [14]. Based upon the results of the questionnaire, MALT items were chosen to be relevant to these daily demands.

For *cognition* the questions were designed to identify certain animals, ability to follow the sequence of a natural phenomenon (e.g., morning-noon-evening-night), and ability to perform simple mathematical calculations needed during daily transactions (e.g., transaction at the shop). For *memory* the questions tested immediate, short term, and long term recall separately. We also tested the ability to recall a visual as well as an auditory experience. The *psychomotor* abilities were tested by asking the patient to copy certain figures on a calibrated graph paper, to build a three-dimensional structure of a wall using building blocks, to cut along a drawn line using a scissor, and to trace along a narrow path (analogous to a line tracing test).

All the three tests were designed using a colorful board, set of printed question cards, plastic building blocks, animal models, an audio device, and an instruction *cum* scoring sheet. For convenience, the three components of neuropsychometric analysis were color coded. Red steps tested memory, green steps tested cognition, and yellow steps tested psycho-motor skills [15].

These tasks were grouped into three different sections:

Section 1: figure the field,

Section 2: home sweet home,

Section 3: road not taken.

Section 1 included steps like identification of animals and vegetables on the countryside/neighborhood, and identification of well-known sequences of events like sowing seeds, transplanting the saplings, harvesting, and finally transporting to the city. In this section, we also asked the patient to build a wall using blocks. The failure to perform this task was considered a sign of psycho-motor impairment.

Table 1: MALT-steps summary.

| Section | Task | Corresponding mental function |
|---|---|---|
| (1) Figure the field | Copy the figures | Visuospatial abilities |
| | Group similar objects | Recognition |
| | Trace the sequence | Executive function |
| | Name the animals | Naming |
| | Build the wall | Constructional ability |
| (2) Home sweet home | Complete the task | Executive function |
| | Remember the arrangement | Immediate visual memory |
| | Cut along the line | Psychomotor skills |
| | Recall the steps | Attention |
| | Identify the sound | Auditory recall |
| (3) The road not taken | Trace the path | Psycho-motor skills |
| | What from shop? | Delayed visual recall |
| | How much to pay? | Calculation |
| | Choose the shortest path. | Decision making |
| | Quiz | Divided attention |
| | Time, space, and reason | Abstraction \| Orientation |

Section 2 included steps like remembering the arrangement of things on the shelves at home and ability to narrate the steps of a task performed at home daily, such as washing a cloth or making tea. Impairment in memory and organization reflected directly on the performance in these steps. In the same section we tested the ability of the patient to identify and remember sounds by using different stimuli, such as a church bell or an ambulance siren. Examinees were also asked to cut paper using a pair of scissors, a measure of psychomotor abilities.

Section 3 included tasks that tested the numerical abilities of the patient (like we asked the patient to perform small transactions at the shop) and tasks that asked them to identify places that they may visit on a daily basis, like a temple, a water pump, or a market place. Short term memory was tested by asking the patient to recall the short list of things to buy from the shop that was narrated to him in Section 2. We included a test analogous to the trail tracing test in Section 3 where the patient had to negotiate a narrow path from the shop back to home, using his index finger along the trail. Performance on this step can be impaired in patients with psycho-motor impairment.

Two other tests were performed on the MALT board, which could affect the daily activities in MHE. These included (a) divided attention: ability to observe images on the board that were not included as a part of the task; (b) judgment ability: to select the shortest of the three shown paths. Table 1 shows the steps included in the three sections of the test that appear on the MALT board (Figure 1) and the corresponding

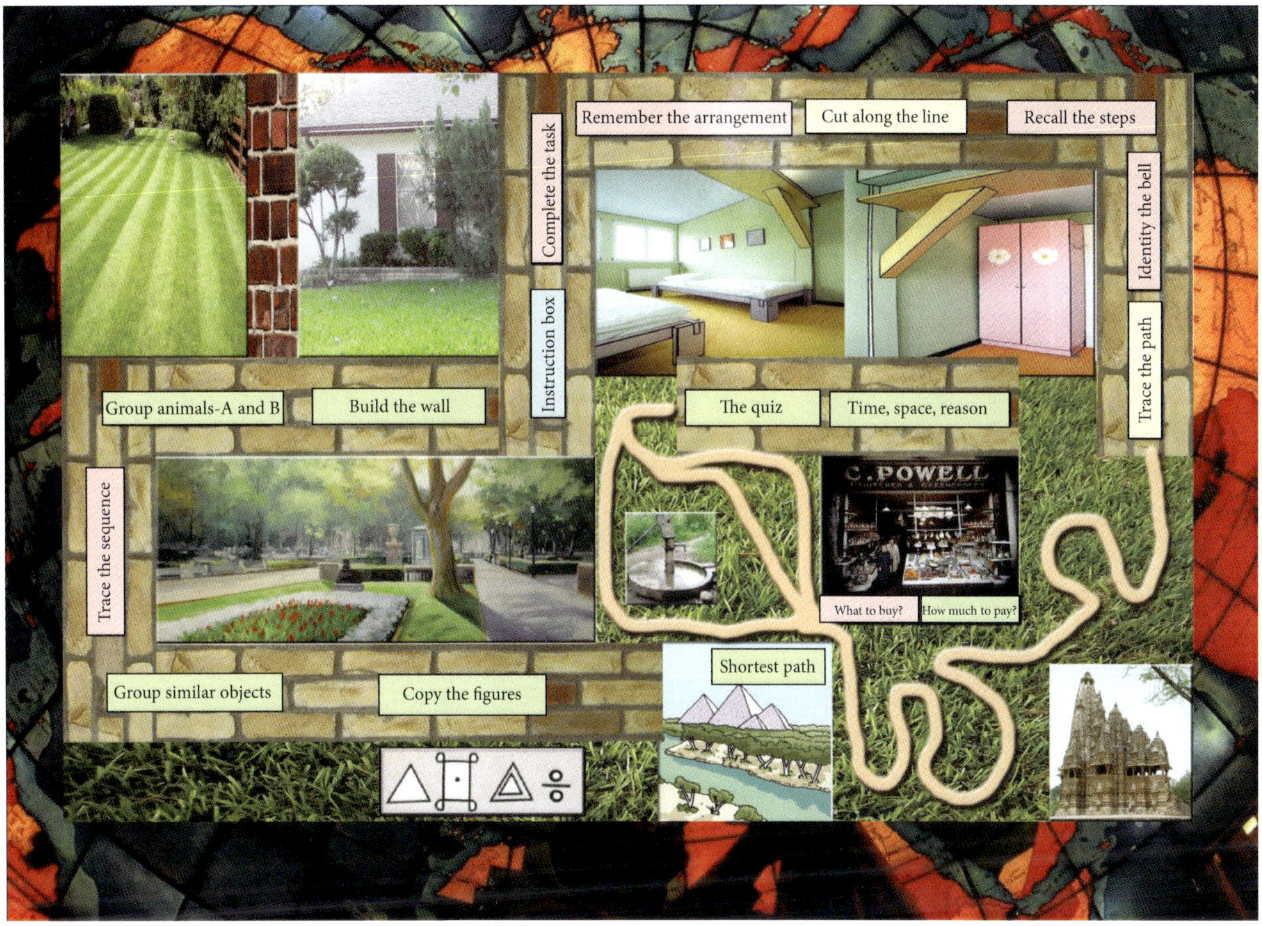


FIGURE 1: MALT test board. The test is administered clock-wise starting from Step 1, "Copy the figures." The red steps test memory, green-cognition, and yellow-psychomotor skills. The scores are noted on instruction cum scoring sheet (Table 2).

mental function that each step evaluates. Table 2 shows the instruction cum scoring sheet.

*2.2. Interpretation of MALT.* To score the performance on MALT, we took into account both accuracy and speed of performance. Based upon the performance of initial 10 controls in the test, we fixed an upper limit of 1 minute for each of steps 3, 5, and 6. The maximum scores on the entire test was 60 and 20 each on cognition, memory, and psychomotor skills. Higher scores implied greater impairment in mental function.

Informed consent was obtained from each patient included in the study and the study protocol conforms to the ethical guidelines of the 1975 Declaration of Helsinki as reflected in a priori approval by the ethics committee of Stanley Medical College and Hospital. The study was conducted at the Department of Medical Gastroenterology, Stanley Hospital. Forty proven cirrhotic patients were recruited as cases from among the out-patients and in-patients registered in our department. The diagnosis was based on clinical presentation and ultrasound findings. Patients with neurological deficit, obvious overt encephalopathy, alcohol abuse 72 hours prior to the test, or those on sedatives or psycho-active drugs in the preceding 24 hours were excluded. Patients with cardiac failure, renal disease, and chronic obstructive airway disease were also excluded. It was ensured that the patients had not received lactulose, lactitol, or antibiotics like rifaximin, neomycin, or quinolones in the past three months. Controls were healthy individuals screened at the Master Health Checkup scheme in the hospital.

All controls and patients had critical flicker frequency test using portable battery-powered Hepatonorm Analyzer, Accelab GmbH, Kusterdingen, Germany. The test was done in a quiet dark room. The analyzer evoked an intrafoveal light stimulus with defined pulses [7, 16]. The frequency of pulsation decreased gradually. The patient was asked to press a hand held switch when the change was apparent. The procedure was repeated 5 times to make the subject familiar with the process and 9 readings were recorded. The mean for each patient was calculated. A value below the 38 Hz mark was considered diagnostic of MHE [5, 7, 16].

The subjects (cases and controls) were then brought into a well lit room and were allowed a relaxation time of 15 minutes after which MALT was administered by two trained medical professionals (SD and SM). The patient and the tester are seated across a table with the test board, question cards,

Table 2: MALT instruction cum scoring sheet.

| Sl | Method of administering the test | Instruction to fill up the next column | Step score | Final count |
|---|---|---|---|---|
| 1 | Copy the figures<br>The subject is asked to draw the shown geometrical figures (printed on the board) onto a provided ruled paper, without altering the size<br>(The original figures cross three units on the same paper) | Symmetrical figure. . .0<br>else. . .1<br>Number of units crossed | . . .<br><br>3-. . . | . . . |
| 2 | Group similar objects<br>The subject is shown one card (of a set of cards) showing the pictures of a few things belonging to two different categories (birds and vegetables, say). The subject is asked to place the blocks of the same color on objects of the same type | Number of objects misgrouped | . . ./2 | . . . |
| 3 | Trace the sequence<br>The subject is shown a card to trace a well known sequence (like seed-sapling-tree-wood log-table)<br>The examiner waits for a maximum of 1 minute, else proceeds to the next step | Score the time in seconds<br>0–10 s. . .0, 11–20 s. . .1, 21–30 s. . .2, 31–40 s. . .3, >40 s. . .4 | . . . | . . . |
| 4 | Name the animals<br>A: the subject is shown an animal (a cow, say) and is asked to name it<br>B: the subject is asked to separate animals of a certain kind from among the toys | Score time in seconds<br><5 s. . .0, 5–15 s. . .1, >15 s. . .2<br><15 s. . .0, else 1 | . . .<br><br>. . . | . . . |
| 5 | Build the wall<br>The subject is asked to build a two layered wall on the given line using the provided blocks The examiner waits for a maximum of 1 minute and then proceeds to the next step<br>Instruction box<br>The subject is made to hear three different bell sounds like the alarm, ambulance, and church bell using the audio device. He is also asked to be vigilant about the things he sees in the rest of the game | A well built wall. . .0<br>Asymmetrical. . .1<br>Unable to build. . .2<br>(Asymmetry is defined as inability to place the blocks linearly either along the line in the game board or inability to stack two layers one over the other) | . . . | . . . |
| 6 | Complete the task<br>The patient is asked to arrange in sequence, the cards depicting the steps of a daily act performed by people at home<br>The examiner waits for a maximum of 1 minute and then proceeds to the next step | Able to complete the task. . .0<br>Else. . .1 | . . . | . . . |
| 7 | Remember the arrangement<br>The subject is shown an arrangement in the shelf (image available on a question card) and it is narrated once for convenience<br>Immediately following this, the subject is asked to recall the arrangement | Number of objects recalled correctly | (6-. . .)/2 | . . . |
| 8 | Cut along the line<br>The subject is asked to cut along a line with both indentation and curve<br>The graph sheet on the reverse is analyzed for deviation | Deviation (in small units)<br>5–10. . .3<br>>10. . .5<br>Time (in seconds)<br>>45. . .5, else. . .0 | . . .<br><br>. . . | . . . |
| 9 | Recall the steps of the game till this point, in no specific order<br>The examiner asks a question pertaining to the sequence of the steps (what comes after X, say) | Number of steps recalled<br>Correct answer. . .0<br>Else. . .1 | 8-. . .<br>. . . | . . . |
| 10 | Identify the sound of the bell<br>One of the three bells sounded in the instruction box is sounded again | Unable to identify. . .1<br>Else. . .0 | . . . | . . . |

Table 2: Continued.

| Sl | Method of administering the test | Instruction to fill up the next column | Step score | Final count |
|---|---|---|---|---|
| 11 | Trace the path<br>Subject is asked to trace a 5 mm thick path to the shop | Time (in seconds)<br>>30 s. . .5, 16–30 s. . .3<br>Else. . .0 | . . . | . . . |
| | | Deviation (in small grids on the graph paper)<br><5. . .0, 5–15. . .3,<br>16–25. . .4, >25. . .5 | . . . | |
| 12 | What from the shop?<br>The subject is asked if he remembers what he had to get for the empty basket on the lowest shelf of the rack (This tests the recall of the question card shown in Step 7) | Incorrect. . .1<br>Else. . .0 | . . . | . . . |
| 13 | How much to pay?<br>The subject is given a simple calculation pertaining to day to day transactions | Incorrect. . .1<br>Else. . .0 | . . . | . . . |
| 14 | Choose the shortest path<br>The subject is asked to choose the shortest path back home | Incorrect. . .1<br>Else. . .0 | . . . | . . . |
| 15 | Quiz<br>The subject is asked if he saw certain things on the game board while tracing the path to the shop | Number of questions answered | 4-. . . | . . . |
| 16 | Time, space, and reason | A wrong answer to the question pertaining to spatial and temporal orientation, and silence in response to the reasoning question would be marked as "D" (for disoriented) | | |

an audio device, and a table clock. The performance of the patient was noted on the instruction/scoring sheet, including time to completion.

Both MALT and CFF were done in the same sitting. Patients were randomly assigned to MALT or CFF as the first test. Both tests were executed by two different persons (SD and SM) who were blinded to the other examiner's results. The performers administering the tests were trained by experienced clinicians so as to minimize the intra- and interobserver variations.

Chi-square test was used to assess differences between qualitative variables. Student's $t$-test was used to compare the mean CFF values and mean MALT scores between the cases and the controls. Preliminary analyses provided data for receiver-operating characteristic curves to determine the optimum cut-off value for MALT score for the diagnosis of MHE. The best sensitivity and specificity was found at a cut-off score of 20. Using the CFF performance as the reference standard, statistical analysis was performed using Student's $t$-test and the receiver-operating characteristic (ROC) curve. The cirrhotics were classified as "cirrhotics with MHE" and "cirrhotics without MHE," based upon their CFF readings. These groups were compared among themselves and with the control groups. SPSS version 10 was used for all statistical analyses and in the generation of the plots.

The test-retest reproducibility was assessed using the Bland-Altman plot. Twenty subjects including 10 cases and 10 controls were administered MALT twice at an interval of a six hours. It was ensured that patients being evaluated were not on lactulose, lactitol, neomycin, or any sedative meanwhile. The test was administered by the same examiner. The scores of the first and the second session of MALT were compared. The report was prepared in accordance with standards for reporting diagnostic accuracy, STARD guidelines (Figure 2) [17].

## 3. Results

*3.1. Demographic and Subject Characteristics.* The study comprised of 40 patients with cirrhosis (hereinafter referred to as "cases") and included 25 males (62.5%). There were 36 healthy controls (hereinafter referred to as "controls") and included 16 males (44.44%). The base line characteristics of controls and cases are shown in Table 3. The mean age of the cases and controls was significantly different ($P = 0.04$). There was no difference in sex distribution ($P = 0.18$), educational status ($P = 0.93$), and monthly income ($P = 0.09$) among the cases and the controls.

The etiology of cirrhosis was alcohol in 15 patients (37.5%), HCV in 13 (32.5%), nonalcoholic fatty liver disease in 6 (17.5%), autoimmune in 1 (2.5%), and cryptogenic in 8 (20%). There were 22 patients (55%) belonging to Child-Pugh class A and 18 (45%) to class B. Among the cirrhotics, there were 18 variceal bleeders (45%) and 2 patients (5%)

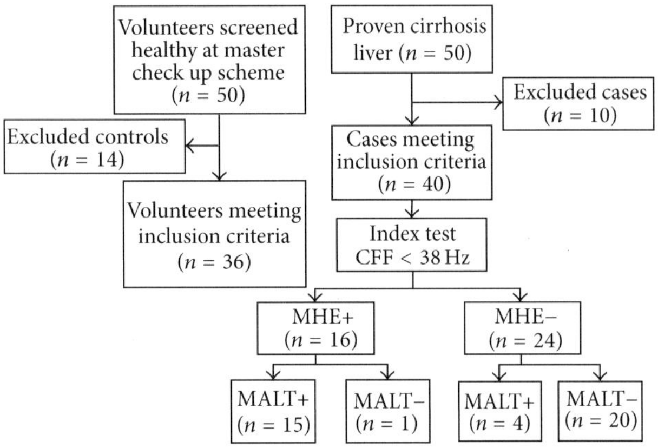


Figure 2: Study design flowchart according to the STARD guidelines.

had coagulopathy. 4 patients (10%) had refractory ascites, 2 patients (5%) had spontaneous bacterial peritonitis, and 8 others (20%) had urosepsis.

*3.2. Critical Flicker Frequency.* Using 38 Hz as CFF cut-off for MHE, 16 out of the 40 cirrhotics had MHE (40%), 8 each (50%) belonged to Child Class A and Child Class B. Among the 24 cirrhotics without MHE, 14 (58.33%) belonged to Child A and 10 (41.66%) to Child B at the time of MHE testing. The mean CFF for the cases was 39 ± 4.2 Hz compared to 42 ± 1.9 Hz among the controls ($P = 0.00$) (Figure 3(a)). The demographic characteristics and the lab parameters of the MHE and non-MHE groups among the cirrhotics or the "cases" are compared in Table 4.

*3.3. MALT.* The cases performed worse than controls on MALT. The controls scored 10 ± 5 compared to the cases, who scored 18 ± 8 (Figure 3(b)). This difference was significant ($P = 0.00$). On plotting the ROC curve (Figure 4(a)), the sensitivity and the specificity were found to be 94% and 83%, respectively, for a cut-off value set at 20. Using ROC with CFF as the gold standard, the AUC for diagnosis of MHE using MALT score was 89%. Figure 3(b) compares the mean MALT scores of MHE, non-MHE cirrhotics, and controls. MHE patients scored higher than the non-MHE and controls using the 20 mark as cut-off.

*3.4. Test-Retest Variability.* The test-retest variability was assessed using the intraclass correlation coefficient, ICC = 0.894 ($P = 0.000$). The Bland-Altman plot (Figure 4(b)) shows that the MALT retest scores of the 10 cases and 10 controls (who were subjected to the same test at an interval of 6 hours) was in agreement with the initial test scores.

*3.5. Other Considerations.* The Hepatonorm analyzer, manufactured in Germany, is an electronic device which runs on a battery that needs to be regularly changed. The price per unit is US$3053 and one day long user training costs US$230. The MALT board and its kit cost approximately US$5. The cost

Table 3: Demographic characteristics of cases and controls.

| Demographic characteristic (Mean ± SD) | Controls ($n$ = 36) | Cases ($n$ = 40) |
|---|---|---|
| Age (years) | 42 ± 9.7* | 46 ± 8.3* |
| Male : female | 16/20 | 25/15 |
| Education (not educated/educated) | 13/23 | 13/27 |
| Income per month (in US dollars) | 15.36 ± 14.51 | 10.77 ± 7.40 |

*$P < 0.05$.

ratio is of the order of $10^5$. The mean time of administration for both MALT and CFF was 10 ± 2 minutes.

## 4. Discussion

The highlights of the study are (a) a significant correlation between CFF and MALT scores in the population under study ($P < 0.05$); (b) the ROC curve and the box-whisker plots indicate that MALT is a highly sensitive and specific test considering CFF as the standard; and (c) the intraclass correlation coefficient was 0.894 on assessment of test-retest variability. The sensitivity and specificity of MALT was found to be 94% and 83%, respectively, compared to earlier reported 72.4% and 77.2% for CFF when the cut-off is set at 38 Hz [18]. Though MALT may be seen to be a time taking procedure, the mean time taken for MALT and CFF did not vary significantly. The former is inexpensive test compared to CFF.

A number of neuropsychological tools have been used to diagnose cognitive deficits in patients with cirrhosis. These include an extended neuropsychological assessment, shorter batteries, and computerized tests. The extended neuropsychological assessment is based upon the expert judgment and is difficult to validate [19]. The two shorter batteries—RBANS (Repeatable Battery for Assessment of Neuropsychological Status) and PHES (Psychometric Hepatic Encephalopathy Score) are primarily paper-pencil tests. The performance on these tests is affected by the level of literacy and on the familiarity of the subject to paper and pencil among the literates. However, these tests have their own advantages. RBANS is validated on a large normative data, it is available in multiple languages and has parallel versions available for repeated testing. However, most studies are in Alzheimer's patients and the studies in cirrhotics are only few [20]. PHES was originally validated in a series of nonalcoholic patients in Germany and has normative data available from some countries. However, our knowledge of MHE has grown since those studies and, now, it is understood that an ideal diagnostic tool should reflect on those daily activities which affect the quality of life, the ability to drive, and so forth, which are often impaired in MHE [21, 22]. To overcome the shortcoming of these short batteries for the use in resource-limited settings including their dependence on the literacy level, the figure connection test (FCT) was reported by a group in India [9]. However, FCT only tests a discrete cognitive domain impaired in MHE. Computerized neuropsychological tests include cognitive drug research (CDR), inhibitory control

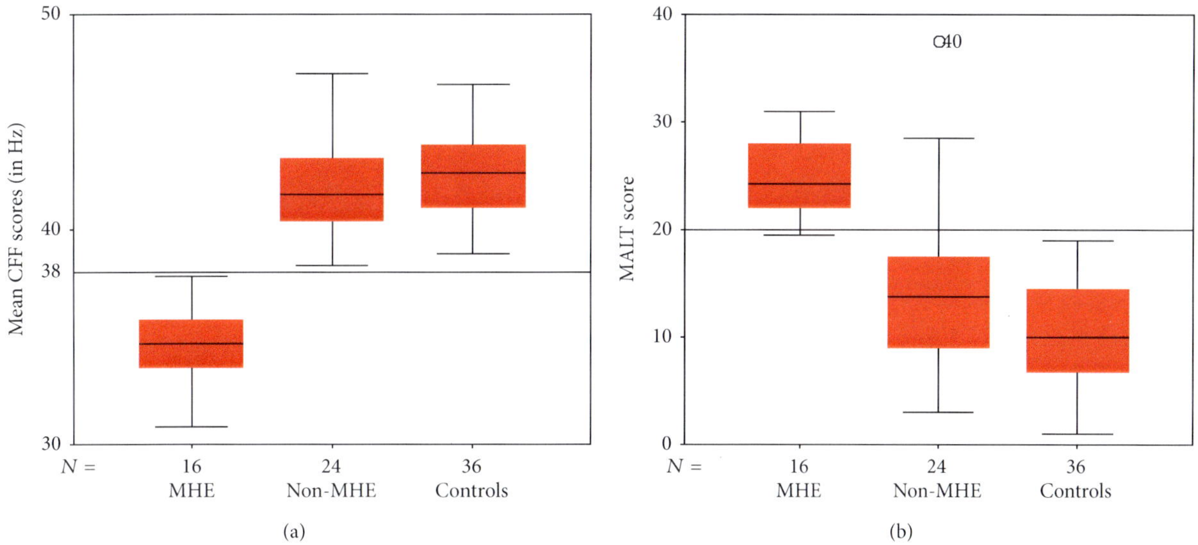


FIGURE 3: Intergroup comparison for CFF reading and MALT scores. The panel (a) compares the CFF readings between the controls, the non-MHE cirrhotics, and MHE (+) cirrhotics. The panel (b) compares the MALT scores between the same groups.

TABLE 4: Demographics within the cirrhosis group.

| | Cirrhotics without MHE (CFF−) ($n = 24$) | Cirrhotics with MHE (CFF+) ($n = 16$) |
|---|---|---|
| Age | $43.5 \pm 8.1^*$ | $50 \pm 7.2^*$ |
| Years of education | $6.4 \pm 4.5^*$ | $3.06 \pm 3.7^*$ |
| Gender (M/F) | 16/8 | 9/7 |
| Cirrhosis etiology (Alcohol/HCV/HCV+Alcohol/NASH/Others) | 09/05/00/04/06 | 03/05/03/02/03 |
| MELD score (median) | 11 | 14 |
| Child score (A/B) | 14/10 | 8/8 |
| Total bilirubin (median) | 1.5 | 1.6 |
| INR (median) | $1.1^*$ | $1.3^*$ |
| Serum creatinine (median, in mg/dL) | $0.73^*$ | $0.86^*$ |
| MALT scores | $14.8 \pm 7.8^\dagger$ | $24.8 \pm 3.5^\dagger$ |

$^*P < 0.05$ between two groups.
$^\dagger P < 0.01$ between two groups.

test (ICT), and the scan test which have been validated in the UK, USA, and Italy, respectively [23–25]. We do not have the validation data for these tests in our population.

The introduction of MALT has been based on the fundamental assumption that the currently available tests for the diagnosis of MHE are designed to test for one or two domains of mental impairment, and are expensive or not widely available [10]. MALT was designed to include tasks performed on a day-to-day routine basis. In the population under study, more than 36% of the participants were illiterate and the remaining who were literate were not used to paper and pencil. This is in line with the "demise of the pencil" reported by Iduru and Mullen [22]. Moreover, age and education correction factors are absent for Psychometric Hepatic Encephalopathy Score (PHES) in our population.

The prevalence of MHE among the cirrhotics in the present study is 40%. It is in agreement with the prevalence of 41% reported in a recent study involving 200 cirrhotics from North India while on the higher side compared to 30% reported in the study from Spain using PHES [18, 26]. It would either signify that MALT included more true positives or that the prevalence is different in our population [27, 28].

MALT is a psychometric test which displays day-to-day activity on a colorful board and disagreement between administrators of the test is significantly less (85% agreement in interobserver studies). Though the tasks on the game board remain the same, the elements of the tasks are not printed on the board but on multiple cards. This is to avoid a memory effect that accompanies any psychometric test. MALT includes steps like "build the wall" and "trace the

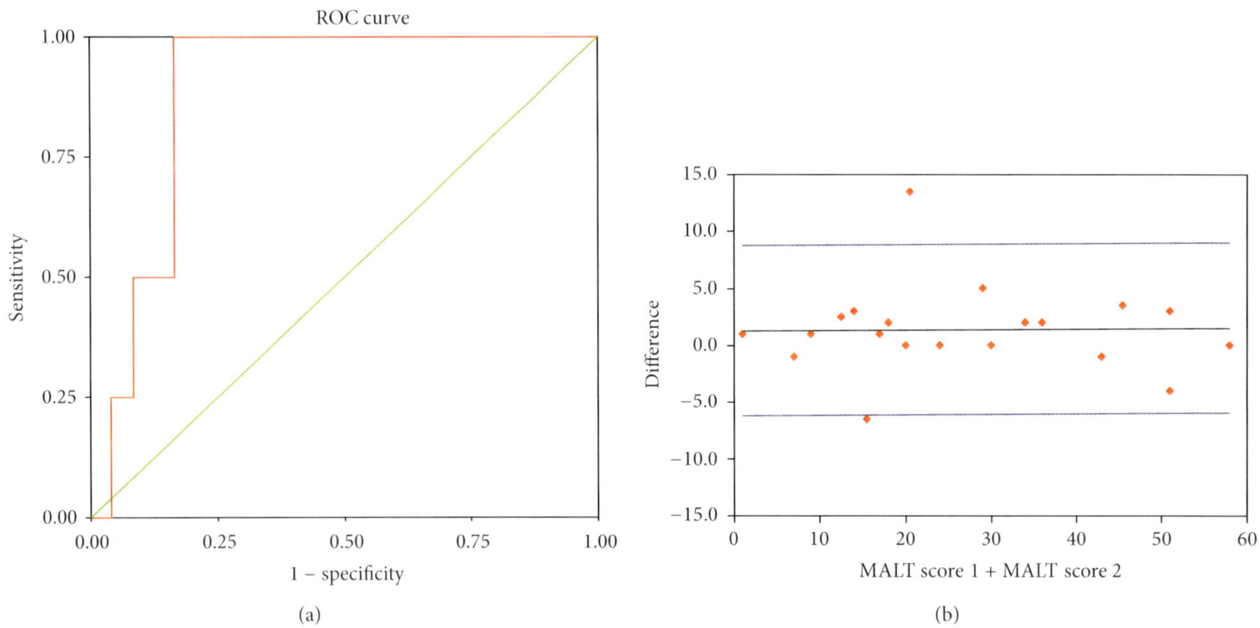


FIGURE 4: (a) ROC curve using CFF as gold standard and MALT score 20 as cut-off for the diagnosis of MHE. (b) Bland-Altman plot for the test-retest agreement of MALT.

path" which are analogous to block design and trail tracing test. In MALT, the subject is not asked to connect numbers, but rather to trace the sequence of a day-to-day event from morning to night, which in true sense does not need a level of literacy.

Although the majority of surveyed hepatologists in Spain and the United States agreed that MHE was a significant problem requiring testing during out-patient visits, only a few were able to actually perform the test during their day-to-day clinical practice [29, 30]. MALT needs validation in large number of patients. In the future, when the test is available in the form of a touch screen audio-visual videogame, the test could be self-administered by the patient during the wait period in the clinic. Moreover, MALT is in the form of a colorful board. It might be interesting to note if administration of such a test has any effect on the mood and affect of the depressed cirrhotic. It will also be of interest to follow up MALT scores of patients on therapy like lactulose for hepatic encephalopathy. Also, to see a head to head analysis of MALT compared to other psychometric tests in future. However, these were beyond the scope of the present study. The choice of CFF as the gold standard in the current study was also to circumvent many problems known to be encountered with administering multiple psychometric tests [2, 31].

This study largely aimed to design a psychometric battery to diagnose MHE in our population, which is useful for the illiterate patients and to check its reliability. The high sensitivity and specificity of MALT, its ease of administration, reproducibility, and cost-effectiveness seen in this pilot beckon further validation studies involving larger sample sizes.

## References


[1] J. S. Bajaj, M. Hafeezullah, Y. Zadvornova et al., "The effect of fatigue on driving skills in patients with hepatic encephalopathy," *The American Journal of Gastroenterology*, vol. 104, no. 4, pp. 898–905, 2009.

[2] P. Sharma, B. C. Sharma, V. Puri, and S. K. Sarin, "Critical flicker frequency: diagnostic tool for minimal hepatic encephalopathy," *Journal of Hepatology*, vol. 47, no. 1, pp. 67–73, 2007.

[3] C. Wein, B. Popp, H. Koch, G. Oehler, and P. Schauder, "Minimal hepatic encephalopathy impairs fitness to drive," *Hepatology*, vol. 39, no. 3, pp. 739–745, 2004.

[4] A. T. Blei and J. Córdoba, "Hepatic encephalopathy," *The American Journal of Gastroenterology*, vol. 96, no. 7, pp. 1968–1976, 2001.

[5] M. Romero-Gómez, F. Boza, M. S. García-Valdecasas, E. García, and J. Aguilar-Reina, "Subclinical hepatic encephalopathy predicts the development of overt hepatic encephalopathy," *The American Journal of Gastroenterology*, vol. 96, no. 9, pp. 2718–2723, 2001.

[6] J. S. Bajaj, M. Hafeezullah, J. Franco et al., "Inhibitory control test for the diagnosis of minimal hepatic encephalopathy," *Gastroenterology*, vol. 135, no. 5, pp. 1591.e1–1600.e1, 2008.

[7] G. Kircheis, W. E. Fleig, R. Görtelmeyer, S. Grafe, and D. Häussinger, "Assessment of low-grade hepatic encephalopathy: a critical analysis," *Journal of Hepatology*, vol. 47, no. 5, pp. 642–650, 2007.

[8] K. Weissenborn, N. Rückert, H. Hecker, and M. P. Manns, "The number connection tests A and B: interindividual variability

and use for the assessment of early hepatic encephalopathy," *Journal of Hepatology*, vol. 28, no. 4, pp. 646–653, 1998.

[9] R. K. Dhiman, V. A. Saraswat, M. Verma, and S. R. Naik, "Figure connection test: a universal test for assessment of mental state," *Journal of Gastroenterology and Hepatology*, vol. 10, no. 1, pp. 14–23, 1995.

[10] S. Iduru, K. Hisamuddin, and K. D. Mullen, "Minimal hepatic encephalopathy: simplifying its diagnosis," *The American Journal of Gastroenterology*, vol. 102, no. 7, pp. 1537–1538, 2007.

[11] J. Bajaj, "Minimal hepatic encephalopathy matters in daily life," *World Journal of Gastroenterology*, vol. 14, no. 23, pp. 3609–3615, 2008.

[12] P. Ferenci, A. Lockwood, K. Mullen, R. Tarter, K. Weissenborn, and A. T. Blei, "Hepatic encephalopathy—definition, nomenclature, diagnosis, and quantification: final report of the Working Party at the 11th World Congresses of Gastroenterology, Vienna, 1998," *Hepatology*, vol. 35, no. 3, pp. 716–721, 2002.

[13] H. Schomerus and W. Hamster, "Quality of life in cirrhotics with minimal hepatic encephalopathy," *Metabolic Brain Disease*, vol. 16, no. 1-2, pp. 37–41, 2001.

[14] N. Kumar, C. Shekhar, P. Kumar, and A. S. Kundu, "Kuppuswamy's socioeconomic status scale-updating for 2007," *The Indian Journal of Pediatrics*, vol. 74, no. 12, pp. 1131–1132, 2007.

[15] D. J. Siegel, "Perception and cognition," in *Kaplan and Sadock's Synopsis of Psychiatry: Behavioral Sciences/Clinical Psychiatry*, B. Kaplan and V. Kaplan, Eds., pp. 45–50, Lippincott Williams & Wilkins, Philadelphia, Pa, USA, 9th edition, 2003.

[16] G. Kircheis, N. Hilger, and D. Häussinger, "Value of critical flicker frequency and psychometric hepatic encephalopathy score in diagnosis of low-grade hepatic encephalopathy," *Gastroenterology*, vol. 146, no. 4, pp. 961.e11–969.e11, 2014.

[17] P. M. Bossuyt, J. B. Reitsma, D. E. Bruns et al., "Towards complete and accurate reporting of studies of diagnostic accuracy: the STARD initiative," *Clinical Chemistry and Laboratory Medicine*, vol. 41, no. 1, pp. 68–73, 2003.

[18] M. Romero-Gómez, J. Córdoba, R. Jover et al., "Value of the critical flicker frequency in patients with minimal hepatic encephalopathy," *Hepatology*, vol. 45, no. 4, pp. 879–885, 2007.

[19] J. Córdoba, "New assessment of hepatic encephalopathy," *Journal of Hepatology*, vol. 54, no. 5, pp. 1030–1040, 2011.

[20] S. Mooney, T. I. Hasssanein, R. C. Hilsabeck et al., "Utility of the Repeatable Battery for the Assessment of Neuropsychological Status (RBANS) in patients with end-stage liver disease awaiting liver transplant," *Archives of Clinical Neuropsychology*, vol. 22, no. 2, pp. 175–186, 2007.

[21] K. Weissenborn, J. C. Ennen, H. Schomerus, N. Rückert, and H. Hecker, "Neuropsychological characterization of hepatic encephalopathy," *Journal of Hepatology*, vol. 34, no. 5, pp. 768–773, 2001.

[22] S. Iduru and K. D. Mullen, "The demise of the pencil? New computer-assisted tests for minimal hepatic encephalopathy," *Gastroenterology*, vol. 135, no. 5, pp. 1455–1456, 2008.

[23] H. Mardini, B. K. Saxby, and C. O. Record, "Computerized psychometric testing in minimal encephalopathy and modulation by nitrogen challenge and liver transplant," *Gastroenterology*, vol. 135, no. 5, pp. 1582–1590, 2008.

[24] J. S. Bajaj, K. Saeian, M. D. Verber et al., "Inhibitory control test is a simple method to diagnose minimal hepatic encephalopathy and predict development of overt hepatic encephalopathy," *The American Journal of Gastroenterology*, vol. 102, no. 4, pp. 754–760, 2007.

[25] P. Amodio, P. Marchetti, F. del Piccolo et al., "Study on the sternberg paradigm in cirrhotic patients without overt hepatic encephalopathy," *Metabolic Brain Disease*, vol. 13, no. 2, pp. 159–172, 1998.

[26] P. Sharma and B. C. Sharma, "Predictors of minimal hepatic encephalopathy in patients with cirrhosis," *Saudi Journal of Gastroenterology*, vol. 16, no. 3, pp. 181–187, 2010.

[27] A. Das, R. K. Dhiman, V. A. Saraswat, M. Verma, and S. R. Naik, "Prevalence and natural history of subclinical hepatic encephalopathy in cirrhosis," *Journal of Gastroenterology and Hepatology (Australia)*, vol. 16, no. 5, pp. 531–535, 2001.

[28] R. K. Dhiman, V. A. Saraswat, B. K. Sharma et al., "Minimal hepatic encephalopathy: consensus statement of a working party of the Indian National Association for Study of the Liver," *Journal of Gastroenterology and Hepatology*, vol. 25, no. 6, pp. 1029–1041, 2010.

[29] J. S. Bajaj, A. Etemadian, M. Hafeezullah, and K. Saeian, "Testing for minimal hepatic encephalopathy in the United States: an AASLD survey," *Hepatology*, vol. 45, no. 3, pp. 833–834, 2007.

[30] M. Vergara-Gómez, M. Flavià-Olivella, M. Gil-Prades, B. Dalmau-Obrador, and J. Córdoba-Cardona, "Diagnosis and treatment of hepatic encephalopathy in Spain: results of a survey of hepatologists," *Gastroenterologia y Hepatologia*, vol. 29, no. 1, pp. 1–6, 2006.

[31] J. Varghese, M. A. Thiravia, B. Natarajan, and J. Venkataraman, "Critical flicker test: yet another tool for minimal hepatic encephalopathy," *European Journal of Gastroenterology and Hepatology*, vol. 19, no. 11, p. 1031, 2007.

# 14

# Evaluation of Serum Cystatin C as a Marker of Early Renal Impairment in Patients with Liver Cirrhosis

**Mahmoud Omar,[1] Wael Abdel-Razek,[1] Gamal Abo-Raia,[2] Medhat Assem,[1] and Gasser El-Azab[1]**

[1]*Department of Hepatology, National Liver Institute, Menoufia University, Shebeen El-Kom, Egypt*
[2]*Department of Clinical Pathology, National Liver Institute, Menoufia University, Shebeen El-Kom, Egypt*

Correspondence should be addressed to Gasser El-Azab; g.elazab@gmail.com

Academic Editor: Daisuke Morioka

*Background.* Serum cystatin C (CysC) was proposed as an effective reflection of the glomerular filtration rate (GFR). However, its role in patients with liver cirrhosis has not been extensively verified especially in the detection of early RI. *Patients and Methods.* Seventy consecutive potential candidates for living donor liver transplantation with serum creatinine (Cr) <1.5 mg/dL were included. CysC, Cr, and estimated GFR [creatinine clearance (CCr), Cockcroft-Gault formula (C-G), MDRD equations with 4 and 6 variables, CKD-EPI-Cr, CKD-EPI-CysC, and CKD-EPI-Cr-CysC] were all correlated to isotopic GFR. Early RI was defined as GFR of 60–89 mL/min/1.73 $m^2$. *Results.* Patients were 25.7% and 74.3% Child-Pugh classes B and C, respectively. GFR was ≥90, 60–89, and 30–59 mL/min/1.73 $m^2$ in 31.4%, 64.3%, and 4.3% of the patients, respectively. All markers and equations, except C-G, were significantly correlated to GFR with CKD-EPI-Cr-CysC formula having the highest correlation ($r = 0.474$) and the largest area under the ROC curve (0.808) for discriminating early RI. At a cutoff value of 1.2 mg/L, CysC was 89.6% sensitive and 63.6% specific in detecting early RI. *Conclusion.* In patients with liver cirrhosis, CysC and CysC-based equations showed the highest significant correlation to GFR and were measures that best discriminated early RI.

## 1. Introduction

Renal impairment is a common finding in patients with chronic liver disease; it has a huge impact on the patients' survival [1]. Moreover, the severity of renal dysfunction increases with the advancement of liver cirrhosis and portal hypertension [2]. Therefore, close follow-up of the renal function in patients with liver cirrhosis is mandatory and markers of early renal impairment are priceless in these patients [2].

Using the current markers and equations of the renal function in cirrhotic patients can be challenging. Serum creatinine, the most widely used marker, may underestimate renal impairment in patients with liver cirrhosis. Decreased hepatic production of creatine, reduced muscle mass, and malnutrition account for an increased gap between serum creatinine levels and the actual renal function [3]. High serum bilirubin levels may also interfere with the analytical methods of serum creatinine measurement, although this is no more a problem after using the modern Jaffe method autoanalyzers [4]. Inulin clearance, the standard method for measuring the glomerular filtration rate (GFR), is costly and impractical as it requires 24-hour urinary catheterization [5]. Isotopic renal scans are not less costly; they cannot be used for repeated measurements that are needed in such patients. Creatinine clearance tends to overestimate the GFR and requires accurate urine volume measurement [6]. Based on serum creatinine, Cockcroft-Gault formula and modification of diet in renal disease (MDRD) equations are of limited value in cirrhotic patients; they overestimate the GFR as well [7].

Serum cystatin C (CysC) has been proposed as a novel biomarker of the renal function [8]. Several studies have reported its value in different sets of patients [9–16]. However, only few studies have evaluated the role of serum CysC in patients with liver cirrhosis [17–19] and none of these studies have studied its role in detecting early renal impairment in

TABLE 1: GFR-estimating equations used in the study.

| | |
|---|---|
| Cockcroft-Gault formula | 140 − age (years) × weight (kg)/(Scr × 72) × 0.85 if female |
| MDRD equations using 4 variables | $186 \times Scr^{-1.154} \times age\ (years)^{-0.203} \times 0.742$ if female × 1.212 if black |
| MDRD equations using 6 variables | $170 \times Scr^{-0.999} \times age\ (years)^{-0.176} \times BUN\ (mg/dL)^{-0.170} \times albumin\ (g/dL)^{0.318} \times 0.762$ if female × 1.180 if black |
| The CKD-EPI creatinine equation | $141 \times \min(Scr/\kappa, 1)^{\alpha} \times \max(Scr/\kappa, 1)^{-1.209} \times 0.993^{Age}$ [×1.018 if female] [×1.159 if black], where $\alpha$ is −0.329 for females and −0.411 for males |
| The CKD-EPI cystatin C equation | $133 \times \min(Scys/0.8, 1)^{-0.499} \times \max(Scys/0.8, 1)^{-1.328} \times 0.996^{Age}$ [×0.932 if female] |
| The CKD-EPI creatinine–cystatin C equation | $135 \times \min(Scr/\kappa, 1)^{\alpha} \times \max(Scr/\kappa, 1)^{-0.601} \times \min(Scys/0.8, 1)^{-0.375} \times \max(Scys/0.8, 1)^{-0.711} \times 0.995^{Age}$ [×0.969 if female] [×1.08 if black], where $\alpha$ is −0.248 for females and −0.207 for males |

$\kappa$ is 0.7 for females and 0.9 for males, max is the maximum of Scr/$\kappa$ or 1, min is the minimum of Scr/$\kappa$ or 1, Scr is serum creatinine in (mg/dL), and Scys is serum cystatin C in (mg/L).

these patients. In our study, we aimed at evaluating the role of serum CysC as a marker of the renal function in patients with liver cirrhosis and, more important, as an indicator of renal impairment at its early stages in such patients. We compared different markers and estimating equations, including serum CysC and CysC-based equations, to the isotopic GFR being used as the gold standard of the actual renal performance.

## 2. Methodology

*2.1. Patients.* This prospective observational study was conducted on seventy consecutive patients with liver cirrhosis who presented to the Liver Transplantation Unit, National Liver Institute, Menoufia University, as potential candidates for liver transplantation. The diagnosis of cirrhosis was based on a combination of clinical, laboratory, and ultrasonographic findings [20]. Patients aged 18–80 years were eligible for the study if they had serum creatinine less than 1.5 mg/dL. Patients were excluded if they had dehydration, sepsis, or gastrointestinal bleeding during the month before enrollment. The local ethics committee approved the study. A written informed consent was obtained from all participating patients prior to inclusion in the study.

*2.2. Baseline Assessment.* Included patients were subjected to history taking, clinical examination, abdominal ultrasonography, and baseline laboratory investigations including liver and renal tests, urine analysis, and complete blood count. Child-Pugh [21, 22] and MELD [23] scores were calculated for all patients.

*2.3. Assessment of the Renal Function.* Enrolled patients underwent $^{99m}$Tc-DTPA renal scan to measure the isotopic GFR. Serum and urine samples were collected on the same day of the renal scan. Serum samples were used to measure serum creatinine, CysC, and blood urea nitrogen (BUN). The Quantikine Human Cystatin C Immunoassay (R&D Systems Inc., Minneapolis, MN, USA), an enzyme-linked immunosorbent assay (ELISA), was used to measure serum CysC on a CX7 analyzer (Beckman, Brea, CA, USA). Creatinine clearance (CCr) was calculated through the following equation: CCr = (urinary creatinine × 24 hours of urine volume)/(serum creatinine × 1440) [24]. GFR was furthermore calculated using six estimating formulae, Cockcroft-Gault formula [25], the modification of diet in renal disease (MDRD) equations using 4 and 6 variables [26, 27], and Chronic Kidney Disease Epidemiology Collaboration (CKD-EPI) equations using creatinine alone (CKD-EPI Cr) [28], CysC alone (CKD-EPI CysC), or both CKD-EPI (Cr-CysC) [29] (Table 1). Isotopic GFR was used as the reference to which all other measures and estimating formulae of the renal function were compared. In this study, the upper limit of normal for serum creatinine was 1.2 mg/dL and early renal impairment was defined as a GFR of 60–89 mL/min.

*2.4. Statistical Analysis.* Data were analyzed using IBM SPSS Statistics for Macintosh, Version 22.0 (IBM Corp., Armonk, NY, USA). Two-tailed $p$ values were considered statistically significant if they were less than 0.05.

Bivariate correlations were tested using Pearson's ($r$) and Spearman's (rho) correlation coefficients for parametric and nonparametric measure of statistical dependence, respectively. The coefficient of determination ($R^2$) was also calculated to measure the percent of variation in one variable which could be predicted by the variation in the other variable. $R^2$ closer to 1 indicates a better model fit.

The ability of the studied tests and formulae to discriminate early renal impairment was evaluated using the area under the receiver operating characteristic (ROC) curve (AUC). A cutoff was then proposed to each test or formula with the most acceptable sensitivity and specificity. The following tests of diagnostic accuracy were calculated for the measures and estimates of the renal function with a 95% confidence interval: sensitivity, specificity, positive predictive value (PPV), and negative predictive value (NPV).

Bland-Altman plot was used to analyze the agreement between isotopic GFR and the other mathematical formulae of GFR. One sample $t$-test was used to test for significance of the difference between each of these formulae and isotopic GFR.

Table 2: Baseline characteristics of the enrolled patients.

| | Mean ± SD | Range |
|---|---|---|
| Age (years) | 47.4 ± 9.3 | 18–75 |
| Weight (kg) | 78.2 ± 14.7 | 48–110 |
| Total bilirubin (mg/dL) | 3.9 ± 3.2 | 0.6–17.5 |
| Albumin (g/dL) | 2.6 ± 0.5 | 1.7–3.5 |
| Isotopic GFR (mL/min) | 84.5 ± 16.6 | 53–133 |
| BUN (mg/dL) | 19.3 ± 10.8 | 4.7–72.3 |
| Creatinine (mg/dL) | 0.8 ± 0.3 | 0.3–1.4 |
| Creatinine clearance (mL/min) | 82.4 ± 31.3 | 24–199 |
| Cystatin C (mg/L) | 1.9 ± 1 | 0.3–4.5 |
| Child-Pugh score | 10.7 ± 1.7 | 7–14 |
| MELD score | 16.2 ± 4.9 | 8–31 |
| MDRD 4 (mL/min) | 119.2 ± 63.5 | 45.7–367 |
| MDRD 6 (mL/min) | 97.4 ± 50.4 | 28.4–291.7 |
| Cockcroft-Gault formula (mL/min) | 132.9 ± 65 | 47.9–421.1 |
| CKD-EPI-Cr (mL/min) | 101.0 ± 26.7 | 47.1–175.6 |
| CKD-EPI-CysC (mL/min) | 52 ± 40 | 11.4–185.9 |
| CKD-EPI-Cr-CysC (mL/min) | 61.5 ± 26.3 | 29.7–154.8 |

BUN, blood urea nitrogen; CKD-EPI, Chronic Kidney Disease Epidemiology Collaboration; GFR, glomerular filtration rate; MDRD, modification of diet in renal disease equation with 4 and 6 variables; MELD, model for end-stage liver disease; SD, standard deviation.

## 3. Results

The baseline characteristics and demographic and clinical data of the enrolled patients are presented in Tables 2 and 3. The study sample had predominance of males (87.1%). Etiology of the liver disease was most commonly chronic hepatitis C infection (72.9%). About 29% of the patients had hepatocellular carcinoma (HCC). Most patients were Child-Pugh class C (74.3%) and had moderate ascites (41.4%). About 64% of the patients had early renal impairment. None of the patients had proteinuria or other urine abnormalities.

Different measures and estimates of the renal function were correlated with the isotopic GFR using Pearson's correlation (Table 4). Serum CysC and CKD-EPI equations using CysC alone or both creatinine and CysC had the highest and most significant correlation coefficient ($r$ = 0.437, 0.473, and 0.474, resp., $p < 0.0001$) (Figure 1). CKD-EPI (Cr-CysC) had the highest $R^2$ among all other measures.

The discriminating ability of the studied measures and estimates of the renal function in detecting early renal impairment was assessed by plotting the ROC curves (Figure 2). Table 5 presents the AUC for each of the measures and formulae. CKD-EPI (Cr-CysC) had the largest AUC (0.808, $p < 0.0001$). We then used the ROC curves' coordinates to define cutoff values with acceptable sensitivity and specificity for the studied tests and formulae. Table 6 shows the sensitivity, specificity, PPV, and NPV for the different measures and formulae in detecting early renal impairment according to these cutoff values. At a cutoff value of 1.2 mg/L, CysC was 89.6% sensitive and 63.6% specific in detecting early renal impairment with PPV of 84.3% and NPV of 73.7%.

Table 3: Demographic and clinical data of the enrolled patients.

| | $n$ (%) |
|---|---|
| Sex | |
| Males | 61 (87.1) |
| Females | 9 (12.9) |
| Etiology of liver disease | |
| Chronic hepatitis C | 51 (72.9) |
| Chronic hepatitis B | 12 (17.1) |
| Budd-Chiari syndrome | 2 (2.9) |
| Unknown etiology | 5 (7.1) |
| HCC | |
| No | 50 (71.4) |
| Yes | 20 (28.6) |
| Ascites | |
| No | 9 (12.9) |
| Mild | 23 (32.8) |
| Moderate | 29 (41.4) |
| Marked | 9 (12.9) |
| Child-Pugh class | |
| B | 18 (25.7) |
| C | 52 (74.3) |
| Renal impairment | |
| No (GFR ≥90 mL/min) | 22 (31.4) |
| Early (GFR 60–89 mL/min) | 45 (64.3) |
| Advanced (GFR 30–59 mL/min) | 3 (4.3) |

GFR, glomerular filtration rate; HCC, hepatocellular carcinoma.

Table 4: Pearson's correlation of the variables with the isotopic GFR.

| | $r$ | $p$ |
|---|---|---|
| 1/creatinine ($mg/dL^{-1}$) | 0.287 | 0.016 |
| Creatinine clearance (mL/min) | 0.367 | 0.002 |
| 1/cystatin C ($mg/L^{-1}$) | 0.437 | <0.0001 |
| MDRD 4 | 0.260 | 0.030 |
| MDRD 6 | 0.286 | 0.017 |
| Cockcroft-Gault formula | 0.198 | 0.100 |
| CKD-EPI-Cr | 0.247 | 0.039 |
| CKD-EPI-CysC | 0.473 | <0.0001 |
| CKD-EPI-Cr-CysC | 0.474 | <0.0001 |

CKD-EPI, Chronic Kidney Disease Epidemiology Collaboration; Cr, creatinine; CysC, cystatin C; MDRD, modification of diet in renal disease equation with 4 and 6 variables; $r$, Pearson's correlation coefficient.

The Bland-Altman plot was used to describe agreement between isotopic GFR and different mathematical formulae (Table 7 and Figure 3). The mean difference with CCr was 2.0429, which was not statistically significant ($p = 0.565$).

## 4. Discussion

This study showed that serum CysC and CysC-based equations were the best measures that correlated with the isotopic GFR, compared to other measures and equations that have been evaluated in the study. This confirms the results of the

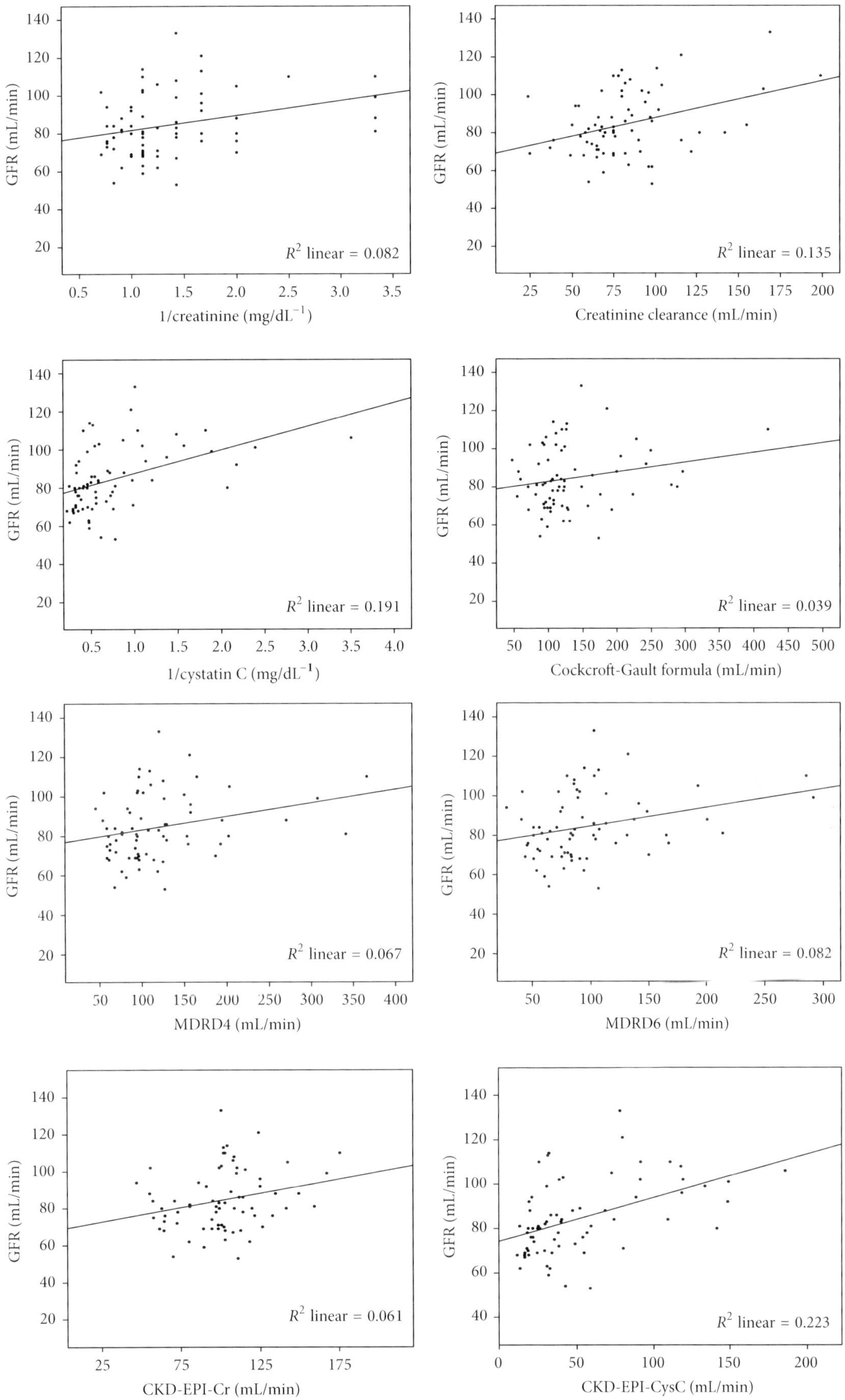


FIGURE 1: Continued.

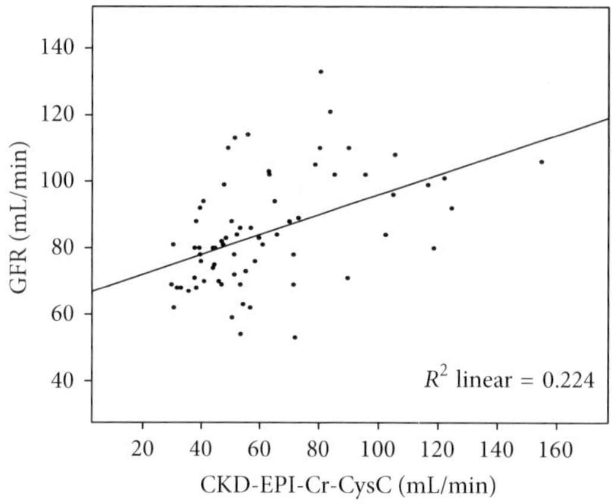


FIGURE 1: Scatter plots of the isotopic glomerular filtration rate (GFR) versus 1/creatinine, creatinine clearance, 1/cystatin C, Cockcroft-Gault formula, MDRD equations with 4 and 6 variables, CKD-EPI-Cr, CKD-EPI-CysC, and CKD-EPI-Cr-CysC.

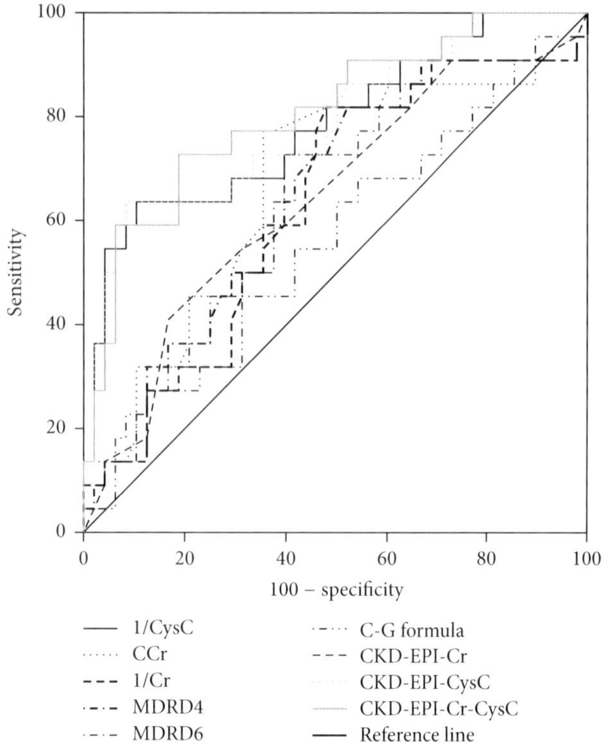


FIGURE 2: ROC curves of 1/creatinine, creatinine clearance, 1/cystatin C, MDRD equations with 4 and 6 variables, Cockcroft-Gault formula, CKD-EPI-Cr, CKD-EPI-CysC, and CKD-EPI-Cr-CysC for detecting early renal impairment.

TABLE 5: Area under the curve for detecting early renal impairment for studied tests and formulae.

| Variable | AUC | 95% CI | $p$ |
|---|---|---|---|
| 1/Cr | 0.642 | 0.500–0.784 | 0.058 |
| CCr | 0.674 | 0.533–0.815 | 0.020 |
| 1/CysC | 0.785 | 0.663–0.907 | <0.0001 |
| MDRD 4 | 0.646 | 0.506–0.787 | 0.051 |
| MDRD 6 | 0.644 | 0.503–0.784 | 0.054 |
| C-G formula | 0.562 | 0.413–0.710 | 0.411 |
| CKD-EPI-Cr | 0.632 | 0.491–0.773 | 0.078 |
| CKD-EPI-CysC | 0.788 | 0.667–0.909 | <0.0001 |
| CKD-EPI-Cr-CysC | 0.808 | 0.695–0.921 | <0.0001 |

AUC, area under the curve; C-G formula, Cockcroft-Gault formula; CKD-EPI, Chronic Kidney Disease Epidemiology Collaboration; CI, confidence interval; Cr, creatinine; CCr, creatinine clearance; CysC, cystatin C; MDRD, modification of diet in renal disease equation with 4 and 6 variables.

previous studies that came up with similar conclusions [18, 30–32]. Several studies have reported the superior diagnostic accuracy of serum CysC and CysC-based formulae over other markers and equations in detecting moderate and severe renal impairment in patients with liver cirrhosis [18, 33, 34]. However, since patients with liver cirrhosis are extremely sensitive to the modest decreases in the GFR that can markedly impact their survival [35], it is of great clinical importance to identify markers that can detect renal impairment at its early stage in these patients. Using Pearson's correlation, our study found that CKD-EPI (Cr-CysC) formula was the most accurate marker, with the largest AUC, in detecting early renal impairment in patients with liver cirrhosis. This finding is novel, putting CysC and CysC-based equations on the top of the list of markers and estimating formulae of the renal function in such patients. The results also showed that serum CysC was the most sensitive (89.6%) measure in detecting early renal impairment at a cutoff value of 1.2 mg/L with acceptable specificity (63.6%).

One strong limitation of serum creatinine and creatinine-based equations is that serum creatinine lags behind a decreasing GFR [36]. So they are not accurately reflecting the present status of the renal function of the patient, a limitation that has been overcome by serum CysC that proved to accurately reflect the early stages of renal impairment according to the results of this study.

However, Bland-Altman plot analysis showed disputing results. Estimated CCr was the only measurement that had significant agreement with isotopic GFR. This contradiction may be explained as a correlation coefficient between two

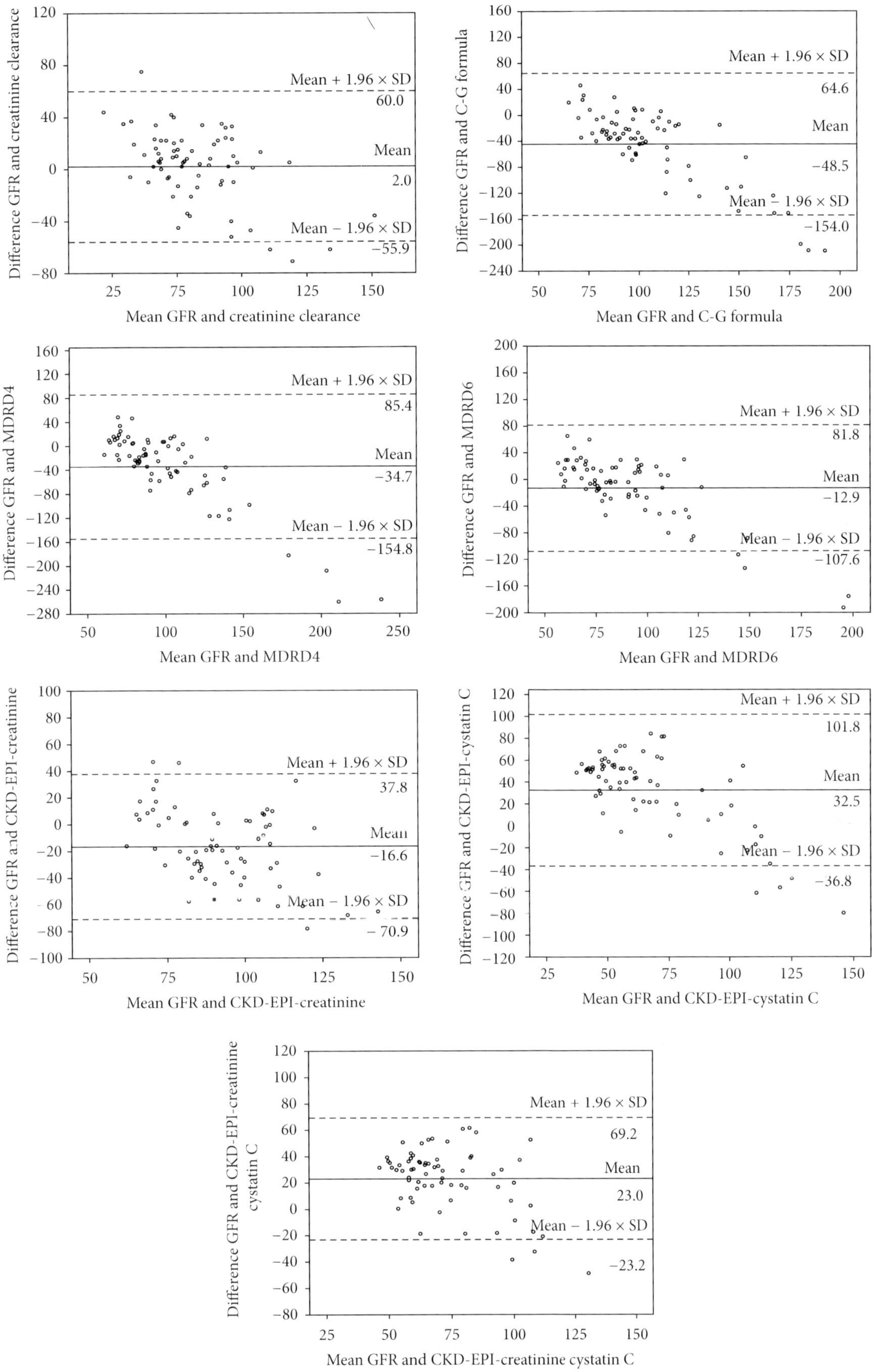


FIGURE 3: Bland-Altman plot for the agreement between isotopic GFR and the other GFR estimating formulae.

Table 6: Cutoffs of measures and estimates for detection of early renal impairment with their measures of diagnostic accuracy.

| | Cutoff of early RI | Sensitivity (%) | Specificity (%) | PPV (%) | NPV (%) |
|---|---|---|---|---|---|
| Cr | 0.75 mg/dL | 68.8 | 54.5 | 76.7 | 44.4 |
| CCr | 77 mL/min | 77.3 | 64.6 | 54.5 | 60.9 |
| CysC | 1.2 mg/L | 89.6 | 63.6 | 84.3 | 73.7 |
| MDRD 4 | 96.8 mL/min | 72.7 | 54.2 | 57.3 | 62.7 |
| MDRD 6 | 85.5 mL/min | 72.7 | 60.4 | 54.6 | 59.2 |
| C-G formula | 119.3 mL/min | 54.5 | 58.3 | 48.3 | 47.8 |
| CKD-EPI-Cr | 99.8 mL/min | 77.3 | 55.2 | 63.3 | 70.9 |
| CKD-EPI-CysC | 38.7 mL/min | 72.7 | 66.7 | 68.6 | 71.0 |
| CKD-EPI-Cr-CysC | 52.8 mL/min | 77.3 | 61.4 | 66.7 | 73.0 |

C-G formula, Cockcroft-Gault formula; CKD-EPI, Chronic Kidney Disease Epidemiology Collaboration; Cr, creatinine; CCr, creatinine clearance; CysC, cystatin C; MDRD, modification of diet in renal disease equation with 4 and 6 variables; NPV, negative predictive value; PPV, positive predictive value; RI, renal impairment.

Table 7: Bland-Altman plot analysis for the agreement between isotopic GFR and the other GFR estimating formulae.

| | Mean ± SD | $p$ | 95% CI |
|---|---|---|---|
| CCr | 2.04 ± 29.6 | 0.565 | −5.0–9.1 |
| C-G formula | −44.7 ± 55.8 | <0.0001 | −58.1–−31.3 |
| MDRD 4 | −34.7 ± 61.3 | <0.0001 | −49.3–−20.1 |
| MDRD 6 | −12.9 ± 48.3 | 0.028 | −24.5–−1.4 |
| CKD-EPI-Cr | −16.6 ± 27.7 | <0.0001 | −23.2–−9.9 |
| CKD-EPI-CysC | 32.5 ± 35.3 | <0.0001 | 24.1–40.9 |
| CKD-EPI-Cr-CysC | 23 ± 23.6 | <0.0001 | 17.4–28.6 |

C-G formula, Cockcroft-Gault formula; CKD-EPI, Chronic Kidney Disease Epidemiology Collaboration; Cr, creatinine; CCr, creatinine clearance; CysC, cystatin C; MDRD, modification of diet in renal disease equation with 4 and 6 variables.

measures might be highly correlated; yet, there could be substantial differences in the two measurements across their range of values. Also, results of Bland-Altman method might be disturbed when there is heterogeneous bias with significant heteroscedastic error [37].

The results of this study are robust even though the sample size was relatively small because we have used the isotopic GFR as the reference to which all other measures and formulae were compared. Therefore, in contrast to some previous studies that used CCr as reference [33, 38], the results of our study can be generalized over a larger scale. Still, we recommend further studies to be designed to confirm and validate the results of this study. Future studies should formulate a general predictive model of the renal function in patients with liver cirrhosis based on serum CysC levels, a model that can make the isotopic GFR dispensable.

In conclusion, finding a good marker of the renal function is crucial to the survival of patients with liver cirrhosis, given the huge impact of the renal impairment on the prognosis of these patients. Our study found that serum CysC and CysC-based formulae were not only the best measures that reflected the actual renal performance in cirrhotic patients, but also the most accurate ones in detecting early stages of renal impairment in these patients.

## References

[1] A. Slack, A. Yeoman, and J. Wendon, "Renal dysfunction in chronic liver disease," *Critical Care*, vol. 14, no. 2, article 214, 2010.

[2] V. Arroyo, J. Fernandez, and P. Ginès, "Pathogenesis and treatment of hepatorenal syndrome," *Seminars in Liver Disease*, vol. 28, no. 1, pp. 81–95, 2008.

[3] T. Takabatake, H. Ohta, Y.-I. Ishida, H. Hara, Y. Ushiogi, and N. Hattori, "Low serum creatinine levels in severe hepatic disease," *Archives of Internal Medicine*, vol. 148, no. 6, pp. 1313–1315, 1988.

[4] A. J. Slack and J. Wendon, "The liver and kidney in critically ill patients," *Blood Purification*, vol. 28, no. 2, pp. 124–134, 2009.

[5] E. Cholongitas, V. Shusang, L. Marelli et al., "Review article: renal function assessment in cirrhosis—difficulties and alternative measurements," *Alimentary Pharmacology and Therapeutics*, vol. 26, no. 7, pp. 969–978, 2007.

[6] N. L. Proulx, A. Akbari, A. X. Garg, A. Rostom, J. Jaffey, and H. D. Clark, "Measured creatinine clearance from timed urine collections substantially overestimates glomerular filtration rate in patients with liver cirrhosis: a systematic review and individual patient meta-analysis," *Nephrology Dialysis Transplantation*, vol. 20, no. 8, pp. 1617–1622, 2005.

[7] J. MacAulay, K. Thompson, B. A. Kiberd, D. C. Barnes, and K. M. Peltekian, "Serum creatinine in patients with advanced liver disease is of limited value for identification of moderate renal dysfunction: are the equations for estimating renal function better?" *Canadian Journal of Gastroenterology*, vol. 20, no. 8, pp. 521–526, 2006.

[8] L. A. Stevens, J. Coresh, T. Greene, and A. S. Levey, "Assessing kidney function—measured and estimated glomerular filtration rate," *The New England Journal of Medicine*, vol. 354, no. 23, pp. 2473–2483, 2006.

[9] Y. Kandasamy, R. Smith, and I. M. R. Wright, "Measuring cystatin C to determine renal function in neonates," *Pediatric Critical Care Medicine*, vol. 14, no. 3, pp. 318–322, 2013.

[10] R. B. Dhia, I. Hellara, O. Harzallah et al., "Evaluation of the renal function in type 2 diabetes: clearance calculation or cystatin C?" *Annales de Biologie Clinique*, vol. 70, no. 3, pp. 287–294, 2012.

[11] H.-X. Guo, C.-H. Wang, Z.-Q. Li et al., "The application of serum cystatin C in estimating the renal function in women with preeclampsia," *Reproductive Sciences*, vol. 19, no. 7, pp. 712–717, 2012.

[12] S. Niemczyk, M. Piotrowska, and K. Szamotulska, "Usefulness of creatinine and cystatin C in the assessment of renal function in chronic kidney disease and coexisting diseases," *Polski Merkuriusz Lekarski*, vol. 32, no. 191, pp. 313–317, 2012.

[13] M. M. Sagheb, S. Namazi, B. Geramizadeh, A. Karimzadeh, M. B. Oghazian, and I. Karimzadeh, "Serum cystatin C as a marker of renal function in critically Ill patients with normal serum creatinine," *Nephro-Urology Monthly*, vol. 6, no. 2, Article ID e15224, 2014.

[14] Y. Suzuki, K. Matsushita, T. Yoshida, Y. Sawabe, and F. Nomura, "Clinical validity of renal function markers including serum cystatin C on chronic kidney disease classification," *Rinsho Byori*, vol. 59, no. 4, pp. 345–351, 2011.

[15] Y. Suzuki, M. Seimiya, T. Yoshida, Y. Sawabe, K. Matsushita, and F. Nomura, "Usefulness of the standardized serum cystatin C reagent in evaluation of renal function," *Rinsho Byori*, vol. 61, no. 8, pp. 665–670, 2013.

[16] K.-S. Woo, J.-L. Choi, B.-R. Kim, J.-E. Kim, and J.-Y. Han, "Clinical usefulness of serum cystatin C as a marker of renal function," *Diabetes and Metabolism Journal*, vol. 38, no. 4, pp. 278–284, 2014.

[17] Đ. Ćulafić, "Role of cystatin C and renal resistive index in assessment of renal function in patients with liver cirrhosis," *World Journal of Gastroenterology*, vol. 20, no. 21, pp. 6573–6579, 2014.

[18] D. J. Kim, H. S. Kang, H. S. Choi et al., "Serum cystatin C level is a useful marker for the evaluation of renal function in patients with cirrhotic ascites and normal serum creatinine levels," *The Korean Journal of Hepatology*, vol. 17, no. 2, pp. 130–138, 2011.

[19] Y. Ustundag, K. Hekimoğlu, S. Ilikhan, G. Zaimoğlu, S. Acikgöz, and S. Aydemir, "Serum glucagon and cystatin C levels with renal doppler sonography findings in non-azotemic liver cirrhosis cases," *Hepato-Gastroenterology*, vol. 58, no. 107-108, pp. 926–931, 2011.

[20] D. Schuppan and N. H. Afdhal, "Liver cirrhosis," *The Lancet*, vol. 371, no. 9615, pp. 838–851, 2008.

[21] C. G. Child and J. G. Turcotte, "Surgery and portal hypertension," *Major problems in clinical surgery*, vol. 1, pp. 1–85, 1964.

[22] R. N. H. Pugh, I. M. Murray Lyon, and J. L. Dawson, "Transection of the oesophagus for bleeding oesophageal varices," *British Journal of Surgery*, vol. 60, no. 8, pp. 646–649, 1973.

[23] R. Wiesner, E. Edwards, R. Freeman et al., "Model for end-stage liver disease (MELD) and allocation of donor livers," *Gastroenterology*, vol. 124, no. 1, pp. 91–96, 2003.

[24] B. A. C. van Acker, G. C. M. Koomen, M. G. Koopman, D. R. de Waart, and L. Arisz, "Creatinine clearance during cimetidine administration for measurement of glomerular filtration rate," *The Lancet*, vol. 340, no. 8831, pp. 1326–1329, 1992.

[25] D. W. Cockcroft and M. H. Gault, "Prediction of creatinine clearance from serum creatinine," *Nephron*, vol. 16, no. 1, pp. 31–41, 1976.

[26] A. S. Levey, J. P. Bosch, J. B. Lewis, T. Greene, N. Rogers, and D. Roth, "A more accurate method to estimate glomerular filtration rate from serum creatinine: a new prediction equation," *Annals of Internal Medicine*, vol. 130, no. 6, pp. 461–470, 1999.

[27] National Kidney Foundation, "K/DOQI clinical practice guidelines for chronic kidney disease: evaluation, classification, and stratification," *American Journal of Kidney Diseases*, vol. 39, no. 2, supplement 1, pp. S1–S266, 2002.

[28] A. S. Levey, L. A. Stevens, C. H. Schmid et al., "A new equation to estimate glomerular filtration rate," *Annals of Internal Medicine*, vol. 150, no. 9, pp. 604–612, 2009.

[29] L. A. Inker, C. H. Schmid, H. Tighiouart et al., "Estimating glomerular filtration rate from serum creatinine and cystatin C," *The New England Journal of Medicine*, vol. 367, no. 1, pp. 20–29, 2012.

[30] H. S. Ahn, Y. S. Kim, S. G. Kim et al., "Cystatin C is a good predictor of hepatorenal syndrome and survival in patients with cirrhosis who have normal serum creatinine levels," *Hepato-Gastroenterology*, vol. 59, no. 116, pp. 1168–1173, 2012.

[31] Y. Ustundag, U. Samsar, S. Acikgoz et al., "Analysis of glomerular filtration rate, serum cystatin C levels, and renal resistive index values in cirrhosis patients," *Clinical Chemistry and Laboratory Medicine*, vol. 45, no. 7, pp. 890–894, 2007.

[32] S. Demirtaş, A. Bozbaş, A. Akbay, Y. Yavuz, and L. Karaca, "Diagnostic value of serum cystatin C for evaluation of hepatorenal syndrome," *Clinica Chimica Acta*, vol. 311, no. 2, pp. 81–89, 2001.

[33] E. Randers, P. Ivarsen, E. J. Erlandsen et al., "Plasma cystatin C as a marker of renal function in patients with liver cirrhosis," *Scandinavian Journal of Clinical and Laboratory Investigation*, vol. 62, no. 2, pp. 129–134, 2002.

[34] M. Adachi, A. Tanaka, M. Aiso, Y. Takamori, and H. Takikawa, "Benefit of cystatin C in evaluation of renal function and prediction of survival in patients with cirrhosis," *Hepatology Research*, 2015.

[35] P. Ginès and R. W. Schrier, "Renal failure in cirrhosis," *The New England Journal of Medicine*, vol. 361, no. 13, pp. 1279–1290, 2009.

[36] S. Herget-Rosenthal, J. Metzger, A. Albalat, V. Bitsika, and H. Mischak, "Proteomic biomarkers for the early detection of acute kidney injury," *Prilozi*, vol. 33, no. 1, pp. 27–48, 2012.

[37] D. P. O'Connor, M. T. Mahar, M. S. Laughlin, and A. S. Jackson, "The Bland-Altman method should not be used in regression cross-validation studies," *Research Quarterly for Exercise and Sport*, vol. 82, no. 4, pp. 610–616, 2011.

[38] A. L. Gerbes, V. Gulberg, M. Bilzer, and M. Vogeser, "Evaluation of serum cystatin C concentration as a marker of renal function in patients with cirrhosis of the liver," *Gut*, vol. 50, no. 1, pp. 106–110, 2002.

15

# IFNL4 ss469415590 Variant Is Associated with Treatment Response in Japanese HCV Genotype 1 Infected Individuals Treated with IFN-Including Regimens

**Tatsuo Miyamura,[1] Tatsuo Kanda,[1] Shingo Nakamoto,[2] Makoto Arai,[1] Masato Nakamura,[1] Shuang Wu,[1] Xia Jiang,[1] Reina Sasaki,[1] Yuki Haga,[1] Shin Yasui,[1] Yoshihiko Ooka,[1] Tetsuhiro Chiba,[1] Fumio Imazeki,[1] Shigeru Mikami,[3] and Osamu Yokosuka[1]**

[1] *Departments of Gastroenterology and Nephrology, Graduate School of Medicine, Chiba University, 1-8-1 Inohana, Chuo-ku, Chiba 260-8677, Japan*
[2] *Department of Molecular Virology, Graduate School of Medicine, Chiba University, Chiba 260-8677, Japan*
[3] *Department of Gastroenterology, Kikkoman General Hospital, Noda 278-0005, Japan*

Correspondence should be addressed to Tatsuo Kanda; kandat-cib@umin.ac.jp

Academic Editor: Shigeru Marubashi

*Aim.* Eradication of hepatitis C virus (HCV) is still challenging even if interferon- (IFN-) free regimens with direct-acting antiviral agents (DAAs) for HCV-infected individuals are available in clinical practice. IFNL4 is a newly described protein, associated with human antiviral defenses. We investigated whether IFNL4 ss469415590 variant has an effect on the prediction of treatment response in HCV-infected patients treated with IFN-including regimens. *Patients and Methods.* In all, 185 patients infected with HCV genotype 1 treated with peg-IFN plus ribavirin, with or without telaprevir, were genotyped for IFNL4 ss469415590. We retrospectively investigated whether the role of IFNL4 ss469415590 variant and other factors could predict sustained virological response (SVR) in Japanese patients infected with HCV genotype 1. *Results.* There were 65.7%, 31.5%, and 2.8% patients in the IFNL4 ss469415590 TT/TT, TT/-G, and -G/-G groups, respectively. SVR rates were 82.1% or 49.3% in patients treated with peg-IFN plus ribavirin with or without telaprevir, respectively. IFNL4 ss469415590 variant and HCV viral loads or IFNL4 ss469415590 variant and early virological response were better predictors of SVR in patients treated with peg-IFN plus ribavirin with or without telaprevir, respectively. *Conclusion.* In the era of DAAs, measurement of IFNL4 ss469415590 variant could help the prediction of SVR in Japanese HCV genotype 1 infected individuals treated with IFN-including regimens.

## 1. Introduction

Chronic hepatitis C virus (HCV) infection is a leading cause of hepatocellular carcinoma (HCC) and end-stage liver disease requiring liver transplantation in the United States [1, 2]. In Japan, HCV infection is still a major cause of HCC [3]. At present, HCV infection is a world health problem.

The former standard treatment with peginterferon (peg-IFN) plus ribavirin led to ~50% and ~80% sustained virological response (SVR) rates in patients infected with HCV genotypes 1 and 2, respectively [4]. Since 2011, peg-IFN plus ribavirin with telaprevir or boceprevir has been available in the United States as well as that with telaprevir in Japan. These treatments resulted in higher SVR rates (~70% and ~80% for treatment-naïve patients and previous treatment relapsers, resp.) in HCV genotype 1 infected patients [5].

Genome-wide association studies (GWAS) [6–8] revealed that several single nucleotide polymorphisms (SNPs) near the IFNL3 (previously called IL28B) coding region, such as rs8099917 and rs12978690, are associated with treatment response to peg-IFN plus ribavirin treatment. We also reported that IFNL3 rs8099917 was useful for the prediction of SVR in patients infected with HCV genotype 1 [9]. However, the mechanism between IFNL3 and clearance of HCV has been unclear despite the extensive work [10–12]. We also reported that IFNL3 induces IFN-stimulated genes (ISGs) such as IFN-$\gamma$-inducible protein (IP-10) that are reportedly associated with the progression of HCV-related pathogenesis and antiviral activities against HCV [12].

A recent study [13] showed that a variant upstream of IFNL3 could create IFNL4, impairing the clearance of HCV. Bibert et al. [14] reported that induction of IL28B and IP-10 mRNA relies on IFNL4 ss469415590 TT/-G variant in peripheral blood mononuclear cells (PBMCs), and this variant would improve the prediction of treatment response to peg-IFN and ribavirin [14, 15].

So far, only a few studies are available about the association between IFNL4 ss469415590 variant and treatment response in Japanese patients infected with HCV genotype 1. Peg-IFN plus ribavirin with telaprevir is also still one of the standard care treatments for chronic hepatitis C genotype 1 patients, at least until IFN-free regimens become generally available in clinical daily practice.

In the present study, the usefulness of IFNL4 ss469415590 variant for the prediction of virological response in chronic hepatitis C patients treated with peg-IFN plus ribavirin with or without telaprevir was investigated.

## 2. Patients and Methods

*2.1. Patients.* The present study comprised a total of 185 patients with chronic hepatitis C treated with peg-IFN plus ribavirin with or without telaprevir at the Department of Gastroenterology, Chiba University Hospital, and the Department of Gastroenterology, Kikkoman General Hospital in Chiba, Japan. Of these patients, 81 patients treated with peg-IFN plus ribavirin had been already included in previous reports [9, 11, 16]. Written informed consent was obtained from all patients, and the study was approved by the Ethics Committee of Chiba University, School of Medicine (number 428). All patients were of Asian origin and infected with HCV genotype 1. They underwent standard antiviral therapy with the combination of peg-IFN plus ribavirin [4] or telaprevir with peg-IFN plus ribavirin [17, 18]. HCV RNA was measured at baseline, at weeks 4 and 12, at the end of treatment, and at 24 weeks after the end of treatment. SVR was defined as undetectable serum HCV RNA at 24 weeks after the end of treatment. Patients with undetectable HCV RNA at 4 and 12 weeks after the commencement of treatment were considered to have had rapid virological response (RVR) and early virological response (EVR), respectively [19]. Relapse was defined as undetectable HCV RNA at the end of treatment, but it reappeared after the end of treatment [20]. Null response was defined as less than 2 $\log_{10}$ decrease in HCV RNA (IU/mL) from baseline after 12 weeks of therapy [20].

*2.2. DNA Extraction and IFNL4 Variant Genotyping.* Blood DNA was extracted by DNA extracted all lysis reagents (Applied Biosystems, Foster City, CA, USA). IFNL4 ss469415590 was determined by TaqMan SNP assay. Primers were purchased from Applied Biosystems. Thermal cycling was performed with the ABI Step One real-time PCR system as previously described [9]. We analyzed IFNL4 ss469415590 TT/TT as major genotype and TT/-G and -G/-G as minor genotypes in the present study.

*2.3. Measurement of HCV RNA in Serum.* HCV RNA was measured by COBAS AMPLICOR HCV Monitor test v. 2.0 (range: 0.5–850 KIU/mL, lower limit of detection: 1.7 log IU/mL) or COBAS TaqMan HCV test with levels ranging from 1.2 to 7.8 log IU/mL (Roche Diagnostics, Tokyo, Japan). In all patients treated with telaprevir with peg-IFN plus ribavirin, HCV RNA was measured by COBAS TaqMan HCV test.

*2.4. Statistical Analysis.* Data are expressed as mean ± SD. Variables with categorical data were compared among groups using chi-square test and Student's $t$-test as indicated. $P < 0.05$ was considered statistically significant. Variables with $P < 0.1$ at univariate analysis were retained for multivariate logistic regression analysis. Statistical analysis was performed using the Excel statistics program for Windows, version 7 (SSRI, Tokyo, Japan).

## 3. Results

IFNL4 ss469415590 variant was determined in 178 of the total 185 patients, and 117 (65.7%) had TT/TT, 56 (31.5%) had TT/-G, and 5 (2.8%) had -G/-G of ss469415590 in the present study (Table 1). In 141 patients treated with peg-IFN plus ribavirin without telaprevir, 93 (66.0%) had TT/TT, 43 (30.5%) had TT/-G, and 5 (3.5%) had -G/-G of ss469415590 (Table 2). In 37 patients treated with peg-IFN, ribavirin, and telaprevir, 24 (64.9%) had TT/TT and 13 (35.1%) had TT/-G of ss469415590 (Table 3). The distribution of IFNL4 ss469415590 variant of both treatment groups was quite similar.

In 24-week follow-up after treatment, 82.1% or 49.3% of patients treated with peg-IFN plus ribavirin with or without telaprevir, respectively, achieved SVR (Table 1). To clarify the predictors of SVR, we compared the baseline characteristics and treatment response between SVR and non-SVR groups of the patients treated with peg-IFN plus ribavirin (Table 4(a)). Univariate analysis showed that previous treatment response, $\gamma$-GTP levels, and platelet count, having RVR, EVR, and IFNL4 ss469415590 variant in the patients treated with peg-IFN plus ribavirin, contributed to the achievement of SVR. Factors associated with SVR by univariate analysis were then subjected to multivariate logistic regression analysis. SVR was attained independently of IFNL4 ss469415590 major genotype and having EVR in these patients treated with peg-IFN plus ribavirin (Table 4(b)).

Next, we compared the baseline characteristics and treatment response between SVR and non-SVR groups of the patients treated with peg-IFN, ribavirin, and telaprevir (Table 5(a)). HCV RNA at baseline was included, as the measurement of HCV RNA detection was uniform in this group

Table 1: Baseline characteristics of patients in the present study.

| | All patients, $n = 185$ | Patients with dual therapy, $n = 146$ | Patients with triple therapy, $n = 39$ | $P$ values (dual therapy versus triple therapy groups) |
|---|---|---|---|---|
| Gender, male/female | 102/83 | 73/73 | 29/10 | 0.011 |
| Age, years | 56.2 ± 10.7 | 55.7 ± 11.2 | 58.2 ± 8.7 | 0.197 |
| Previous treatment: naïve/relapse/null | 119/45/21 | 102/26/18 | 17/19/3 | 0.0043 (naïve versus non-naïve) |
| AST, IU/L | 57.1 ± 48.0 | 58.0 ± 48.7 | 53.9 ± 45.9 | 0.630 |
| ALT, IU/L | 70.4 ± 64.7 | 71.0 ± 64.9 | 68.1 ± 64.8 | 0.800 |
| $\gamma$-GTP, IU/L | 57.0 ± 66.7 | 56.4 ± 68.6 | 59.2 ± 59.8 | 0.816 |
| Hemoglobin, g/dL | 14.1 ± 1.3 | 14.0 ± 1.2 | 14.6 ± 1.3 | 0.0070 |
| Platelets, $\times 10^4$/mm$^3$ | 16.6 ± 5.6 | 16.8 ± 5.8 | 16.0 ± 5.1 | 0.434 |
| Treatment response | | | | |
| RVR, $n$ | 42 | 15 | 27 | <0.0001 |
| EVR, $n$ | 99 | 65 | 34 | <0.0001 |
| SVR/relapse/null | 104/39/42 | 72/37/37 | 32/2/5 | <0.0001 |
| IFNL4, ss469415590, major/minor/ND | 117/61/7 | 93/48/5 | 24/13/2 | 0.944 |

Peginterferon plus ribavirin with or without telaprevir therapy was defined as triple or dual therapy, respectively. Null: null response; AST: aspirate aminotransferase; ALT: alanine aminotransferase; $\gamma$-GTP: $\gamma$-glutamyltransferase; RVR: rapid virological response; EVR: early virological response; SVR: sustained virological response.

Table 2: Baseline characteristics and treatment response in 141 patients treated with peginterferon plus ribavirin according to IFNL4 ss469415590 variant.

| | IFNL4 major, $n = 93$ | IFNL4 minor, $n = 48$ | $P$ values (major versus minor groups) |
|---|---|---|---|
| Gender, male/female | 46/47 | 25/23 | 0.900 |
| Age, years | 56.1 ± 11.7 | 54.7 ± 10.6 | 0.488 |
| Previous treatment: naïve/relapse/null | 68/19/6 | 29/7/12 | 0.0042 |
| AST, IU/L | 53.4 ± 48.5 | 65.0 ± 44.0 | 0.167 |
| ALT, IU/L | 65.1 ± 64.9 | 82.0 ± 63.3 | 0.14 |
| $\gamma$-GTP, IU/L | 40.9 ± 39.2 | 87.5 ± 98.9 | 0.000107 |
| Hemoglobin, g/dL | 13.9 ± 1.2 | 14.2 ± 1.2 | 0.16 |
| Platelets, $\times 10^4$/mm$^3$ | 16.8 ± 5.7 | 16.8 ± 6.1 | 1.00 |
| Treatment response | | | |
| RVR, $n$ | 15 | 0 | 0.0079 |
| EVR, $n$ | 59 | 5 | <0.0001 |
| SVR/relapse/null | 60/23/10 | 10/12/25 | <0.0001 |

Null: null response; AST: aspirate aminotransferase; ALT: alanine aminotransferase; $\gamma$-GTP: $\gamma$-glutamyltransferase; RVR: rapid virological response; EVR: early virological response; SVR: sustained virological response.

(see Section 2). Univariate analysis showed that having RVR and EVR in the patients treated with peg-IFN, ribavirin, and telaprevir contributed to achievement of SVR. Factors associated with SVR by univariate analysis were then subjected to multivariate logistic regression analysis. SVR was attained independently of lower HCV RNA at baseline, and IFNL4 ss469415590 major genotype in these patients was treated with peg-IFN plus ribavirin and telaprevir (Table 5(b)).

## 4. Discussion

The present study confirmed previous studies that IFNL4 ss469415590 variant plays an important role in eradicating HCV genotype 1 from patients treated with peg-IFN plus ribavirin with or without telaprevir [14, 21–23]. Multivariate analysis revealed that IFNL4 ss469415590 major genotype was statistically associated with achieving SVR in patients treated with peg-IFN plus ribavirin as well as those treated with peg-IFN, ribavirin, and telaprevir.

IFNL3-associated SNPs were strongly associated with treatment response to peg-IFN plus ribavirin without telaprevir treatment [6–9]. Although there have been several reports on the mechanism involving IFNL3 [10, 11], the exact mechanism or function of IFNL3 has yet to be clarified. Bibert et al. [14] reported that induction of IL28B and IP-10 mRNA relied on ss469415590 TT/-G but not rs12979860, making

Table 3: Baseline characteristics and treatment response in 37 patients treated with peginterferon, ribavirin, and telaprevir according to IFNL4 ss469415590 variant.

| | IFNL4 major, $n = 24$ | IFNL4 minor, $n = 13$ | $P$ values (major versus minor groups) |
|---|---|---|---|
| Gender, male/female | 19/5 | 9/4 | 0.78 |
| Age, years | 59.5 ± 7.7 | 55.2 ± 10.2 | 0.15 |
| Previous treatment: naïve/relapse/null | 10/13/1 | 7/4/2 | 0.71 |
| AST, IU/L | 50.9 ± 48.9 | 59.8 ± 44.2 | 0.58 |
| ALT, IU/L | 63.8 ± 60.5 | 77.9 ± 77.2 | 0.54 |
| $\gamma$-GTP, IU/L | 51.8 ± 52.2 | 78.6 ± 73.3 | 0.25 |
| Hemoglobin, g/dL | 14.6 ± 1.2 | 14.5 ± 1.3 | 0.81 |
| Platelets, $\times10^4/mm^3$ | 15.9 ± 5.2 | 16.5 ± 5.3 | 0.74 |
| HCV RNA (log IU/mL) | 6.70 ± 0.54 | 6.18 ± 0.87 | 0.0309 |
| Treatment response | | | |
| RVR, $n$ | 17 | 8 | 0.83 |
| EVR, $n$ | 22 | 10 | 0.45 |
| SVR/relapse/null | 22 | 8 | 0.0727 |

Null: null response; AST: aspirate aminotransferase; ALT: alanine aminotransferase; $\gamma$-GTP: $\gamma$-glutamyltransferase; RVR: rapid virological response; EVR: early virological response; SVR: sustained virological response.

Table 4: Comparison of SVR and non-SVR patients treated with peginterferon and ribavirin by univariate analysis (a) and multivariate analysis (b).

(a) Univariate analysis

| | SVR, $n = 72$ | Non-SVR, $n = 74$ | $P$ values (SVR versus non-SVR groups) |
|---|---|---|---|
| Gender, male/female | 39/33 | 34/40 | 0.40 |
| Age, years | 54.4 ± 12.7 | 57.0 ± 9.3 | 0.15 |
| Previous treatment: naïve/relapse/null | 59/12/1 | 43/14/17 | 0.00020 |
| AST, IU/L | 54.1 ± 54.3 | 61.8 ± 42.5 | 0.34 |
| ALT, IU/L | 69.0 ± 71.5 | 73.0 ± 58.2 | 0.71 |
| $\gamma$-GTP, IU/L | 42.7 ± 41.3 | 70.0 ± 85.7 | 0.0158 |
| Hemoglobin, g/dL | 13.9 ± 1.1 | 14.1 ± 1.3 | 0.31 |
| Platelets, $\times10^4/mm^3$ | 17.8 ± 5.4 | 15.7 ± 5.9 | 0.0265 |
| Treatment response | | | |
| RVR, $n$ | 15 | 0 | 0.000107 |
| EVR, $n$ | 53 | 12 | <0.0001 |
| IFNL4, ss469415590, major/minor/ND | 60/10/2 | 33/38/3 | <0.0001 |

Null: null response; AST: aspirate aminotransferase; ALT: alanine aminotransferase; $\gamma$-GTP: $\gamma$-glutamyltransferase; RVR: rapid virological response; EVR: early virological response; SVR: sustained virological response.

(b) Factors associated with SVR among patients treated with peginterferon plus ribavirin by multivariate analysis

| Factor | Category | Odds ratio | 95% CI | $P$ values |
|---|---|---|---|---|
| IFNL4, ss469415590 | major/minor | 2.56 | 1.005–6.557 | 0.0486 |
| EVR | +/− | 10.16 | 4.28–24.10 | <0.0001 |

EVR: early virological response.

ss469415590 TT/-G the only functional variant identified, although there are contrary opinions [24, 25].

Prokunina-Olsson et al. [13] found that several novel transcripts and ss469415590 are specific for the region upstream of IFNL3. Their global protein BLAST search [13] showed that 179 amino acids (p179) from transcripts with the ss469415590-G allele have only homology with 29.1% amino acid identity and 40.8% amino acid similarity with IFNL3 among predictive proteins from the 10 novel transcripts. IFNL3 and these p179 (IFNL4) proteins are most related within the sequences, corresponding to the A and F helices of IFNL3, which constitute the core area for interaction of IFNL3 with its primary receptor, IFNLR1 (IL28R1) [13]. The beneficial insertion ss469415590-TT allele could abrogate IFNL4. IFNL4 signaling via IFN$\lambda$ receptor could regulate antiviral activity against coronaviruses as well as HCV [26]. Manuel et al. [27] also reported that polymorphisms in the IFNL3/4 region influence susceptibility to CMV replication

Table 5: Comparison of SVR and non-SVR patients treated with peginterferon, ribavirin, and telaprevir by univariate analysis (a) and multivariate analysis (b).

(a) Univariate analysis

| | SVR, $n$ = 32 | Non-SVR, $n$ = 7 | $P$ values (SVR versus non-SVR groups) |
|---|---|---|---|
| Gender, male/female | 24/8 | 5/2 | 0.77 |
| Age, years | 57.8 ± 9.3 | 59.8 ± 5.6 | 0.58 |
| Previous treatment: naïve/relapse/null | 14/17/1 | 3/2/2 | 0.13 |
| AST, IU/L | 55.9 ± 50.1 | 44.7 ± 16.0 | 0.56 |
| ALT, IU/L | 71.9 ± 70.6 | 51.1 ± 19.9 | 0.44 |
| $\gamma$-GTP, IU/L | 62.1 ± 64.7 | 46.2 ± 27.9 | 0.53 |
| Hemoglobin, g/dL | 14.6 ± 1.3 | 14.4 ± 1.6 | 0.72 |
| Platelets, $\times 10^4/\text{mm}^3$ | 16.4 ± 5.2 | 14.3 ± 4.6 | 0.33 |
| HCV RNA (log IU/mL) | 6.45 ± 0.68 | 6.81 ± 0.75 | 0.220 |
| Treatment response | | | |
| RVR, $n$ | 27 | 0 | <0.0001 |
| EVR, $n$ | 32 | 2 | <0.0001 |
| IFNL4, major/minor/ND | 22/8/2 | 2/5/0 | 0.0727 |

Null: null response; AST: aspirate aminotransferase; ALT: alanine aminotransferase; $\gamma$-GTP: $\gamma$-glutamyltransferase; RVR: rapid virological response; EVR: early virological response; SVR: sustained virological response.

(b) Factors associated with SVR among patients treated with peginterferon, ribavirin, and telaprevir by multivariate analysis

| Factor | Category | Odds ratio | 95% CI | $P$ values |
|---|---|---|---|---|
| HCV RNA (log IU/mL) | <6.4/6.4≤ | 13.74 | 1.014–186.30 | 0.048 |
| IFNL4 ss469415590 | major/minor | 17.54 | 1.980–156.25 | 0.010 |

in solid-organ transplant recipients, suggesting that IFNL4 as well as IFNL3 play important roles in human antiviral defenses.

Our results indicated that IFNL4 ss469415590 variant is useful for prediction of the treatment response to IFN-including regimens. A recent study [28] showed that IFNL4 ss469415590 minor genotype was associated with slower early viral decay, due to slower loss of free virus and decreased drug efficacy in patients treated with the DAA sofosbuvir against HCV NS5B, along with RBV, suggesting that IFNL4 variant might be useful in the DAA era. In IFN-free DAA therapies, it is unclear whether these variants play a role or not, although it is possible that certain DAAs could have effects on IFN signaling such as ISGs of host cells.

## 5. Conclusions

Measurement of IFNL4 ss469415590 variant is another option for prediction of the treatment response to IFN-including regimens in Japanese HCV genotype 1 infected individuals. Together, the mechanism of the interaction between treatment response and IFNL4 as well as IFNL3 in HCV-infected patients should be further explored.

## Authors' Contribution

Tatsuo Miyamura, Tatsuo Kanda, and Shingo Nakamoto contributed equally to the paper.

## Acknowledgments

The authors thank all their colleagues at the liver units of their hospitals who cared for the patients described herein. This work was supported by Research Grants for Scientific Research from the Ministry of Education, Culture, Sports, Science, and Technology, Japan.

## References

[1] A. M. Di Bisceglie, "Hepatitis C and hepatocellular carcinoma," *Hepatology*, vol. 26, no. 3, supplement 1, pp. 34S–38S, 1997.

[2] J. W. Ward, "The epidemiology of chronic hepatitis C and one-time hepatitis C virus testing of persons born during 1945 to

1965 in the United States," *Clinics in Liver Disease*, vol. 17, no. 1, pp. 1–11, 2013.

[3] I. Saito, T. Miyamura, A. Ohbayashi et al., "Hepatitis C virus infection is associated with the development of hepatocellular carcinoma," *Proceedings of the National Academy of Sciences of the United States of America*, vol. 87, no. 17, pp. 6547–6549, 1990.

[4] T. Kanda, F. Imazeki, and O. Yokosuka, "New antiviral therapies for chronic hepatitis C," *Hepatology International*, vol. 4, no. 3, pp. 548–561, 2010.

[5] T. Kanda, O. Yokosuka, and M. Omata, "Treatment of hepatitis C virus infection in the future," *Clinical and Translational Medicine*, vol. 2, article 9, 2013.

[6] D. Ge, J. Fellay, A. J. Thompson et al., "Genetic variation in IL28B predicts hepatitis C treatment-induced viral clearance," *Nature*, vol. 461, no. 7262, pp. 399–401, 2009.

[7] V. Suppiah, M. Moldovan, G. Ahlenstiel et al., "IL28B is associated with response to chronic hepatitis C interferon-$\alpha$ and ribavirin therapy," *Nature Genetics*, vol. 41, no. 10, pp. 1100–1104, 2009.

[8] Y. Tanaka, N. Nishida, M. Sugiyama et al., "Genome-wide association of IL28B with response to pegylated interferon-$\alpha$ and ribavirin therapy for chronic hepatitis C," *Nature Genetics*, vol. 41, no. 10, pp. 1105–1109, 2009.

[9] T. Miyamura, T. Kanda, S. Nakamoto et al., "Roles of ITPA and IL28B genotypes in chronic hepatitis C patients treated with peginterferon plus ribavirin," *Viruses*, vol. 4, no. 8, pp. 1264–1278, 2012.

[10] M. Sugiyama, Y. Tanaka, T. Wakita, M. Nakanishi, and M. Mizokami, "Genetic variation of the *IL-28B* promoter affecting gene expression," *PLoS ONE*, vol. 6, no. 10, Article ID e26620, 2011.

[11] T. Miyamura, T. Kanda, S. Nakamoto et al., "Hepatic STAT1-nuclear translocation and interleukin 28B polymorphisms predict treatment outcomes in hepatitis C virus genotype 1-infected patients," *PLoS ONE*, vol. 6, no. 12, Article ID e28617, 2011.

[12] T. Kanda, X. Jiang, S. Nakamoto et al., "Different effects of three interferons L on toll-like receptor related gene expression in HepG2 cells," *Cytokine*, vol. 64, no. 2, pp. 577–583, 2013.

[13] L. Prokunina-Olsson, B. Muchmore, W. Tang et al., "A variant upstream of *IFNL3* (*IL28B*) creating a new interferon gene *IFNL4* is associated with impaired clearance of hepatitis C virus," *Nature Genetics*, vol. 45, no. 2, pp. 164–171, 2013.

[14] S. Bibert, T. Roger, T. Calandra et al., "IL28B expression depends on a novel TT/-G polymorphism which improves HCV clearance prediction," *Journal of Experimental Medicine*, vol. 210, no. 6, pp. 1109–1116, 2013.

[15] Y. Nozawa, T. Umemura, Y. Katsuyama et al., "Genetic polymorphism in IFNL4 and response to pegylated interferon-$\alpha$ and ribavirin in Japanese chronic hepatitis C patients," *Tissue Antigens*, vol. 83, no. 1, pp. 45–48, 2014.

[16] S. Nakamoto, T. Kanda, F. Imazeki et al., "Simple assay based on restriction fragment length polymorphism associated with IL28B in chronic hepatitis C patients," *Scandinavian Journal of Gastroenterology*, vol. 46, no. 7-8, pp. 955–961, 2011.

[17] H. Kumada, J. Toyota, T. Okanoue, K. Chayama, H. Tsubouchi, and N. Hayashi, "Telaprevir with peginterferon and ribavirin for treatment-naive patients chronically infected with HCV of genotype 1 in Japan," *Journal of Hepatology*, vol. 56, no. 1, pp. 78–84, 2012.

[18] T. Hara, N. Akuta, F. Suzuki et al., "A pilot study of triple therapy with telaprevir, peginterferon and ribavirin for elderly patients with genotype 1 chronic hepatitis C," *Journal of Medical Virology*, vol. 85, no. 10, pp. 1746–1753, 2013.

[19] T. Kanda, F. Imazeki, Y. Yonemitsu et al., "Quantification of hepatitis C virus in patients treated with peginterferon-alfa 2a plus ribavirin treatment by COBAS TaqMan HCV test," *Journal of Viral Hepatitis*, vol. 18, no. 7, pp. e292–e297, 2011.

[20] M. Omata, T. Kanda, M.-L. Yu et al., "APASL consensus statements and management algorithms for hepatitis C virus infection," *Hepatology International*, vol. 6, no. 2, pp. 409–435, 2012.

[21] Y. Nozawa, T. Umemura, Y. Katsuyama et al., "Genetic polymorphism in IFNL4 and response to pegylated interferon-$\alpha$ and ribavirin in Japanese chronic hepatitis C patients," *Tissue Antigens*, vol. 83, no. 1, pp. 45–48, 2014.

[22] H. Fujino, M. Imamura, Y. Nagaoki et al., "Predictive value of the IFNL4 polymorphism on outcome of telaprevir, peginterferon, and ribavirin therapy for older patients with genotype 1b chronic hepatitis C," *Journal of Gastroenterology*, 2013.

[23] Y. Nagaoki, M. Imamura, Y. Kawakami et al., "Interferon lambda 4 polymorphism affects on outcome of telaprevir, pegylated interferon and ribavirin combination therapy for chronic hepatitis C," *Hepatology Research*, 2014.

[24] A. F. Stättermayer, R. Strassl, A. Maieron et al., "Polymorphisms of interferon-$\lambda$4 and IL28B-effects on treatment response to interferon/ribavirin in patients with chronic hepatitis C," *Alimentary Pharmacology and Therapeutics*, vol. 39, no. 1, pp. 104–111, 2014.

[25] L. M. Real, K. Neukam, R. Herrero et al., "IFNL4 ss469415590 variant shows similar performance to rs12979860 as predictor of response to treatment against hepatitis C virus genotype 1 or 4 in Caucasians," *PLoS ONE*, vol. 9, no. 4, Article ID e95515, 2014.

[26] O. J. Hamming, E. Terczyńska-Dyla, G. Vieyres et al., "Interferon lambda 4 signals via the IFN$\lambda$ receptor to regulate antiviral activity against HCV and coronaviruses," *EMBO Journal*, vol. 32, no. 23, pp. 3055–3065, 2013.

[27] O. Manuel, A. Wójtowicz, S. Bibert et al., "Influence of IFNL3/4 polymorphisms on the incidence of cytomegalovirus infection after solid-organ transplantation," *The Journal of Infectious Diseases*, 2014.

[28] E. G. Meissner, D. Bon, L. Prokunina-Olsson et al., "*IFNL4*-$\Delta$G genotype is associated with slower viral clearance in Hepatitis C, genotype-1 patients treated with sofosbuvir and ribavirin," *Journal of Infectious Diseases*, vol. 209, no. 11, pp. 1700–1704, 2014.

# 16

# Central Portalization Correlates with Fibrosis but Not with Risk Factors for Nonalcoholic Steatohepatitis in Steatotic Chronic Hepatitis C

**Hwajeong Lee,[1,2] Sanaz Ainechi,[1] Karen Dresser,[2] and Elizabeth M. Kurian[2,3]**

[1] *Anatomic Pathology, Albany Medical College, 47 New Scotland Avenue, MC81, Albany, NY 12208, USA*
[2] *Anatomic Pathology, University of Massachusetts, 1 Innovation Drive, Biotech 3, Worcester, MA 01605, USA*
[3] *Anatomic Pathology, University of Texas Southwestern Medical Center, 5323 Harry Hines Boulevard, Dallas, TX 75390-9234, USA*

Correspondence should be addressed to Hwajeong Lee; leeh5@mail.amc.edu

Academic Editor: Daisuke Morioka

Concomitant steatosis in chronic hepatitis C is associated with fibrosis and unfavorable treatment outcome. Central zone injury in nonalcoholic steatohepatitis (NASH) manifests as central portalization, with centrizonal microvessels and ductular reaction. We investigated whether central portalization in steatotic HCV biopsies would identify patients with metabolic risk factors for NASH. Liver biopsies with chronic hepatitis C and >10% steatosis ($n = 65$) were evaluated for the degree of steatosis, zonation of steatosis, fibrosis, and nonalcoholic fatty liver disease (NAFLD) activity score. The presence of centrizonal microvessels, sinusoidal capillarization, ductular reaction, and CK7 positive intermediate-phenotype hepatocytes were evaluated by CD34 and CK7 immunostain. The degree of steatosis and fibrosis showed a positive correlation. Additional positive correlations were noted between centrizonal angiogenesis and NAFLD activity score and central portalization and fibrosis. However, neither central portalization nor zonation of steatosis identified patients with metabolic risk factors for NASH. Therefore, central portalization cannot be used as a surrogate marker to identify patients with metabolic risk factors for NASH in steatotic HCV biopsies. The mechanism of centrizonal injury in steatotic HCV hepatitis is not solely attributable to the metabolic risk factors for NASH.

## 1. Introduction

In chronic hepatitis C, steatosis is a common histologic finding. Studies have categorized the steatosis of chronic HCV into viral type versus metabolic type. The "viral" type of steatosis is well demonstrated in HCV genotype 3; these liver biopsies show a greater amount of steatosis compared to those of non-3 genotypes [1–4]. Experimental studies suggest that the HCV viral core protein impairs lipid oxidation and induces accumulation of triglyceride in the hepatocytes [5–7]. Furthermore, the degree of steatosis is related to the viral load [4–6, 8, 9], and the amount of steatosis decreases following treatment [10–12]. In the setting of liver transplantation, the hepatic steatosis is an early indicator of HCV reinfection [13]. The second type of "metabolic" steatosis is usually demonstrated in non-3 genotypes and is associated with risk factors of nonalcoholic fatty liver disease, such as high body mass index (BMI) [1, 4, 14–16]. In these patients, insulin resistance enhances peripheral lipolysis and hepatic lipogenesis [17], while impairing the export of triglycerides from the hepatocytes [6]. Thus, insulin resistance appears to play a key role in the development of metabolic steatosis [14]. Since chronic hepatitis C patients are also at risk for impaired glucose metabolism and demonstrate a higher homeostatic model assessment (HOMA-IR; a surrogate marker of insulin resistance), viral and metabolic factors are not mutually exclusive in the pathogenesis of steatosis [6, 18–21].

Retrospective and longitudinal studies show that the degree of steatosis in chronic hepatitis C is positively correlated with the degree of fibrosis [1, 4, 6, 16, 22, 23], and steatosis/fibrosis negatively affects the likelihood of achieving a sustained virologic response following treatment [6, 10, 15, 23–26]. Similarly, hepatitis C biopsies with concomitant

NASH were more frequently associated with advanced fibrosis compared to those without NASH [2, 7, 15]. Moreover, superimposed hepatic steatosis in chronic hepatitis C appears to pose an increased risk of hepatocellular carcinoma [27, 28]. The current literature suggests that management of metabolic risk factors for NASH, such as obesity and type 2 diabetes mellitus (DM), may alter the disease progression in chronic hepatitis C [3, 21, 29–33].

A recent study showed that biopsies of NASH exhibit increased vascular channels and ductular reaction in central zones, termed central portalization, and it was more common in advanced fibrosis [34]. We investigated whether the central portalization in steatotic HCV biopsies would identify a subset of patients with metabolic risk factors for NASH. If the groups with or without risk factors for NASH demonstrate a difference in the degree of vascular proliferation and ductular reaction in the central zone, the histologic findings may be used as a surrogate marker to identify a subset of chronic hepatitis C patients at risk for superimposed NASH with its adverse outcome.

## 2. Materials and Methods

*2.1. Study Group and Control Groups.* The study was approved by the institutional review board. Liver biopsies from HCV hepatitis with concurrent macrovesicular steatosis (ranging from 10% to 80%), during the period of 2006–2008, constituted the study group ($n = 65$). Demographic and clinical data including the presence of type 2 diabetes mellitus (DM), obesity (body mass index (BMI) $\geq 30\ kg/m^2$), hyperlipidemia, history of alcohol use, HCV genotypes, and treatment history were obtained from the electronic medical records.

For control groups, 22 cases of nonalcoholic steatohepatitis (NASH) biopsies with no history of HCV and 20 cases of HCV hepatitis biopsies with ≤10% of steatosis were retrieved. Relevant demographic and clinical data were obtained from the electronic medical records.

*2.2. H&E and Trichrome Stain Review.* Each liver biopsy was evaluated for the amount of steatosis and fibrosis. Ishak's fibrosis staging system was used for the study group and HCV control group [35]. Fibrosis staging system by NASH Clinical Research Network (CRN) was used for NASH control group [36]. The central zones around terminal hepatic veins were defined as previously published [37], and the number of central zones was recorded for each biopsy. For the study group, the zonation of steatosis (zone 3 or random) was evaluated. In addition, NAFLD activity score was calculated using the published criteria—degree of steatosis (5–33%: 1, >33–66%: 2, >66%: 3), ballooning (few: 1, many: 2), and lobular inflammation (<2 foci: 1, 2–4 foci: 2, >4 foci: 3; counted in 20x fields)—for the study group and NASH control group [36]. The presence of arterioles with muscular vessel wall in the central zone was evaluated on H&E stain.

*2.3. Immunohistochemical Stain.* The immunohistochemical stain for CK7 (1 : 200, Dako M7018, mouse monoclonal, clone OV-TL 12/20), CK19 (1 : 50, Dako M0888, mouse monoclonal, clone RCK108), and CD34 (1 : 160, Dako M7165, mouse monoclonal, clone QBEnd 10) was performed on the 5-micrometer thick tissue sections of paraffin-embedded tissue blocks. Antigen retrieval was carried out with 0.01 M citrate buffer at pH 6.0. The slides were stained on the Dako Autostainer (Dako Corporation, Carpinteria, CA).

Sections of various control tissues (breast for CK7, liver for CK19, and colon for CD34) with known positivity for the target proteins were used as positive stain controls. Positive staining was defined as dark brown staining pattern. Scant or fine granular background staining or no staining at all was considered negative.

*2.4. Evaluation of Central Portalization.* Microvessel and ductular reaction in the central zone was evaluated by CD34 and CK7, respectively. As described previously [38], microvessels are defined as small lumen-forming vascular channels with CD34 positive endothelial lining, without a visible muscular wall. Ductular reaction is defined as the presence of CK7 positive biliary-type cells arranged in ductular configuration [38]. Sinusoidal CD34 staining without complete lumen-forming channels was interpreted as sinusoidal capillarization. CK7 positive hepatocytes in the central zone, without morphologic ductule formation, were considered intermediate-phenotype hepatocytes [38]. Initially, the number of central zones with microvessels, sinusoidal capillarization, ductular reaction, and intermediate-type hepatocytes were evaluated, respectively. However, the distinction between microvessels and sinusoidal capillarization was difficult in some cases. Since the results of statistical analyses did not differ when sinusoidal capillarization was combined with microvessels, no distinction was made for the purpose of scoring, and sinusoidal capillarization was included in the count of microvessels (see below $M$ score). For the same reasons, the intermediate-phenotype hepatocytes were included in the count of ductular reaction (see below $D$ score).

Any zone with CK19 positivity was excluded from enumeration. The CK19 positive areas represent portal tracts or tangentially sectioned extensions of fibrous septa surrounding portal tracts, which may mimic central zones (see Section 4). The $M$ score is defined as the number of central zones with microvessels and sinusoidal capillarization divided by the total number of central zones—the ratio of central zones with angiogenesis to the total number of central zones, within a biopsy. For example, in a biopsy with 10 central zones, if 2 central zones show microvessels and 3 central zones show sinusoidal capillarization, the $M$ score is $(2 + 3)$ divided by $10 = 0.5$. The $D$ score is defined as the number of central zones showing ductular reaction (including intermediate-type hepatocytes) divided by the total number of central zones in a biopsy. Cases displaying less than 4 central zones were considered inadequate for evaluation and were excluded from the statistical analysis ($n = 18$).

*2.5. Statistical Analysis.* Fisher's exact test was used when determining whether there are nonrandom associations between two categorical variables. Student's $t$-test was used when comparing the means of two groups. Pearson's correlation coefficient was used for correlation of two parameters.

Table 1: Clinical data, steatosis, and fibrosis of steatotic HCV (>10% steatosis) study group and two control groups—$^{*}P < 0.05$ by Fisher's exact test, statistically significant; the information regarding risk factors was unavailable or incomplete in 9 patients of the study group. #HCV genotype was known in 44 cases in the study group and 17 cases in HCV control group. M: male; F: female; DM: diabetes mellitus; obesity: body mass index (BMI) of ≥30 kg/m$^2$; n/a: not applicable; Ishak: Ishak's fibrosis staging system [35]; NASH CRN: NASH Clinical Research Network's fibrosis staging system for NASH [36].

| | Study group | Control group | |
|---|---|---|---|
| | HCV with >10% steatosis | HCV with ≤10% steatosis | NASH, no HCV |
| Number of cases | 65 | 20 | 22 |
| Age | 48 | 47 | 43 |
| M : F | 49 : 16 | 17 : 3 | 13 : 9 |
| Type 2 DM | 14 (22%) | 1 (5%) ($P = 0.11$) | 5 (23%) ($P = 1.00$) |
| Obesity | 33 (51%) | 5 (25%) ($P = 0.07$) | 20 (91%) ($P = 0.001^{*}$) |
| Alcohol | 32 (49%) | 8 (40%) ($P = 0.61$) | 4 (18%) ($P = 0.01^{*}$) |
| HCV genotype# | | | |
| 1a/1b | 34 (77%) | 17 (100%) ($P = 0.049^{*}$) | n/a |
| 2a/2b | 3 (7%) | 0 ($P = 0.55$) | n/a |
| 3 | 7 (16%) | 0 ($P = 0.17$) | n/a |
| Steatosis | | | |
| <33% | 22 (34%) | 20 (100%) | 10 (46%) ($P = 0.44$) |
| 33–66% | 30 (46%) | 0 | 3 (14%) ($P = 0.01^{*}$) |
| >66% | 13 (20%) | 0 | 9 (41%) ($P = 0.09$) |
| Fibrosis | Ishak | Ishak | NASH CRN |
| | 0–2: 23 (35%) | 0–2: 13 (65%) ($P = 0.04^{*}$) | 0-1: 14 (64%) |
| | 3-4: 23 (35%) | 3-4: 6 (30%) ($P = 0.79$) | 2: 4 (18%) |
| | 5-6: 19 (29%) | 5-6: 1 (5%) ($P = 0.03^{*}$) | 3: 2 (9%) |
| | | | 4: 2 (9%) |

A $P$ value of less than 0.05 was considered statistically significant.

## 3. Results

*3.1. Study Group: Clinical Data and Review of Histology.* Thirty-four (52%) patients had one or more risk factors, and 21 (32%) patients had no risk factors for NASH. The most common risk factor for NASH was obesity (Table 1). When only patients with one or more metabolic risk factors were considered, 97% (33/34) of them had obesity. The HCV genotype was available in 44 patients; all genotype 3 cases belonged to the study group (Table 1). Thirteen patients had been treated for HCV hepatitis prior to the biopsies. Clinical follow-up for twelve months or longer was available in 55 patients, with a mean follow-up period of 48 months (12–72 months). During the follow-up period, 6 (11%) subsequently developed clinical NASH or type 2 DM, and 16 (29%) experienced adverse outcomes, including relapse after treatment ($n = 2$), no response to treatment ($n = 3$), discontinuation of treatment due to side effects ($n = 5$), progression of fibrosis, hepatic decompensation, and development of hepatocellular carcinoma ($n = 6$).

On histologic review, the zonation of steatosis (zone 3 steatosis) was appreciated in 6 cases, of which 4 had metabolic risk factors for NASH. When the fibrosis, steatosis, and NAFLD activity score were compared between the subgroups with and without clinical parameters (categorical variables) among the study group, only the degree of steatosis between the obese and nonobese group showed a statistically significant difference (Table 2). Combination of the study group and HCV control group with ≤10% steatosis showed an even greater difference, with an average steatosis of 48% in the obesity group and 29% in the nonobese group ($P = 0.001$ by Student's $t$-test).

On average, 6 (range 1–22) central zones were identified per biopsy. The mean Ishak's fibrosis stage was 2.9 for the biopsies with adequate number of central zones (>3) and 4.3 for the biopsies with inadequate number (≤3) of central zones ($P = 0.019$ by Student's $t$-test). Similarly, the number of central zones showed an inverse relationship to fibrosis by Pearson's correlation test (Table 3). No statistically significant correlation was found between the fibrosis and steatosis in the study group. However, when the control HCV group with ≤10% of steatosis was combined with the steatotic HCV study group, there was a positive correlation between the degree of steatosis and Ishak's fibrosis stage ($r = 0.26$ by Pearson's correlation coefficient; $P = 0.046$).

Two cases showed arterioles in the central zone.

*3.2. Study Group: Evaluation of Central Portalization.* A total of forty-seven cases were studied, after excluding cases with less than 4 central zones. All 47 (100%) cases showed microvessels and/or sinusoidal capillarization, with the average $M$ score of 0.5 (range 0.1–1) (Figures 1(a) and 1(b)). Thirty-four (72%) of 47 cases showed ductular reaction and/or

TABLE 2: Clinical parameters versus fibrosis, steatosis, and nonalcoholic fatty liver disease (NAFLD) activity score [36] in the study group by Student's $t$-test. Present: with the clinical parameter; absent: without the clinical parameter; Ishak: Ishak's fibrosis staging system [35]; *statistically significant ($P < 0.05$); type 2 DM: type 2 diabetes mellitus.

| | Clinical parameter | Present | Absent | $P$ value |
|---|---|---|---|---|
| Fibrosis (Ishak) | Obesity | 2.9 | 3.9 | $P = 0.058$ |
| | Type 2 DM | 3.3 | 3.3 | $P = 0.918$ |
| | Alcohol | 3.6 | 3.0 | $P = 0.193$ |
| Steatosis (%) | Obesity | 56% | 45% | $P = 0.030$* |
| | Type 2 DM | 49% | 50% | $P = 0.880$ |
| | HCV genotype 3 | 50% | 48% | $P = 0.776$ |
| NAFLD activity score | Obesity | 5.3 | 4.7 | $P = 0.09$ |
| | Type 2 DM | 4.9 | 5.0 | $P = 0.76$ |
| | Hyperlipidemia | 5.8 | 4.9 | $P = 0.08$ |
| | Alcohol | 4.8 | 5.2 | $P = 0.25$ |

TABLE 3: Pearson's correlation coefficient ($r$) and $P$ values for histologic parameters. NASH: nonalcoholic steatohepatitis; NS: not statistically significant ($P \geq 0.05$); *$P < 0.05$: statistically significant; NAFLD: nonalcoholic fatty liver disease [36]; $M$ score and $D$ score: see Section 2.4 for definition.

| | Parameters | $r$ | $P$ value |
|---|---|---|---|
| **Study group** HCV with steatosis >10% | Central zone versus fibrosis | −0.38 | 0.0018* |
| | Central zone versus steatosis | | NS |
| | Fibrosis versus steatosis | | NS |
| | Fibrosis versus NAFLD activity score | | NS |
| | $M$ score versus fibrosis | 0.38 | 0.008* |
| | $D$ score versus fibrosis | 0.36 | 0.013* |
| | $M$ score versus steatosis | | NS |
| | $D$ score versus steatosis | | NS |
| | $M$ score versus NAFLD activity score | 0.30 | 0.041* |
| | $D$ score versus NAFLD activity score | | NS |
| **HCV control group** HCV with ≤10% steatosis | $M$ score versus fibrosis | | NS |
| | $D$ score versus fibrosis | 0.54 | 0.036* |
| | $M$ score versus $D$ score | 0.49 | 0.06 |
| **NASH control group** NASH, no HCV | $M$ score versus fibrosis | | NS |
| | $M$ score versus NAFLD activity score | | NS |
| | $M$ score versus steatosis | | NS |

intermediate-phenotype hepatocytes, with the average $D$ score of 0.3 (range 0-1) (Figures 1(a) and 1(c)). The $M$ score showed a positive correlation with Ishak's fibrosis stage and NAFLD activity score. Similarly, the $D$ score showed a positive correlation with fibrosis. Neither $M$ nor $D$ score showed statistically significant correlation with steatosis (Table 3).

No statistically significant difference was found in the $M$ and $D$ scores between the groups: with and without obesity, type 2 DM, hyperlipidemia, history of alcohol use, history of treatment, and HCV genotype 3. The result remained unchanged when the cutoff of steatosis was increased to 33% for the study group.

*3.3. Control Groups.* In the HCV control group, 15 cases were adequate for evaluation, and the $D$ score showed a positive correlation with Ishak's fibrosis stage (Table 3). No statistically significant correlation was found between the $M$ score and fibrosis, and the result remained unchanged when the cases with advanced fibrosis were only evaluated.

In the NASH control group without HCV, 64% of the biopsies showed low NASH CRN's fibrosis stage (0: 4 cases, 1a: 9 cases, 1b: 1 case, and 1c: 0 cases). No correlation was found between the $M$ score and fibrosis, NAFLD activity score, and/or steatosis (Table 3). Ductular reaction was seen in only 3 of 15 cases; hence, statistical analysis was not performed.

## 4. Discussion

Chronic hepatitis C affects about 160 million worldwide [21] and is a significant cause of liver-related mortality [39, 40]. Hence, the staging liver biopsy for HCV hepatitis is a very common liver sample encountered in routine surgical pathologists' practice. Steatosis in HCV liver biopsies is common and is seen in approximately 74% of genotype 3 and 48% of

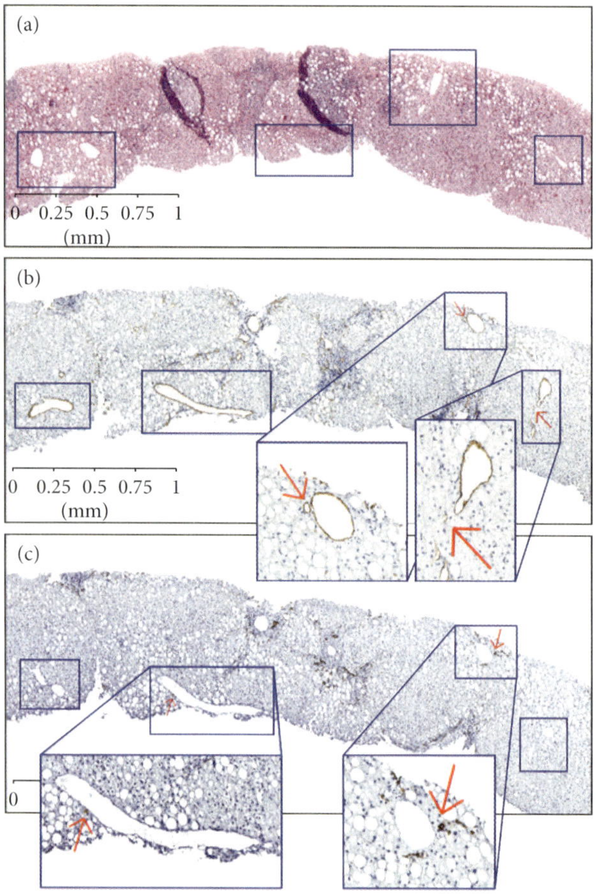


FIGURE 1: (a) Low magnification view of steatotic HCV liver biopsy with 4 central zones marked by squares (H&E, ×50). (b) Level section of the same liver biopsy demonstrates two central zones with microvessel and sinusoidal capillarization. In this case, the *M* score is 2/4 = 0.5. Insets: high magnification of microvessel/sinusoidal capillarization highlighted by CD34 immunostain and arrows (CD34, ×50; insets: CD34, ×200). (c) Level section of the same liver biopsy demonstrates two central zones with ductular reaction and intermediate-phenotype hepatocytes (CK7, ×50). In this case, the *D* score is 2/4 = 0.5. Insets: high magnification of ductular reaction/intermediate-phenotype hepatocytes highlighted by CK7 immunostain and arrows (CK7, ×50; insets: CK7, ×200).

nongenotype 3 biopsies [1]. Concomitant steatosis in chronic hepatitis C confers a worse prognosis in the progression of fibrosis, treatment outcome, and risk of hepatocellular carcinoma [1, 4, 6, 10, 15, 16, 22–33]. Moreover, nonalcoholic steatohepatitis (NASH) and its risk factors superimposed on chronic hepatitis C are associated with progression of fibrosis, suggesting that modification of the metabolic risk factors for NASH might be beneficial for these patients [2, 3, 15, 21].

The current study confirms that obesity is a dominating metabolic risk factor in steatotic HCV biopsies, and the biopsies from patients with obesity demonstrate a higher degree of steatosis than those without obesity. All genotype 3 biopsies demonstrated more than 10% of steatosis, supporting the role of a viral factor in steatosis.

Our results also confirm the previous findings that steatosis and fibrosis are positively correlated in chronic hepatitis C [1, 4, 6, 16, 22–25]. Furthermore, the study group contained more fibrosis than the HCV control group. However, when HCV biopsies with >10% steatosis are only considered, the degree of steatosis does not correlate with fibrosis.

All the study groups showed either microvessels or sinusoidal capillarization in the central zone, and the *M* score showed a positive correlation with the NAFLD score and fibrosis. This result suggests the role of central zone injury and angiogenesis in the progression of fibrogenesis in steatotic HCV hepatitis, similar to NASH [34]. The association between angiogenesis, steatosis, and chronic hepatitis C was addressed in prior studies [41–43]. Kukla et al. studied 35 steatotic liver biopsies of chronic hepatitis C in comparison to 37 nonsteatotic biopsies and showed that higher grade of steatosis was associated with advanced fibrosis and angiogenesis [41]. Their study excluded genotype 3 and patients with risk factors for NASH, and the central zone was not separately evaluated. However, the authors observed higher CD34 expression in the "lobules" and "fibrous septa in the lobules" of the biopsies with >66% of steatosis. Thus, the result seems to suggest a positive correlation between steatosis and centrizonal angiogenesis in steatotic HCV biopsies in the absence of risk factors for NASH [41].

There are two possible mechanisms for angiogenesis in chronic liver diseases. Preexisting vasculature may grow and branch as a part of tissue repair in response to inflammation by recruitment of proangiogenic markers. This process is visualized as predominantly periportal vasculature with inflammatory activity and fibrosis in chronic hepatitis C biopsies [42]. In contrast, in conditions of centrizonal ischemia, angiogenesis may be induced by tissue hypoxia, via intrahepatic vascular remodeling and sinusoidal capillarization, and upregulation of proangiogenesis in extracellular matrix-producing cells, including hepatic stellate cells [43–48]. This ischemia-driven centrizonal angiogenesis has been postulated in the pathogenesis of central portalization in NASH [34]. The positive correlation between the *M* score and NAFLD activity score and the fact that leptin, a circulating peptide hormone mainly produced by adipose tissue, leads to upregulation of proinflammatory and proangiogenic cytokines in human hepatic stellate cells [45] raise a possibility that the latter mechanism may be involved in the angiogenesis of steatotic chronic hepatitis C. Future correlation studies between the distribution of the hepatic stellate cells and angiogenesis in steatotic chronic hepatitis C may be insightful.

Centrizonal ductular reaction and intermediate-phenotype hepatocytes seem to correlate with fibrosis in chronic hepatitis C biopsies, regardless of steatosis. This is shown by the positive correlation between the *D* score and fibrosis in the study group, as well as the HCV control group. Centrizonal ductular reaction is speculated to represent an end-product of metaplasia or dedifferentiation of parenchymal hepatocytes in response to tissue hypoxia. Similarly, intermediate-phenotype hepatocytes, which may constitute an intermediate stage of dedifferentiation of centrizonal hepatocytes, were reported in conditions demonstrating centrilobular scarring, such as chronic venous outflow obstruction and NASH [34, 38, 49, 50]. Thus, our result is in keeping with a prior study [49] and supports that centrizonal ischemic injury is involved in the fibrogenesis of chronic hepatitis C.

In our NASH control group, no correlation between the *M* score and fibrosis was found, contradicting Gill et al.'s study [34]. In their study, cases with low fibrosis stage (NASH CRN stages 0 and 1a) were excluded, while 13 of 22 (59%) cases were NASH CRN stage 0 or 1a in our study. The predominance of low stage fibrosis and low case number may have contributed to the discrepant result in our study.

We evaluated the utility of central portalization as a histologic marker to identify metabolic risk factors in steatotic HCV biopsies. However, neither *M* nor *D* score identified patients with obesity, type 2 DM, and hyperlipidemia in the study group. Therefore, central portalization cannot be used as a surrogate marker to identify patients with risk factors for NASH in steatotic HCV biopsies. Neither the history of treatment nor HCV genotype 3 correlated with *M* or *D* scores. Likewise, neither the *M* score nor *D* score predicted adverse outcome.

The negative result might be due to insufficient clinical data; the information was inconsistent or unavailable in the electronic medical records in some cases. For example, 6 patients subsequently developed clinical NASH and type 2 DM during the follow-up period, suggesting that the biopsies may have been performed at the subclinical stage of insulin resistance. Or, the negative result may be due to the confounding alcohol history, which may have contributed to centrizonal injury. However, neither *M* score nor *D* score differed between the patients with and without alcohol history, making this possibility unlikely. An alternative and more reasonable explanation is that the mechanism of central zone injury in steatotic chronic hepatitis C is not simply attributable to the risk factors for NASH.

NASH biopsies tend to show accentuated steatosis in zone 3, in contrast to randomly distributed steatosis of HCV biopsies. Hence, zonation of steatosis may be used as a histologic marker to identify HCV patients with concomitant metabolic risk factors. In this study, the zonation of steatosis was evaluated without prior knowledge of the clinical information. However, only 6 cases showed zonation of steatosis in our study group. Moreover, the evaluation of zonation was challenging in cases of advanced fibrosis and marked steatosis, which preclude a standardized approach. This observation suggests that the utility of zonation as a surrogate histologic marker to detect metabolic risk factors is limited.

Our study is not without limitations. Many cases of advanced fibrosis were excluded from the statistical analysis due to low number of recognizable central zones. The inverse correlation between the number of central zones and fibrosis clearly demonstrates the interpretational challenge. Also, any zone with CK19 positivity was excluded from the central zone count. In brief, lobular CK19 positive cells may originate from the adjacent portal tracts by branching and migration of portal cholangiocytes, in conditions of predominant portal injury, such as chronic hepatitis C [38, 51]. Alternatively, the lobular CK19 positive cells may represent dedifferentiating centrizonal hepatocytes, expressing progenitor cell phenotype via CK19 expression, as seen in conditions of predominant centrizonal injury [34, 38]. Regardless, all CK19 positive zones were excluded to minimize the chance of counting portal tracts as central zones, further reducing the number of central zones. Lastly, higher stage fibrosis was overrepresented in the study group compared to the HCV control group, and the case number was low in the HCV control group. These factors may have contributed to the lack of correlation between the *M* score and fibrosis in the HCV control group.

## 5. Conclusions

In summary, our study demonstrates that central zone injury represented by central portalization is positively correlated with fibrosis in steatotic chronic hepatitis C biopsies. The mechanism of central zone injury and fibrogenesis in steatotic chronic hepatitis C does not appear to be solely attributable to the metabolic risk factors for NASH; thus, central portalization cannot be used as a surrogate marker to identify these patients.

## References

[1] A. Lonardo, P. Loria, L. E. Adinolfi, N. Carulli, and G. Ruggiero, "Hepatitis C and steatosis: a reappraisal," *Journal of Viral Hepatitis*, vol. 13, no. 2, pp. 73–80, 2006.

[2] J. A. Solis-Herruzo, M. Pérez-Carreras, E. Rivas et al., "Factors associated with the presence of nonalcoholic steatohepatitis in patients with chronic hepatitis C," *The American Journal of Gastroenterology*, vol. 100, no. 5, pp. 1091–1098, 2005.

[3] Z. M. Younossi, A. J. McCullough, J. P. Ong et al., "Obesity and non-alcoholic fatty liver disease in chronic hepatitis C," *Journal of Clinical Gastroenterology*, vol. 38, no. 8, pp. 705–709, 2004.

[4] L. E. Adinolfi, M. Gambardella, A. Andreana, M.-F. Tripodi, R. Utili, and G. Ruggiero, "Steatosis accelerates the progression of liver damage of chronic hepatitis C patients and correlates with specific HCV genotype and visceral obesity," *Hepatology*, vol. 33, no. 6, pp. 1358–1364, 2001.

[5] K. Moriya, H. Fujie, Y. Shintani et al., "The core protein of hepatitis C virus induces hepatocellular carcinoma in transgenic mice," *Nature Medicine*, vol. 4, no. 9, pp. 1065–1067, 1998.

[6] S. J. Hwang and S. D. Lee, "Hepatic steatosis and hepatitis C: still unhappy bedfellows?" *Journal of Gastroenterology and Hepatology (Australia)*, vol. 26, no. 1, pp. 96–101, 2011.

[7] G. Perlemuter, A. Sabile, P. Letteron et al., "Hepatitis C virus core protein inhibits microsomal triglyceride transfer protein activity and very low density lipoprotein secretion: a model of viral-related steatosis," *FASEB Journal*, vol. 16, no. 2, pp. 185–194, 2002.

[8] L. Rubbia-Brandt, R. Quadri, K. Abid et al., "Hepatocyte steatosis is a cytopathic effect of hepatitis C virus genotype 3," *Journal of Hepatology*, vol. 33, no. 1, pp. 106–115, 2000.

[9] L. Rubbia-Brandt, G. Leandro, L. Spahr et al., "Liver steatosis in chronic hepatitis C: a morphological sign suggesting infection

with HCV genotype 3," *Histopathology*, vol. 39, no. 2, pp. 119–124, 2001.

[10] D. Kumar, G. C. Farrell, C. Fung, and J. George, "Hepatitis C virus genotype 3 is cytopathic to hepatocytes: reversal of hepatic steatosis after sustained therapeutic response," *Hepatology*, vol. 36, no. 5, pp. 1266–1272, 2002.

[11] K. R. Reddy, S. Govindarajan, P. Marcellin et al., "Hepatic steatosis in chronic hepatitis C: baseline host and viral characteristics and influence on response to therapy with peginterferon $\alpha$-2a plus ribavirin," *Journal of Viral Hepatitis*, vol. 15, no. 2, pp. 129–136, 2008.

[12] L. Castéra, C. Hézode, F. Roudot-Thoraval et al., "Effect of antiviral treatment on evolution of liver steatosis in patients with chronic hepatitis C: indirect evidence of a role of hepatitis C virus genotype 3 in steatosis," *Gut*, vol. 53, no. 3, pp. 420–424, 2004.

[13] L. Baiocchi, G. Tisone, G. Palmieri et al., "Hepatic steatosis: a specific sign of hepatitis C reinfection after liver transplantation," *Liver Transplantation and Surgery*, vol. 4, no. 6, pp. 441–447, 1998.

[14] T. J. S. Cross, M. M. Rashid, P. A. Berry, and P. M. Harrison, "The importance of steatosis in chronic hepatitis C infection and its management: a review," *Hepatology Research*, vol. 40, no. 3, pp. 237–247, 2010.

[15] J. P. Ong, Z. M. Younossi, C. Speer, A. Olano, T. Gramlich, and N. Boparai, "Chronic hepatitis C and superimposed nonalcoholic fatty liver disease," *Liver*, vol. 21, no. 4, pp. 266–271, 2001.

[16] A. Monto, J. Alonzo, J. J. Watson, C. Grunfeld, and T. L. Wright, "Steatosis in chronic hepatitis C: relative contributions of obesity, diabetes mellitus, and alcohol," *Hepatology*, vol. 36, no. 3, pp. 729–736, 2002.

[17] K. L. Donnelly, C. I. Smith, S. J. Schwarzenberg, J. Jessurun, M. D. Boldt, and E. J. Parks, "Sources of fatty acids stored in liver and secreted via lipoproteins in patients with nonalcoholic fatty liver disease," *The Journal of Clinical Investigation*, vol. 115, no. 5, pp. 1343–1351, 2005.

[18] J. M. Hui, A. Sud, G. C. Farrell et al., "Insulin resistance is associated with chronic hepatitis C and virus infection fibrosis progression," *Gastroenterology*, vol. 125, no. 6, pp. 1695–1704, 2003.

[19] L.-K. Chen, S.-J. Hwang, S.-T. Tsai, J.-C. Luo, S.-D. Lee, and F.-Y. Chang, "Glucose intolerance in Chinese patients with chronic hepatitis C," *World Journal of Gastroenterology*, vol. 9, no. 3, pp. 505–508, 2003.

[20] M. Sougleri, C. Labropoulou-Karatza, P. Paraskevopoulou, H. Fragopanagou, and T. Alexandrides, "Chronic hepatitis C virus infection without cirrhosis induces insulin resistance in patients with $\beta$-thalassaemia major," *European Journal of Gastroenterology and Hepatology*, vol. 13, no. 10, pp. 1195–1199, 2001.

[21] J. Jaroszewicz and R. Flisiak, "Metabolic syndrome and hepatitis C infection—brothers in arms," *Liver International*, vol. 33, no. 8, pp. 1135–1137, 2013.

[22] S.-J. Hwang, J.-C. Luo, C.-W. Chu et al., "Hepatic steatosis in chronic hepatitis C virus infection: prevalence and clinical correlation," *Journal of Gastroenterology and Hepatology*, vol. 16, no. 2, pp. 190–195, 2001.

[23] L. Castéra, C. Hézode, F. Roudot-Thoraval et al., "Worsening of steatosis is an independent factor of fibrosis progression in untreated patients with chronic hepatitis C and paired liver biopsies," *Gut*, vol. 52, no. 2, pp. 288–292, 2003.

[24] T. Poynard, V. Ratziu, J. McHutchison et al., "Effect of treatment with peginterferon or interferon alfa-2b and ribavirin on steatosis in patients infected with hepatitis C," *Hepatology*, vol. 38, no. 1, pp. 75–85, 2003.

[25] H. M. Patton, K. Patel, C. Behling et al., "The impact of steatosis on disease progression and early and sustained treatment response in chronic hepatitis C patients," *Journal of Hepatology*, vol. 40, no. 3, pp. 484–490, 2004.

[26] T. J. S. Cross, A. Quaglia, J. Nolan, S. Hughes, and P. M. Harrison, "Do steatosis and steatohepatitis impact on sustained virological response (SVR) rates in patients receiving pegylated interferon and ribavirin for chronic hepatitis C infection?" *Journal of Medical Virology*, vol. 82, no. 6, pp. 958–964, 2010.

[27] A. Tanaka, S. Uegaki, H. Kurihara et al., "Hepatic steatosis as a possible risk factor for the development of hepatocellular carcinoma after eradication of hepatitis C virus with antiviral therapy in patients with chronic hepatitis C," *World Journal of Gastroenterology*, vol. 13, no. 39, pp. 5180–5187, 2007.

[28] K. Ohata, K. Hamasaki, K. Toriyama et al., "Hepatic steatosis is a risk factor for hepatocellular carcinoma in patients with chronic hepatitis C virus infection," *Cancer*, vol. 97, no. 12, pp. 3036–3043, 2003.

[29] A. D. Clouston, J. R. Jonsson, D. M. Purdie et al., "Steatosis and chronic hepatitis C: analysis of fibrosis and stellate cell activation," *Journal of Hepatology*, vol. 34, no. 2, pp. 314–320, 2001.

[30] I. J. Hickman, A. D. Clouston, G. A. Macdonald et al., "Effect of weight reduction on liver histology and biochemistry in patients with chronic hepatitis C," *Gut*, vol. 51, no. 1, pp. 89–94, 2002.

[31] M. Romero-Gómez, M. Diago, R. J. Andrade et al., "Treatment of insulin resistance with metformin in naïve genotype 1 chronic hepatitis C patients receiving peginterferon alfa-2a plus ribavirin," *Hepatology*, vol. 50, no. 6, pp. 1702–1708, 2009.

[32] I. A. Hanouneh, A. E. Feldstein, R. Lopez et al., "Clinical significance of metabolic syndrome in the setting of chronic hepatitis C virus infection," *Clinical Gastroenterology and Hepatology*, vol. 6, no. 5, pp. 584–589, 2008.

[33] S. Bondini and Z. M. Younossi, "Non-alcoholic fatty liver disease and hepatitis C infection," *Minerva Gastroenterologica e Dietologica*, vol. 52, no. 2, pp. 135–143, 2006.

[34] R. M. Gill, P. Belt, L. Wilson, N. M. Bass, and L. D. Ferrell, "Centrizonal arteries and microvessels in nonalcoholic steatohepatitis," *The American Journal of Surgical Pathology*, vol. 35, no. 9, pp. 1400–1404, 2011.

[35] K. Ishak, A. Baptista, L. Bianchi et al., "Histological grading and staging of chronic hepatitis," *Journal of Hepatology*, vol. 22, no. 6, pp. 696–699, 1995.

[36] D. E. Kleiner, E. M. Brunt, and M. Van Natta, "Nonalcoholic steatohepatitis clinical research network. Design and validation of a histological scoring system for nonalcoholic fatty liver disease," *Hepatology*, vol. 41, no. 6, pp. 1313–1321, 2005.

[37] A. R. Crawford, X. I.-Z. Lin, and J. M. Crawford, "The normal adult human liver biopsy: a quantitative reference standard," *Hepatology*, vol. 28, no. 2, pp. 323–331, 1998.

[38] G. Krings, B. Can, and L. Ferrell, "Aberrant centrizonal features in chronic hepatic venous outflow obstruction: centrilobular mimicry of portal-based disease," *American Journal of Surgical Pathology*, vol. 38, no. 2, pp. 205–214, 2014.

[39] V. Calvaruso and A. Craxì, "2011 European Association of the Study of the Liver hepatitis C virus clinical practice guidelines," *Liver International*, vol. 32, no. 1, pp. 2–8, 2012.

[40] L. B. Seeff, "Natural history of chronic hepatitis C," *Hepatology*, vol. 36, no. 5, pp. S35–S46, 2002.

[41] M. Kukla, A. Gabriel, D. Sabat et al., "Association between liver steatosis and angiogenesis in chronic hepatitis C," *Polish Journal of Pathology*, vol. 61, no. 3, pp. 154–160, 2010.

[42] A. Gabriel, M. Kukla, M. Wilk, Ł. Liszka, M. Petelenz, and J. Musialik, "Angiogenesis in chronic hepatitis C is associated with inflammatory activity grade and fibrosis stage," *Pathology Research and Practice*, vol. 205, no. 11, pp. 758–764, 2009.

[43] M. Fernández, D. Semela, J. Bruix, I. Colle, M. Pinzani, and J. Bosch, "Angiogenesis in liver disease," *Journal of Hepatology*, vol. 50, no. 3, pp. 604–620, 2009.

[44] J. Medina, A. G. Arroyo, F. Sánchez-Madrid, and R. Moreno-Otero, "Angiogenesis in chronic inflammatory liver disease," *Hepatology*, vol. 39, no. 5, pp. 1185–1195, 2004.

[45] S. Aleffi, I. Petrai, C. Bertolani et al., "Upregulation of proinflammatory and proangiogenic cytokines by leptin in human hepatic stellate cells," *Hepatology*, vol. 42, no. 6, pp. 1339–1348, 2005.

[46] E. Novo, S. Cannito, E. Zamara et al., "Proangiogenic cytokines as hypoxia-dependent factors stimulating migration of human hepatic stellate cells," *American Journal of Pathology*, vol. 170, no. 6, pp. 1942–1953, 2007.

[47] V. Ankoma-Sey, M. Matli, K. B. Chang et al., "Coordinated induction of VEGF receptors in mesenchymal cell types during rat hepatic wound healing," *Oncogene*, vol. 17, no. 1, pp. 115–121, 1998.

[48] Y. Q. Wang, J. M. Luk, K. Ikeda et al., "Regulatory role of vHL/HIF-1$\alpha$ in hypoxia-induced VEGF production in hepatic stellate cells," *Biochemical and Biophysical Research Communications*, vol. 317, no. 2, pp. 358–362, 2004.

[49] S. Matsukuma, H. Takeo, T. Kono, Y. Nagata, and K. Sato, "Aberrant cytokeratin 7 expression of centrilobular hepatocytes: a clinicopathological study," *Histopathology*, vol. 61, no. 5, pp. 857–862, 2012.

[50] R. K. Pai and J. A. Hart, "Aberrant expression of cytokeratin 7 in perivenular hepatocytes correlates with a cholestatic chemistry profile in patients with heart failure," *Modern Pathology*, vol. 23, no. 12, pp. 1650–1656, 2010.

[51] V. J. Desmet, "Ductal plates in hepatic ductular reactions. Hypothesis and implications. I. Types of ductular reaction reconsidered," *Virchows Archiv*, vol. 458, no. 3, pp. 251–259, 2011.

# 17

# Quantification of Pregenomic RNA and Covalently Closed Circular DNA in Hepatitis B Virus-Related Hepatocellular Carcinoma

**Fugui Bai,[1] Yoshihiko Yano,[1,2] Takumi Fukumoto,[3] Atsushi Takebe,[3] Motofumi Tanaka,[3] Kaori Kuramitsu,[3] Nungki Anggorowati,[1] Hanggoro Tri Rinonce,[1] Dewiyani Indah Widasari,[1] Masaya Saito,[2] Hirotaka Hirano,[2] Takanobu Hayakumo,[2] Yasushi Seo,[2] Takeshi Azuma,[2] Yonson Ku,[3] and Yoshitake Hayashi[1]**

[1] *Center for Infectious Diseases, Kobe University Graduate School of Medicine, Kobe 650-0017, Japan*
[2] *Department of Gastroenterology, Kobe University Graduate School of Medicine, Kobe 650-0017, Japan*
[3] *Department of Hepato-Biliary-Pancreatic Surgery, Kobe University Graduate School of Medicine, Kobe 650-0017, Japan*

Correspondence should be addressed to Yoshihiko Yano; yanoyo@med.kobe-u.ac.jp

Academic Editor: Daisuke Morioka

Pregenomic RNA (pgRNA) is generated from covalently closed circular DNA (cccDNA) and plays important roles in viral genome amplification and replication. Hepatic pgRNA and cccDNA expression levels indicate viral persistence and replication activity. This study was aimed to measure hepatic pgRNA and cccDNA expression levels in various states of hepatitis B virus (HBV) infection. Thirty-eight hepatocellular carcinoma (HCC) patients, including 14 positive for hepatitis B surface antigen (HBsAg) and 24 negative for HBsAg but positive for anti-hepatitis B core (anti-HBc) antibody, were enrolled in this study. In HBsAg-negative but anti-HBc-positive group, HBV-DNA was detected in 20 of 24 (83%) noncancerous liver tissues for at least two genomic regions based on polymerase chain reaction (PCR) analysis. pgRNA and cccDNA expression levels in occult HBV-infected patients were significantly lower than those in HBsAg-positive patients ($P < 0.001$). pgRNA and cccDNA in cancerous tissues were also detected without significant difference from those in noncancerous tissues. In conclusion, cccDNA and pgRNA are detected and represented HBV replication not only in noncancerous but also in cancerous liver tissues. In addition, the replication is shown in not only patients with HBsAg-positive but also occult HBV-infected patients, suggesting the contribution to HCC development.

## 1. Introduction

Hepatitis B virus (HBV) infection remains a major health problem, even though methods for preventing vertical transmission and treatment guidelines have been introduced. Approximately, 2 billion people worldwide are infected with HBV. Three hundred fifty million of them have chronic infection. HBV is particularly endemic in sub-Saharan Africa, the Pacific, and Asia [1]. It frequently causes chronic hepatitis, which, subsequently, progresses to liver cirrhosis and hepatocellular carcinoma (HCC). HBV is responsible for most of the worldwide attributable risk of liver cirrhosis and HCC. The risk is even higher in endemic regions [2].

HBV is an incomplete double-stranded circular DNA virus, with a DNA length of approximately 3,200 bp. After HBV infects the liver cells, the relaxed-circular DNA is transferred into the nucleus and is repaired to covalently closed circular DNA (cccDNA) by DNA polymerase. The cccDNA plays a key role in the life cycle of the virus. It acts as a template for the generation of mRNAs, including pregenomic RNA (pgRNA) [3–5]. The transcription of cccDNA generates four kinds of mRNA: PreC/C (3.5 kb), PreS1 (2.4 kb), S (2.1 kb), and X (0.7 kb). The transcription of cccDNA is a critical step for viral genomic amplification and replication. PgRNA is also generated during the transcription from cccDNA and works as a template of viral genomic DNA.

The cccDNA is detected in various phases of chronic hepatitis, and its levels reflect viral replication in the infected cells. HBV-DNA is sometimes detected in patients negative for hepatitis B surface antigen (HBsAg) but positive for anti-hepatitis B core (anti-HBc) antibody and/or anti-hepatitis B surface (anti-HBs) antibody, which is often called occult HBV infection [4]. Recent studies revealed that cccDNA was expressed in HCC without HBs antigen [5]. However, it is still debated whether HBV-DNA is responsible for the development of HCC in patients with occult HBV infection.

In this study, we measured the levels of cccDNA and pgRNA in cancerous and contiguous noncancerous liver tissues of HCC patients with overt and occult HBV infection to examine the viral existence and replication. We also determined the nucleotide variations and amino acid mutations in patients with occult HBV infection.

## 2. Materials and Methods

*2.1. Patients.* Cancerous and contiguous noncancerous liver tissues were obtained from 38 HCC patients (mean ± SD, 63.37 ± 12.01 years; male-female ratio, 34/4) who underwent surgical resection at Kobe University Hospital, Japan, between April 2010 and December 2011. HBsAg-positive carriers ($n = 14$) and HBsAg-negative/HBcAb-positive patients ($n = 24$) were enrolled in this study. Hepatitis C virus (HCV) infected patients who were detected by anti-HCV positivity were excluded. Tissue samples were rapidly frozen in liquid nitrogen and stored at –80°C after resection.

The demographic and clinical data, including age, sex, body mass index (BMI), results of standard test for HBV-related HCC, and stage of the disease, were collected from medical record after institutional review board approval was obtained.

Written informed consent was obtained from each patient before all the procedures in this study were done. This study was reviewed and approved by the Ethics Committee at Kobe University.

*2.2. Detection of HBV-DNA, cccDNA, and pgRNA in Tissue Samples.* Total DNA and RNA from cancerous and contiguous noncancerous tissues were extracted from about 20 mg of liver tissues using a QIAamp DNA Mini Kit (QIAGEN Sciences, Germantown, MD) and Isogen (Nippon Gene, Tokyo, Japan). The DNA and RNA concentrations were measured spectrophotometrically. The cDNA was synthesized from five $\mu$g of total RNA using the Oligo (dT) 15 primer (Promega, Madison, WI) and M-MLV Reverse Transcriptase (Invitrogen, Carlsbad, CA) according to the manufacturers' instructions.

To detect intrahepatic HBV-DNA, a nested polymerase chain reaction (PCR) was carried out using the specific primers for amplifying S, precore-core, polymerase, and X region. The primers used are listed in Table 1. The first and second round PCRs were performed under the same condition described previously [5]. Appropriate controls were included in each PCR. The PCR products were resolved on 2% agarose gels and visualized under ultraviolet illumination with ethidium bromide staining. Patients, who were serologically negative for HBsAg but positive for intrahepatic HBV-DNA at least in two regions of HBV genome based on PCR assays, were defined as having occult infections.

We further performed quantitative real-time PCR using an Applied Biosystems 7500 RT-PCR System (Applied Biosystems, Foster City, CA). Briefly, 2 $\mu$L of HBV-cccDNA or pgRNA was amplified using TaqMan Gene Expression Master Mix (Applied Biosystems, Foster City, CA), primers for cccDNA (CCC and BC1) or pgRNA (PGP and BC1), and FRET hybridization probes (hbvLC and hbvFL) as listed in Table 1. The amplification was performed under conditions described previously [8].

To avoid cross-contamination between samples, standard precautions were used for all procedures. Reagents, samples, and amplified products were stored in separate areas.

*2.3. Determination of HBV Genotypes and Subgenotypes.* HBV genotypes and subgenotypes were determined by phylogenetic analysis based on the S region. Part of S region was amplified in PCR using HB2F and HB2R primer (Table 1) with condition described previously [7]. The amplified fragments were purified using ExoSAP-IT (USB, Cleveland, OH) and directly sequenced using BigDye Terminator v3.1. Cycle Sequencing Kit (Applied Biosystems, Foster City, CA). The sequencing was performed in an ABI PRISM 3100-*Avant* Genetic Analyzer (Applied Biosystems, Foster City, CA). The sequences were edited manually and subsequently aligned using Clustal X version 2.0.12 software (http://www.clustal.org/). A phylogenetic tree was constructed by the neighbor-joining method using the Molecular Evolutionary Genetic Analysis (MEGA) version 4.0.2 software (http://megasoftware.net/) [9]. To show the reliability of this analysis, bootstrap resampling and reconstruction were performed 1,000 times [10].

*2.4. Detection of Amino Acid Substitutions in the "a" Determinant Region and Mutations in the Core Promoter and Precore Region.* Some amino acid substitutions in the "a" determinant region are thought to result in detectable HBV-DNA in HBsAg-negative patients. Therefore, the sequences within this region were aligned and analyzed to identify amino acid substitutions among HBV strains obtained from patients positive for HBV-DNA. We used the previously described primer pairs as shown in Table 1 [7] to amplify the "a" determinant region. Core promoter and precore region were also amplified using primers and condition described previously (Table 1) [7].

Those amplified fragments were directly sequenced, and the obtained sequences from each region were aligned with reference sequences retrieved from GenBank databases to identify the substitutions or mutations.

*2.5. Statistical Analyses.* Statistical analyses were performed using IBM SPSS Statistics version 21.0 (IBM, Armonk, NY). The categorical variables were analyzed using the $\chi^2$ test or Fisher's exact test, whereas continuous variables were analyzed using independent $t$-tests or the Mann-Whitney test. Differences were considered statistically significant at $P < 0.05$.

Table 1: Sequences and positions of primers and probes used in this study.

| Primer and probe | Region | Position | Polarity | Sequence (5′ to 3′) | Reference |
|---|---|---|---|---|---|
| Occult case determination | | | | | |
| HBV 1 | PreS-S | 2815–2834 | Sense | GGTCACCATATTCTTGGGAA | [6] |
| HBV 2 | PreS-S | 690–671 | Antisense | AATGGCACTAGTAAACTGAG | [6] |
| HBV 17 | PreS-S | 3037–3057 | Sense | AATCCAGATTGGGACTTCAA | [6] |
| HBV 4 | PreS-S | 459–440 | Antisense | CCTTGATAGTCCAGAAGAAC | [6] |
| HBV 5 | Precore-core | 2021–2040 | Sense | GCCTTAGAGTCTCCTGAGCA | [6] |
| HBV 6 | Precore-core | 2464–2448 | Antisense | GTCCAAGGAATACTAAC | [6] |
| HBV 7 | Precore-core | 2048–2066 | Sense | CCTCACCATACTGCACTCA | [6] |
| HBV 8 | Precore-core | 2385–2366 | Antisense | GAGGGAGTTCTTCTTCTAGG | [6] |
| Pol 1 S | Polymerase | 2412–2430 | Sense | CGCGTCGCAGAAGATCTCA | [5] |
| Pol 1 AS | Polymerase | 256–237 | Antisense | CGAGTCTAGACTCTGTGGTA | [5] |
| Pol 2 S | Polymerase | 2452–2476 | Sense | GTATYCCTTGGACTCATAAGGTGGG | [5] |
| Pol 2 AS | Polymerase | 2838–2814 | Antisense | CTTGTTCCCAAGAATATGGTGACCC | [5] |
| X 1 S | X | 1100–1121 | Sense | CGCCAACTTACAAGGCCTTTCT | [5] |
| HBV 19 | X | 1550–1529 | Antisense | CGTTCACGGTGGTCTCCAT | [6] |
| HBV 15 | X | 1380–1400 | Sense | GCTAGGCTGTGCTGCCAACTG | [6] |
| HBV 21 | X | 1518–1497 | Antisense | GGTCGGTCGGAACGGCAGACGG | [6] |
| Genotyping and amplification of "a" determinant region | | | | | |
| HB2F | S | 414–433 | Sense | TGCTGCTATGCCTCATCTTC | [7] |
| HB2R | S | 989–970 | Antisense | CATACTTTCCAATCAATAGG | [7] |
| Amplification of core promoter and precore regions | | | | | |
| HB7F | C | 1611–1630 | Sense | GAGACCACCGTGAACGCCCA | [7] |
| HB7R | C | 2072–2048 | Antisense | CCTGAGTGCTGTATGGTGAGG | [7] |
| cccDNA and pgRNA quantification | | | | | |
| CCC | X/C | 1555–1573 | Sense | GTGCCTTCTCATCTGCCGG | [8] |
| PGP | X/C | 1826–1843 | Sense | CACCTCTGCCTAATCATC | [8] |
| BC1 | X/C | 1974–1955 | Antisense | GGAAAGAAGTCAGAAGGCAA | [8] |
| hbvLC | C | 1874–1848 | Antisense | GGAGGCTTGAACAGTAGGACATGAAC | [8] |
| hbvFL | C | 1897–1876 | Antisense | CYAAAGCCACCCAAGGCACAGC | [8] |

## 3. Results

*3.1. Clinical Characteristics of the Patients.* The clinical characteristics of HBsAg-negative/HBcAb-positive patients were compared with those of HBsAg-positive carriers (Table 2). The HBsAg-positive carriers were significantly younger than HBsAg-negative/HBcAb-positive patients (55.7 ± 12.0 versus 68.7 ± 9.3 years; $P = 0.002$). The complication of diabetes mellitus is significantly higher in HBsAg-negative/HBcAb-positive patients. It was indicated by higher level of HbA1c in this group (5.96 ± 0.87 versus 5.04 ± 0.33; $P < 0.001$). Ten of them (42%) were treated by oral medication and/or insulin injection therapy for diabetes. In addition, four patients had massive alcohol consumption and had been diagnosed as alcoholic cirrhosis. The average body mass index (BMI) in HBsAg-negative/HBcAb-positive patients tended to be high compared with those in HBsAg-positive carriers (23.1 ± 3.4 versus 20.5 ± 3.7; $P = 0.079$) although not significant statistically. Four HBsAg-positive patients were treated by nucleotide analogue for more than one year, and HBV-DNA was undetectable in their sera. A significantly greater proportion of HBsAg-positive carriers had an HBV viral load of >4 log copies/mL as compared with HBsAg-negative/HBcAb-positive patients (42.9% versus 0%; $P = 0.012$). Thirty-two HBV strains could be genotyped. Almost all (96.9%) patients were infected by genotype C2. Only one patient (3.1%) was infected by genotype B1 (Table 2 and Figure 2).

*3.2. Detection of HBV-DNA, cccDNA, and pgRNA in the Tissue.* Based on the nested PCR analysis, HBV-DNA was detected in all cancerous and noncancerous tissues of HBsAg-positive carriers. On the other hand, at least two HBV

TABLE 2: Clinical characteristics of patients.

| | HBsAg-positive carriers ($n$ = 14) | HBsAg−/HBcAb+ patients ($n$ = 24) | $P$ value |
|---|---|---|---|
| Male/female | 13/1 | 21/3 | NS |
| Age (years) | 55.7 ± 12.0 | 68.7 ± 9.3 | 0.002 |
| BMI | 20.5 ± 3.7 | 23.1 ± 3.4 | NS |
| Prevalence of BMI >22 | 3/14 (21%) | 14/24 (58%) | 0.03* |
| Platelet count (/mm$^3$) | 18.1 ± 4.0 | 19.3 ± 8.4 | NS |
| Albumin (g/dL) | 4.2 ± 0.6 | 3.9 ± 0.6 | NS |
| AST (IU/L) | 30.3 ± 5.9 | 74.0 ± 59.6 | NS |
| HbA1c | 5.04 ± 0.33 | 5.96 ± 0.87 | <0.001 |
| ICG-R 15 (%) | 9.54 ± 2.76 | 11.15 ± 5.22 | NS |
| Child-Pugh (A/B/C) | 13/1/0 | 18/3/0 | NS |
| HBV-DNA > 4 log copies/mL | 6 (42.9) | 0 (0.0) | 0.012 |
| Genotype B/C | 1/13 | 0/17 | NS |
| AFP > 200 (ng/mL) | 7 (50%) | 8 (33.3%) | NS |
| PIVKA-II > 400 (mAU/mL) | 9 (64.3%) | 14 (58.3%) | NS |
| Stage I/II/III/IV | 1/4/2/3 | 1/6/2/9 | NS |

AST: aspartate aminotransferase; AFP: $\alpha$-fetoprotein; PIVKA-II: protein induced by vitamin K absence or antagonist II; NS: not significant.
*Mann-Whitney's $U$ test.

TABLE 3: Detection of HBV-DNA in 24 HCC patients with HBsAg-negative and HBcAb-positive patients.

| | Cancerous tissue | Noncancerous tissue | $P$ value |
|---|---|---|---|
| S region | 9 (38%) | 17 (71%) | 0.020 |
| Precore-core region | 4 (17%) | 4 (17%) | NS |
| Polymerase region | 14 (58%) | 10 (42%) | NS |
| X region | 12 (50%) | 21 (88%) | 0.005 |
| Positive in ≥2 regions | 10 (42%) | 20 (83%) | 0.003 |

NS: not significant.

genomic regions were detected in 20 of 24 (83%) noncancerous tissues from HBsAg-negative/HBcAb-positive patients ($P$ = 0.003). Those patients were classified as having occult HBV infection. The S (71% versus 38%, $P$ = 0.02) and X (88% versus 50%, $P$ = 0.005) regions were detected more frequent in noncancerous tissues than in cancerous tissues (Table 3). Twenty patients with occult HBV infection were compared with 14 HBsAg-positive carriers. The mean pgRNA and cccDNA expression levels in noncancerous tissues were significantly lower in occult HBV-infected patients (5.72 ± 1.22 log copies/$\mu$g of extracted RNA and 7.52 ± 1.48 log copies/$\mu$g of extracted DNA, resp.) than in HBsAg-positive carriers (7.55 ± 1.50 log copies/$\mu$g of extracted RNA and 10.37 ± 1.15 log copies/$\mu$g of extracted DNA, resp.; both, $P$ < 0.001). In addition, pgRNA and cccDNA expression levels in cancerous tissues were lower in occult HBV-infected patients (6.11±1.08 log copies/$\mu$g of extracted RNA and 7.84±1.91 log copies/$\mu$g of extracted DNA, resp.) than in HBsAg-positive patients (8.10 ± 1.77 log copies/$\mu$g of extracted RNA and 10.02 ± 4.28 log copies/$\mu$g of extracted DNA, resp.; $P$ = 0.004 and $P$ = 0.201, resp.; Figure 1). The pgRNA and cccDNA in HBsAg-positive patients were also compared in relation with nucleotide analogue therapy. However, no significant difference was detected between undertreated patients and naïve patients (pgRNA, 7.58 ± 1.48 versus 7.45 ± 1.62 log copies/$\mu$g of extracted RNA; cccDNA, 10.13 ± 0.98 versus 10.15 ± 1.34 log copies/$\mu$g of extracted DNA, resp.). The ratio of pgRNA/cccDNA in noncancerous tissues was also examined, but no difference was detected between HBsAg-positive patients and occult HBV-infected patients (0.75 ± 0.18 versus 0.85 ± 0.19, resp.).

*3.3. Amino Acid Substitutions in the "a" Determinant Region and Mutations in the Core Promoter and Precore Region.* Table 4 shows the distribution of amino acid substitutions in the "a" determinant region in HBsAg-positive patients and occult HBV-infected patients. Two specific substitutions (I126T and I126V) were detected in the occult HBV infection group. However, all of the occult infected patients had the viral loads less than 4 log copies/mL. Substitutions in I126T and T131P were also detected in HBsAg-positive patients.

The A1762T/G1764A, T1846A, C1858, and G1896A mutations were detected in HBsAg-positive carriers and in occult HBV-infected patients, without significant differences in their prevalence rates. However, the T1753C mutation was only found in HBsAg-positive carriers (29%), and it was statistically significant ($P$ = 0.033; Table 5).

## 4. Discussion

HBV is a major cause of HCC in most Asian countries. Chronic HCV infection is the leading cause and HBV infection is the second most common cause of HCC in Japan [11]. However, approximately 10% of HCC patients were serologically negative for HBsAg and HCV-Ab [12]. Chronic forms of hepatitis, particularly alcoholic hepatitis, steatohepatitis, and autoimmune hepatitis, may induce HCC in the absence of hepatitis viral infection. The number of cases of HCC without hepatitis viral infection has increased

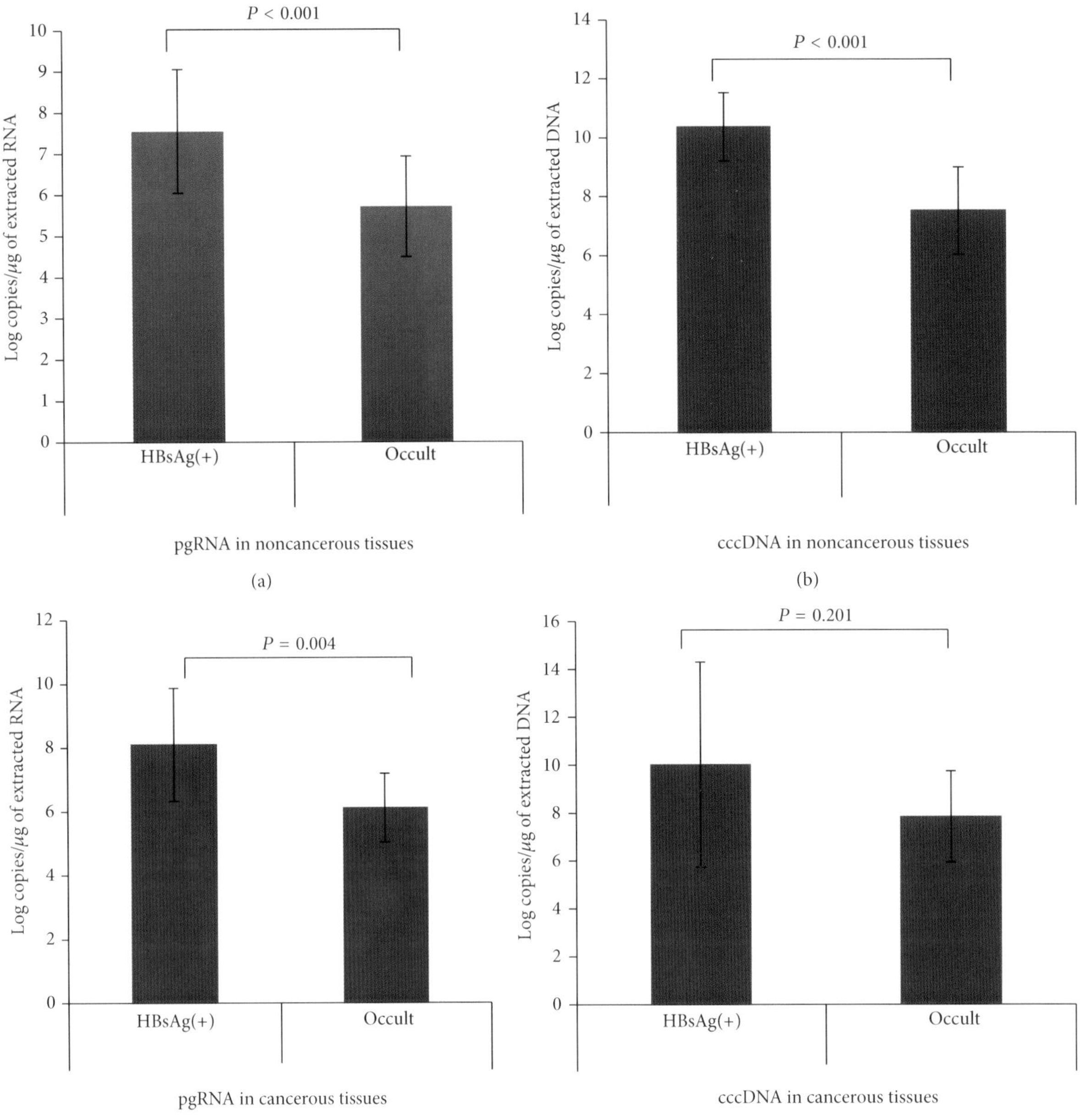


FIGURE 1: Quantitative analysis of pgRNA (a, c) and cccDNA (b, d) in noncancerous and cancerous liver tissues. The pgRNA and cccDNA expression levels were significantly higher in HBsAg-positive patients than in occult HBV-infected patients.

in recent years because of the introduction of vaccination programmes aimed at preventing vertical transmission of HBV and screening systems to prevent HCV infection from transfusion and transmission [13].

Occult HBV infection is diagnosed when serum is negative for HBsAg, but serum or liver is positive for HBV-DNA, regardless of anti-HBc status [14]. Several studies have assessed HBV-DNA status in HBsAg-negative HCC patients [6, 15]. However, it is still controversial whether occult HBV infection is associated with liver damage. In particular, although it was reported that occult HBV infection did not progress to severe liver disease [16], other studies showed that occult HBV infection caused liver disease progression in patients with chronic HCV infection [17].

Earlier studies suggested that individuals could recover from self-limited acute hepatitis because of the role of cytotoxic or memory T cells. However, these patients might carry the HBV genome for a long time without showing clinical signs of hepatic injury [18]. Furthermore, histopathological examination of such patients showed mild necroinflammation after decades of recovery [19]. In the immunocompetent state, occult HBV is not destructive, but progressive liver dysfunction may occur if other deleterious factors are present [20]. In this study, the HBsAg-negative/HBcAb-positive

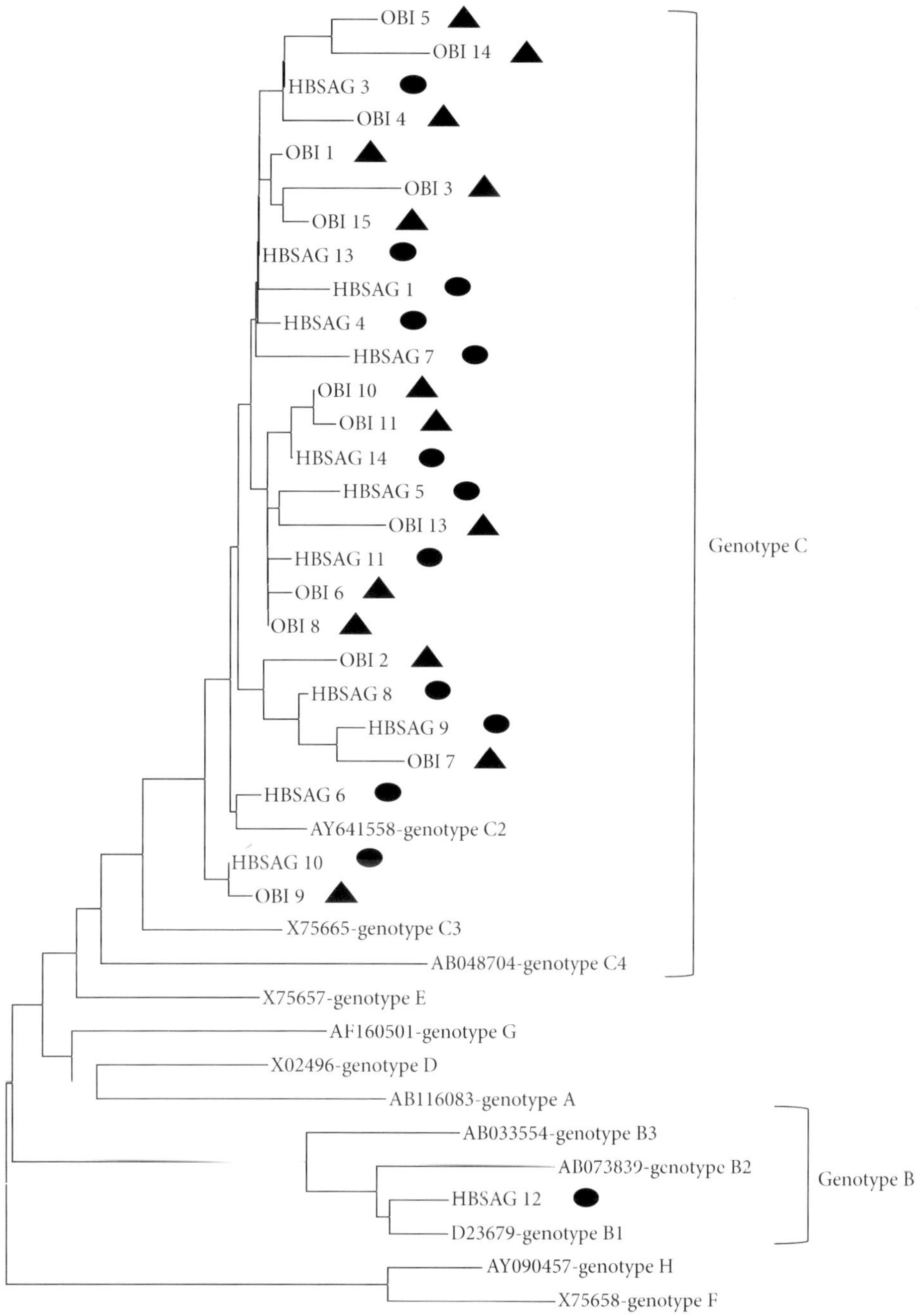


FIGURE 2: Phylogenetic tree analysis of the S gene sequences of strains isolated in this study. The HBV strains from different genotypes (A to H) are obtained from GenBank. The GenBank HBV sequences are indicated with their accession number followed by genotypes. The sequences determined in this study are indicated by isolate number, starting with HBSAG or OBI, and are labelled with black circles and triangles for HBsAg-positive patients and patients with occult HBV infection, respectively.

patients were significantly older than the HBsAg-positive carriers, suggesting that the hepatocarcinogenesis between these two groups was different.

The association of occult HBV infection with HCC has been extensively reviewed [21]. It was also reported that cryptic HBV infection had a pro-oncogenic role in chronic HCV carriers and in cryptogenic liver diseases [6]. In animal studies, for woodchucks and ground squirrels infected with woodchuck or ground-squirrel hepatitis virus, liver cancer progression was apparent, even after elimination of these viruses [22]. A previous study showed that occult HBV was strongly associated with liver cancer, independently of age, sex, cirrhosis, and contemporary HCV infection. Aside from indirect oncogenic mechanisms (e.g., mild necroinflammation), direct oncogenic mechanisms, including viral integration into the host genome and maintenance of transcriptional

Table 4: The alignment of "a" determinant amino acid sequences.

| Sample number or GenBank accession numbers | Genotype | Amino acids alignment (124–147) in the "a" determinant region |
|---|---|---|
| Consensus sequences | | |
| D23684 | C2 | CTIPAQGTSMFPSCCCTKPSDGNC |
| D23678 | B1 | -------------------T---- |
| Occult HBV infection | | |
| OBI-1 | C2 | ------------------------ |
| OBI-2 | C2 | --V--------------------- |
| OBI-4 | C2 | ------------------------ |
| OBI-5 | C2 | ------------------------ |
| OBI-6 | C2 | ------------------------ |
| OBI-7 | C2 | ------------------------ |
| OBI-8 | C2 | ------------------------ |
| OBI-9 | C2 | ------------------------ |
| OBI-10 | C2 | ------------------------ |
| OBI-11 | C2 | ------------------------ |
| OBI-12 | C2 | --T--------------------- |
| OBI-13 | C2 | ------------------------ |
| OBI-14 | C2 | ------------------------ |
| OBI-15 | C2 | ------------------------ |
| OBI-16 | C2 | ------------------------ |
| OBI-17 | C2 | ------------------------ |
| OBI-18 | C2 | ------------------------ |
| HBsAg-positive patients | | |
| HBSAG-1 | C2 | -------P---------------- |
| HBSAG-2 | C2 | ------------------------ |
| HBSAG-3 | C2 | ------------------------ |
| HBSAG-4 | C2 | ------------------------ |
| HBSAG-5 | C2 | ------------------------ |
| HBSAG-6 | C2 | --T--------------------- |
| HBSAG-7 | C2 | ------------------------ |
| HBSAG-8 | C2 | ------------------------ |
| HBSAG-9 | C2 | ------------------------ |
| HBSAG-10 | C2 | ------------------------ |
| HBSAG-11 | C2 | ------------------------ |
| HBSAG-12 | B1 | ------------------------ |
| HBSAG-13 | C2 | ------------------------ |
| HBSAG-14 | C2 | ------------------------ |

activity, allow the production of potential pro-oncogenic factors, such as X protein, which may contribute to the development of cirrhosis and liver cancer [6].

In the present study, cccDNA and pgRNA in cancerous tissues were higher than those in noncancerous tissues, and this was supported by previous data [5]. However, several reports showed that cccDNA levels in cancerous tissues were lower than those in noncancerous tissues [23]. The controversial result might be dependent on the difference of the necroinflammation and liver fibrosis [24]. It was also reported that cccDNA in the liver was correlated with serum HBV-DNA viral load and decreased during antiviral therapy [25]. In the present study, four HBsAg-positive patients were treated by nucleotide analogue therapy more than one year. However, cccDNA was not different regardless of therapy. It might be partly caused by sample number and therapeutic duration.

This study revealed that intrahepatic cccDNA and pgRNA levels in cancerous and noncancerous tissues were low in occult HBV-infected patients and were lower than those in HBsAg-positive carriers. These results suggest that transcriptional activity was low in occult HBV-infected HCC patients. Even though transcriptional activity and replication were lower in HCC patients with occult HBV infection, it might still be sufficient to induce HCC [5].

Other studies have detected cccDNA and pgRNA in cancerous and noncancerous tissues in patients with occult HBV infection [5, 6]. HBV cccDNA is formed from relaxed circular-DNA and enters the nuclei of the host's cells. This stable nonintegrated minichromosome is used as a template

TABLE 5: Mutations in the core promoter and precore regions in patients divided by serological status.

| | HBsAg-positive carriers ($n$ = 14) | Occult HBV-infected patients ($n$ = 9) | $P$ value |
|---|---|---|---|
| T1753C | 4 (29%) | 0 (0%) | 0.033 |
| A1762T/G1764A | 11 (79%) | 5 (56%) | NS |
| T1846A | 3 (21%) | 3 (33%) | NS |
| G1896A | 8 (57%) | 4 (44%) | NS |

NS: not significant.

for the transcription of viral mRNAs and pgRNA. In turn, viral mRNA is used to generate viral proteins and replication factors. The pgRNA is then encapsidated and reverse-transcribed into HBV-DNA. Animal experiments revealed that 1–50 cccDNA molecules gather in the nucleus, but the viral and host factors that regulate cccDNA are still poorly defined [26].

Some studies of duck hepatitis B virus revealed a negative feedback mechanism by which large surface protein suppresses cccDNA production [27]. In the present study, the S and X regions were detected in significantly more noncancerous tissues than in cancerous tissues. A previous study reported that a decrease in HBsAg expression in the cancer may contribute to an increase in intrahepatic HBV-DNA in the form of cccDNA in cancerous tissues, suggesting that viral replication is minimal within cancer cells and that the majority of intrahepatic HBV-DNA is in the form of cccDNA [6]. In the present study, the expression levels of cccDNA and pgRNA in HCC patients with occult HBV infection were similar or slightly lower in noncancerous tissues than in cancerous tissues, although more studies are needed to confirm these findings. However, the present results suggest that HBV persisted and was continuously replicated in cancerous and noncancerous cells.

Mutations in the S gene may alter HBsAg antigenicity and anti-HBs production. It was reported that a single amino acid mutation in the "a" determinant region (amino acids 124–147) of HBsAg could lead to a change in the immunologic epitope [28], and mutations or deletion in the S gene disrupted HBsAg production [29]. In the present study, two specific substitutions (I126T and I126V) were detected in occult HBV-infected patients. However, the HBV-DNA titre was <4 log copies/mL in all of the occult HBV-infected patients. Therefore, it is still unclear whether these substitutions are related to viral replication.

In conclusion, the present study confirmed that HBV persisted and was continuously replicated in cancerous and noncancerous tissues. In addition, cccDNA and pgRNA levels were thought to represent HBV replication in the liver and might contribute to the development of HCC in HBsAg carriers and occult HBV-infected patients.

## Acknowledgments

This study was supported by a Grant-in-Aid from the Japan Initiative for Global Research Network on Infectious Disease (J-GRID) supported by the Ministry of Education, Culture, Sports, Science and Technology, Japan, and a SATREPS Grant from Japan Science and Technology Agency and Japan International Cooperation Agency.

## References

[1] D. Lavanchy, "Hepatitis B virus epidemiology, disease burden, treatment, and current and emerging prevention and control measures," *Journal of Viral Hepatitis*, vol. 11, no. 2, pp. 97–107, 2004.

[2] E. Tabor, "Hepatocellular carcinoma: global epidemiology," *Digestive and Liver Disease*, vol. 33, no. 2, pp. 115–117, 2001.

[3] J. Beck and M. Nassal, "Hepatitis B virus replication," *World Journal of Gastroenterology*, vol. 13, no. 1, pp. 48–64, 2007.

[4] G. Raimondo, T. Pollicino, I. Cacciola, and G. Squadrito, "Occult hepatitis B virus infection," *Journal of Hepatology*, vol. 46, no. 1, pp. 160–170, 2007.

[5] D. K. H. Wong, F. Y. Huang, C. L. Lai et al., "Occult hepatitis B infection and HBV replicative activity in patients with cryptogenic cause of hepatocellular carcinoma," *Hepatology*, vol. 54, no. 3, pp. 829–836, 2011.

[6] T. Pollicino, G. Squadrito, G. Cerenzia et al., "Hepatitis B virus maintains its pro-oncogenic properties in the case of occult HBV infection," *Gastroenterology*, vol. 126, no. 1, pp. 102–110, 2004.

[7] F. Sugauchi, M. Mizokami, E. Orito et al., "A novel variant genotype C of hepatitis B virus identified in isolates from Australian Aborigines: complete genome sequence and phylogenetic relatedness," *Journal of General Virology*, vol. 82, no. 4, pp. 883–892, 2001.

[8] A. Laras, J. Koskinas, E. Dimou, A. Kostamena, and S. J. Hadziyannis, "Intrahepatic levels and replicative activity of covalently closed circular hepatitis B virus DNA in chronically infected patients," *Hepatology*, vol. 44, no. 3, pp. 694–702, 2006.

[9] N. Saitou and M. Nei, "The neighbor-joining method: a new method for reconstructing phylogenetic trees," *Molecular Biology and Evolution*, vol. 4, no. 4, pp. 406–425, 1987.

[10] K. Tamura, J. Dudley, M. Nei, and S. Kumar, "MEGA4: Molecular Evolutionary Genetics Analysis (MEGA) software version 4.0," *Molecular Biology and Evolution*, vol. 24, no. 8, pp. 1596–1599, 2007.

[11] H. Nordenstedt, D. L. White, and H. B. El-Serag, "The changing pattern of epidemiology in hepatocellular carcinoma," *Digestive and Liver Disease*, vol. 42, no. 3, pp. 206–214, 2010.

[12] A. Zidan, H. Scheuerlein, S. Schule, U. Settmacher, and F. Rauchfuss, "Epidemiological pattern of hepatitis B and hepatitis C as etiological agents for hepatocellular carcinoma in Iran and worldwide," *Hepatitis Monthly*, vol. 12, no. 10, Article ID e6894, 2012.

[13] S. G. Lim, R. Mohammed, M.-F. Yuen, and J.-H. Kao, "Prevention of hepatocellular carcinoma in hepatitis B virus infection," *Journal of Gastroenterology and Hepatology*, vol. 24, no. 8, pp. 1352–1357, 2009.

[14] G. Raimondo, J.-P. Allain, M. R. Brunetto et al., "Statements from the Taormina expert meeting on occult hepatitis B virus

infection," *Journal of Hepatology*, vol. 49, no. 4, pp. 652–657, 2008.

[15] C. Brechot, M. Hadchouel, and J. Scotto, "State of hepatitis B virus DNA in hepatocytes of patients with hepatitis B surface antigen-positive and -negative liver diseases," *Proceedings of the National Academy of Sciences of the United States of America*, vol. 78, no. 6, pp. 3906–3910, 1981.

[16] J.-H. Kao, P.-J. Chen, M.-Y. Lai, and D.-S. Chen, "Occult hepatitis B virus infection and clinical outcomes of patients with chronic hepatitis C," *Journal of Clinical Microbiology*, vol. 40, no. 11, pp. 4068–4071, 2002.

[17] A. Tamori, "Possible contribution to hepatocarcinogenesis of X transcript of hepatitis b virus in Japanese patients with hepatitis C virus," *Hepatology*, vol. 29, no. 5, pp. 1429–1434, 1999.

[18] B. Rehermann, C. Ferrari, C. Pasquinelli, and F. V. Chisari, "The hepatitis B virus persists for decades after patients' recovery from acute viral hepatitis despite active maintenance of a cytotoxic T-lymphocyte response," *Nature Medicine*, vol. 2, no. 10, pp. 1104–1108, 1996.

[19] N. Yuki, T. Nagaoka, M. Yamashiro et al., "Long-term histologic and virologic outcomes of acute self-limited hepatitis B," *Hepatology*, vol. 37, no. 5, pp. 1172–1179, 2003.

[20] G. Raimondo, T. Pollicino, and G. Squadrito, "What is the clinical impact of occult hepatitis B virus infection?" *The Lancet*, vol. 365, no. 9460, pp. 638–640, 2005.

[21] M. Torbenson and D. L. Thomas, "Occult hepatitis B," *Lancet Infectious Diseases*, vol. 2, no. 8, pp. 479–486, 2002.

[22] B. E. Korba, F. V. Wells, B. Baldwin et al., "Hepatocellular carcinoma in woodchuck hepatitis virus-infected woodchucks: presence of viral DNA in tumor tissue from chronic carriers and animals serologically recovered from acute infections," *Hepatology*, vol. 9, no. 3, pp. 461–470, 1989.

[23] L. C. Faria, M. Gigou, A. M. Roque-Afonso et al., "Hepatocellular carcinoma is associated with an increased risk of hepatitis B virus recurrence after liver transplantation," *Gastroenterology*, vol. 134, no. 7, pp. 1890–1899, 2008.

[24] Q. Wang, M. I. Fiel, W. Luan et al., "Impact of intrahepatic hepatitis B DNA and covalently closed circular DNA on survival after hepatectomy in HBV-associated hepatocellular carcinoma patients," *Annals Surgical Oncology*, vol. 20, no. 12, pp. 3761–3770, 2013.

[25] M. Abu-Amara and J. J. Feld, "Does antiviral therapy for chronic hepatitis B reduce the risk of hepatocellular carcinoma?" *Seminars in Liver Disease*, vol. 33, no. 2, pp. 157–166, 2013.

[26] M. Levrero, T. Pollicino, J. Petersen, L. Belloni, G. Raimondo, and M. Dandri, "Control of cccDNA function in hepatitis B virus infection," *Journal of Hepatology*, vol. 51, no. 3, pp. 581–592, 2009.

[27] R. J. Lenhoff and J. Summers, "Coordinate regulation of replication and virus assembly by the large envelope protein of an avian hepadnavirus," *Journal of Virology*, vol. 68, no. 7, pp. 4565–4571, 1994.

[28] K. Yamamoto, M. Horikita, F. Tsuda et al., "Naturally occurring escape mutants of hepatitis B virus with various mutations in the S gene in carriers seropositive for antibody to hepatitis B surface antigen," *Journal of Virology*, vol. 68, no. 4, pp. 2671–2676, 1994.

[29] M. Cabrerizo, J. Bartolomé, C. Caramelo, G. Barril, and V. Carreño, "Molecular analysis of hepatitis B virus DNA in serum and peripheral blood mononuclear cells from hepatitis B surface antigen-negative cases," *Hepatology*, vol. 32, no. 1, pp. 116–123, 2000.

# 18

# Newer Oral Anticoagulants in the Treatment of Acute Portal Vein Thrombosis in Patients with and without Cirrhosis

**P. Priyanka,[1] J. T. Kupec,[2] M. Krafft,[2] N. A. Shah,[3] and G. J. Reynolds[2]**

[1]*Department of Medicine, West Virginia University Hospitals, Morgantown, WV, USA*
[2]*Department of Medicine, Section of Digestive Diseases, West Virginia University Hospitals, Morgantown, WV, USA*
[3]*Department of Medicine, Section of Hematology, West Virginia University Hospitals, Morgantown, WV, USA*

Correspondence should be addressed to P. Priyanka; priyanka.priyanka@hsc.wvu.edu

Academic Editor: Dirk Uhlmann

*Background.* Newer oral anticoagulants (NOACs) are being utilized increasingly for the treatment of venous thromboembolism (VTE). NOAC use is the standard of care for stroke prophylaxis in nonvalvular atrial fibrillation and treatment of acute VTE involving extremities and pulmonary embolism. In contrast, most guidelines in the literature support the treatment of acute portal vein thrombosis (PVT) with low molecular weight heparin (LMWH) and vitamin K antagonists (VKA). Literature evaluating NOAC use in the treatment of acute portal vein thrombosis is sparse. This review focuses on the safety and efficacy of the use of NOACs in the treatment of acute PVT in patients, with or without concomitant cirrhosis, based on the most recent data available in the current literature. *Methods.* A systematic review was conducted through a series of advanced searches in the following medical databases: PubMed, BioMed Central, Cochrane, and Google Scholar. Keywords utilized were as follows: NOAC, DOAC (direct oral anticoagulants), portal vein thrombosis, rivaroxaban, apixaban, dabigatran, and edoxaban. Articles related to newer anticoagulant use in patients with portal vein thrombosis were included. *Results.* The adverse events, including bleeding events (major and minor) and the failure of anticoagulation (propagation of thrombus or recurrence of PVT), are similar between the NOACs and traditional anticoagulants for the treatment of acute PVT, irrespective of the presence of cirrhosis. *Conclusions.* Newer oral anticoagulants are safe and efficacious alternatives to traditional anticoagulation with low molecular weight heparin and vitamin K antagonists in the treatment of acute portal vein thrombosis with or without cirrhosis.

## 1. Introduction

Portal vein thrombosis (PVT) is defined as thrombosis within the portal vein trunk and intrahepatic portal branches. The presence of PVT in cirrhosis varies with a reported incidence of 8.4% to 11.2% and prevalence nearing 26% [1]. The benefits of anticoagulation are seen in both cirrhotic and noncirrhotic patients. These benefits include a higher rate of recanalization (42-100%), a lower thrombus extension rate, a lower incidence of hepatic decompensation, and improved survival [2–7].

Historically, patients with liver dysfunction were advised to avoid newer oral anticoagulants due to the risk of excess bleeding and reduced effectiveness. However, increasing evidence suggests that oral anticoagulants are not only safe but also efficacious when compared to the traditional anticoagulation [8–12].

Although the exact duration of anticoagulation for acute portal vein thrombosis remains controversial, the American Association for the Study of Liver Disease (AASLD) recommends at least three months of anticoagulant use in the treatment of PVT, irrespective of the presence of cirrhosis [13]. Most trials of treatment of PVT have effectively used low molecular weight heparin and warfarin [5, 14, 15]. Far fewer studies have examined the safety and efficacy of newer oral anticoagulants (NOACs) in the treatment of this disease process.

NOACs are one of the landmark advances in the recent practice of medicine as they overcome numerous drawbacks of traditional anticoagulants. NOACs are currently approved for stroke prophylaxis in nonvalvular atrial fibrillation, venous thromboembolism (VTE) prophylaxis in orthopedic surgery patients, and the treatment of VTE involving the extremities and acute pulmonary embolism (PE) [16]. Despite this progress, anticoagulation of portal vein thrombosis with NOACs has remained controversial. Traditionally, low molecular weight heparin (LMWH) and vitamin K antagonists (VKAs) have been used mainly due to lower costs, more physician experience with these agents, and easy reversibility in case of severe bleeding [5, 6]. The role of NOACs for the PVT treatment is still undefined in the current literature.

The complications of PVT (gastrointestinal bleeding, including variceal, intestinal infarction and development of portal hypertension, portal cholangiopathy, and subsequent hepatic decompensation) can be quite serious [1]. Recanalization of the thrombus occurs more frequently with the aid of anticoagulation thereby reducing complications mentioned above. Additionally, the development of PVT is associated with higher morbidity and mortality after liver transplantation, complicating treatment strategies [17]. As supported by animal data, another proposed benefit of anticoagulation in PVT is the suggestion that fibrogenesis may be reduced by thrombin antagonism [17, 18].

Patients with cirrhosis have been excluded *ipso facto* in clinical trials of NOACs mostly due to concerns of severe bleeding in the absence of reversal agents. Off-label use of NOACs in VTE involving atypical sites like splanchnic vein thrombosis, cerebral venous thrombosis, and renal and ovarian vein thrombosis has been evaluated with excellent efficacy and safety profile [19]. Despite the ever-increasing evidence, NOACs have not yet found mainstream success as an alternative for the treatment of PVT [13].

The purpose of this review is to evaluate the existing literature on the use of NOACs for PVT in patients with and without cirrhosis.

## 2. Methods

A comprehensive, systematic search of the PubMed, Biomed Central, Cochrane Library, and Google Scholar was performed. Relevant English language articles were identified up to February 28, 2018. Manual searching for relevant publications from the reference section of extracted articles was also performed.

A total of 53 manuscripts were identified after searching the above databases. Duplicate studies were removed. Of these articles, 43 were discarded as they were not relevant to the topic and 10 were included (Table 1).

Of the selected 10 articles, four studies were original manuscripts and six were case reports. Only one study was prospective and three were retrospective. Six studies involved patients with cirrhosis, three articles included only noncirrhotic patients, and one study included patients both with and without cirrhosis. In all, a total of 119 patients, across all studies, were included.

Recanalization rates and thrombus recurrence rates served as efficacy endpoints. Bleeding events were utilized as the complication endpoint.

## 3. Drawbacks of Traditional Anticoagulants Use in PVT with Cirrhosis

Despite their acceptance as the standard of care for many thromboembolic events, there are some disadvantages of using LMWH and VKAs in the treatment of PVT.

For example, in patients with cirrhosis, the efficacy of unfractionated heparin (UFH) and LMWH may be significantly decreased (up to 40%) due to lower levels of antithrombin synthesis by the liver [24]. Additionally, LMWH has limited use in concurrent renal impairment.

Coagulopathy from liver disease frequently results in an elevated INR and thus utilizing the INR to guide dosing of VKAs is particularly challenging. Following the INR as a monitoring parameter was only studied in noncirrhotic population and is being used by extrapolation for VKA monitoring in patients with cirrhosis [8]. Elevated INR levels associated with cirrhosis can offer a false measure of the therapeutic efficacy. Conversely, when VKAs artificially elevate the INR, this can directly affect the model for end-stage liver disease (MELD) score, impacting transplantation eligibility. Protein C, a vitamin K dependent anticoagulant factor, is reduced in cirrhosis and may decrease the efficacy of VKAs [8].

VKAs have a narrow therapeutic window as well as numerous drug and dietary interactions and need frequent coagulation testing and dose adjustments. Despite their efficacy, VKAs are far from an easy means of anticoagulation.

## 4. Advantages of NOACs for VTE

There are benefits to considering NOACs for the treatment of thromboembolic events. These medications can be cost-effective and convenient. Unlike LMWH, they do not require daily subcutaneous injections, and since their pharmacokinetics and pharmacodynamics are predictable, they do not require routine dose monitoring like warfarin. In contrast to the strict dietary precautions VKA users have to follow, NOACs pharmacodynamics are not affected by dietary intake [25]. In addition, NOACs act faster than VKAs. Rivaroxaban's onset of action is 30 minutes, faster than the 36-72 hours for warfarin (which requires overlap with heparin therapy). Interactions of NOACs with other drugs are rare, with the exception of a few antibiotics and antifungals, which may be significant for patients with malignancy [26].

Systemic clearance upon discontinuation of NOACs is faster (5-9 hours in young adults and 11-13 hours in older adults) and more reliable when compared to warfarin (20-60 hours) [27]. Clinically this is significant as rivaroxaban can be stopped much closer to an elective surgery or invasive procedure than warfarin. All of these properties combine to increase patient compliance, reliability, and effectiveness.

## 5. Rivaroxaban Is the Most Studied NOAC for the Treatment of PVT

Rivaroxaban has been consistently used in the most studies examining the role of NOACs in the treatment of PVT either

TABLE 1

| Author | Study design | Number of patients (n) | Duration | Agent | Response | Bleeding events |
|---|---|---|---|---|---|---|
| Janczak [19] (2018) | Prospective, non-cirrhotic, Atypical sites | Total N=36 PVT N= 16 | | Rivaroxaban Apixaban | Recurrence rate 7.3 % (n=2) (both had malignancy) | Minor N=1 (3.6%) Major N=2 (7.2%) |
| Qi [20] (2017) | Case report, cirrhotic, CPT not specified | SMV, splenic vein, N=1 | 11 weeks | Rivaroxaban | Recanalization | Melena and hematemesis |
| Nery [21] (2017) | Case report Non-cirrhotic | N=1 | >6m | Rivaroxaban 20 mg daily | Complete recanalization L branch, partial recanalization right branch | None |
| De Gottardi [10] (2016) | Retrospective, Both cirrhotic and non-cirrhotic, Splanchnic | Total, N= 94 PVT N= 80 (Non cirrh- N=38 Cirrh- N=22) | Non-cirrhotic 13.1 m cirrhotic 9.6 m | Rivaroxaban Apixaban Dabigatran | Not studied | Cirrhosis: Minor, n=7, Major, n=2 Non-cirrh: Minor, n= 4 Major, n=1 |
| Hum [9] (2016) | Retrospective, Cirrhotic, CPT A, B & C All indications | Total, N= 27 PVT N=4 | | Rivaroxaban 15 mg bid +/- 20 mg daily load, Apixaban 5mg bid +/- 10mg bid load, No bridging | Recurrence rate 4% (n=1) | Major N=1 (4%) Minor, N=7 |
| Yang [12] (2016) | Case report, cirrhotic CPT A | N=1 | 6 m | Rivaroxaban 15 mg bid x 3 wks, then 20 mg/d | Complete recanalization | None |
| Intagliata [8] (2015) | Retrospective, cirrhotic, CPT A and B | Total N= 20 PVT, N=12 | 10.6 m | Apixaban Rivaroxaban | Not studied | Major, n=1 |
| Martinez [22] (2014) | Case report, Cirrhotics, CPT A | N=1 | 6 m | Rivaroxaban 20 mg /d | Complete recanalization | None |
| Lenz [11] (2014) | Case report, Cirrhotic CPT A | N=1 | 5 m | Rivaroxaban 10 mg daily | Complete recanalization | None |
| Pannach [23] (2013) | Case report, Non-cirrhotic | N=1 | >4 weeks | Rivaroxaban 20 mg daily | Complete recanalization | None |

CPT: Child Pugh Turcotte; Cirrh: cirrhosis.

as a single agent or in combination with a second agent such as apixaban or dabigatran [8–12, 19, 21–23]. Similarly, the studies evaluating the pharmacodynamics and hepatotoxicity of NOACs in patients with cirrhosis were mainly performed with rivaroxaban [28, 29].

## 6. Summary of the Data Supporting Treatment of PVT with NOACs (Table 1)

There is little scientific evidence regarding the use of NOACs in PVT, and well-designed prospective studies are even fewer. Recently, a prospective study involving patients from the Mayo Clinic thrombophilia registry for initial treatment of acute venous thromboembolism of atypical location (VTE-AL) was published [19]. Outcomes, recurrence of PVT, and bleeding rates were similar for rivaroxaban and apixaban for patients with VTE in a typical location (VTE-TL) treated with NOACs compared to VTE-AL treated with enoxaparin in 623 patients without cirrhosis. In this study group, 29 had PVT and 63 patients had VTE-AL. Another multicenter, retrospective European study with 94 patients from 17 centers looked at NOAC use for splanchnic vein thrombosis, cardiac arrhythmias, peripheral deep vein thrombosis (DVT), and PE [19]. They concluded that NOACs were an effective and safe alternative to LMWH and VKAs, including patients with PVT with and without underlying cirrhosis.

Smaller studies aimed at evaluating the risk of bleeding in patients with PVT treated with NOACs show near equal complications to those treated with LMWH and VKAs [8, 9]. It must be noted, however, that patients with decompensated cirrhosis were mostly excluded from these studies with only a few Child Pugh Turcotte (CPT) class C patients included in just one study [9].

## 7. Special Considerations of NOACs in PVT

PVT can be associated with thrombosis of the mesenteric vein. Mesenteric vein thrombosis may cause impaired drug absorption due to reduced mesenteric perfusion resulting from severe venous congestion [19]. This could interfere with the efficacy of NOACs. It is important to be aware of this possibility while initiating treatment with NOACs in patients with PVT.

Given the progressive nature of cirrhosis, hepatic function may change over time. During long-term treatment with NOACs, this progression could potentially be missed as routine coagulation testing is not recommended with NOACs. This emphasizes the need for detailed testing of the liver function prior to initiation of treatment and also supports periodic monitoring of coagulation parameters while on NOACs [30].

A recent study suggests reduced in vitro anticoagulant potency of rivaroxaban in patients with CPT B and C cirrhosis and increased anticoagulant effect of dabigatran proportional to the severity of liver disease [31]. This may result in overanticoagulation or even undertreatment. Measurement of factor X levels for rivaroxaban and factor II levels in dabigatran may be necessary in cirrhosis patients to ensure the therapeutic efficacy. This highlights the need for agent-specific dose adjustments in the presence of liver cirrhosis.

## 8. Local Anticoagulant Action of Factor Xa Inhibitors in PVT

It has been postulated that reduced flow rates in the portal vein in PVT or cirrhosis may be associated with severe protein C deficiency contributing to a locally prothrombotic milieu [32]. Due to the very high bioavailability of rivaroxaban and other factor Xa inhibitors, local anticoagulant action of these agents compared to systemic anticoagulants has been proposed, as the metabolites of rivaroxaban have no anticoagulant activity [11]. This could support the use of even lower doses (2.5 mg once or twice daily) of rivaroxaban in PVT.

## 9. Agent-Specific Considerations in NOACs

*9.1. Rivaroxaban, Apixaban, and Edoxaban.* Rivaroxaban, apixaban, and edoxaban are direct factor Xa inhibitors with half-lives of 5-9 hours, 12 hours, and 10-15 hours, respectively. Rivaroxaban and apixaban are metabolised in the liver (67%) and kidneys (33%) and are extensively bound to plasma proteins. Edoxaban is metabolised hepatically and renally equally. Each of these agents is well absorbed in gastrointestinal (GI) tract and has high bioavailability. Rivaroxaban absorption occurs only in the stomach making it the better choice for patients with gastric tubes. Apixaban is absorbed through the entire length of GI tract, predominantly in the distal small bowel and ascending colon. As a result, apixaban administration may not be suitable for patients with a proximal colectomy or a distal small bowel resection. Edoxaban is absorbed mainly in the small intestine; therefore it can be given effectively to patients with previous colectomy [33–37].

## 10. Dabigatran

Unlike the factor Xa inhibitors, dabigatran has unique pharmacodynamics. Dabigatran has poor absorption in the gastrointestinal tract, limited hepatic metabolism, minimal binding to plasma proteins, and a longer half-life (12-14 hours) and is eliminated almost entirely through the kidneys (80%) [38]. Additionally, dabigatran has a different mechanism of action; it is a direct thrombin inhibitor [39, 40]. It is known to cause significant dyspepsia due to high concentrations in the colon secondary to poor GI absorption and tartaric acid content of the capsule [41]. It becomes clinically significant as simultaneous administration of pantoprazole reduces dabigatran's effective therapeutic area under curve (AUC) by 22%. At this time, dose modification of dabigatran in CPT A and B cirrhosis patients is not indicated due to limited data available on its use in these patients.

## 11. Efficacy of NOACs in Acute PVT

Anticoagulant efficacy can be defined as both the rate of recanalization of the thrombus in the portal vein and reduction in recurrent thrombi formation. NOACs appear to perform as well as traditional anticoagulants in achieving recanalization and have similar thrombus recurrence rates [9, 19]. In the aforementioned Mayo oncology study, recurrence of VTE-AL was 7.3% in patients with underlying malignancy treated with rivaroxaban [19]. This was not different from recurrence rates noted in VTE-TL. NOAC use in splanchnic vein thrombosis, a study by the Vascular Liver Disease Group (VALDIG) consortium that included patients with and without cirrhosis, showed thrombotic events in two of 58 treated patients (3.4 %), including a case of progression of PVT [10]. No anticoagulation failure was reported in the cirrhosis group in this study. In another study, only one failure of anticoagulation in both the NOAC and the traditional anticoagulant groups was observed in 27 patients with cirrhosis treated for various indications [9]. Additionally, no progression of PVT was noted. Complete recanalization of PVT has been noted in case reports; one report describes partial recanalization [11, 12, 20–22].

## 12. Monitoring of NOACs

In 2014 guidelines from the Australasian Society of Thrombosis and Hemostasis, prothrombin time prolongation was thought to be most sensitive test for rivaroxaban and edoxaban, while activated partial thromboplastin time (aPTT) and thrombin time (TT) were markers of dabigatran [42]. HEMOCLOT® direct thrombin inhibitors assay (HYPHEN BioMed, France, CK002K) is the recommended confirmatory test for drug levels of dabigatran. Drug-specific anti-factor Xa assays are recommended for apixaban, edoxaban, and rivaroxaban for confirmation. The assays for these agents are not currently commercially available and they are of little use in emergent situations. Furthermore, it is important to note that a normal aPTT with dabigatran or normal PT with apixaban, edoxaban, or rivaroxaban does not exclude the presence of active drug [43].

## 13. Indications and Duration of NOAC Treatment in PVT

AASLD guidelines recommend at least three months of anticoagulation with traditional anticoagulants for all patients with acute PVT irrespective of presence of symptoms. Long-term treatment should be considered in patients with permanent risk factors for thrombosis and concomitant mesenteric vein thrombosis, due to the risk of mesenteric infarction [40].

The American College of Chest Physicians recommends a minimum of three months of anticoagulation for symptomatic patients only and no anticoagulation for asymptomatic patients [16]. Indefinite anticoagulation should be considered in patients with permanent risk factors such as cirrhosis, malignancy, or autoimmune disorders.

The duration of anticoagulation with NOACs has not been addressed in any guideline as NOACs are still not the standard of care in PVT treatment. In the studies discussed in this review, the duration of treatment varies from 5 to 13 months in duration and longer in some cases.

## 14. Adverse Events Noted in the Studies Involving NOACs in PVT

*14.1. Bleeding.* As with any form of anticoagulation, the risk of bleeding should be balanced with the potential benefit of treatment. A few studies have evaluated the overall risk of bleeding when utilizing newer oral anticoagulants. Major bleeding was defined as overt bleeding with a drop in the hemoglobin greater than or equal to 2 g/dl, transfusion of two or more units of packed red blood cells, or intracranial, intraspinal, intraocular, retroperitoneal, pericardial, or fatal bleeding.

Any bleeding events not meeting the above criteria, but requiring medical attention, were categorized as nonmajor bleeding.

*14.2. Major Bleeding.* In the available studies, the rate of major bleeding with NOACs was not higher than with traditional anticoagulants. In patients treated with apixaban and rivaroxaban from the Mayo Thrombophilia Registry, two patients out of 36 treated with NOACs (5.55%) with underlying malignancy had a major bleeding event [19]. In the VALDIG study, major bleeding requiring discontinuation of NOAC was seen in two of 258 (0.71%) patients without cirrhosis and one of 36 (2.7%) patients with cirrhosis [10]. These included bleeding after variceal band ligation and after hysterectomy in the noncirrhosis cohort and lower GI bleeding in the cirrhosis group. These rates are not higher than major bleeding rates with traditional anticoagulants. No excessive major bleeding rates were noted in two other studies specifically designed to investigate the risk of bleeding in cirrhotic patients with NOACs when compared to traditional anticoagulants [8, 9]. Due to differences in the dosing regimens and indications for anticoagulation, investigators could not ascertain if the risk of bleeding was uniform in their cohort. Some data actually suggests that the risk of major bleeding was higher with traditional anticoagulant use (28%) than NOACs (4%) in patients with cirrhosis [9]. This reduced risk was specifically noted for central nervous system (CNS) bleeds, as no CNS bleeding was noted with NOAC therapy compared to three (17%) cases for traditional anticoagulants. Only one case report recorded hematemesis and melena but no other major bleeding events were noted in any case reports [11, 12, 20–23].

*14.3. Nonmajor Bleeding.* Nonmajor bleeding rates were actually lower in patients with VTE-TL treated with NOAC (8.7%) in the Mayo study than the nonmajor bleeding rate in patients with VTE-AL treated with enoxaparin (15.6%) [19]. The VALDIG study showed similar nonmajor bleeding rates in patients with cirrhosis (11.1%) and without cirrhosis (12%). These bleeding events included epistaxis, gingival bleeding, GI bleeding in the noncirrhotic group and bleeding from portal hypertensive gastropathy, lower GI bleeding, epistaxis, and bleeding after band ligation in the cirrhosis cohort. In another study, minor bleeding events included vaginal bleeding and GI bleeding [8].

A recent meta-analysis from 43 randomized controlled trials has concluded that there is an increased risk of gastrointestinal bleeding with NOACs use with an incidence of 1.4% [44]. Furthermore, this risk was found to be more for rivaroxaban and dabigatran and less for edoxaban and apixaban. Concurrent antiplatelet therapy can further increase the bleeding risk by five times. Currently, although there is no evidence in literature to suggest that anticoagulation increases the risk of variceal bleeding, studies recommend screening for varices and initiating or optimizing beta blocker therapy or perform endoscopic variceal ligation (EVL) before starting anticoagulation [45, 46].

## 15. Other Side Effects

While much of the risk-benefit discussion with the patients centers on the risk of bleeding, additional adverse effects (AEs) of NOAC treatment should be considered. As these drugs are relatively new, the amount of data available is limited. Some of these AEs were elucidated by VALDIG investigators. In patients without cirrhosis, leukopenia (n=1) was a rare event but was not severe enough to discontinue treatment. However, dizziness (n=1) did require discontinuation of the medication [10].

## 16. Other Limitations of NOACs

*16.1. Higher Cost.* New medications often face challenges with respect to insurance coverage and overall costs to the patients and NOACs are no exception. Higher costs are a concern with NOACs, but it has been shown that these costs can be offset by reduced costs of monitoring, less healthcare provider time, and an increased convenience to the patient. As such, some data supports the idea that rivaroxaban can be more cost-effective than warfarin in the prevention of recurrent VTE [47].

*16.2. Hepatotoxicity.* Interestingly, no cases of hepatotoxicity were noted in the studies focusing on NOAC use in PVT, possibly due to smaller size of these studies. Liver toxicity of NOACs, particularly rivaroxaban, more so than dabigatran or apixaban, has been reported in the literature. The incidence of hepatotoxicity in patients with chronic advanced liver disease is estimated to be 0.1-1% and appears to be idiosyncratic in nature [28, 29]. Liver dysfunction is usually reversible after stopping the treatment. Though infrequent, patients should be made aware of the possible symptoms of liver dysfunction.

*16.3. Cautious Use in Liver Dysfunction.* Moderate or severe hepatic impairment can reduce NOAC clearance and augment their pharmacodynamic effects to varying degrees. Significantly increased exposure was noted in CPT B cirrhosis patients compared to CPT A patients for rivaroxaban [48]. In patients with CPT B cirrhosis, the area under the plasma concentration or AUC of rivaroxaban and apixaban is increased (2.27 times and 1.09 times, respectively) and decreased (4.8% and 5.6%) for edoxaban and dabigatran, respectively [30]. In comparison, there was no difference in the drug exposure between patients with mild and moderate hepatic dysfunction after administration of a single 15 mg dose of edoxaban, indicating more consistent drug pharmacokinetics [49]. Currently, rivaroxaban and edoxaban are recommended to be avoided in patients with CPT B and C cirrhosis and apixaban in patients with CPT C cirrhosis [33–35]. There are risks of higher doses of NOACs, particularly in prolonged exposure in patients with liver dysfunction, but the data is limited with respect to recommending a dose adjustment in moderate to severe liver dysfunction with any of these drugs [11]. These factors should be considered when choosing a NOAC in patients with cirrhosis.

*16.4. Cautious Use in Renal Impairment.* Since all NOACs are excreted through kidneys to some degree, caution needs to be exercised in utilizing NOACs in the presence of renal impairment. The Food and Drug Administration (FDA) has approved a lower dose of dabigatran (75 mg bid), apixaban (5 mg bid or 2.5 mg bid), and rivaroxaban (15 mg od) for patients with renal insufficiency and creatinine clearance of 15-30 ml/min [33, 34, 38]. NOACs are not indicated at this time in end-stage renal disease (ESRD) and patients on hemodialysis.

*16.5. Reversal.* One of the notable advantages of the traditional anticoagulants is the availability of reversal agents. This is significant in the context of NOACs where a lack of a cost-effective, widely available reversal agent hampers their use with respect to major bleeding events. To reduce the risk of excessive bleeding during surgery, adequate reversal of NOACs is of paramount importance in patients awaiting liver transplantation.

A recent review supported the superiority of four-factor prothrombin complex concentrate (4F-PCC) over fresh frozen plasma (FFPs) as a reversal agent [50]. Determining the appropriate dose of 4F-PCC remains a challenge as excessive use may result in a higher risk of thrombosis. Idarucizumab, a monoclonal antibody for dabigatran reversal, used as a single intravenous dose has been shown to be effective. Though available in many countries, use of both PCC and idarucizumab remains limited as they may be cost prohibitive [51]. Andexanet alfa, a recombinant modified human factor Xa decoy protein, though not yet approved, has shown potential as a possible reversal of factor Xa inhibitors. Ciraparantag binds directly to factor Xa inhibitors, dabigatran, LMWH, and unfractionated heparin and is under evaluation for reversal of both direct thrombin inhibitors and factor Xa inhibitors [51].

In addition, dabigatran is amenable to neutralization with gastric lavage soon after ingestion and, due to its low protein binding and lipophilic nature, hemodialysis in severe cases.

## 17. Dosing of NOACs for PVT Patients

The presence of cirrhosis may affect the dosing of NOACs. Yet current data is unclear in determining the appropriate dose. In the VALDIG study, the median daily dose of all NOACs (rivaroxaban, apixaban, and dabigatran) in patients without cirrhosis was 25% higher than patients with cirrhosis [10]. In another study, involving 20 patients with VTE, including 12 patients with splanchnic vein thrombosis, 75% were treated with therapeutic dose of rivaroxaban (20 mg daily) and apixaban (5 mg twice a day), and 25% were treated with lower dose (rivaroxaban 10 mg daily and apixaban 5 mg daily) successfully without excessive bleeding episodes and recurrence rates [8]. Other studies were performed without dose modification [9]. Case reports support a standard dose of rivaroxaban, even in the presence of cirrhosis, without any effect on efficacy and bleeding events [11, 12]. At this time, there is no clear guidance in the literature about the effect of dose modification on the efficacy and possible benefit for cirrhosis patients.

## 18. Bridging NOACs with Traditional Anticoagulants before the Initiation of PVT Treatment

Traditionally, VKAs are bridged with unfractionated heparin (UFH) or LMWH for five days. For treatment of VTE in typical locations, NOACs do not routinely require heparin bridging. At this time, the data regarding bridging NOACs with UFH/LMWH is limited and is currently subject to the physician preference.

The available studies and case reports support several approaches to potentially utilizing another agent to bridge patients before starting NOAC, and some of them do not address bridging at all [8, 19]. NOAC was used as the initial anticoagulant in one-third of patients without cirrhosis while two-thirds were previously treated with traditional anticoagulants, without any mention of bridging [8]. Other studies did not bridge their patients with traditional anticoagulants [9]. There are case reports in this review where patients were bridged with heparin and some in which heparin was not used [11, 23].

## 19. Limitations

There are some limitations to the studies included in this review. First, it is significant heterogeneity which makes comparison between studies difficult. There are differences in baseline patient characteristics, the indications for anticoagulation, the anticoagulant agents used, the doses given, and the primary endpoints. It is difficult to standardize a review when such parameters do not align. The second major limitation is the quality of the studies available. None of the included studies were randomized controlled trials, and, barring one study, all were retrospective. The study sizes were small. These were not controlled studies as the anticoagulation prescribing (initiation, choice of the agents, discontinuation, and transitioning to and from traditional anticoagulants due to intolerance or adverse effects) was not under the investigators' control. Many studies did not have a control group. Additionally, patients with CPT C cirrhosis were largely excluded. Patients with mesenteric ischemia or renal impairment were also excluded from these studies limiting our insight into management of these subgroups with NOACs.

## 20. Conclusions and Future Directions

Although the current literature does not conclusively establish the role of NOACs in treatment of PVT in the presence or absence of cirrhosis, it extends the armamentarium of safe and efficacious options available for anticoagulation of these patients.

This review establishes that NOACs can be used effectively and safely without any risk of increased bleeding events in the treatment of PVT, even in patients with CPT class A and B cirrhosis. This review also presents the evidence that NOACs are already being increasingly used off label for this indication despite the lack of robust data on their safety and efficacy. This preliminary data may prompt better quality studies in the future comparing traditional and newer anticoagulants.

## Authors' Contributions

P. Priyanka was responsible for topic selection, study concept and design, acquisition of data, analysis and interpretation of data, drafting of the manuscript, literature search, writing, editing, and submitting the manuscript. J. T. Kupec contributed to analysis and interpretation of data, drafting of the manuscript, critical revision of the manuscript for important intellectual content, and editing. M. Krafft was responsible for analysis and interpretation of data, drafting of the manuscript, critical revision of the manuscript for important intellectual content, and editing. N. A. Shah contributed to critical revision of the manuscript for important intellectual content and editing. G. J. Reynolds contributed to critical revision of the manuscript for important intellectual content.

## References

[1] L. Amitrano, M. A. Guardascione, V. Brancaccio et al., "Risk factors and clinical presentation of portal vein thrombosis in patients with liver cirrhosis," *Journal of Hepatology*, vol. 40, no. 5, pp. 736–741, 2004.

[2] X. Qi, V. de Stefano, H. Li, J. Dai, X. Guo, and D. Fan, "Anticoagulation for the treatment of portal vein thrombosis in liver cirrhosis: a systematic review and meta-analysis of observational studies," *European Journal of Internal Medicine*, vol. 26, no. 1, pp. 23–29, 2015.

[3] L. Loffredo, D. Pastori, A. Farcomeni, and F. Violi, "Effects of Anticoagulants in Patients With Cirrhosis and Portal Vein Thrombosis: A Systematic Review and Meta-analysis," *Gastroenterology*, vol. 153, no. 2, pp. 480–487.e1, 2017.

[4] H. Chen, F. Turon, V. Hernández-Gea et al., "Nontumoral portal vein thrombosis in patients awaiting liver transplantation," *Liver Transplantation*, vol. 22, no. 3, pp. 352–365, 2016.

[5] M. G. Delgado, S. Seijo, and I. Yepes, "Efficacy and safety of anticoagulation on patients with cirrhosis and portal vein thrombosis," *Clinical Gastroenterology and Hepatology*, vol. 10, no. 7, pp. 776–783, 2012.

[6] M. Senzolo, T. M. Sartori, V. Rossetto et al., "Prospective evaluation of anticoagulation and transjugular intrahepatic portosistemic shunt for the management of portal vein thrombosis in cirrhosis," *Liver International*, vol. 32, no. 6, pp. 919–927, 2012.

[7] E. Villa, C. Cammà, M. Marietta et al., "Enoxaparin prevents portal vein thrombosis and liver decompensation in patients with advanced cirrhosis," *Gastroenterology*, vol. 143, no. 5, pp. 1253–1260, 2012.

[8] N. M. Intagliata, Z. H. Henry, H. Maitland et al., "Direct Oral Anticoagulants in Cirrhosis Patients Pose Similar Risks of Bleeding When Compared to Traditional Anticoagulation," *Digestive Diseases and Sciences*, vol. 61, no. 6, pp. 1721–1727, 2016.

[9] J. Hum, J. J. Shatzel, J. H. Jou, and T. G. Deloughery, "The efficacy and safety of direct oral anticoagulants vs traditional anticoagulants in cirrhosis," *European Journal of Haematology*, vol. 98, no. 4, pp. 393–397, 2017.

[10] A. De Gottardi, J. Trebicka, C. Klinger et al., "Antithrombotic treatment with direct-acting oral anticoagulants in patients with splanchnic vein thrombosis and cirrhosis," *Liver International*, vol. 37, no. 5, pp. 694–699, 2017.

[11] K. Lenz, B. Dieplinger, R. Buder, P. Piringer, M. Rauch, and M. Voglmayr, "Successful treatment of partial portal vein thrombosis (PVT) with low dose rivaroxaban," *Zeitschrift für Gastroenterologie*, vol. 52, no. 10, pp. 1175–1177, 2014.

[12] H. Yang, S. R. Kim, and M. J. Song, "Recurrent acute portal vein thrombosis in liver cirrhosis treated by rivaroxaban," *Clinical and Molecular Hepatology*, vol. 22, no. 4, pp. 499–502, 2016.

[13] L. D. DeLeve, D.-C. Valla, and G. Garcia-Tsao, "Vascular disorders of the liver," *Hepatology*, vol. 49, no. 5, pp. 1729–1764, 2009.

[14] B. Condat, F. Pessione, S. Hillaire et al., "Current outcome of portal vein thrombosis in adults: risk and benefit of anticoagulant therapy," *Gastroenterology*, vol. 120, no. 2, pp. 490–497, 2001.

[15] W. Ageno, N. Riva, S. Schulman et al., "Long-term clinical outcomes of splanchnic vein thrombosis results of an international registry," *JAMA Internal Medicine*, vol. 175, no. 9, pp. 1474–1480, 2015.

[16] W. Ageno, A. S. Gallus, A. Wittkowsky, M. Crowther, E. M. Hylek, and G. Palareti, "Oral anticoagulant therapy: antithrombotic therapy and prevention of thrombosis, 9th ed: American College of Chest Physicians evidence-based clinical practice guidelines," *CHEST*, vol. 141, no. 2, supplement, pp. e44S–e88S, 2012.

[17] K. I. Rodríguez-Castro, R. J. Porte, E. Nadal, G. Germani, P. Burra, and M. Senzolo, "Management of nonneoplastic portal vein thrombosis in the setting of liver transplantation: a systematic review," *Transplantation*, vol. 94, no. 11, pp. 1145–1153, 2012.

[18] S. Seijo and J. C. Garcia-Pagan, "Anticoagulation in cirrhosis: Ready ... set ... wait!," *Hepatology*, vol. 58, no. 3, pp. 1175-1176, 2013.

[19] D. T. Janczak, M. K. Mimier, R. D. McBane et al., "Rivaroxaban and Apixaban for Initial Treatment of Acute Venous Thromboembolism of Atypical Location," *Mayo Clinic Proceedings*, vol. 93, no. 1, pp. 40–47, 2018.

[20] X. Qi, E. M. Yoshida, N. Mendez-Sanchez, and X. Guo, "Rivaroxaban recanalized occlusive superior mesenteric vein thrombosis, but increased the risk of bleeding in a cirrhotic patient," *Liver International*, vol. 37, no. 10, pp. 1574-1575, 2017.

[21] F. Nery, D. Valadares, S. Morais, M. T. Gomes, and A. De Gottardi, "Efficacy and Safety of Direct-Acting Oral Anticoagulants Use in Acute Portal Vein Thrombosis Unrelated to Cirrhosis," *Gastroenterology Research*, vol. 10, no. 2, pp. 141–143, 2017.

[22] M. Martinez, A. Tandra, and R. Vuppalanchi, "Treatment of acute portal vein thrombosis by nontraditional anticoagulation," *Hepatology*, vol. 60, no. 1, pp. 425-426, 2014.

[23] S. Pannach, J. Babatz, and J. Beyer-Westendorf, "Successful treatment of acute portal vein thrombosis with rivaroxaban," *Thrombosis and Haemostasis*, vol. 110, no. 4, pp. 626-627, 2013.

[24] W. Potze, F. Arshad, J. Adelmeijer et al., "Routine coagulation assays underestimate levels of antithrombin-dependent drugs but not of direct anticoagulant drugs in plasma from patients with cirrhosis," *British Journal of Haematology*, vol. 163, no. 5, pp. 666–673, 2013.

[25] M. A. Smythe, J. Fanikos, M. P. Gulseth et al., "Rivaroxaban: Practical considerations for ensuring safety and efficacy," *Pharmacotherapy*, vol. 33, no. 11, pp. 1223–1245, 2013.

[26] A. M. Morrill, D. Ge, and K. C. Willett, "Dosing of Target-Specific Oral Anticoagulants in Special Populations," *Annals of Pharmacotherapy*, vol. 49, no. 9, pp. 1031–1045, 2015.

[27] S. M. Bates and J. S. Ginsberg, "Clinical practice. Treatment of deep-vein thrombosis," *The New England Journal of Medicine*, vol. 351, no. 3, pp. 268–277, 2004.

[28] E. Liakoni, A. E. Rätz Bravo, and S. Krähenbühl, "Hepatotoxicity of New Oral Anticoagulants (NOACs)," *Drug Safety*, vol. 38, no. 8, pp. 711–720, 2015.

[29] D. Caldeira, M. Barra, A. T. Santos et al., "Risk of drug-induced liver injury with the new oral anticoagulants: Systematic review and meta-analysis," *Heart*, vol. 100, no. 7, pp. 550–556, 2014.

[30] J. Graff and S. Harder, "Anticoagulant therapy with the oral direct factor Xa inhibitors rivaroxaban, apixaban and edoxaban and the thrombin inhibitor dabigatran etexilate in patients with hepatic impairment," *Clinical Pharmacokinetics*, vol. 52, no. 4, pp. 243–254, 2013.

[31] W. Potze, J. Adelmeijer, and T. Lisman, "Decreased in vitro anticoagulant potency of Rivaroxaban and Apixaban in plasma from patients with cirrhosis," *Hepatology*, vol. 61, no. 4, pp. 1435-1436, 2015.

[32] M. A. Zocco, E. di Stasio, R. de Cristofaro et al., "Thrombotic risk factors in patients with liver cirrhosis: correlation with MELD scoring system and portal vein thrombosis development," *Journal of Hepatology*, vol. 51, no. 4, pp. 682–689, 2009.

[33] *Xarelto (rivaroxaban) [package insert]*, Janssen Pharmaceuticals Inc. Titusville, http://www.xareltohcp.com/shared/product/prescribing-information.pdf.

[34] *Eliquis(apixaban) [package insert]*, Bristol-Myers Squibb, New York, NY, USA, http://packageinserts.bms.com/pi/pi_eliquis.pdf.

[35] *Savaysa (edoxaban) [package insert]*, Daiichi Sankyo, Tokyo, Japan, http://www.accessdata.fda.gov/drugsatfda_docs/label/2015/206316lbl.pdf.

[36] T. A. Dewald and R. C. Becker, "The pharmacology of novel oral anticoagulants," *Journal of Thrombosis and Thrombolysis*, vol. 37, no. 2, pp. 217–233, 2014.

[37] D. A. Parasrampuria, T. Kanamaru, A. Connor et al., "Evaluation of regional gastrointestinal absorption of edoxaban using the enterion capsule," *Clinical Pharmacology and Therapeutics*, vol. 55, no. 11, pp. 1286–1292, 2015.

[38] *Pradaxa (dabigatran) [package insert]*, Boehringer Ingelheim Pharmaceuticals, Inc, 2015.

[39] J. van Ryn, J. Stangier, S. Haertter et al., "Dabigatran etexilate—a novel, reversible, oral direct thrombin inhibitor: interpretation

of coagulation assays and reversal of anticoagulant activity," *Thrombosis & Haemostasis*, vol. 103, no. 6, pp. 1116–1127, 2010.

[40] S. J. Connolly, M. D. Ezekowitz, S. Yusuf et al., "Dabigatran versus warfarin in patients with atrial fibrillation," *The New England Journal of Medicine*, vol. 361, no. 12, pp. 1139–1151, 2009.

[41] J. Stangier, B. I. Eriksson, O. E. Dahl et al., "Pharmacokinetic profile of the oral direct thrombin inhibitor dabigatran etexilate in healthy volunteers and patients undergoing total hip replacement," *Clinical Pharmacology and Therapeutics*, vol. 45, no. 5, pp. 555–563, 2005.

[42] H. Tran, J. Joseph, L. Young et al., "New oral anticoagulants: A practical guide on prescription, laboratory testing and peri-procedural/bleeding management," *Internal Medicine Journal*, vol. 44, no. 6, pp. 525–536, 2014.

[43] J. W. Eikelboom, D. J. Quinlan, J. Hirsh, S. J. Connolly, and J. I. Weitz, "Laboratory monitoring of non-Vitamin K antagonist oral anticoagulant use in patients with atrial fibrillation: A review," *JAMA Cardiology*, vol. 2, no. 5, pp. 566–574, 2017.

[44] I. L. Holster, V. E. Valkhoff, E. J. Kuipers, and E. T. T. L. Tjwa, "New oral anticoagulants increase risk for gastrointestinal bleeding: a systematic review and meta-analysis," *Gastroenterology*, vol. 145, no. 1, pp. 105.e15–112.e15, 2013.

[45] C. Francoz, J. Belghiti, V. Vilgrain et al., "Splanchnic vein thrombosis in candidates for liver transplantation: usefulness of screening and anticoagulation," *Gut*, vol. 54, no. 5, pp. 691–697, 2005.

[46] L. Amitrano, M. A. Guardascione, A. Menchise et al., "Safety and efficacy of anticoagulation therapy with low molecular weight heparin for portal vein thrombosis in patients with liver cirrhosis," *Journal of Clinical Gastroenterology*, vol. 44, no. 6, pp. 448–451, 2010.

[47] C. D. Seaman, K. J. Smith, and M. V. Ragni, "Cost-effectiveness of rivaroxaban versus warfarin anticoagulation for the prevention of recurrent venous thromboembolism: A U.S. perspective," *Thrombosis Research*, vol. 132, no. 6, pp. 647–651, 2013.

[48] D. Kubitza, A. Roth, M. Becka et al., "Effect of hepatic impairment on the pharmacokinetics and pharmacodynamics of a single dose of rivaroxaban—an oral, direct Factor Xa inhibitor," *British Journal of Clinical Pharmacology*, vol. 76, no. 1, pp. 89–98, 2013.

[49] J. Mendell, L. Johnson, and S. Chen, "An open-label, phase 1 study to evaluate the effects of hepatic impairment on edoxaban pharmacokinetics and pharmacodynamics," *Clinical Pharmacology and Therapeutics*, vol. 55, no. 12, pp. 1395–1405, 2015.

[50] M. Tornkvist, J. G. Smith, and A. Labaf, "Current evidence of oral anticoagulant reversal: A systematic review," *Thrombosis Research*, vol. 162, pp. 22–31, 2018.

[51] T. Y. Hu, V. R. Vaidya, and S. J. Asirvatham, "Reversing anticoagulant effects of novel oral anticoagulants: Role of ciraparantag, andexanetalfa, and idarucizumab," *Vascular Health and Risk Management*, vol. 12, pp. 35–44, 2016.

# 19

# Sofosbuvir Based Regimens in the Treatment of Chronic Hepatitis C with Compensated Liver Cirrhosis in Community Care Setting

**Vijay Gayam,[1] Amrendra Kumar Mandal,[1] Mazin Khalid,[1] Osama Mukhtar,[1] Arshpal Gill,[1] Pavani Garlapati,[1] Mowyad Khalid,[2] and Mohammed Mansour[1]**

[1] *Department of Medicine and Gastroenterology, Interfaith Medical Center, 1545 Atlantic Avenue, Brooklyn, NY 11213, USA*
[2] *Department of Medicine, Wayne State University/Detroit Medical Center, Detroit, Michigan, USA*

Correspondence should be addressed to Vijay Gayam; vgayam@interfaithmedical.com

Academic Editor: Dirk Uhlmann

*Background.* Direct-acting antiviral (DAA) drugs have been highly effective in the treatment of chronic hepatitis C (CHC) infection. We aim to evaluate the treatment response of Sofosbuvir based DAA in CHC patients with compensated liver cirrhosis as limited data exists in the real-world community setting. *Methods.* All the CHC patients with compensated liver cirrhosis treated with Sofosbuvir based DAAs between January 2014 and December 2017 in a community clinic setting were retrospectively analyzed. Pretreatment baseline patient characteristics, treatment efficacy with the sustained virologic response at 12 weeks posttreatment (SVR12), and adverse reactions were assessed. *Results.* One hundred and twelve patients with CHC infection and concurrent compensated cirrhosis were included in the study. Black patients represented the majority of the study population (64%). Eighty-seven patients were treated with Ledipasvir/Sofosbuvir (LDV/SOF) ±Ribavirin and 25 patients were treated with Sofosbuvir/Velpatasvir (SOF/VEL). Overall, SVR 12 after treatment was achieved in 90% in patients who received one of the two DAA regimens (89.7% in LDV/SOF group and 92% in SOF/VEL group). SVR 12 did not vary based on age, sex, body mass index, baseline HCV viral load, HCV/HIV coinfection, type of genotype, and prior treatment status. Apart from a low platelet count, there were no other factors associated with a statistical difference in SVR 12($p$=0.002) between the two regimens. Fatigue (35%) was the most common adverse effect and no patients discontinued treatment due to adverse effects. *Conclusion.* In the community care setting, Sofosbuvir based DAAs are safe, effective with high overall SVR, and well tolerated in patients with CHC patients with compensated liver cirrhosis.

## 1. Introduction

Anywhere between 3.2 and 5 million people in the United States have a chronic hepatitis C (CHC) infection which if untreated can develop into cirrhosis, hepatocellular carcinoma, and death [1, 2]. CHC is the most common indication for a liver transplantation and a more common cause of death than all other notifiable infectious etiologies combined in the United States [3, 4].

Successful treatment of CHC, also described as a sustained virological response (SVR), is defined as an absence of detectable HCV RNA 12 weeks after the completion of treatment. CHC patients who achieve SVR have both lower rates of complications and lower overall mortality [5]. Until recently, CHC treatment was primarily based on interferon-based regimens, but disappointing response rates, particularly amongst patients with advanced liver disease, necessitated the need for a new regimen [6].

Newer drugs that directly inhibit the virus replication cycle have led to the advent of oral HCV treatment regimens known as direct-acting antiviral (DAAs) [7]. In existing clinical trials, DAA regimens have demonstrated cures rates over 90% of patients who have chronic CHC infection and concurrent cirrhosis.

Due to the relative novelty of DAA regimens, there is a paucity of literature establishing safety, tolerability, and efficacy of DAA in the real-world community care setting. As a result, we aim to analyze DAA's safety, tolerability, and efficacy in an inner-city community care setting with an emphasis on the most commonly used DAA in patients with cirrhosis.

## 2. Materials and Methods

The study protocol was approved by the Institutional Review Board (IRB) and the patients were recruited from a community hospital: Interfaith Medical Center

*2.1. Patients.* The 112 consecutive patients with CHC treated between January 2015 and December 2017 were included in this retrospective cohort study and received at least twelve weeks of treatment with one of the recommended combination regimens in standard doses for chronic HCV infection. Two different treatment regimens were used in our study, Ledipasvir (LDV) 90 mg/day+ Sofosbuvir (SOF) 400 mg/day ±Ribavirin (RBV) 1000 mg/day if <75kg and 1200 mg/day if ≥75kg, and Sofosbuvir (SOF) 400 mg/day+ Velpatasvir (VEL) 100 mg/day. Duration of treatment ranged from 12 weeks (n=98) to 24 weeks (n=14) depending on prior treatment status and existing cirrhosis.

*2.2. Study Assessments.* Treatment safety and tolerability were assessed by reviewing documented adverse events, treatment completion rates, reduction in the dosage, and discontinuation of medications. Laboratory studies were conducted both pretreatment and posttreatment. Laboratory values were then compared to look for any abnormalities associated with antiviral therapy. A diagnosis of liver cirrhosis was based on the amalgamation of clinical symptoms, laboratory parameters including FibroSure score ≥ 0.75, imaging modalities (ultrasonography and or computed tomography scan), and histopathology when indicated. We included compensated cirrhosis, defined as the absence of ascites, jaundice, hepatic encephalopathy and variceal bleeding according to the American Association for the Study of Liver Diseases, in this study.

Treatment response was assessed with HCV RNA viral load (IU/ mL) at each of 4 weeks after initiation of treatment, completion of treatment, and 12 weeks after completion of treatment. Viral load was assessed using COBAS® AmpliPrep/COBAS® TaqMan® HCV Quantitative Test, v2.0 (Roche molecular diagnostics) with the lower limit of quantification (LLOQ) of HCV RNA 15 IU/ml. SVR 12 was defined as an undetectable viral load 12 weeks after the completion of treatment.

*2.3. Statistical Analysis.* The SPSS® statistics software package (IBM SPSS® statistics version 21, USA) was used for statistical analysis. Values were expressed as mean ± SD and mean quantitative values were analyzed using Student's t-test. Differences in qualitative values were analyzed by Chi-square test. All $p$ values were two-tailed and $p$-value < 0.05 was considered significant. One-way analysis of variance (ANOVA) was used to determine whether there were differences among the group means. Multivariable logistic regression was performed only in variables with a $p$-value < 0.05 in univariate analysis.

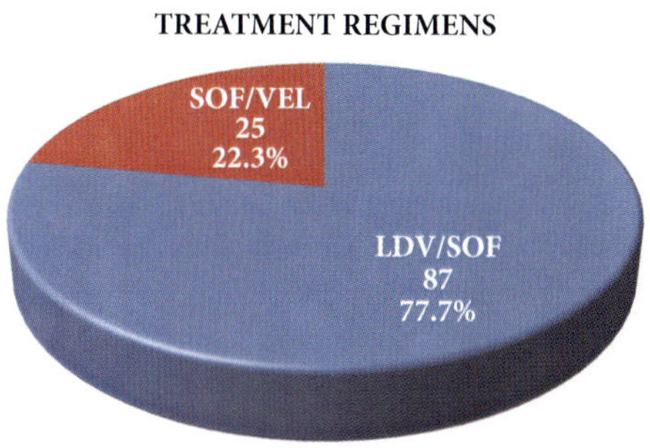


FIGURE 1: Treatment regimens.

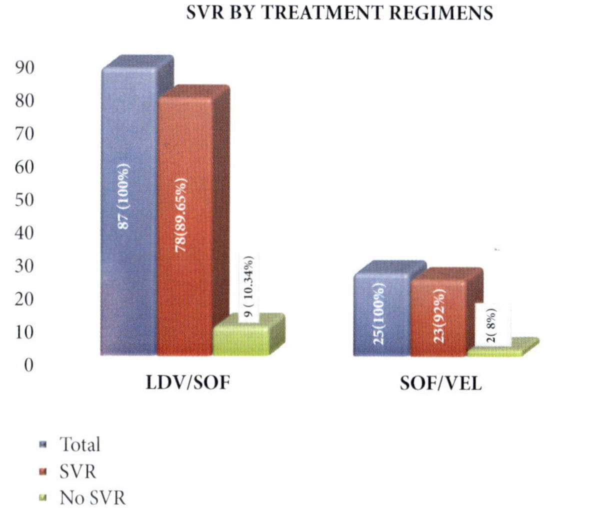


FIGURE 2: Treatment response in both groups by overall SVR 12.

## 3. Results

*3.1. Baseline Characteristics.* Baseline characteristics are shown in Table 1. Mean age of the patients in the study was 60.7 years with age, ranging from 28 to 82 years. The majority of the patients were males 67 (75%), black 71(63.4%), and treatment-naive (76.8%). Genotype 1 was predominant, consisting of over 89.3% of the study population. Nine (23.2%) patients had received prior treatment. Thirty-five patients (31.3%) had a history of diabetes; 51 (45.5%) had hypertension; 12 (10.7%) patients had coronary artery disease, 24 patients had HCV/HIV coinfection. None of the patients had a hepatocellular carcinoma, previous liver transplant, or decompensated cirrhosis.

*3.2. Treatment Regimens.* Among the 112 patients with CHC infection, 87(77.7%) patients were treated with Ledipasvir/Sofosbuvir, and 25 (22.3%) were treated with Sofosbuvir/Velpatasvir (Figure 1).

*3.3. Overall Virologic Response to Treatments.* The overall sustained virological response (SVR) on completion of treatment was 90 %. SVR 12 in the two treatment groups is depicted in Figure 2. In the univariate analysis, there were characteristics noted in the patients who achieved SVR12 as

Table 1: Demographic and clinical characteristics of patients at baseline by treatment regimen.

| Characteristics | All patients ($n$ = 112) | Treatment Regimens LDV/SOF ($n$ = 87) | SOF/VEL ($n$ = 25) | $p$-value |
|---|---|---|---|---|
| **Sex** | | | | |
| Male | 67 (59.8) | 51 (58.6) | 16 (64.0) | 0.629 |
| Female | 45 (40.2) | 36 (41.4) | 9 (36.0) | |
| **Age** (years) | 60.7 (28-82) | 61.6 (28-82) | 57.2 (34-73) | 0.076 |
| **Age group** (Years) | | | | |
| < 65 | 74 (66.1) | 55 (63.2) | 19 (76.0) | 0.234 |
| ≥ 65 | 38 (33.9) | 32 (36.8) | 6 (24.0) | |
| **BMI** (Kg/m$^2$) | 29.0 (18.5-47.0) | 28.7 (18.5-47.0) | 30.2 (20-43) | 0.242 |
| **BMI** (Kg/m$^2$) | | | | |
| < 30 | 65 (58.0) | 52 (59.8) | 13 (52.0) | 0.488 |
| ≥ 30 | 47 (42.0) | 35 (40.2) | 12 (48.0) | |
| **HCV Genotype** | | | | |
| 1a | 66 (58.9) | 52 (59.8 | 14 (56.0) | |
| 1b | 34 (30.4) | 28 (32.2) | 6 (24.0) | 0.131 |
| 2 | 5 (4.5) | 4 (4.6) | 1 (4.0) | |
| 3 | 3 (2.7) | 2 (2.3) | 1 (4.0) | |
| 4 | 4 (3.6) | 1 (1.1) | 3 (12.0) | |
| **HCV RNA** (IU/mL) | | | | |
| < 800,000 | 31 (27.7) | 26 (29.9) | 5 (20.0) | 0.330 |
| ≥ 800,000 | 81 (72.3) | 61 (70.1) | 20 (80.0) | |
| **Prior treatment** | | | | |
| Naïve | 86 (76.8) | 70 (80.5) | 16 (64.0) | 0.086 |
| Experienced | 26 (23.2) | 17 (19.5) | 9 (36.0) | |
| **Comorbidities** | | | | |
| Diabetes | 35 (31.3) | 25 (28.7) | 10 (40.0) | 0.284 |
| Hypertension | 51 (45.5) | 37 (42.5) | 14 (56.0) | 0.233 |
| Coronary artery disease | 12 (10.7) | 9 (10.3) | 3 (12.0) | 0.728 |
| Kidney disease | 9 (8.0) | 8 (9.2) | 1 (4.0) | 0.681 |
| Chronic anemia | 5 (4.5) | 2 (2.3) | 3 (12.0) | 0.073 |
| HIV seropositive | 24 (21.4) | 21 (24.1) | 3 (12.0) | 0.192 |
| **MELD score** | | | | |
| < 10 | 62 (55.4) | 51 (58.6) | 11 (44.0) | 0.195 |
| ≥ 10 | 50 (44.6) | 36 (41.4) | 14 (56.0) | |
| **Laboratory tests** | | | | |
| Hemoglobin (g/dL) | 13.4 (9.2-17.5) | 13.5 (9.2-17.5) | 13.0 (10.0-16.0) | 0.278 |
| Platelets (x1000/mL) | 140.7 (23-316) | 143.4 (43-316) | 131.5 (23-216) | 0.371 |
| Albumin (g/dL) | 3.5 (1.3-4.7) | 3.5 (1.3-4.7) | 3.5 (2.2-4.5) | 0.899 |
| AST (IU/L) | 82.3 (16-210) | 83.3 (16-210) | 78.9 (20-179) | 0.639 |
| ALT (IU/L) | 77.8 (12-264) | 79.5 (12-264) | 72.1 (13-200) | 0.510 |
| Bilirubin (mg/dL) | 1.2 (0.3-4.9) | 1.2 (0.3-4.9) | 1.1 (0.5-3.2) | 0.752 |

Data are presented as mean (range) or number (percentage).
BMI, body mass index; HCV, hepatitis C virus; RNA, ribonucleic acid; APRI, AST-to-platelet ratio index; MELD, model for end-stage liver disease; AST, aspartate transaminase; and ALT, alanine transaminase.

compared to those who did not achieve SVR. Higher mean BMI, higher Child-Pugh score, low mean platelet count, low mean albumin, and low mean bilirubin level were all more likely to be seen in patients who achieved SVR 12 in the univariate analysis. After adjusting baseline characteristics in multivariable logistic regression models, only low platelet count was found as a significant predictor of treatment response ($p$-value =0.020). Interestingly, SVR was not affected by HCV RNA levels or previous treatment status (Table 2).

*3.4. Virologic Response in LDV/SOF Group.* In this group, 78(89.7%) achieved SVR 12. HCV viral load and type of HCV genotype did not have any impact on overall SVR. Additional comorbidities including diabetes mellitus, chronic kidney disease, and HIV seropositivity did not impact SVR rates as shown in Table 3.

*3.5. Virologic Response in SOF/VEL Group.* In this treatment group, 23 (92%) achieved SVR (Table 4). Although this value is encouraging, it may not be truly significant due to a small sample size. HCV viral load and type of HCV genotype did not have any impact on overall SVR. Additional comorbidities including diabetes mellitus, chronic kidney disease, and HIV seropositivity did not impact SVR rates as shown in Table 4.

*3.6. Safety.* Only a small percentage of patients developed minor side effects from DAA treatment, and none required discontinuation of therapy. Fatigue, headache, rash, and thrombocytopenia were the most common adverse events observed. Anemia was seen only in patients treated with LDV/SOF + Ribavirin combination. There were no serious adverse events seen amongst all regimens. There was no statistically significant difference of adverse events noted between the two treatment groups. A complete list of adverse events is shown in Table 5.

## 4. Discussion

Antiviral therapy has rapidly evolved for the treatment of chronic HCV infection. The primary endpoint is to achieve SVR 12, which in turn diminishes the risk of decompensation, hepatocellular carcinoma, and death.

DAAs offer the most effective regimens for the majority of HCV infected patients. Selection of regimens is primarily based on the genotype, cirrhosis status, and other various individual patient factors. The efficacy of DAAs for patients with compensated cirrhosis is now well validated [8–10]. We studied the two most commonly used regimens, LDV/SOF and SOF/VEL.

We noted an SVR of 89.7% in LDV/SOF group which is comparable to ION-2 trial where SVR of 86% was reported in patients with cirrhosis [8]. Another trial (SIRIUS trial) reported a higher SVR of 97% (HCV genotype 1) in compensated cirrhosis. This discrepancy may be explained by the difference in duration of therapy; the SIRIUS trial patients each received 24 weeks of therapy versus our study in which patients received only 12 weeks of therapy [11].

Our second regimen was SOF/VEL which is currently approved for the treatment of all genotypes (as per AASLD guidelines). In the present study, 23 patients (92%) achieved SVR in SOF/VEL which is similar to the study by Asselah et al. They reported SVR in 96% of patients with HCV related cirrhosis after 12 weeks of treatment [12]. Our study also showed SVR rates consistent with ASTRAL-3 and ASTRAL-1 trial. These trials also used SOF/VEL regimen in a similar group of patients with overall SVR rate of 88% and 98%, respectively [12, 13]. Our study also exhibited similar response rates to the recent POLARIS-3 trial in which cirrhotic patients were given SOF/VEL for 12 weeks. They demonstrated an excellent SVR of 96 % in HCV genotype 3 infections [14].

Thrombocytopenia was associated with a lower SVR ($p$=0.02) in our study. Several studies have documented that chronic HCV infection is strongly associated with thrombocytopenia. Between 64% and 76% of patients with fibrosis and cirrhosis related to chronic HCV infections exhibited thrombocytopenia, as compared to only 6% in noncirrhotic patients [15, 16]. Thrombocytopenia is strongly related to the degree of liver fibrosis owing to low thrombopoietin levels and splenic sequestration of blood cells as a direct result of elevated portal pressure, especially among patients with advance fibrosis or cirrhosis [17–19]. Thrombocytopenia has also been associated with a higher risk for cirrhosis-related morbidity and mortality [20, 21]. Thus, early treatment of HCV infection before the development of thrombocytopenia may improve overall treatment outcomes.

Our study was supported by Suwantarat et al. who reported that thrombocytopenia was associated with lower SVR ($P$=0.05) [22]. In contrast to our study, they used interferon-based therapy and greater cytopenia was hypothesized to be a marker for greater TNF activity, which translated into a significant SVR variation. Importantly, several studies including Coverdale et al. and Taniguchi et al. reported that improvement in platelet count correlated with the regression of hepatic fibrosis following SVR 12 among patients with chronic HCV infection [23, 24].

The present study had a high HIV/HCV coinfection rate of 21.4%, but there was still a high overall SVR. This is consistent with the literature, as Osinusi et al. also demonstrated an overall high SVR (97%) in patients with HIV/HCV coinfection [25].

There were no major adverse effects in our study leading to a discontinuation of therapy, which was also noted in the ION-1 trial in which no patient discontinued LDV/SOF. Common adverse events in the present study were fatigue, headache, insomnia, and nausea. ASTRAL-1, 2, and 3 with SOF/VEL also had similar adverse effects [12, 13].

We noted an excellent sustained virological response rate in patients with compensated cirrhosis irrespective of genotypes in both treatment groups, and these results are consistent with the landmark literature described above. Our study is distinct from most studies in current literature as it establishes real-world effectiveness, tolerability, and safety of Sofosbuvir based regimens in CHC patients with compensated cirrhosis. This is in contrast to the literature, which still relies heavily on clinical trials. Limitations of the study are the small sample size and retrospective nature.

TABLE 2: Demographic and clinical characteristics of patients at baseline by treatment response.

| Characteristics | All patients ($N$ =112) | Treatment Response SVR ($n$ =101) | No SVR ($n$ =11) | Univariate Analysis $p$-value | Multivariate Analysis $p$-value |
|---|---|---|---|---|---|
| **Age** (years) | 60.7 (28-82) | 60.7 (28-82) | 60.0 (45-67) | 0.797 | NA |
| **Age group** | | | | | |
| < 65 | 74 (66.1) | 66 (65.3) | 8 (72.7) | 0.747 | NA |
| ≥ 65 | 38 (33.9) | 35 (34.7) | 3 (27.3) | | |
| **Sex** | | | | | |
| Male | 67 (59.8) | 58 (57.4) | 9 (81.8) | 0.194 | NA |
| Female | 45 (40.2) | 43 (42.6) | 2 (18.2) | | |
| **BMI** (Kg/m$^2$) | 29.0 (18.5-47.0) | 29.4 (19.0-47.0) | 25.8 (18.5-32.5) | 0.050* | 0.085 |
| **BMI** (Kg/m$^2$) | | | | | |
| < 30 | 65 (58.0) | 57 (56.4) | 8 (72.7) | 0.353 | NA |
| ≥ 30 | 47 (42.0) | 44 (43.6) | 3 (27.3) | | |
| **HCV Genotype** | | | | | |
| 1a | 66 (58.9) | 57 (56.4) | 9 (81.8) | | |
| 1b | 34 (30.4) | 34 (33.7) | 0 | 0.150 | NA |
| 2 | 5 (4.5) | 4 (4.0) | 1 (9.1) | | |
| 3 | 3 (2.7) | 3 (3.0) | 0 | | |
| 4 | 4 (3.6) | 3 (3.0) | 1 (9.1) | | |
| **HCV RNA** (IU/mL) | | | | | |
| < 800,000 | 31 (27.7) | 28 (27.7) | 3 (27.3) | 1.000 | NA |
| ≥ 800,000 | 81 (72.3) | 73 (72.3) | 8 (72.7) | | |
| **Prior treatment** | | | | | |
| Naïve | 86 (76.8) | 77 (76.2) | 9 (81.8) | 1.000 | NA |
| Experienced | 26 (23.2) | 24 (23.8) | 2 (18.2) | | |
| **Comorbidities** | | | | | |
| Diabetes | 35 (31.3) | 31 (30.7) | 4 (36.4) | 0.738 | NA |
| Hypertension | 51 (45.5) | 46 (45.5) | 5 (45.5) | 0.995 | NA |
| Coronary artery disease | 12 (10.7) | 12 (11.9) | 0 | 0.604 | NA |
| Kidney disease | 9 (8.0) | 8 (7.9) | 1 (9.1) | 1.000 | NA |
| Chronic anemia | 5 (4.5) | 4 (4.0) | 1 (9.1) | 0.410 | NA |
| HIV Seropositive | 24 (21.4) | 20 (19.8) | 4 (36.4) | 0.245 | NA |
| **MELD score** | | | | | |
| < 10 | 62 (55.4) | 59 (58.4) | 3 (27.3) | 0.060 | NA |
| ≥ 10 | 50 (44.6) | 42 (41.6) | 8 (72.7) | | |
| **Laboratory tests** | | | | | |
| Hemoglobin (g/dL) | 13.4 (9.2-17.5) | 13.3 (9.2-17.5) | 13.9 (11.6-15.9) | 0.276 | NA |
| Platelets (x1000/mL) | 140.7 (23-316) | 146.4 (23-316) | 88.6 (43-177) | 0.002* | 0.020 |
| Albumin (g/dL) | 3.5 (1.3-4.7) | 3.6 (1.3-4.7) | 3.2 (2.2-4.1) | 0.042* | 0.873 |
| AST (IU/L) | 82.3 (16-210) | 81.6 (16-198) | 88.7 (42-210) | 0.585 | NA |
| ALT (IU/L) | 77.8 (12-264) | 77.2 (12-204) | 83.9 (27-264) | 0.666 | NA |
| Bilirubin (mg/dL) | 1.2 (0.3-4.9) | 1.1 (0.3-3.9) | 1.6 (0.8-4.9) | 0.043* | 0.821 |

Data are presented as mean (range) or number (percentage).

*Only variables with the $p$-value < 0.05 in univariate analysis were assessed.

BMI, body mass index; HCV, hepatitis C virus; RNA, ribonucleic acid; APRI, AST-to-platelet ratio index; MELD, model for end-stage liver disease; AST, aspartate transaminase; and ALT, alanine transaminase.

TABLE 3: SVR 12 rates in patients receiving LDV/SOF by population subgroup.

| Response | SVR 12 Rate | Univariate Analysis *p*-value | Multivariate Analysis *p*-value |
|---|---|---|---|
| **Overall** | 78/87 (89.7) | | |
| **Age group** | | | |
| < 65 | 49/55 (89.1) | 1.000 | NA |
| ≥ 65 | 29/32 (90.6) | | |
| **Sex** | | | |
| Male | 44/51 (86.3) | 1.000 | NA |
| Female | 34/36 (94.4) | | |
| **BMI** ($Kg/m^2$) | | | |
| < 30 | 45/52 (86.5) | 0.304 | NA |
| ≥ 30 | 33/35 (94.3) | | |
| **HCV Genotype** | | | |
| 1a | 45/52 (86.5) | 0.009* | 0.983 |
| 1b | 28/28 (100) | | |
| 2 | 3/4 (75.0) | | |
| 3 | 2/2 (100) | | |
| 4 | 0/1 (0) | | |
| **HCV RNA** (IU/mL) | | | |
| < 800,000 | 23/26 (88.5) | 1.000 | NA |
| ≥ 800,000 | 55/61 (90.2) | | |
| **Prior treatment** | | | |
| Naïve | 62/70 (88.6) | 0.682 | NA |
| Experienced | 16/17 (94.1) | | |
| **Comorbidities** | | | |
| Diabetes | 21/25 (84.0) | 0.272 | NA |
| Hypertension | 33/37 (89.2) | 1.000 | NA |
| CAD | 9/9 (100) | 0.589 | NA |
| Kidney disease | 7/8 (87.5) | 1.000 | NA |
| Chronic anemia | 2/2 (100) | 1.000 | NA |
| HIV Seropositive | 18/21 (85.7) | 0.681 | NA |
| **MELD Score** | | | |
| < 10 | 48/51 (94.1) | 0.154 | NA |
| ≥ 10 | 30/36 (83.3) | | |
| **ALT** (IU/L) | | | |
| < 40 | 17/18 (94.4) | 0.678 | NA |
| ≥ 40 | 61/69 (88.4) | | |

Data presented as number/total number (percent).
*Only variables with the $p$-value < 0.05 in univariate analysis were assessed.
BMI, body mass index; HCV, hepatitis C virus; RNA, ribonucleic acid; APRI, AST-to-platelet ratio index; MELD, model for end-stage liver disease; and ALT, alanine transaminase

TABLE 4: SVR 12 rates in patients receiving SOF/VEL by population subgroup.

| Response | SVR 12 Rate | Univariate Analysis *p*-value | Multivariate Analysis *p*-value |
|---|---|---|---|
| **Overall** | 23/25 (92.0) | | |
| **Age group** | | | |
| < 65 | 17/19 (89.5) | 1.000 | NA |
| ≥ 65 | 6/6 (100) | | |
| **Sex** | | | |
| Male | 14/16 (87.5) | 0.520 | NA |
| Female | 9/9 (100) | | |
| **BMI** ($Kg/m^2$) | | | |
| < 30 | 12/13 (92.3) | 1.000 | NA |
| ≥ 30 | 11/12 (91.7) | | |
| **HCV Genotype** | | | |
| 1a | 12/14 (85.7) | 0.789 | NA |
| 1b | 6/6 (100) | | |
| 2 | 1/1 (100) | | |
| 3 | 1/1 (100) | | |
| 4 | 3/3 (100) | | |
| **HCV RNA** (IU/mL) | | | |
| < 800,000 | 5/5 (100) | 1.000 | NA |
| ≥ 800,000 | 18/20 (90.0) | | |
| **Prior treatment** | | | |
| Naïve | 15/16 (93.8) | 1.000 | NA |
| Experienced | 8/9 (88.9) | | |
| **Comorbidities** | | | |
| Diabetes | 10/10 (100) | 0.500 | NA |
| Hypertension | 13/14 (92.9) | 1.000 | NA |
| CAD | 3/3 (100) | 1.000 | NA |
| Kidney disease | 1/1 (100) | 1.000 | NA |
| Chronic anemia | 2/3 (66.7) | 0.230 | NA |
| HIV Seropositive | 2/3 (66.7) | 0.230 | NA |
| **MELD Score** | | | |
| < 10 | 11/11 (100) | 0.487 | NA |
| ≥ 10 | 12/14 (85.7) | | |
| **ALT** (IU/L) | | | |
| < 40 | 4/4 (100) | 1.000 | NA |
| ≥ 40 | 19/21 (90.5) | | |

Data presented as number/total number (percent).
BMI, body mass index; HCV, hepatitis C virus; RNA, ribonucleic acid; APRI, AST-to-platelet ratio index; MELD, model for end-stage liver disease; and ALT, alanine transaminase.

## 5. Conclusion

In the community care setting, Sofosbuvir based DAAs remain a safe, effective, and well tolerated in patients with chronic CHC patients with compensated liver cirrhosis.

## Abbreviations

CHC: Chronic hepatitis C
HCV: Hepatitis C virus
HCC: Hepatocellular cancer
DAAs: Direct-acting antivirals
GT: Genotype

TABLE 5: Treatment adverse events.

| Adverse event | Treatment Regimen LDV/SOF | Treatment Regimen SOF/VEL | $p$-value |
|---|---|---|---|
| Fatigue | 26 (29.9) | 9 (36.0) | 0.561 |
| Insomnia | 1 (1.1) | 1 (4.0) | 0.398 |
| Headache | 6 (6.9) | 0 | 0.335 |
| Nausea | 5 (5.7) | 3 (12.0) | 0.374 |
| Abdominal pain | 1 (1.1) | 0 | 1.000 |
| Skin rash | 7 (8.0) | 0 | 0.346 |
| Arthralgia | 3 (3.4) | 2 (8.0) | 0.310 |
| Thrombocytopenia | 6 (6.9) | 2 (8.0) | 1.000 |

Data presented as number (percent).

SOF: Sofosbuvir
RBV: Ribavirin
LDV: Ledipasvir
VEL: Velpatasvir
SVR12: Sustained virologic response at 12 weeks posttreatment
APRI: Aspartate aminotransferase-to-platelet ratio index
ESLD: End stage liver disease.

## Disclosure

An abstract of this article is presented as a poster at NY Department of Health Viral Hepatitis Symposium, May 2018.

## Authors' Contributions

Vijay Gayam, M.D., made substantial contribution to conception and design of the study, data acquisition, analysis, interpretation of the data, and drafting of the manuscript, performed critical reviews, communicated with the journal, and addressed comments from the reviewers. Amrendra Kumar Mandal, M.D., and Mazin Khalid, M.D., performed data acquisition and provided assistance with interpretation of data and drafting of the manuscript. Osama Mukhtar, M.D., and Mowyad Khalid, M.D., made substantial contribution to statistical data analysis and interpretation of the data. Pavani Garlapati and Arshpal Gill have contributed in the acquisition of the patient data. Dr. Mohammed Mansour made substantial contribution to critical review of the abstract. All the authors vouch for the veracity and completeness of the data presented and agreed to submit the manuscript for publication.

## References

[1] M. M. Denniston, R. B. Jiles, J. Drobeniuc et al., "Chronic hepatitis C virus infection in the United States, national health and nutrition examination survey 2003 to 2010," *Annals of Internal Medicine*, vol. 160, no. 5, pp. 293–300, 2014.

[2] G. L. Armstrong, A. Wasley, E. P. Simard, G. M. McQuillan, W. L. Kuhnert, and M. J. Alter, "The prevalence of hepatitis C virus infection in the United States, 1999 through 2002," *Annals of Internal Medicine*, vol. 144, no. 10, pp. 705–714, 2006.

[3] K. N. Ly, E. M. Hughes, R. B. Jiles, and S. D. Holmberg, "Rising mortality associated with Hepatitis C virus in the United States, 2003-2013," *Clinical Infectious Diseases*, vol. 62, no. 10, pp. 1287-1288, 2016.

[4] O. Mitchell and A. Gurakar, "Management of hepatitis C post-liver transplantation: a comprehensive review," *Journal of Clinical and Translational Hepatology*, vol. 3, no. 2, article 140, 2015.

[5] S. Bruno, P. M. Battezzati, G. Bellati et al., "Long-term beneficial effects in sustained responders to interferon-alfa therapy for chronic hepatitis C," *Journal of Hepatology*, vol. 34, no. 5, pp. 748–755, 2001.

[6] E. Vezali, A. Aghemo, and M. Colombo, "A review of the treatment of chronic hepatitis C virus infection in cirrhosis," *Clinical Therapeutics*, vol. 32, no. 13, pp. 2117–2138, 2010.

[7] T. J. Liang and M. G. Ghany, "Current and future therapies for hepatitis C virus infection," *The New England Journal of Medicine*, vol. 368, no. 20, pp. 1907–1917, 2013.

[8] N. Afdhal, S. Zeuzem, P. Kwo et al., "Ledipasvir and sofosbuvir for untreated HCV genotype 1 infection," *The New England Journal of Medicine*, vol. 370, no. 20, pp. 1889–1898, 2014.

[9] N. Afdhal, K. R. Reddy, D. R. Nelson et al., "Ledipasvir and sofosbuvir for previously treated HCV genotype 1 infection," *The New England Journal of Medicine*, vol. 370, no. 16, pp. 1483–1493, 2014.

[10] D. R. Nelson, J. N. Cooper, J. P. Lalezari et al., "All-oral 12-week treatment with daclatasvir plus sofosbuvir in patients with hepatitis C virus genotype 3 infection: ALLY-3 phase III study," *Hepatology*, vol. 61, no. 4, pp. 1127–1135, 2015.

[11] M. Bourlière, J. Bronowicki, V. de Ledinghen et al., "Ledipasvir-sofosbuvir with or without ribavirin to treat patients with HCV genotype 1 infection and cirrhosis non-responsive to previous protease-inhibitor therapy: a randomised, double-blind, phase 2 trial (SIRIUS)," *The Lancet Infectious Diseases*, vol. 15, no. 4, pp. 397–404, 2015.

[12] J. J. Feld, I. M. Jacobson, C. Hézode et al., "Sofosbuvir and velpatasvir for HCV genotype 1, 2, 4, 5, and 6 infection," *The New England Journal of Medicine*, vol. 373, no. 27, pp. 2599–2607, 2015.

[13] G. R. Foster, N. Afdhal, S. K. Roberts et al., "Sofosbuvir and velpatasvir for HCV Genotype 2 and 3 infection," *The New England Journal of Medicine*, vol. 373, no. 27, pp. 2608–2617, 2015.

[14] I. M. Jacobson, E. Lawitz, E. J. Gane et al., "Efficacy of 8 Weeks of Sofosbuvir, Velpatasvir, and Voxilaprevir in Patients With Chronic HCV Infection: 2 Phase 3 Randomized Trials," *Gastroenterology*, vol. 153, no. 1, pp. 113–122, 2017.

[15] F. N. Bashour, J. C. Teran, and K. D. Mullen, "Prevalence of peripheral blood cytopenias (hypersplenism) in patients with nonalcoholic chronic liver disease," *American Journal of Gastroenterology*, vol. 95, no. 10, pp. 2936–2939, 2000.

[16] E. G. Giannini, "Review article: Thrombocytopenia in chronic liver disease and pharmacologic treatment options," *Alimentary Pharmacology & Therapeutics*, vol. 23, no. 8, pp. 1055–1065, 2006.

[17] A. Pohl, C. Behling, D. Oliver, M. Kilani, P. Monson, and T. Hassanein, "Serum aminotransferase levels and platelet counts as predictors of degree of fibrosis in chronic hepatitis C virus infection," *American Journal of Gastroenterology*, vol. 96, no. 11, pp. 3142–3146, 2001.

[18] T. Poynard and P. Bedossa, "Age and platelet count: a simple index for predicting the presence of histological lesions in patients with antibodies to hepatitisC virus," *Journal of Viral Hepatitis*, vol. 4, no. 3, pp. 199–208, 1997.

[19] C. Pilette, F. Oberti, C. Aubé et al., "Non-invasive diagnosis of esophageal varices in chronic liver diseases," *Journal of Hepatology*, vol. 31, no. 5, pp. 867–873, 1999.

[20] T. R. Morgan, M. G. Ghany, H.-Y. Kim et al., "Outcome of sustained virological responders with histologically advanced chronic hepatitis C," *Hepatology*, vol. 52, no. 3, pp. 833–844, 2010.

[21] A. J. van der Meer, B. J. Veldt, J. J. Feld et al., "Association between sustained virological response and all-cause mortality among patients with chronic hepatitis C and advanced hepatic fibrosis," *The Journal of the American Medical Association*, vol. 308, no. 24, pp. 2584–2593, 2012.

[22] N. Suwantarat, A. D. Tice, T. Khawcharoenporn, and D. C. Chow, "Weight loss, leukopenia and thrombocytopenia associated with sustained virologic response to hepatitis C treatment," *International Journal of Medical Sciences*, vol. 7, no. 1, pp. 36–42, 2010.

[23] S. A. Coverdale, D. A. Samarasinghe, R. Lin et al., "Changes in antipyrine clearance and platelet count, but not conventional liver tests, correlate with fibrotic change in chronic hepatitis C: Value for predicting fibrotic progression," *American Journal of Gastroenterology*, vol. 98, no. 6, pp. 1384–1390, 2003.

[24] H. Taniguchi, Y. Iwasaki, A. Fujiwara et al., "Long-term monitoring of platelet count, as a non-invasive marker of hepatic fibrosis progression and/or regression in patients with chronic hepatitis C after interferon therapy," *Journal of Gastroenterology and Hepatology*, vol. 21, no. 1, pp. 281–287, 2006.

[25] A. Osinusi, K. Townsend, A. Kohli et al., "Virologic response following combined ledipasvir and sofosbuvir administration in patients with HCV genotype 1 and HIV Co-infection," *The Journal of the American Medical Association*, vol. 313, no. 12, pp. 1232–1239, 2015.

# 20

# Video Capsule Endoscopy in the Assessment of Portal Hypertensive Enteropathy

**Yasir Al-Azzawi,[1] Lidia Spaho,[2] Mohammed Mahmoud,[2] Joan Kheder,[2] Anne Foley,[2] and David Cave[2]**

[1] *University of Massachusetts School of Medicine, 55 North Lake Ave, Worcester, MA 01606, USA*
[2] *University of Massachusetts School of Medicine, USA*

Correspondence should be addressed to Yasir Al-Azzawi; yasiralazzawi@gmail.com

Academic Editor: Heather Francis

*Background.* The features of the portal hypertension enteropathy (PHE) vary from mild mucosal changes to varices with or without bleeding. The prevalence and the development are not fully understood. *Aim.* Our aim is to examine the prevalence and the different manifestations of PHE using video capsule endoscopy (VCE). *Methods.* It is a single center retrospective study of patients with cirrhosis, who had VCE. Based on the published literature, we divided the PHE lesions into vascular lesions and mucosal lesions. *Results.* Of the 100 patients with cirrhosis that had a VCE study, the mean age was 62.82 years. Male gender was predominant (64%), while Caucasians represented 82% of the cohort. The most common etiology of cirrhosis was chronic alcohol abuse followed by chronic hepatitis C virus and nonalcoholic steatohepatitis. VCE detected small bowel lesions in 71% of the patients while the features of PHE were found in 65% from the total cohort. AVMs and inflammatory changes were the most common findings, followed by bleeding. More than 50% of the lesions were vascular in nature. The risk of finding PHE in decompensated cirrhosis is twice that in compensated cirrhosis. Forty-five patients had negative EGD exam for any active bleeding, esophageal varices, portal hypertensive gastropathy, or gastric varices. Of these, 69% had features of PHE in their VCE. *Conclusions.* VCE detected small bowel lesions in 71% of our cohort. There is a high prevalence of PHE in decompensated cirrhosis. Vascular lesions are the most common finding in the small bowel of this population.

## 1. Introduction

Cirrhosis or end-stage liver disease is defined as a late stage of scarring and fibrosis of the liver and characterized by alteration of the hepatic architecture as well as the development of regenerative nodules; these changes can lead to a multitude of complications. Cirrhosis can be most commonly attributed to excessive alcohol consumption, viral hepatitis, or nonalcoholic fatty liver disease [1]. Reports from the Centers for Disease Control (CDC) estimate that 75,766 deaths and 2.3 million years of potential life lost during 2001 were attributable to excessive alcohol abuse, which also contributed to 60-70% of the cirrhosis in the USA. It is the 12$^{th}$ leading cause of death in USA and it is the leading cause of morbidity [2]. A recent population-based study showed that, per 2-year interval, cirrhotic patients have 26.4% mortality rate as compared to propensity matched controls who had a mortality rate of 8.4% [3].

The pathophysiology behind developing portal hypertension (PH) is believed to be related to scarring in the liver parenchymal disease, the increased production of vasoconstrictor (endothelins, angiotensin II, norepinephrine, and thromboxane A2), and a decrease in secretion of endothelial vasodilators. As a result, dysregulation of the extrahepatic vascular beds occurs in the splanchnic and systemic circulations causing the blood flow inside the portal veins to increase and the portal vein pressure to rise. Approximately 50% of the patients develop esophageal varices while a small percentage develops complications in the other part of the gastrointestinal tract like ectopic varices in the small bowel [4, 5].

With the availability of VCE in the last two decades, the evaluation of the small bowel has become easy. The ramifications of PH in the small bowel are referred to as portal hypertensive enteropathy (PHE). Multiple studies have attempted to define PHE and identify the major components that it encompasses. Originally in 2005, De Palma et al. had noted that PHE included mucosal inflammatory changes such as edema, erythema, granularity, friability, and spontaneous bleeding as well as vascular lesions such as cherry red spots, telangiectasias, angiodysplasia, and varices [6]. Later in 2008, Kodama et al. used double balloon enteroscopy to classify PHE into villous lesions and vascular lesions [7]. Despite the classifications, there is no gold standard scoring system to differentiate the severity of endoscopic abnormalities found [8].

With the current definitions as stated above, the prevalence of PHE has been noted to vary between 18% and 100% in patients with cirrhosis. The majority of data, when using a broad definition of PHE, indicates that prevalence is >60%. However, not all patients with cirrhosis have PHE; but there are several risk factors that increase the likelihood of PHE: CTP B and C, portosystemic shunts, ascites, portal thrombosis, esophageal varices, and portal hypertensive gastropathy [6, 9].

These patients are at a high risk of GI bleeding, especially small intestinal bleeding that cannot be identified by EGD and colonoscopies. Video capsule endoscopy has been used more frequently in the last decade to identify the bleeding source. VCE serves as the road map to allow for further interventions that need to be taken to evaluate and treat gastrointestinal bleeding.

## 2. Materials and Methods

We retrospectively reviewed the medical record of 100 consecutive patients who were found to be cirrhotic and to have complete video capsule studies between 2010 and 2016 at the University of Massachusetts, UMass Medical Center. Approval was obtained from the University of Massachusetts Institutional Review Board (IRB). By using the ICD codes of cirrhosis and the procedure code of the video capsule endoscope, we were able to identify our patient's cohort. The chart of each patient was reviewed, and the extracted data included the general demographic features of the cohort: the age, gender, and the race of the patients. The diagnosis of cirrhosis was made by histological findings or compatible typical radiographic features, clinical presentations, and laboratory tests. The severity of cirrhosis was classified using two classifications: Child-Pugh classification and the model for end-stage liver disease (MELD) score classification.

Two generations of Given Imaging capsules were used during the study period including the consecutive generations of PillCam SB2 and SB3 (Medtronic, Minneapolis, MN). Reading software was Rapid v 6-8. Video capsule endoscopy studies were read by experienced gastroenterologists and the findings were documented in in Provation (Provation, Minneapolis, MN). The findings used in this study included the indications for the video capsule evaluation as documented in the charts of the patients which were obscure GI bleed, anemia, and/or abnormal findings on the cross-sectional imaging studies.

## 3. Classification

Our classification of the PHE was based on the published studies reported by De Palma et al., Kodama et al., and Abdelaal et al. [6, 7, 10]. The first classification of the PHE was reported by De Palma et al. in 2005. We divided PHE into two grades: Grade 1 which includes edema, erythema, granularity, friability, and/or spontaneous bleeding and Grade 2 which includes cherry-red spots, telangiectasias, angiodysplasia-like lesions, and varices.

Kodama et al. divided PHE into villous lesions and vascular lesions. Villous lesions include either edema, atrophy, or erythematous changes of the villi while vascular lesions include varices, red spots, vascular spiders, and lymphoid follicles with dilated vessels and dilated/proliferated vessels. Lastly, Abdelaal et al. diagnosed PHE based on his scoring system which depended on four main types of mucosal lesions of the small intestine: red spots, angioectasias, varices, and inflammatory-like lesions.

In our study, we divided the PHE lesions into two types of lesions: vascular and mucosal lesions. Vascular lesions included arteriovenous malformation (AVM), red spots, bleeding, or varices while the mucosal lesions included mild inflammatory changes such as erythematous changes and edema or severe inflammatory changes including mosaic-like pattern or snakeskin mucosal changes, and congested and friable mucosa.

We also divided our cohort based on their Child-Turcotte-Pugh (CTP) classification into classes A, B, and C using the patients' clinical presentations of ascites and hepatic encephalopathy, in addition to their laboratory findings.

## 4. Statistical Analysis

Comparisons were performed using the unpaired chi-square test for quantitative data and the chi-squared test for categorical data. A Yates correction or Fisher's exact test was used when required. P-value < 0.05 was considered statistically significant. Odds ratios (ORs) and 95% confidence intervals (95% CIs) were used in the analyses.

## 5. Results

One hundred patients with cirrhosis had a VCE study between 2010 and 2016. The mean age of the cohort was 62.82±2 years and the mean/MELD score was 13.86±0.66. Male gender was predominant with 64% of the cohort while the Caucasians represented 82% (Table 1). The most common etiologies of the cirrhosis in our cohort were chronic alcohol abuse followed by chronic hepatitis C virus (HCV) and nonalcoholic steatohepatitis (NASH) with percentages of 37%, 22%, and 18%, respectively (Figure 1).

Small intestine evaluation by VCE detected small intestinal lesions in 71% of the patients while 29% patients had normal study. The features of PHE were found in 65% of the cohort. Vascular lesions were found in 43% of the cohort and inflammatory lesions were found in 33%. 11 patients were found to have more than one type of PHE types with vascular lesions comprising more than 50% of the PHE lesions. AVMs and inflammatory changes were the most common findings, followed by bleeding with percentages of 18%, 18%, and 15%, respectively (Figure 2).

Our cohort had more decompensated cirrhosis defined by CTP B and C than compensated cirrhosis which is defined as

Table 1: Demographic MELD: model for end-stage liver disease.

| Demographic | Number & (%) |
|---|---|
| Total number of patients | 100 |
| Age | 62.82±2 |
| MELD score | 13.86(±0.66) |
| Demographics: | |
| Male | 64(64%) |
| Female | 36(36%) |
| Whites | 82(82%) |
| Asian | 2(2%) |
| African-American | 1(1%) |
| Others | 15(15%) |

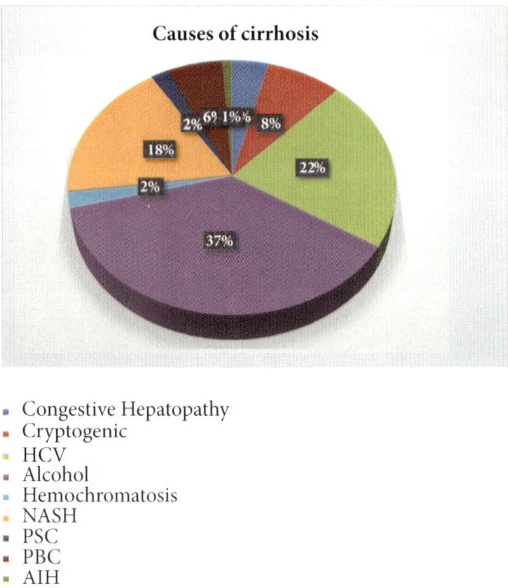


Figure 1: Causes of cirrhosis. HCV: hepatitis C virus, NASH: nonalcoholic steatohepatitis, PSC: primary sclerosing cholangitis, PBC: primary biliary cirrhosis, and AIH: autoimmune hepatitis.

CTP A. Decompensated cirrhosis (CTP B and C) represented 54% of the cohort while compensated cirrhosis (CTP A) represented 46% of the cohort.

When the two groups were compared, compensated cirrhosis versus decompensated cirrhosis, our data showed that the risk of having PHE in decompensated cirrhosis (CTP B and C) is two times the risk in compensated cirrhosis with an odd ratio of 2 and P-value of 0.01. Our study found that there was no correlation between thrombocytopenia and PHE. The risk of PHE is double that in patients with thrombocytopenia when compared with patients with normal platelet count but did not reach statistically significant value with P-value 0.09 (Table 2).

There was no correlation between the presence of PHE and patients' gender in this study. In addition, there was no correlation between the etiology of cirrhosis and PHE. We evaluated the correlation between PHE and other endoscopic features of portal hypertension like esophageal varices, portal hypertension gastropathy, and gastric varices. Of the 45 patients which had negative EGD exam for any esophageal varices (EV), portal hypertensive gastropathy (PHG), or gastric varices (GV), 31 patients (69%) had features of portal hypertension enteropathy in their VCE. 55 patients had features of portal hypertension through the EGD exam including EV, portal hypertension gastropathy, or gastric varices, and 34 of them (61%) had PHE. Our study also showed that the presence of PHE does not correlate with the presence or the absence of the EV, portal hypertension gastropathy, or gastric varices in cirrhotic patients (Table 2).

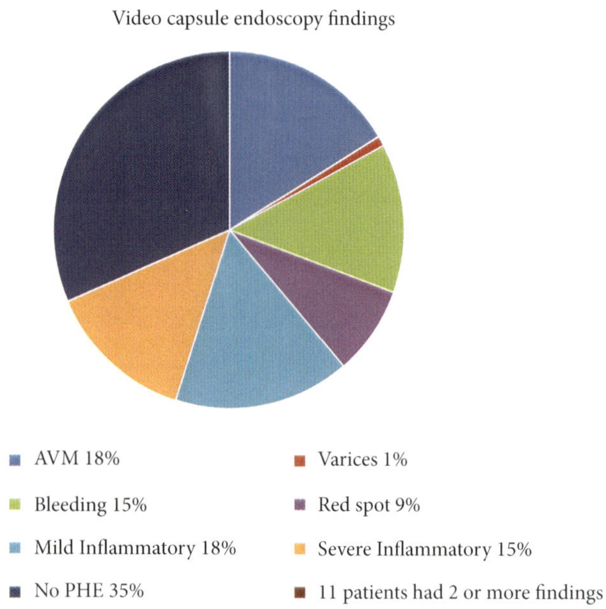


Figure 2: Video capsule endoscopy findings.

Table 2: The predictor factors of PHE. CTP-A: Child-Turcotte-Pugh score A, CTP-B+C: Child-Turcotte-Pugh score B and C, HCV: hepatitis C virus, NASH: nonalcoholic steatohepatitis, PSC: primary sclerosing cholangitis, PBC: primary biliary cirrhosis, EV: esophageal varices, PHG: portal hypertension gastropathy, GV: gastric varices, PHE: portal hypertension enteropathy, and OR: odd ratio.

| Predictor factors | Number | PHE | No PHE | OR | P-value |
|---|---|---|---|---|---|
| CTP-A | 46 | 26 | 20 | 0.5 | 0.01 |
| CTP-B+C | 54 | 39 | 15 | 2.0 | 0.01 |
| Alcohol | 37 | 20 | 17 | 0.4 | 0.04 |
| HCV | 22 | 13 | 9 | 0.4 | 0.02 |
| NASH | 18 | 14 | 4 | 2.1 | 0.1 |
| Cholestatic liver disease (PSC+PBC) | 8 | 6 | 2 | 1.6 | 0.4 |
| Thrombocytopenia | 69 | 48 | 21 | 1.8 | 0.09 |
| Male | 64 | 42 | 22 | 1.1 | 0.7 |
| Female | 36 | 23 | 13 | 0.9 | 0.7 |
| EGD + (EV, PHG, or GV) | 55 | 34 | 21 | 0.7 | 0.5 |
| EGD - | 45 | 31 | 14 | 1.3 | 0.5 |

## 6. Discussion

The features of portal hypertension in the small intestine vary from normal mucosa to bleeding ectopic varices that can lead to death. It can involve any part of the gastrointestinal tract: esophageal varices, gastropathy, small intestine enteropathy, and/or colopathy [11]. Historically, the first article describing portal hypertension features in the small intestine was reported by Jonas et al. who studied those changes in rats. They described portal hypertension enteropathy as changes in the small intestinal mucosa that includes erythema, decreased duodenal villous perfusion, and an increased susceptibility to injuries [12].

The features of portal hypertension enteropathy were first described endoscopically by Thiruvengadam as an erythematous change in the small intestinal mucosa that resembled the features of gastropathy and both changes had been called portal hypertension gastroenteropathy [13]. The introduction of video capsule endoscopy and small intestine enteroscopy devices helped in better estimating the prevalence of PHE. More data was published in the last decade describing the features of the portal hypertension enteropathy (PHE). Most of these published reports as mentioned above classified the PHE into two categories: vascular lesions (arteriovenous malformation (AVM), red spots, bleeding, and varices) and inflammatory lesions (mild: erosions, erythema or severe: edema, congested, granular, and friable mucosa) [6, 7, 10].

Most of the information that we have about PHE is from relatively small size studies, both retrospective and prospective. These studies estimated the prevalence to have a wide range between 18% and 100% but the majority of these studies specially the one with large sample size have a narrower range of 65% to 69% [8]. Our cohort is the largest cohort study in the USA including 100 cirrhotic patients showing that the prevalence of the PHE is 65%, which is similar to the previously published reports [5–8]. Vascular lesions were detected more than the inflammatory lesions with percentages of 43% and 33%, respectively.

We found no association between the PHE and the age, gender, and the etiology of cirrhosis which is similar to the findings of other published studies. The association of PHE and the presence of esophageal varices and/or portal hypertension gastropathy was documented by both Goulas et al. and Aoyama et al. [11, 14]. This association was found to be in accordance with a study reported by De Palma et al., which showed a strong association between the portal hypertension enteropathy with larger esophageal varices, portal hypertension, gastropathy, and colopathy.

In our study, 45 patients had a negative EGD study for any active bleeding or signs of portal hypertension: esophageal varices, gastric varices, or portal hypertension gastropathy. Thirty-one of them (67%) had features of portal hypertension enteropathy in their VCE evaluation of the small intestine. Therefore, no association was found between the PHE and EV, portal hypertension gastropathy, or gastric varices.

The prevalence of each type of PHE is different between the published studies. The prevalence of vascular types of PHE like AVMs, red spots, and varices ranged within 24%-55%, 22%-62%, and 8%-38%, respectively [9, 15]. In our study, the prevalence is lower than the published studies: the prevalence of the vascular AVMs, red spots, and varices was 18%, 15%, and 1%, respectively.

The reported prevalence of inflammatory lesions ranges between 5% and 13% [9, 10, 16, 17]. Our cohort had a higher prevalence of mild and severe inflammatory changes of 15-18%, respectively.

The correlation between PHE and the liver function demonstrated by Child-Turcotte-Pugh (CTP) classification is still controversial. The Child-Pugh classification system takes into consideration the synthetic function of the liver (albumin, INR, and bilirubin) and the clinical presentations of the portal hypertension (ascites and hepatic encephalopathy). Misra et al., Alessandro et al., Pennazio et al., and Goulas et al. found that there is no association between the CTP score and the presence of PHE [14, 16–18].

In contrast, Aoyama et al. found that PHE is associated with higher CTP score [11]. De Palma et al. and Abdulaal et al. both confirmed the association between PHE and the CTP score as a linear correlation [6, 10]. Our study supports that correlation as we found a strong association between the CTP score and the presence of PHE. The risk of having PHE in decompensated cirrhosis is twice the risk in the compensated cirrhosis with an odd ratio of 2.0 with CI 95% ($P<0.05$).

The absence of the features of portal hypertension in the esophagus and stomach did not exclude the presence of PHE. Therefore, the absence of association between PHE and portal hypertension features in the stomach and esophagus should not preclude the evaluation of the small intestine as source of bleeding in the cirrhotic patient and VCE might be warranted regardless the existence of gastroesophageal portal hypertension features.

These findings provide further insight to the role of the VCE that can assess in management of these populations, though our study has its limitation, being a single center, being retrospective in design, and including a high percentage of Caucasians, but it is the first to evaluate such findings in cirrhotic patients.

## 7. Conclusion

We conclude that one-third of cirrhotic patients with suspect GI bleed/anemia have treatable PHE lesions. AVMs, varices, and bleeding lesions are all treatable lesions that can be evaluated by video capsule endoscopy and treated by small bowel enteroscopy, single balloon enteroscopy, double balloon enteroscopy, or trans-jugular intrahepatic-portosystemic shunting. Hepatologists and gastroenterologists should not be hesitant to pursue this investigative modality in this population, when no active bleeding is found by traditional EGD and colonoscopic evaluation.

## 8. Summary

Portal hypertension enteropathy is prevalent in cirrhotic patient and carries the risk of obscure GI bleeding. The published data regards the small samples sizes which suggested the prevalence, and our cohort, the largest cohort in the US, supported the previous facts. Our data supports the fact that PHE was associated with decompensated cirrhosis. The absence of varices in the stomach or esophagus should not distract the gastroenterologist from further investigating the small intestine for features of portal hypertension.

## Disclosure

This abstract was presented as a poster presentation at the United European week in Barcelona, Spain, and it was published as an abstract in United European Gastroenterology Journal.

## Authors' Contributions

Lidia Spaho and Mohamed Mahmoud helped with the data collection. Joan Kheder was responsible for data analysis. Anne Foley was responsible for writing and editing for the Institutional Review Board (IRB). Yasir Al-Azzawi was responsible for data collection, data analysis, and writing the manuscript. Dave Cave supervised the study project and edited the manuscript.

## References

[1] R. J. Wong, M. Aguilar, R. Cheung et al., "Nonalcoholic steatohepatitis is the second leading etiology of liver disease among adults awaiting liver transplantation in the United States," *Gastroenterology*, vol. 148, no. 3, pp. 547–555, 2015.

[2] J. J. Heidelbaugh and M. Bruderly, "Cirrhosis and chronic liver failure: part I. Diagnosis and evaluation," *American Family Physician*, vol. 74, pp. 756–762, 2006.

[3] S. Scaglione, S. Kliethermes, G. Cao et al., "The epidemiology of cirrhosis in the United States a population-based study," *Journal of Clinical Gastroenterology*, vol. 49, no. 8, pp. 690–696, 2015.

[4] J.-C. García-Pagán, J. Gracia-Sancho, and J. Bosch, "Functional aspects on the pathophysiology of portal hypertension in cirrhosis," *Journal of Hepatology*, vol. 57, no. 2, pp. 458–461, 2012.

[5] D. Schuppan and N. H. Afdhal, "Liver cirrhosis," *The Lancet*, vol. 371, no. 9615, pp. 838–851, 2008.

[6] G. D. De Palma, M. Rega, S. Masone et al., "Mucosal abnormalities of the small bowel in patients with cirrhosis and portal hypertension: a capsule endoscopy study," *Gastrointestinal Endoscopy*, vol. 62, no. 4, pp. 529–534, 2005.

[7] M. Kodama, H. Uto, M. Numata et al., "Endoscopic characterization of the small bowel in patients with portal hypertension evaluated by double balloon endoscopy," *Journal of Gastroenterology*, vol. 43, no. 8, pp. 589–596, 2008.

[8] S. R. Jeon and J.-O. Kim, "Capsule endoscopy for portal hypertensive enteropathy," *Gastroenterology Research and Practice*, vol. 2016, 2016.

[9] P. Mekaroonkamol, R. Cohen, and S. Chawla, "Portal hypertensive enteropathy," *World Journal of Hepatology*, vol. 7, no. 2, pp. 127–138, 2015.

[10] U. M. Abdelaal, E. Morita, S. Nouda et al., "Evaluation of portal hypertensive enteropathy by scoring with capsule endoscopy: is transient elastography of clinical impact?" *Journal of Clinical Biochemistry and Nutrition*, vol. 47, no. 1, pp. 37–44, 2010.

[11] T. Aoyama, S. Oka, H. Aikata et al., "Small bowel abnormalities in patients with compensated liver cirrhosis," *Digestive Diseases and Sciences*, vol. 58, no. 5, pp. 1390–1396, 2013.

[12] G. Jonas, R. A. Erickson, and T. Morgan, "Effect of portal hypertension on In Vivo bile acid-mediated small intestinal mucosal injury in the rat," *Digestive Diseases and Sciences*, vol. 35, no. 6, pp. 743–748, 1990.

[13] R. Thiruvengadam and C. J. Gostout, "Congestive gastroenteropathy—an extension of nonvariceal upper gastrointestinal bleeding in portal hypertension," *Gastrointestinal Endoscopy*, vol. 35, no. 6, pp. 504–507, 1989.

[14] Spyros Goulas, Konstantina Triantafyllidou, Stephanos Karagiannis et al., "Capsule Endoscopy in the Investigation of Patients with Portal Hypertension and Anemia," *Canadian Journal of Gastroenterology & Hepatology*, vol. 22, Article ID 534871, 6 pages, 2008.

[15] E. Rondonotti, F. Villa, C. Signorelli, and R. de Franchis, "Portal hypertensive enteropathy," *Gastrointestinal Endoscopy Clinics of North America*, vol. 16, no. 2, pp. 277–286, 2006.

[16] S. P. Misra, M. Dwivedi, V. Misra, and M. Gupta, "Ileal varices and portal hypertensive ileopathy in patients with cirrhosis and portal hypertension," *Gastrointestinal Endoscopy*, vol. 60, no. 5, pp. 778–783, 2004.

[17] R. Alessandro, P. Marco, O. Antonio et al., "Capsule Endoscopy in Cirrhotic Patients: Prevalence and Spectrum of Small Bowel Lesions," *Gastrointestinal Endoscopy*, vol. 61, no. 5, p. AB158, 2005.

[18] M. Pennazio, "Capsule endoscopy," *Endoscopy*, vol. 37, no. 11, pp. 1073–1078, 2005.

21

# HCV Integrated Care: A Randomized Trial to Increase Treatment Initiation and SVR with Direct Acting Antivirals

**Erik J. Groessl,[1,2] Lin Liu,[1,2] Marisa Sklar,[1,2] and Samuel B. Ho[1,2]**

[1] *VA San Diego Healthcare System, San Diego, CA, USA*
[2] *University of California, San Diego, San Diego, CA, USA*

Correspondence should be addressed to Erik J. Groessl; egroessl@ucsd.edu

Academic Editor: Maria Buti

*Background and Aims.* Psychiatric or substance use disorders are barriers to successful HCV antiviral treatment. In a randomized, controlled trial (RCT), the effects of HCV Integrated Care (IC) for increasing treatment rates and sustained viral response (SVR) were studied with direct acting antivirals (DAA). *Methods.* In 2012-13, VA patients, whose screening was positive for depression, PTSD, or substance use ($N = 79$), were randomized to IC or Usual Care (UC). IC consisted of brief psychological interventions and case management. The primary endpoint was SVR among patients followed for an average of 16.6 months. *Results.* 42% of the study participants were previously homeless and 79% had HCV genotype 1. Twice as many IC participants (45%) initiated treatment compared with UC participants (23%) ($\chi^2 = 4.59$, $p = 0.032$). Among those treated, SVR rates did not significantly differ (IC: 12/18 = 67%; UC: 5/9 = 55%; $p = 0.23$). Among all randomized participants, IC participants trended toward better SVR rates (30.0% versus 12.8% in UC; $p = 0.07$). *Conclusions.* Although first-generation DAAs are no longer used, this smaller RCT helps confirm the results of a larger multisite RCT showing that Integrated Care results in higher treatment initiation and SVR rates among HCV-infected persons with comorbid psychological disorders. Integrated mental health services can facilitate treatment among the most challenging HCV patients, many of whom have not been successfully treated. This trial is registered with ClinicalTrials.gov number NCT00722423.

## 1. Introduction

Almost three million people remain chronically infected with hepatitis C virus (HCV) in the US [1, 2] with 80 million infected globally [3]. The medical consequences of HCV are still increasing because of the 20–40-year lag time between initial infection and health complications [4]. Thus, it is a crucial time for both identifying undetected HCV cases and treating large numbers of HCV-infected people with antiviral treatments [5–7].

High SVR rates (>90%) in clinical trials [8] and reduced side effect profiles of the latest direct acting antiviral (DAA) regimens have led some to declare this as a "golden era" in the fight to eradicate HCV [5]. In the past, however, SVR rates found in HCV antiviral treatment clinical trials are often diminished outside of controlled trial settings [9] and among patients who face more barriers to successful treatment [10]. Evidence suggests that psychiatric comorbidity and/or substance use disorders (SUD) continue to be barriers to treating more people. A recent VA medical center study found that 45% of current HCV patients were deemed poor candidates for interferon-free treatment based on their comorbidity profiles (psychiatric and substance use disorders) [11]. Similarly, another medical center reported that 30% of treatment-eligible, high priority HCV patients most at risk for advanced fibrosis were unable or unwilling to engage in HCV care despite outreach efforts. In that study, homelessness, substance use disorder, and other comorbidities were associated with nonengagement in care [12]. Finally, some HCV-infected persons with active or recent SUDs have been considered ineligible for Medicaid payments for interferon-free medications [13, 14].

To address ongoing barriers to treatment success with more efficacious DAA treatments [15], researchers have developed various interventions designed to improve care access, educate patients, improve treatment adherence, increase treatment initiation and completion rates, and ultimately improve treatment success. One study used patient navigators and multidisciplinary teams to assess risk, educate and prepare patients for treatment, and coordinate medications to improve adherence among HCV-infected patients with greater needs [16]. Treatment initiation increased 2- to 3-fold and on-site patients receiving more services had higher odds of initiating treatment [16]. Another recent study used a multidisciplinary team focused on educating patients before antiviral treatment and facilitating medication adherence in an HMO setting [17]. The study lacked a comparison group but obtained SVR rates in an outpatient HMO setting similar to those found in highly controlled clinical trials.

These recent studies build upon previous research on HCV self-management [18–21] and the Hepatitis C Integrated Care Program [22–25]. Integrated Care (IC) emphasizes patient-provider collaboration and involves the delivery of case management, education, and brief psychological interventions within the HCV clinic, promoting access and improved care. Our prior multisite RCT demonstrated that the HCV Integrated Care Program resulted in significant increases in treatment initiation and SVR rates with pegylated interferon plus ribavirin regimens [24]. The objective of the current study was to determine if the prior multisite trial results could be replicated with *first-generation* DAA triple therapy regimens (boceprevir/telaprevir, pegylated interferon, and ribavirin) in a small RCT. We hypothesized that HCV patients receiving Integrated Care would have higher treatment initiation and SVR rates than patients receiving care as usual.

## 2. Methods

The study was approved by the University of California, San Diego institutional review board. All project activities comply with Ethical Principles for Medical Research Involving Human Subjects outlined in the Helsinki Declaration.

*2.1. Study Design.* The study was conducted at a single VA medical center with an established HCV clinic staffed by experienced physicians. Patients attending this HCV clinic were screened and recruited from January 2012 through February 2013 (Figure 1). Eligible patients were consented and randomized with a 1 : 1 ratio using online random assignment tools. The blocked randomization sequence with 20 subjects per block was concealed from the project staff that enrolled and randomized participants. A detailed description of the intervention has been published with the prior study methods [22]. A sample of 88 subjects was initially targeted, providing power of 80% to detect a difference between the groups on overall SVR rates. It was assumed that 35% and 60% of participants would be treated in the Usual Care and Integrated Care groups, respectively, and that 60% of treated patients in each group would achieve an SVR, producing 16 and 9 SVRs.

*2.2. Study Participants.* Participants were VA patients with confirmed active HCV infection (HCV PCR positive) whose screening was positive for substance use or psychiatric risk factors that were viewed as relative contraindications to antiviral treatment [26]. As part of clinical care, all patients attending the HCV clinic are asked to complete a standardized screening form. The self-administered form screened for symptoms of depression (scores $\geq 10$) on the Beck Depression Inventory (BDI), posttraumatic stress disorder (endorsement $\geq 3$ items) on VA Primary Care PTSD Screen (PTSD), alcohol use (AUDIT-C) (scores $\geq 4$), and self-reported active drug use in prior 6 months on the Drug Use Questionnaire (excluding marijuana). In addition, clinic staff checked medical records for positive urine toxicology in 6 months prior to baseline (excluding marijuana). Criteria for exclusion included participation in the previous multisite trial of HCV Integrated Care, decompensated cirrhosis, and other significant life-threatening diseases (serious or incapacitating cancer or cardiac, renal, pulmonary, or autoimmune medical disease). Patients with prior treatment experience and patients who were nonresponders or had significant adverse events were also excluded. More details on criteria have been published previously [22].

### 2.3. Interventions

*2.3.1. Usual Care (UC).* Usual Care (UC) was consistent with current VA treatment guidelines for required "standard of care" [27]. The HCV clinic had a gastroenterologist and a hepatologist physician coordinating care with clinical nursing, internal medicine physicians, and a clinic psychiatrist.

The team weighed the severity of risk factors (screening measures, compliance history, and medical history) for each patient and either (a) referred them to mental health and/or substance use clinics for further assessment and treatment or (b) managed risk factors within the HCV clinic (primarily medication management) and prepared them for antiviral treatment.

*2.3.2. Integrated Care (IC).* Integrated Care (IC) followed a manualized protocol delivered by a mental health provider (MHP) who had a Master's degree in Marriage and Family Therapy. The MHP provided ongoing brief psychological interventions (cognitive behavioral and motivational interviewing) designed to address the specific risk factors identified at screening. Through regular individual appointments, the MHP facilitated a complete treatment evaluation, encouraged the initiation of antiviral treatment, and served as a regular contact and case manager both before and during antiviral treatment. The MHP met regularly with clinic physicians, nurses, and other mental health providers to discuss progress toward treatment. Details of the IC intervention and protocol have been published [22, 24].

*2.4. Antiviral Treatment.* Participants in both intervention arms were offered antiviral treatment following VA hepatitis C treatment guidelines [27]. The guidelines indicated that treatment candidates should demonstrate compliance with healthcare recommendations, stable psychiatric disease, and abstinence from substance use for a time period established

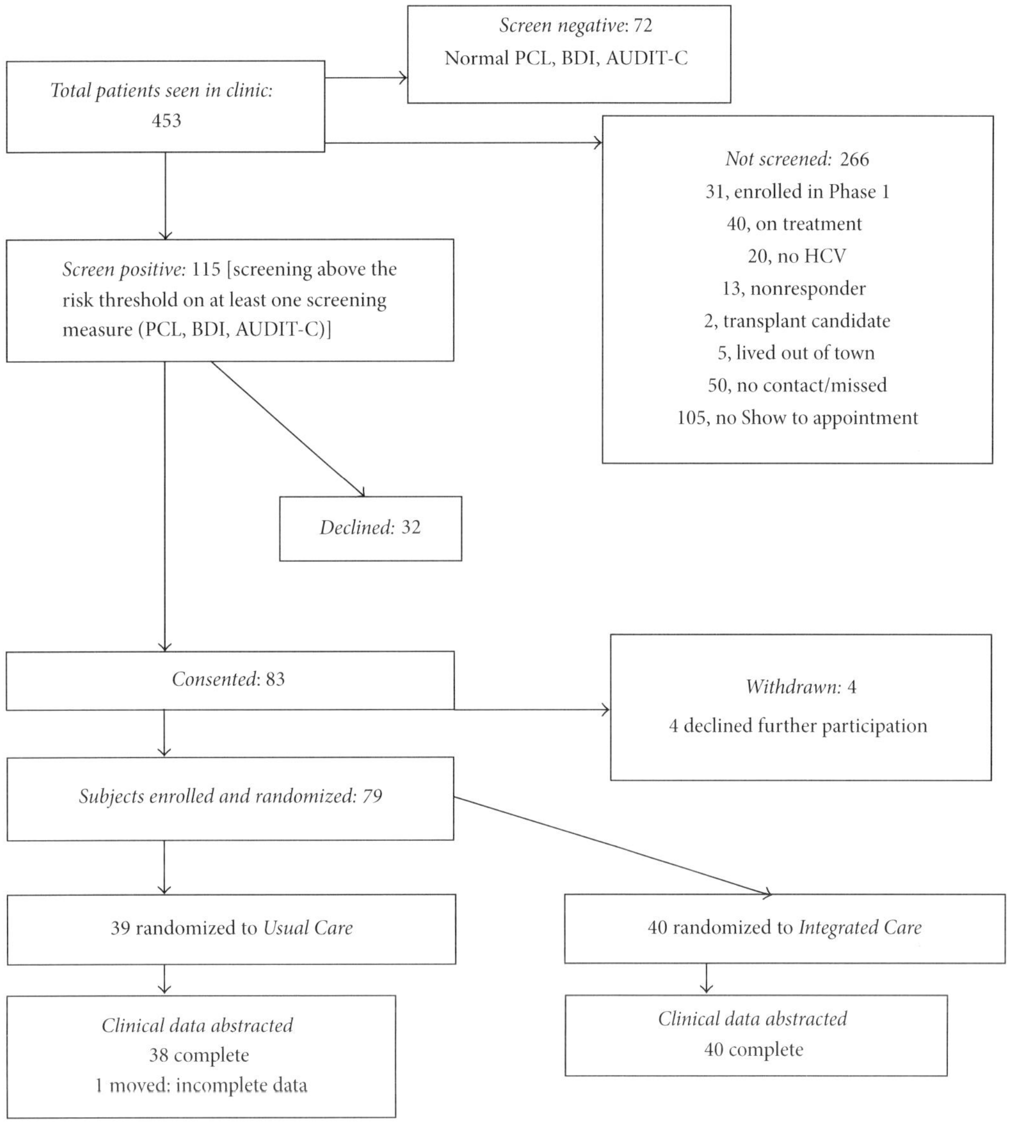


Figure 1: Patient enrollment and randomization.

by the clinic. All participants that initiated antiviral treatment were monitored using standard protocols for each medication regimen. The standard HCV genotype 1 antiviral medication regimens were boceprevir or telaprevir, in combination with pegylated interferon alfa and ribavirin (PR). The standard HCV genotype 2/3 antiviral medication regimen remained PR since no DAA were available for these genotypes at the time. To promote generalizability, the specific type or length of antiviral treatment was left to the discretion of the HCV clinical team or to local clinical trials in which participants enrolled. All participants receiving antiviral treatment were monitored for significant adverse events that could lead to early termination of treatment.

*2.5. Measures.* The primary outcomes were treatment initiation and SVR, defined as "undetectable" outcomes of viral testing conducted at 12 weeks (or more) after the end of treatment [28, 29]. A secondary outcome was the proportion of patients completing 100% of planned treatment duration and the proportion of treatment weeks completed (0–100%). All antiviral treatment data was abstracted from participant medical records by a trained research assistant and 100% confirmed by the study data manager. Abstracted data included medication type and dose, treatment duration recommended, and treatment duration attained.

Serious adverse events were also assessed and were defined as any hospitalization, emergency room visit, and/or death. All patients were followed for treatment initiation status through June 2013 at which time the intervention ended. Treatment completion outcomes were followed through December 2013 and the primary outcome of SVR was followed until March 2014.

*2.6. Statistical Analysis.* "Intent-to-treat" analysis was performed for all clinical outcomes. The univariate association between SVR and covariates was examined using simple logistic regression. Despite a limited sample size, multivariable logistic regression was used to study the difference in SVR between intervention and control groups adjusting for baseline covariates. Only variables that were significantly unbalanced between groups and significantly associated with the outcome ($p < 0.05$) were considered as potential covariates for multivariable analysis and were kept in the final model if the $p$ value $< 0.05$. Treatment initiation differences were compared using the log-rank chi-square test and visualized with a Kaplan–Meier curve. Cox proportional hazard model was used for multivariable analysis to adjust for covariates. The actual treatment completion percentage, the proportion of subjects completing 80% of treatment, and adverse events were summarized by treatment group and compared using Wilcoxon rank sum and Fisher's exact test.

## 3. Results

*3.1. Study Participants.* The flow of patients through the screening, enrollment, and randomization process is shown in Figure 1. Of the 83 participants that provided initial consent, 4 participants refused further participation, were not randomized, and were withdrawn. Thus, 79 participants were randomized, 39 to Usual Care and 40 to Integrated Care. Patients were enrolled over 14 months, and the mean patient follow-up period was 16.6 months (range = 10.3–21.9 months).

Table 1 shows the baseline characteristics for study participants by intervention arm. Participants were 40.5% non-White and had a high frequency of known barriers to access (72% unemployed or disabled, 42% homeless within the prior 5 years, 63% with prior psychiatric illness, and 47% with a prior substance use diagnosis). When considering substance use as a whole, 32% of participants reported active drug use within one year and/or active alcohol abuse based on positive AUDIT-C score. The mean BDI score was 15.5, and 71% met criteria for depression at enrollment. The UC group had a higher mean age ($p = 0.01$) than the IC group. The two intervention groups were not significantly different on any other baseline characteristics.

*3.2. Treatment Initiation and Time to Treatment Initiation.* Almost twice as many IC participants (18/40 or 45%) initiated treatment compared with subjects in Usual Care (9/39 or 23%) ($\chi^2 = 4.59$, $p = 0.032$, Figure 2). In multivariate analysis, age was the only variable initially identified for inclusion in multivariable analysis, but, to replicate our prior analysis, we included genotype which was identified as a significant predictor for treatment initiation in our previous study [24]. When age and genotype were added to the model as covariates, time to treatment initiation was not significantly different between IC and UC participants (HR = 1.88, 95% CI = 0.82–4.27, $p = 0.13$). Participants with type 2–4 genotype (HR = 3.24, $p = 0.01$) and younger subjects with (HR = 0.95, $p = 0.01$) started treatment earlier. Of patients that initiated treatment, six patients had genotype 2 or 3 in IC and two patients had genotype 2 in UC; and 1 patient in both IC and UC received experimental DAA therapy.

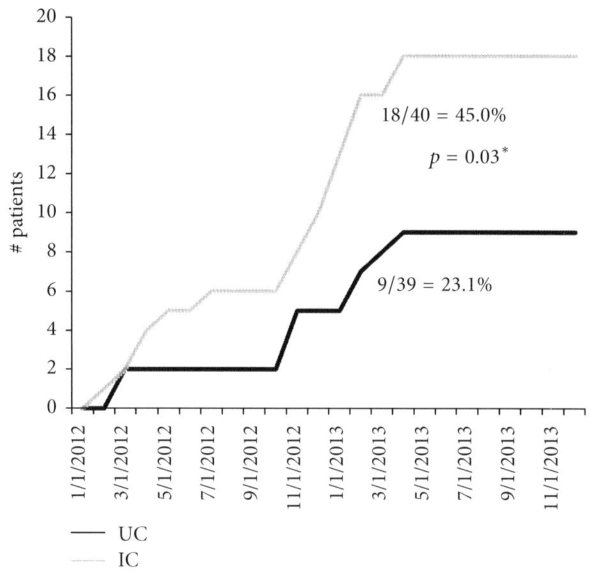


FIGURE 2: Antiviral treatment initiation over time in Integrated Care (IC) versus Usual Care (UC) groups.

*3.3. Sustained Viral Response (SVR).* For patients that initiated antiviral therapy, the rate of SVR was not significantly different (IC: 12/18 = 67%; UC: 5/9 = 55%; $p = 0.23$). When looking only at genotype 1, 7/12 had an SVR in IC, while 4/7 had an SVR in UC.

*3.4. Intent-to-Treat Sustained Viral Response (SVR).* Among all randomized patients, including those that never initiated treatment, the rate of SVR was 2.3 times greater in the IC group (12/40; 30%) than in the UC group (5/39; 13%). The difference trended toward significance but was not statistically significant at $p < 0.05$ (OR = 2.91, $p = 0.07$) in univariate analysis (Figure 3). Age was the only variable identified for inclusion in multivariable analysis but was not significant in the final model (OR = 0.94, $p = 0.07$) (see Table 2).

*3.5. Treatment Completion.* Among patients that initiated antiviral treatment, no significant differences were found between the proportions of IC (14/18 = 78%) and UC participants (5/9 = 56%) completing 100% of planned treatment duration.

*3.6. Adverse Events.* There were no significant differences between IC and UC groups in the number of serious adverse events, measured by hospitalizations, hospital days, emergency room visits, and deaths (Table 3).

## 4. Discussion

Study results indicate that IC participants were twice as likely to initiate antiviral treatment. The proportion of treated participants obtaining an SVR and competing the full duration of planned treatment was not significantly different between groups. When viewing SVR from an intent-to-treat

TABLE 1: Patient characteristics.

| | | Total ($n$ = 79) $n$ (%) | Integrated Care ($n$ = 40) $n$ (%) | Usual Care ($n$ = 39) $n$ (%) | $p$ value |
|---|---|---|---|---|---|
| Demographics | | | | | |
| Age | Mean (SD) | 55.7 (8.4) | 54.0 (8.7) | 57.4 (7.7) | 0.01 |
| BMI | Mean (SD) | 28.8 (5.5) | 29.0 (5.8) | 28.6 (5.3) | 0.79 |
| Gender | Male | 75 (94.9) | 37 (92.5) | 38 (97.4) | 0.62 |
| Race/ethnicity | African American or Black | 19 (24.1) | 7 (17.5) | 12 (30.8) | 0.36 |
| | White | 47 (59.5) | 25 (62.5) | 22 (56.4) | |
| | Native American | 1 (1.3) | 0 (0) | 1 (2.6) | |
| | Hispanic | 11 (13.9) | 7 (17.5) | 4 (10.3) | |
| | Asian/Pacific Islander | 1 (1.3) | 1 (2.5) | 0 (0) | |
| Marital status | Single | 20 (25.3) | 11 (27.5) | 9 (23.1) | 0.69 |
| | Married or widowed | 25 (31.6) | 11 (27.5) | 14 (35.9) | |
| | Separated or divorced | 33 (41.8) | 18 (45.0) | 15 (38.5) | |
| | Missing | 1 (1.3) | 0 (0) | 1 (2.6) | |
| Education | Grades 1 to 8 | 1 (1.3) | 0 (0) | 1 (2.6) | 0.61 |
| | Grades 9 to 11 | 4 (5.1) | 2 (5.0) | 2 (5.1) | |
| | High school/GED | 18 (22.8) | 12 (30.0) | 6 (15.4) | |
| | Some college | 43 (54.4) | 21 (52.5) | 22 (56.4) | |
| | College grad | 6 (7.6) | 2 (5.0) | 4 (10.2) | |
| | Post-grad | 1 (1.3) | 0 (0) | 1 (2.6) | |
| | Missing | 6 (7.6) | 3 (7.5) | 3 (7.7) | |
| Employment | Full- and part-time | 9 (11.4) | 4 (10.0) | 5 (12.8) | 0.92 |
| | Unemployed | 28 (35.4) | 13 (32.5) | 15 (38.5) | |
| | Disabled | 29 (36.7) | 15 (37.5) | 14 (35.9) | |
| | Retired or volunteer | 11 (13.9) | 7 (17.5) | 4 (10.2) | |
| | Missing | 2 (2.5) | 1 (2.5) | 1 (2.6) | |
| Homeless in last 5 years | Negative | 38 (48.1) | 18 (45.0) | 20 (51.3) | 0.51 |
| | Positive | 33 (41.8) | 19 (47.5) | 14 (35.9) | |
| | Missing | 8 (10.1) | 3 (7.5) | 5 (12.8) | |
| Clinical characteristics | | | | | |
| Primary genotype | Type 1 | 62 (78.5) | 29 (72.5) | 33 (84.6) | 0.27 |
| | Types 2, 3, and 4 | 17 (21.5) | 11 (27.5) | 6 (15.4) | |
| Fibrosis level | Mean (SD) | 2.2 (1.8) | 2.1 (1.8) | 2.3 (1.9) | 0.84 |
| Prior liver biopsy | | 36 (45.6) | 18 (45) | 18 (46.2) | 0.99 |
| Biopsy after enrollment | | 18 (22.8) | 8 (20) | 10 (25.6) | 0.60 |
| Prior HCV treatment | | 14 (17.7) | 7 (17.5) | 7 (17.9) | 0.96 |
| Prior psychiatric illness | | 50 (63.3) | 27 (67.5) | 23 (59) | 0.49 |
| Prior substance abuse | | 37 (46.8) | 19 (47.5) | 18 (46.2) | 0.99 |
| Other prior comorbidity | | 34 (43%) | 16 (40%) | 18 (46.2) | 0.65 |
| Number of comorbid disorders | Mean (SD) | 0.59 (0.81) | 0.6 (0.9) | 0.59 (0.72) | 0.73 |
| Eligibility screen measures | | | | | |
| Depression (BDI) screen[a] | Negative | 22 (27.8) | 14 (35.0) | 8 (20.5) | 0.21 |
| | Positive | 56 (70.9) | 26 (65.0) | 30 (78.9) | |
| | Missing | 1 (1.3) | 0 (0) | 1 (2.6) | |
| Depression (BDI score) | Mean (SD) | 15.5 (9.2) | 15.4 (9.5) | 15.7 (9.0) | 0.96 |
| PTSD risk screen[b] | Positive | 36 (53.7) | 21 (56.8) | 18 (52.9) | 0.81 |
| Alcohol (AUDIT-C) screen[c] | Positive | 15 (19.0) | 7 (17.5) | 8 (20.5) | 0.78 |
| AUDIT-C screen score | Mean (SD) | 1.5 (2.9) | 1.4 (2.5) | 1.7 (3.2) | 0.83 |
| Active drug use screen[d] | Positive | 13 (16.5) | 5 (12.5) | 8 (20.5) | 0.38 |
| Active alcohol risk *or* drug use (past 6 months) | Positive | 25 (31.6) | 12 (30.0) | 13 (33.3) | 0.81 |

[a]BDI screen positive score includes scores ≥ 10; [b]VA Primary Care PTSD screen score ≥ 3; [c]AUDIT-C screen positive score ≥ 4 at baseline; [d]self-reported active drug use and/or positive urine toxicology in 6 months prior to baseline (excluding marijuana).

Table 2: Multivariable regression analysis.

(a) Association between time to treatment initiation and intervention group

| Variables | Hazard ratio | 95% confidence interval | $p$ value |
|---|---|---|---|
| Intervention group, IC* versus UC† | 1.88 | (0.82, 4.27) | 0.13 |
| Age | 0.95 | (0.92, 0.99) | 0.01 |
| Genotype (type 2, 3, and 4 versus type 1) | 3.24 | (1.43, 7.37) | 0.01 |

(b) Association between SVR and intervention group

| Variables | Odds ratio | 95% confidence interval | $p$ value |
|---|---|---|---|
| Intervention group, IC* versus UC† | 2.91 | (0.92, 9.27) | 0.07 |

*IC = Integrated Care; †UC = Usual Care.

Table 3: Adverse event outcomes.

| | Integrated Care ($n$ = 40) Mean (SD) | Usual Care ($n$ = 39) Mean (SD) | $p$ value |
|---|---|---|---|
| Number of hospitalization events/patient | 0.35 (0.83) | 0.31 (0.80) | 0.81 |
| Number of hospital days/patient | | | |
| Subjects with hospital event[a] | 14.3 (23.6) | 11.5 (9.01) | 0.65 |
| All subjects[b] | 2.85 (11.6) | 1.77 (5.32) | 0.82 |
| Number of ER visits/patient | 0.78 (1.12) | 0.74 (1.29) | 0.71 |
| Number of deaths, $n$ (%) | 1 (2.5) | 3 (7.7) | 0.36 |

[a]14 (8 IC and 6 UC) subjects with hospitalization events; [b]number of hospital days is 0 for subjects without hospitalization event; IC = Integrated Care; UC = Usual Care.

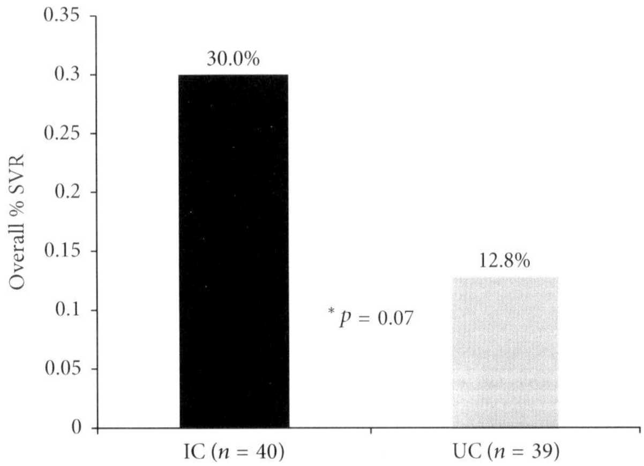


Figure 3: Cumulative probability of treatment initiation by intervention group over time (months). Patients are censored at end of study follow-up. ne = number of events (treatment initiation).

perspective, 30% of all IC participants versus 13% of all UC participants obtained an SVR.

Although new antiviral treatments are demonstrating high SVR rates in clinical trials [1, 2], the treatments are expensive and SVR rates may be lower in clinical practices providing care to patients who face additional challenges [10, 15]. HCV-infected persons who are homeless, lack resources, and/or have ongoing substance use and psychiatric disorders may not readily engage in care or be adequately prepared to adhere to antiviral regimens without interventional assistance. For example, one recent VA study found that almost half of the HCV patients reviewed were poor candidates for interferon-free treatment based on psychiatric and substance use comorbidity [11]. Recently, a study tried to engage 481 consecutive HCV patients at high risk for advanced stage 3-4 fibrosis (FIB4 score > 2.4) in HCV care. Of these, 379 patients were considered medically eligible for antiviral treatment. Within this group, 32% (123/379) were unwilling or unable to engage in HCV-related care after repeated outreach attempts or clinic visits. Factors associated with nonengagement included history of homelessness, substance use disorder, and other comorbidities [12]. In addition, Medicaid payments have been restricted in many states for treating HCV patients with active or recent SUDs with the most efficacious and expensive regimens [14]. Thus, there remains a clear need for programs to better prepare or engage HCV-infected persons with psychiatric and substance use comorbidity for antiviral treatment in the DAA era.

The current study sought to confirm the results of a previous multisite study that demonstrated that HCV Integrated Care could more than double treatment rates and SVR in this population [24]. The previous study was conducted from 2009 to 2012 when the majority of treatments were pegylated IFN plus ribavirin. The current data were collected from 2012 to 2013 as part of a smaller RCT during the era of first-generation DAA triple therapy (telaprevir or boceprevir plus pegylated interferon and ribavirin). The current results were very similar to those of the larger study, with almost twice as many Integrated Care participants initiating treatment with DAA triple therapy regimens, when compared to Usual Care, and 2.3 times as many Integrated

Care participants achieving an SVR. Despite the large effects size, the group differences in treatment initiation and SVR did not quite reach statistical significance in multivariate analyses, because of a limited sample size and a smaller than expected increase in treatment rates with first-generation DAAs. However, when viewed as a follow-up to and in combination with the results of our large multisite trial [24], and given the size of effects found in the current study, we conclude that the HCV Integrated Care Program remains an effective tool for boosting treatment rates and SVR in persons with psychiatric and substance use disorders with DAA treatments.

The overall treatment rates with the new first-generation DAA treatments were only slightly higher than those found in the previous study, which is consistent with national VA data showing that treatment rates did not increase significantly with the advent of DAA triple therapies [30]. This likely results from even more challenging side effects when adding a DAA to standard pegylated interferon and ribavirin. For those receiving antiviral therapy, treatment adherence rates and SVR rates tended to be higher for IC participants, but differences were not statistically significant given the relatively small patient numbers. The SVR rates are comparable to those reported from VA national data (50%) for genotype 1 patients treated with first-generation DAA therapies [9]. Thus, although not statistically significant here, these data along with fewer deaths in the UC group follow the same trend found previously, making it unlikely that study effects resulted from healthcare providers simply treating more IC patients. For example, combining data from both studies, we find 9 deaths among 222 IC patients and 17 deaths among 220 UC patients ($p = 0.04$). For veterans with HCV and with a history of substance use and psychiatric disorders, working closely with a mental health case manager may provide more than motivation and support to start antiviral treatment, inclining them to better adhere to treatment and other healthcare recommendations.

A limitation of the current study was the overall sample size. In 2011, a modification to a previous larger multisite study was obtained to conduct the current smaller RCT, capitalizing on existing infrastructure. At that time, there were expectations that treatment rates would increase dramatically given the increased efficacy of the new triple therapies. Thus, the power calculations assumed higher treatment rates. The effect found in the current study would have been statistically significant had the treatment rates been as expected. The lower treatment rates were evident during the current RCT but additional time and resources were not available to extend enrollment. The current sample size also limited efforts to conduct subgroup analyses for patients with substance use disorders versus other comorbidities, or with specific genotypes. An additional limitation is that patients and providers were not blinded to intervention assignment. It is possible that cross-contamination between experimental groups occurred. However, the IC practitioner never interacted with UC comparison group participants, and if physician contact with the IC interventionist influenced care of UC participants, an increase in antiviral treatment would be expected in the UC group, biasing the study toward the null hypothesis and strengthening conclusions.

Overall, the concept of integrated or collaborative care for patients with multiple comorbidities has been shown to be effective in a number of clinical settings [31]. After the initial surge in interferon-free DAA treatment initiation for HCV patients with better access, less comorbidity, or cirrhosis, medical practices may need to focus on patients with additional barriers to care. As demonstrated recently, a significant percentage of patients with HCV most at risk for advanced fibrosis remain reluctant or unable to engage in care with interferon-free treatments [12]. The principles of Integrated Care include colocation of critical resources, multidisciplinary team members, patient activation, and coordination of care targeted to the needs of individual patients. Although the ongoing need for HCV Integrated Care interventions may currently be more limited to subgroups that are difficult to treat, the results presented support the use of Integrated Care strategies for optimizing the numbers of patients that successfully complete antiviral therapy while conserving limited resources. With many HCV-infected persons still needing treatment, efforts to implement Integrated Care can facilitate initiation and completion of interferon-free DAA regimens.

In conclusion, further study of the benefits of HCV Integrated Care interventions is warranted, especially among hard-to-treat subgroups such as IV drug users. The current study confirms the results of a previous multisite study, yet the lack of adequate power was a limitation. Thus, it is important for future studies to ensure the recruitment of a sample size providing adequate power.

## Disclosure

Samuel B. Ho, M.D., is a member of the Advisory Board of Janssen Pharmaceuticals, Inc., and of Speakers Bureau of Prime Education, Inc.

## Acknowledgments

Research funding was provided by VA Health Services Research and Development (HSR&D), Grant IIR-07-101-3. Samuel B. Ho, M.D., received research and grant support from Genentech, Inc., and Gilead Sciences.

## References

[1] M. M. Denniston, R. B. Jiles, J. Drobeniuc et al., "Chronic hepatitis C virus infection in the United States, national health and nutrition examination survey 2003 to 2010," *Annals of Internal Medicine*, vol. 160, no. 5, pp. 293–300, 2014.

[2] S. D. Holmberg, P. R. Spradling, A. C. Moorman, and M. M. Denniston, "Hepatitis C in the United States," *The New England Journal of Medicine*, vol. 368, no. 20, pp. 1859–1861, 2013.

[3] Polaris Observatory HCVC, "Global prevalence and genotype distribution of hepatitis C virus infection in 2015: a modelling study," *Lancet Gastroenterol Hepatol*, vol. 2, pp. 161–176, 2017.

[4] G. L. Davis, M. J. Alter, H. El-Serag, T. Poynard, and L. W. Jennings, "Aging of hepatitis C virus (HCV)-infected persons in the United States: a multiple cohort model of HCV prevalence and disease progression," *Gastroenterology*, vol. 138, no. 2, pp. 513–e6, 2010.

[5] M. Colombo, "Interferon-free therapy for hepatitis C: the hurdles amid a golden era," *Digestive and Liver Disease*, vol. 47, no. 9, pp. 727–733, 2015.

[6] B. D. Smith, R. L. Morgan, G. A. Beckett et al., "Recommendations for the identification of chronic hepatitis C virus infection among persons born during 1945–1965," *MMWR Recommendations and Reports*, vol. 61, pp. 1–32, 2012.

[7] B. D. Smith, R. L. Morgan, G. A. Beckett, Y. Falck-Ytter, D. Holtzman, and J. W. Ward, "Hepatitis C virus testing of persons born during 1945–1965: recommendations from the centers for disease control and prevention," *Annals of Internal Medicine*, vol. 157, no. 11, pp. 817–822, 2012.

[8] J. A. Gutierrez, E. J. Lawitz, and F. Poordad, "Interferon-free, direct-acting antiviral therapy for chronic hepatitis C," *Journal of Viral Hepatitis*, vol. 22, no. 11, pp. 861–870, 2015.

[9] G. N. Ioannou, L. A. Beste, and P. K. Green, "Similar effectiveness of boceprevir and telaprevir treatment regimens for hepatitis C virus infection on the basis of a nationwide study of veterans," *Clinical Gastroenterology and Hepatology*, vol. 12, no. 8, pp. 1371–1380, 2014.

[10] L. Henry and Z. Younossi, "Patient-reported and economic outcomes related to sofosbuvir and ledipasvir treatment for chronic hepatitis C," *Expert Review of Pharmacoeconomics and Outcomes Research*, vol. 16, no. 6, pp. 659–665, 2016.

[11] S. Judd, A. M. Liubakka, A. Pavle, S. Patel, Z. Hakim, and F. Antaki, "Assessing key barriers to treatment of chronic hepatitis C virus (HCV) with next generation agents in a veteran population," *Gastroenterology*, vol. 146, no. S-737, 2014.

[12] J. Dever, J. Ducom, A. Ma et al., "Engagement in care of high risk hepatitis C patients with interferon-free therapies," *Hepatology*, vol. 62, no. 483A, 2015.

[13] S. Barua, R. Greenwald, J. Grebely, G. J. Dore, T. Swan, and L. E. Taylor, "Restrictions for medicaid reimbursement of sofosbuvir for the treatment of hepatitis C virus infection in the United States," *Annals of Internal Medicine*, vol. 163, no. 3, pp. 215–223, 2015.

[14] W. Venteicher, "Medicaid patients denied new hepatitis C cures," 2014, Chicago Tribune.

[15] J. P. Meyer, Y. Moghimi, R. Marcus, J. K. Lim, A. H. Litwin, and F. L. Altice, "Evidence-based interventions to enhance assessment, treatment, and adherence in the chronic Hepatitis C care continuum," *International Journal of Drug Policy*, vol. 26, no. 10, pp. 922–935, 2015.

[16] M. M. Ford, N. Johnson, P. Desai, E. Rude, and F. Laraque, "From care to cure: demonstrating a model of clinical patient navigation for hepatitis C care and treatment in high-need patients," *Clinical Infectious Diseases*, vol. 64, no. 5, pp. 685–691, 2017.

[17] J. M. Levin, S. Dabirshahsahebi, and M. Bauer, "Retrospective analysis of hepatitis C infected patients treated through an integrated care model," *World Journal of Gastroenterology*, vol. 22, no. 38, pp. 8558–8567, 2016.

[18] E. J. Groessl, S. B. Ho, S. M. Asch, C. J. Stepnowsky, D. Laurent, and A. L. Gifford, "The hepatitis C self-management program: sustainability of primary outcomes at 1 year," *Health Education and Behavior*, vol. 40, no. 6, pp. 730–740, 2013.

[19] E. J. Groessl, M. Sklar, D. D. Laurent, K. Lorig, T. G. Ganiats, and S. B. Ho, "Cost-effectiveness of the hepatitis C self-management program," *Health Education & Behavior*, vol. 44, no. 1, pp. 113–122, 2017.

[20] E. J. Groessl, K. R. Weingart, A. L. Gifford, S. M. Asch, and S. B. Ho, "Development of the hepatitis C self-management program," *Patient Education and Counseling*, vol. 83, no. 2, pp. 252–255, 2011.

[21] E. J. Groessl, K. R. Weingart, C. J. Stepnowsky, A. L. Gifford, S. M. Asch, and S. B. Ho, "The hepatitis C self-management programme: a randomized controlled trial," *Journal of Viral Hepatitis*, vol. 18, no. 5, pp. 358–368, 2011.

[22] E. J. Groessl, M. Sklar, R. C. Cheung, N. Bräu, and S. B. Ho, "Increasing antiviral treatment through integrated hepatitis C care: a randomized multicenter trial," *Contemporary Clinical Trials*, vol. 35, no. 2, pp. 97–107, 2013.

[23] S. B. Ho, "Hepatitis C: clinical management," *Federal Practitioner*, pp. 17–21, 2003.

[24] S. B. Ho, N. Bräu, R. Cheung et al., "Integrated care increases treatment and improves outcomes of patients with chronic hepatitis C virus infection and psychiatric illness or substance abuse," *Clinical Gastroenterology and Hepatology*, vol. 13, no. 11, pp. 2005–2014, 2015.

[25] S. B. Ho, E. Groessl, A. Dollarhide, S. Robinson, D. Kravetz, and E. Dieperink, "Management of chronic hepatitis c in veterans: the potential of integrated care models," *American Journal of Gastroenterology*, vol. 103, no. 7, pp. 1810–1823, 2008.

[26] F. Kanwal, T. Hoang, B. M. R. Spiegel et al., "Predictors of treatment in patients with chronic hepatitis C infection - role of patient versus nonpatent factors," *Hepatology*, vol. 46, no. 6, pp. 1741–1749, 2007.

[27] H. S. Yee, S. L. Currie, J. M. Darling, and T. L. Wright, "Management and treatment of hepatitis C viral infection: recommendations from the department of veterans affairs hepatitis C resource center program and the national hepatitis C program office," *American Journal of Gastroenterology*, vol. 101, no. 10, pp. 2360–2378, 2006.

[28] E. Lawitz and E. J. Gane, "Sofosbuvir for previously untreated chronic hepatitis C infection," *New England Journal of Medicine*, vol. 369, no. 7, pp. 678-679, 2013.

[29] M. Martinot-Peignoux, C. Stern, S. Maylin et al., "Twelve weeks posttreatment follow-up is as relevant as 24 weeks to determine the sustained virologic response in patients with hepatitis c virus receiving pegylated interferon and ribavirin," *Hepatology*, vol. 51, no. 4, pp. 1122–1126, 2010.

[30] L. A. Beste and G. N. Ioannou, "Prevalence and treatment of chronic hepatitis C virus infection in the us department of veterans affairs," *Epidemiologic Reviews*, vol. 37, no. 1, pp. 131–143, 2015.

[31] E. Woltmann, A. Grogan-Kaylor, B. Perron, H. Georges, A. M. Kilbourne, and M. S. Bauer, "Comparative effectiveness of collaborative chronic care models for mental health conditions across primary, specialty, and behavioral health care settings: systematic review and meta-analysis," *American Journal of Psychiatry*, vol. 169, no. 8, pp. 790–804, 2012.

# 22

# The Use of Thrombopoietin Receptor Agonists for Correction of Thrombocytopenia prior to Elective Procedures in Chronic Liver Diseases: Review of Current Evidence

**Kamran Qureshi,[1] Shyam Patel,[2] and Andrew Meillier[2]**

[1]*Department of Medicine, Section of Gastroenterology, Temple University Lewis Katz School of Medicine, Philadelphia, PA, USA*
[2]*Department of Medicine, Internal Medicine Residency Program, Temple University Hospital, Philadelphia, PA, USA*

Correspondence should be addressed to Kamran Qureshi; kamran.qureshi@temple.edu

Academic Editor: Maria Buti

Patients with chronic liver diseases (CLD) undergo a range of invasive procedures during their clinical lifetime. Various hemostatic abnormalities are frequently identified during the periprocedural work-up; including thrombocytopenia. Thrombocytopenia of cirrhosis is multifactorial in origin, and decreased activity of thrombopoietin has been identified to be a major cause. Liver is an important site of thrombopoietin production and its levels are decreased in patients with cirrhosis. Severe thrombocytopenia (platelet counts < 60–75,000/$\mu$L) is associated with increased risk of bleeding with invasive procedures. In recent years, compounds with thrombopoietin receptor agonist activity have been studied as therapeutic options to raise platelet counts in CLD. We reviewed the use of Eltrombopag, Romiplostim, and Avatrombopag prior to various invasive procedures in patients with CLD. These agents seem promising in raising platelet counts before elective procedures resulting in reduction in platelet transfusions, and they also enabled more patients to undergo the procedures. However, these studies were not primarily aimed at comparing bleeding episodes among groups. Use of these agents had some adverse consequences, importantly being the occurrence of portal vein thrombosis. This review highlights the need of further studies to identify reliable methods of safely reducing the provoked bleeding risk linked to thrombocytopenia in CLD.

## 1. Introduction

The prevalence of thrombocytopenia in chronic liver disease (CLD) is 6% and is noticed to be as high as 70% in patients with liver cirrhosis [1]. The level of thrombocytopenia is associated with the severity of liver disease and the degree of portal hypertension [2]. Multiple theories are proposed to suggest the etiology of thrombocytopenia in CLD. It is believed that there is increased sequestration of platelets in the spleen that occurs as a consequence of splenomegaly [3], which is oftentimes seen in patients with cirrhosis and portal hypertension. The toxic effects of alcohol [4], viral-induced thrombocytopathy [5], and bone marrow suppression are also known to cause thrombocytopenia. The treatment of Hepatitis B Virus (HBV) or Hepatitis C Virus (HCV) infection with interferon causes bone marrow suppression and, subsequently, thrombocytopenia in such patients with CLD [6]. Autoantibodies have been identified in HCV infection and it is thought that these antibodies enhance the removal of platelets by the splenic and hepatic reticuloendothelial system [7]. Thrombopoietin (TPO), also known as Megakaryocyte Growth and Development Factor (MGDF) or c-MpL ligand, is a hormone which is synthesized in the liver and dominantly regulates the process of megakaryocytopoiesis [8]. TPO acts on c-MpL receptor on the surface of megakaryocytes and stimulates various steps of platelet production within the bone marrow [9]. TPO generation in turn is regulated by the rate of platelet cycling (production and destruction), as well as the synthetic function of liver [10]. Several studies have argued about the relative majority influence on this multifactorial etiology of thrombocytopenia in CLD [11].

Platelets play a critical role in hemostasis; however, thrombocytopenia in cirrhosis does not significantly increase the risk of spontaneous bleeding [12]. Though the number of circulating platelets is reduced, there is an increased expression of endothelium-derived von Willebrand factor, which makes the platelets more adherent to the endothelium and maintains the primary hemostasis at the site of bleeding [13]. Platelets also influence secondary hemostasis by participating in thrombin generation alongside the coagulation system. In in vitro studies, thrombin generation was found to be within the normal range despite mild to moderate thrombocytopenia in liver cirrhosis [14]. The threshold of 60,000/$\mu$L platelet count was able to secure values of thrombin generation equal to the lower limit of the normal range [14]. In vivo evidence came from the post hoc analysis of the Hepatitis C Antiviral Long-term Treatment against Cirrhosis (HALT-C) trial. The complication rates in the 2740 liver biopsies that were performed in patients with bridging fibrosis and cirrhosis due to chronic HCV infection were assessed [15]. There were only 16 cases reported with the complication of bleeding; the bleeding rate was higher among patients with platelet counts less than 60,000/$\mu$L [15]. This observation has led to a general acceptance that the platelet count above 50–60,000/$\mu$L range is considered safe before most invasive procedures in patients with liver cirrhosis.

Management of periprocedural bleeding risk is a common clinical scenario in CLD. CLD patients frequently require invasive diagnostic and therapeutic procedures, such as liver biopsies, variceal band ligation, or percutaneous procedures for hepatocellular carcinoma (HCC). Traditionally, the treatment options for thrombocytopenia in CLD have been platelet transfusions, splenic artery embolization, splenectomy, and Transjugular Intrahepatic Portosystemic Stent (TIPS) placement [16–19]. Since its identification, TPO and its receptor have been pursued for the development of pharmacological agents to correct thrombocytopenia of CLD. TPO receptor agonists appear to be a good choice and have been routinely used in the treatment of chronic Idiopathic Thrombocytopenic Purpura (ITP), but their use in the treatment of thrombocytopenia prior to invasive procedures in CLD patients is relatively recent [20].

This paper reviews the only 4 clinical studies reported so far that have evaluated TPO receptor agonists for the correction of thrombocytopenia prior to elective procedures in CLD patients. Table 1 summarizes these studies details and outcomes.

## 2. Rationale of Use of TPO Agonists in CLD

In a study done by Koruk et al. in 2002 [21], it was shown that serum TPO levels decreased as the degree of cirrhosis progressed. This study included 18 patients with chronic hepatitis infection, 48 with liver cirrhosis, and 27 control patients with no liver disease. Serum TPO levels were measured in each of these three cohorts. The mean serum TPO level in the chronic hepatitis group was 100.9 pg/mL, which was very similar to the mean TPO level in the control group (97.6 pg/mL). However, the mean TPO level in cirrhotic group was found to be 69.6 pg/mL, which was significantly lower when compared to the other two groups. In addition, as the degree of cirrhosis progressed (measured by the Child-Pugh score), the level of serum TPO was lower. Thrombocytopenia was seen more commonly in the cirrhosis group (65%). It was thus concluded that impaired production of TPO may contribute to the development of thrombocytopenia in advanced stage liver disease [21].

These findings led to the investigation of agents that act on the TPO receptor in order to correct thrombocytopenia in various clinical situations. Among the recombinant TPO agonists which have been developed for the use in humans, Eltrombopag, Romiplostim (first generation), and Avatrombopag (first and second generation) have shown to increase platelet production in humans. These agents act via c-MpL ligand mediated activation of the JAK-STAT and MAP kinase pathways [22, 23].

## 3. Experience of Use of TPO Agonists in CLD Patients

Eltrombopag is a small nonpeptide molecule that is taken orally, leads to a sustained increase in the platelet count by interacting with the transmembrane domain of the human TPO receptor, and initiates signaling cascades that induce proliferation and differentiation from bone marrow progenitor cells. The human use experience of Eltrombopag in CLD patients followed its utilization in chronic refractory ITP population [28]. Its efficacy and safety for the treatment of thrombocytopenia in patients with CLD was first evaluated in large randomized, double-blind, placebo-controlled trials, Eltrombopag to Initiate and Maintain Interferon Antiviral Treatment to Benefit Subjects with Hepatitis C-Related Liver Disease (ENABLE 1 and ENABLE 2), where it was used to increase platelet counts in thrombocytopenic patients prior to HCV treatment with interferon based therapies [29]. The use of Eltrombopag increased platelet numbers in thrombocytopenic patients with HCV and advanced fibrosis and cirrhosis, thus allowed otherwise ineligible or marginal patients to begin and maintain antiviral therapy, and led to significantly increased rates of HCV cure. The median time to achieve the target platelet count was approximately 2 weeks and 95% percent of patients were able to initiate antiviral therapy. The majority of patients treated with Eltrombopag (76%) maintained a platelet count greater than or equal to 50,000/$\mu$L compared with 19% for placebo. Also a greater proportion of patients on Eltrombopag did not require any antiviral dose reduction as compared with placebo (45% versus 27%) [29]. The differences in SVR could be attributed to greater peginterferon exposure in the Eltrombopag arm as study investigators were required to lower peginterferon doses according to the product labels rather than clinical judgment. However, the study confirmed that Eltrombopag has potent platelet stimulatory effects in humans with liver disease.

Romiplostim is a recombinant fusion TPO mimetic protein that is administered intravenously or subcutaneously and leads to a dose-dependent increase in the platelet count. Through binding and activation of the TPO receptor, it activates intracellular transcriptional pathways, leading to

Table 1: Studies evaluating TPO agonists in CLD patients.

| Study medication (route of administration) | Dosing regimen | Study population | Procedures performed | Primary outcome | Secondary outcomes | Adverse effects |
|---|---|---|---|---|---|---|
| Eltrombopag (oral)<br>Afdhal et al. [24] | 75 mg/day for 2 weeks versus placebo for 2 weeks prior to procedure | $N$ = 292 subjects with CLD and platelet count of <50,000/$\mu$L and a planned elective procedure<br>Cirrhosis: 86% (10% Child-Pugh C)<br>Etiology: 80% viral hepatitis | Majority: 59% low bleeding risk procedures (endoscopy, interventions, and paracentesis)<br>Also 15% mild bleeding risk procedures (liver biopsy, laparoscopy, and HCC ablation) | Subjects in whom a platelet transfusion was avoided before, during, and up to 7 days after the elective invasive procedure: 72% (104/145) in the study group compared with 19% (28/147) in the placebo group did not require platelet transfusion ($p < 0.001$) | Rate of bleeding episodes: nonsignificant for noninferiority (23% in the placebo group and 17% in the study group)<br>Quantity of platelets units transfused: median of 3 units in the study group was lower than 4 units in placebo group<br>Side effects: similar in both groups (headache, pyrexia, and abdominal pain, being most common) | Deaths: 3 in study group (with 1 due to sepsis and possibly related to therapy) versus 2 in placebo group<br>Hepatic decompensation: similar in both groups, most common being hepatic encephalopathy<br>PVT: 9 events identified (7 in study group versus 2 in placebo, OR 3.04) |
| Romiplostim (SC)<br>Moussa and Mowafy [25] | 2 $\mu$g/kg SC every 1 week for a maximum of 4 weeks or until 2 consecutive platelet counts of >70,000/$\mu$L were observed prior to procedure | $N$ = 35 subjects with refractory thrombocytopenia and platelet count of <50,000/$\mu$L and a planned surgical procedure<br>Cirrhosis: 100% (all with Child-Pugh score of 10 and above)<br>Etiology: HCV | Cataract, hernia repair, joint replacement, and fracture fixation | The number of subjects achieving a platelet count >70,000/$\mu$L and thereby eligible for surgery: 94% achieved this end point and underwent procedure | Platelet response: 33/35 achieved the desired goal in 9–30 days. All subjects showed rapid response and 7/35 showed positive long-term response (a platelet count > 50,000/$\mu$L at 3-month follow-up)<br>Safety: no serious adverse effects reported | Deaths: none<br>Bleeding episodes: none<br>Hepatic decompensation: none<br>PVT: none identified |

Table 1: Continued.

| Study medication (route of administration) | Dosing regimen | Study population | Procedures performed | Primary outcome | Secondary outcomes | Adverse effects |
|---|---|---|---|---|---|---|
| Romiplostim (SC)<br>versus<br>Eltrombopag (oral)<br>versus<br>platelet transfusion<br>Basu et al. [26] | 500 mcg SC (as a 1 time dose) given 2 weeks prior to the procedure<br>versus<br>75 mg/day for 2 weeks till the day of procedure<br>versus<br>7 units of platelet transfused the night prior to procedure | $N = 65$ subjects with baseline platelet count of <60,000/$\mu$L prior to study<br>Cirrhosis: 100% (mean MELD score 20)<br>Etiology: 57% HCV, 15% HBV, and other diseases | Outpatient percutaneous liver biopsy | Platelet response: Romiplostim group had significantly higher prebiopsy and postbiopsy platelet counts as compared to the other groups | Cost effectiveness: Romiplostim single dose is cost-effective approach<br>Adverse effects: injection site erythema (39%) being most common | Death: not available<br>Postbiopsy bleeding: none<br>Hepatic decompensation: not available<br>PVT: not available |
| Avatrombopag: first-generation and second-generation formulation (oral)<br>Terrault et al. [27] | Cohort A (first-generation Avatrombopag group): 100 mg loading dose followed by 20, 40, or 80 mg/day on days 2–7 in three parallel arms and also Cohort B (second-generation Avatrombopag group): 80 mg loading dose followed by 10 mg/day for days 2–7 or 20 mg/day for days 2–4 in two parallel arms<br>versus<br>placebo with each study cohort | $N = 130$ subjects with CLD and thrombocytopenia (baseline platelet count of <50,000/$\mu$L) who were scheduled to undergo elective procedure<br>Cirrhosis: 100% (13% Child-Pugh class C)<br>Etiology: 80% viral hepatitis | Majority had endoscopic procedures<br>Also dental procedure, liver biopsy, and paracentesis | An increase in platelet count >20,000/$\mu$L above baseline and at least one platelet count >50,000/$\mu$L within days 4–8 was achieved by 49% of treated subjects in Cohort A and 47.6% in Cohort B compared to 6.3% and 9.5% in placebo<br>The proportion of subjects achieving a platelet count >75,000/$\mu$L or >100,000/$\mu$L at least once within days 4–8: each Avatrombopag regimen had a higher proportion of responders compared with their respective cohort placebo arms ($p < 0.01$) | Platelets response: the maximum median platelet count increase from baseline in all study subjects occurred within 10–13 days. A platelet count >100,000/$\mu$L prior to procedure occurred in 17.6% in subjects with Avatrombopag and none in placebo group<br>Safety: overall similar rate of adverse events in combined study (29%) and combined placebo group (29.7%) | Death: 1 in study (80/10 mg) arm possibly related to study drug<br>Hepatic decompensation: constituted mainly serious adverse effects and were similar in combined study (17.9%) and placebo (10.8%) groups ($p = 0.36$)<br>Bleeding episodes: only 4 subjects had gastrointestinal bleeding episodes<br>PVT: 1 in 100/80 mg arm |

increased platelet production. Majority experience of Romiplostim comes from clinical studies in chronic ITP population [30]. Only anecdotal case reports are available regarding its utility in CLD patients with thrombocytopenia [31].

Avatrombopag is an orally administered, small nonpeptide TPO receptor agonist that is shown to mimic the biological effects of TPO both in vitro and in vivo [32]. It is being utilized in clinical trials including patients with chronic ITP [33] and in CLD (NCT01972529) [34].

*3.1. Eltrombopag.* Eltrombopag was shown to safely increase platelet counts in patients with thrombocytopenia associated with cirrhosis due to chronic HCV infection in a phase II study [35]. Afdhal et al. [24] conducted an international, phase III, double-blinded, randomized, placebo-controlled clinical trial (Eltrombopag Evaluated for Its Ability to Overcome Thrombocytopenia and Enable Procedures, ELEVATE) that assessed the utility of Eltrombopag to increase platelet counts and reduce the need for platelet transfusions in patients with thrombocytopenia and CLD who were undergoing an elective invasive procedure. 292 adult subjects were enrolled between June 2008 and September 2009 and, among those, 252 (86%) had clinically or biopsy proven cirrhosis (10% had Child-Pugh C with score of 10–12 and Model for End-stage Liver Disease, MELD, score $\leq$ 24) with a platelet count of less than 50,000/$\mu$L. All of the subjects otherwise needed a platelet transfusion before the procedure, according to local guidelines at each site. Exclusion criteria included pregnancy, abdominal imaging evidence of Portal Venous Thrombosis (PVT) within the 3 months prior to enrollment, presence of risk factors or a prior history of arterial or venous thrombosis, any condition associated with World Health Organization (WHO) grade 3 or 4 bleeding, or an active infection. The subjects were randomized 1 : 1 to receive either Eltrombopag (75 mg orally daily) or a placebo for 14 days and platelet counts were measured on day 8 and day 15. Invasive procedures were scheduled within 5 days after the patient received the last dose of Eltrombopag. On the day of the procedure, patients with a platelet count of more than 80,000/$\mu$L did not receive a platelet transfusion and those with a platelet count of less than 50,000/$\mu$L received a platelet transfusion before the procedure. The subjects with platelet counts between 50,000/$\mu$L and 80,000/$\mu$L received transfusion per the protocol at their respective centers. The primary end point was the number of subjects who did not require a platelet transfusion prior to, during, and up to 7 days after the procedure. On day 1 of the study, 94% of subjects in the placebo group and 92% of those receiving Eltrombopag had platelet counts of less than 50,000/$\mu$L. On day 15, 59% of the subjects treated with Eltrombopag (compared with 5% in the placebo group) had a platelet count of more than 80,000/$\mu$L. The majority of the subjects in both arms underwent various invasive procedures with similar bleeding risk profiles. The primary end point (avoidance of platelet transfusions) was achieved in 72% (104/145) of the subjects who received Eltrombopag, compared with 19% (28/147) in the placebo group ($p < 0.001$). The most common adverse effects were headache, pyrexia, and abdominal pain, which were observed equally in the treatment and placebo groups. Eight subjects had 10 thrombotic events: 6 subjects from the treatment group and 2 subjects from the placebo group. Nine of the 10 events involved the portal venous system (PVT) and none of the events occurred during the therapy. Of the 6 subjects in the Eltrombopag group who had PVT, 5 had a platelet count higher than 200,000/$\mu$L. No significant difference was observed between the treatment (17%) and placebo (23%) groups in terms of bleeding episodes of WHO grade 2 or higher. The median number of platelets units administered to patients during each transfusion episode was lower in the Eltrombopag group compared with the placebo group (3.0 versus 4.0, resp.). Rates of bleeding episodes were nonsignificant for noninferiority (23% in the placebo group and 17% in the study group). Thus, the daily use of 75 mg of oral Eltrombopag for 14 days raised platelet counts and appreciably reduced the proportion of patients requiring a platelet transfusion prior to elective procedure. Analyses of secondary efficacy end points showed that fewer platelet units were transfused in the Eltrombopag group than in the placebo group and that the bleeding episodes observed in the Eltrombopag group were statistically noninferior to those in the placebo. Of note, the practice with regard to the use of platelet transfusions for thrombocytopenia was not standardized across the centers in this study for those with preprocedure platelet counts less than 80,000/$\mu$L. In total, 20% of CLD patients with thrombocytopenia had WHO grade 2 or higher degree of spotted bleeding, and Eltrombopag did not reduce the events despite improving the platelet numbers. About 4% of the patients who received Eltrombopag were discovered to have PVT. The authors theorized that the sustained increase in platelet count and the predisposing injury from the procedure contributed to the development of the thrombosis. However, it should be noted that Doppler ultrasonography of the abdomen was not a prerequisite during the screening period, so it can be expected that some of the patients at study entry had a subclinical partial PVT or a low flow state, which could contribute to the development or persistence of thrombosis during the study. In the post hoc analysis, an increase in the platelet count to 200,000/$\mu$L or higher was associated with an increased risk of thrombotic events [24]. In clinical practice, a use of different dosing regimen (a decreased dose, less-frequent dosing, or a shorter duration of dosing) could minimize the proportion of patients who have a platelet count of 200,000/$\mu$L or higher and thus reduce the risk of PVT with Eltrombopag.

*3.2. Romiplostim.* Moussa and Mowafy [25] conducted single arm, open label study to evaluate the efficacy of Romiplostim in subjects with HCV cirrhosis and thrombocytopenia who had failed to respond to standard treatment to correct thrombocytopenia prior to an elective procedure by enrolling patients from March 2009 to March 2010 in a single center. All of the 35 included subjects had documented chronic HCV with cirrhosis, classified as Child-Pugh score C, with platelet counts of less than 50,000/$\mu$L, and had failed standard treatments (such as platelet transfusion, antioxidants, and/or folic acid). All of the subjects had a planned nonemergent surgical procedure scheduled. Those with the presence of bone marrow fibrosis, acute leukemia, myelodysplasia, or a history of thromboembolic conditions were excluded from the study. All subjects received a fixed dose of 2 μg/kg subcutaneously (SC) every week for a maximum of 4 weeks or until 2 consecutive platelet counts of above 70,000/μL were observed. The primary end point of the study was defined as the number of subjects achieving a platelet count of more than 70,000/μL; the platelet count was assessed on day 0 and every 3 days for 90 days. A rapid response to Romiplostim therapy was observed, and 33/35 subjects achieved platelet counts above 70,000/μL (mostly between day 12 and day 18) and, thus, underwent surgery without any bleeding complication. Seven of the 35 subjects experienced positive long-term effects of the Romiplostim, defined as a platelet count remaining above 50,000/μL after the end of the platelet count peak (day 42). Although no serious adverse events were observed in this study, headaches were reported among patients receiving the placebo and the study drug. None of the patients had a thromboembolic event, which was evaluated by sonographic and portal duplex imaging. Importantly, none of the patients had a bleeding episode postoperatively. Thus, it was shown that treatment with Romiplostim for correction of severe thrombocytopenia in patients with liver cirrhosis resulted in an increase in the platelet count to a level needed for these patients; thus, they were able to undergo a nonemergent procedure without any significant complications [25]. The Romiplostim product label recommends an initial dose of 1 μg/kg body weight, increasing by increments of 1 μg/kg to a maximum of 10 μg/kg, and indicates vigilant use in patients with CLD, in the presence of platelet counts above the normal range or other risk factors for thromboembolic events. A more conservative treatment dosing regimen was administered in this present study and, thus, no serious adverse events were reported without any episode of postoperative bleeding. In addition, none of the patients experienced a thrombotic event. More than 90% of the patients achieved a suitable platelet count for them to undergo their elective surgical procedure. In addition, it was shown that the use of Romiplostim cost about $500–600 less when compared to the cost of platelet transfusions [25].

*3.3. Romiplostim versus Eltrombopag versus Platelet Transfusion.* Basu et al. [26] conducted a single center, prospective, randomized, double-blind study in which 65 subjects with CLD and thrombocytopenia (baseline platelet count of <60,000/μL) received a TPO agonist or platelets transfusion prior to undergoing a percutaneous liver biopsy. The study evaluated the single use of Romiplostim two weeks prior to a liver biopsy procedure as compared with Eltrombopag and platelet transfusions per center protocol. All of the subjects in this study had liver cirrhosis (mean MELD score 20) secondary to HCV (57%), HBV (15%), NASH, and alcoholic or primary biliary cirrhosis. The exclusion criteria were as follows: patients with ITP, drug induced thrombocytopenia, HIV, HCC, hemangiomas, autoimmune thrombocytopenia, use of steroids, and/or myelodysplastic syndrome. The randomization was performed as follows: Group A with 18 subjects to receive 7 pools of platelets prior to the night prior to the procedure, Group B with 23 subjects to receive a single dose of SC Romiplostim 500 mcg two weeks prior to the procedure, and Group C with 24 subjects to receive oral Eltrombopag 75 mg daily each day for 2 weeks prior to the procedure. All of the subjects had a baseline mean platelet count of less than 60,000/μL prior to enrollment. A platelet count was repeated the day of biopsy and 4 weeks after the procedure. In Group A, the prebiopsy platelet count after transfusions was 183,800/μL and returned to baseline at 4 weeks after the biopsy. In Group B, the prebiopsy platelet count rose to 232,000/μL (significantly higher than Group A and Group C) and stayed significantly elevated 4 weeks after procedure at 366,200/μL ($p < 0.001$ versus Group A and Group C). In Group C, the prebiopsy platelet count was increased to 189,900/μL (no statistical difference compared to Group A); however, 4 weeks after procedure, it was significantly higher at 173,600/μL compared to Group A only. The single dose of Romiplostim was the least expensive method, costing $2284, compared to $7500 for the platelet transfusion and $2991 for the Eltrombopag administration. The adverse effects observed in this study were postinjection site erythema (39%), arthralgia (15%), headache (13%), and/or nausea (8.8%). In addition, no postbiopsy bleeding or hematoma was noted. Although occurrence of PVT, hepatic decompensation, and death was not available in the preliminary study report, the results suggested that the single use of 500 mcg of SC Romiplostim was efficacious, cost-effective, and safe with minimal adverse effects when compared to platelet transfusions and Eltrombopag in patients with cirrhosis and thrombocytopenia needing a liver biopsy.

*3.4. Avatrombopag.* Terrault et al. [27] conducted an international, phase II, randomized placebo-controlled, double-blind trial to evaluate the utility of Avatrombopag in correcting thrombocytopenia in 130 cirrhotic subjects prior to an elective procedure. The included subjects with chronic liver disease were mainly from viral hepatitis (80%), NASH, or alcoholic liver disease; and their MELD scores were less than 24. All of the subjects had clinically proven cirrhosis and 13% of the included subjects had Child-Pugh C disease. All had 2 independent baseline platelet counts ranging from 10 to 58,000/μL and underwent an elective procedure 1 to 4 days after the completion of the dosing schedule of Avatrombopag or the placebo. Those with primary hematologic disorder, ITP of any cause, and/or a history of arterial or venous thrombosis were excluded. Subjects were scheduled to undergo a wide variety of procedures including colonoscopy with or without polypectomy, esophagogastroduodenoscopy with or without banding, bronchoscopy, dental procedure, transarterial chemoembolization of HCC, right heart catheterization, radiofrequency ablation of HCC, liver biopsy, paracentesis, TIPS placement, and hernia repair. Subjects were randomized to two control arms along with Avatrombopag in two intervention cohorts as Cohort A (4 arms) who received either a placebo or 1 of 3 different doses of first-generation oral Avatrombopag formulation (100 mg loading dose followed by 20, 40, or 80 mg/day on days 2–7) and Cohort B (3 arms) who received either a placebo or 1 of 2 different doses of second-generation oral Avatrombopag formulation (80 mg loading dose followed by 10 mg/day for days 2–7 or 20 mg/day for days 2–4). In phase I studies, the second-generation formulation produced about 1.6 times the exposure relative to the first-generation formulation. Thus, dosing was adjusted for study arms. Study's primary end point was defined as an increase in platelet count by 20,000/$\mu$L above baseline and at least one platelet count of above 50,000/$\mu$L from days 4 to 8. This was achieved by 49% of the treated subjects in Cohort A (compared to 6.3% in the control arm) and 47.6% in Cohort B (compared to 9.5% in the control arm). Excluding the 100/40 mg arm in Cohort A ($p = 0.17$), each of the Avatrombopag subcohorts had a high percentage of responders (subjects achieving a platelet count >75,000/$\mu$L or >100,000/$\mu$L at least once within days 4–8) compared with their respective placebo arm ($p < 0.01$). Nausea, fatigue, and headache were among the most common adverse effects, which were noted in the treatment and placebo group. Serious adverse events occurred in 10.8% of placebo and 17.9% of Avatrombopag treated group ($p = 0.36$); most of these events were complications of underlying cirrhosis, such as ascites and hepatic encephalopathy. Hepatic decompensation constituted the main serious adverse effect and was similar in combined study (17.9%) and placebo (10.8%) groups ($p = 0.36$) [27]. There was 1 death after the planned procedure in Cohort B (80/10 mg arm); the death was thought to be possibly related to the study drug, but the patient also had preexisting cardiopulmonary disease. A single case of PVT was identified in Cohort A (100/80 mg arm) that was diagnosed on study day 34. This PVT was then successfully managed with a portal vein thrombectomy, followed by warfarin anticoagulation. Bleeding episodes as a procedure related adverse event were not assessed in this study; however, only 4 episodes of GI bleeding were observed. Thus, this study showed that the use of Avatrombopag achieved significant increases in platelet counts 3–7 days after treatment in approximately 50% of subjects and in up to 75% of those receiving the highest dose, thus suggesting a potential treatment for thrombocytopenia in patients with advanced CLD undergoing elective invasive procedures in a week's time. The dose-dependent rise in platelet count prior to procedure was not evaluated as a marker of reduced risk of bleeding. This study started off using the first-generation formulation of Avatrombopag and subsequently included a separate cohort and dosing regimen to use second-generation formulation of this TPO agent (thus completed phase II analysis for the ongoing phase III study with second-generation Avatrombopag). The patient who developed a PVT had peak platelet count reaching 199,000/$\mu$L, with a platelet count at time of diagnosis of 55,000/$\mu$L and Doppler sonography scan performed three months prior to study entry demonstrated evidence of a very low portal vein flow. This study used Doppler scans and/or MRI and CT imaging only in Cohort B and thus removed patients with PVT at screening. Of note, platelet transfusion was not standardized or evaluated in this study as an end point [27]. Phase III studies will utilize Avatrombopag to evaluate the rate of platelet transfusion as a primary end point in order to confirm and extend the finding of correction of thrombocytopenia prior to the procedures in cirrhosis patients.

## 4. Conclusion

Thrombocytopenia is frequently present in the patients with CLD who require an invasive procedure as part of their routine clinical care. In the study evaluating the bleeding risk among patients with severe thrombocytopenia (platelet count less than 75,000/$\mu$L), it was found that 31% of the patients had bleeding complication related to procedure [36]. Platelet transfusions are often used to increase patient's platelet count—to reduce the anticipated risk of bleeding, in either the setting prior to a procedure or an elective surgery. In addition, platelet transfusions were routinely done prior to initiation of interferon therapy in patients with HCV and thrombocytopenia to minimize the dose adjustments or therapy interruptions. Platelet transfusions have many drawbacks, including transfusion reactions, short efficacy, and the development of refractory thrombocytopenia due to the development of anti-platelet antibodies from receiving multiple transfusions. The use of TPO agonists seems to have merits of avoiding transfusion related complications and have shown relative efficacy in improving platelet counts in CLD in various clinical scenarios [29, 35]. To date, limited data is available for studying the use of such agents to improve platelet number and thus reduce the bleeding complications related to invasive procedures in CLD patients.

Analysis of large phase III ELEVATE trial [24] delineated the need for further experience with the use of Eltrombopag therapy and assessment of risk factors for development of PVT for careful patient selection. Until further studies are performed, the clinical use of Eltrombopag is not recommended in CLD patients with thrombocytopenia prior to an elective invasive procedure. Based on the evidence provided by Moussa and Mowafy [25] with regard to Romiplostim therapy, further larger studies with a longer follow-up period are needed to define an optimal dosing schedule. More durable clinical outcome data is needed prior to the utilization of this agent in clinical practice. Further, Basu et al. [26] showed that single Romiplostim was efficacious, cost-effective, and safe with minimal adverse effects when compared to platelet transfusions and Eltrombopag in cirrhotic patients undergoing a liver biopsy with platelets less than 60,000/$\mu$L. However, the data regarding mortality, hepatic decompensation, and thrombotic events was missing from this preliminary report on this study. The most recent clinical trial completed by Terrault et al. [27] elucidated that oral Avatrombopag increased platelet counts in a generally dose-dependent manner in patients with cirrhosis and thrombocytopenia; however, this effect was not assessed in relation to platelet transfusions or reduction in bleeding risks. At least 2 clinical trials are currently underway which will evaluate the efficacy of Avatrombopag in reducing the proportion of participants who require platelet transfusions or as a rescue therapy to reduce the bleeding risk before and after an elective procedure in patients with liver cirrhosis.

## Additional Points

*Key Messages.* (1) Severe thrombocytopenia is a frequent hemostatic abnormality seen in chronic liver disease patients and is associated with increased bleeding risk with invasive procedures. (2) Impaired production of thrombopoietin is considered to contribute to the development of thrombocytopenia in chronic liver disease. (3) Platelet transfusions, splenic artery embolization, splenectomy, and Transjugular Intrahepatic Portosystemic Stent placement are invasive methods to correct thrombocytopenia in chronic liver disease patients. (4) Initial studies have shown thrombopoietin receptor agonists to be beneficial in these patients especially to improve platelet counts prior to elective invasive procedures. More studies are needed to evaluate the efficacy of thrombopoietin receptor agonists to correct thrombocytopenia in chronic liver disease patients, specifically in regard to the reduction in bleeding risks related to invasive procedures and minimizing the complications (such as portal vein thrombosis) among different agents.

## Competing Interests

The authors declare that they have no competing interests.

## References

[1] N. Afdhal, J. McHutchison, R. Brown et al., "Thrombocytopenia associated with chronic liver disease," *Journal of Hepatology*, vol. 48, no. 6, pp. 1000–1007, 2008.

[2] S.-N. Lu, J.-H. Wang, S.-L. Liu et al., "Thrombocytopenia as a surrogate for cirrhosis and a marker for the identification of patients at high-risk for hepatocellular carcinoma," *Cancer*, vol. 107, no. 9, pp. 2212–2222, 2006.

[3] R. H. Aster, "Pooling of platelets in the spleen: role in the pathogenesis of 'hypersplenic' thrombocytopenia," *The Journal of Clinical Investigation*, vol. 45, no. 5, pp. 645–657, 1966.

[4] H. S. Ballard, "Hematological complications of alcoholism," *Alcoholism: Clinical and Experimental Research*, vol. 13, no. 5, pp. 706–720, 1989.

[5] T. Nagamine, T. Ohtuka, K. Takehara, T. Arai, H. Takagi, and M. Mori, "Thrombocytopenia associated with hepatitis C viral infection," *Journal of Hepatology*, vol. 24, no. 2, pp. 135–140, 1996.

[6] M. PeckRadosavljevic, M. Wichlas, M. Homoncik-Kraml et al., "Rapid suppression of hematopoiesis by standard or pegylated interferon-$\alpha$," *Gastroenterology*, vol. 123, no. 1, pp. 141–151, 2002.

[7] T. Doi, H. Homma, S. Mezawa et al., "Mechanisms for increment of platelet associated IgG and platelet surface IgG and their implications in immune thrombocytopenia associated with chronic viral liver disease," *Hepatology Research*, vol. 24, no. 1, pp. 23–33, 2002.

[8] K. Kaushansky, "Thrombopoietin," *The New England Journal of Medicine*, vol. 339, no. 11, pp. 746–754, 1998.

[9] J. Chen, L. Herceg-Harjacek, J. E. Groopman, and J. Grabarek, "Regulation of platelet activation in vitro by the c-Mpl ligand, thrombopoietin," *Blood*, vol. 86, no. 11, pp. 4054–4062, 1995.

[10] F. J. de Sauvage, P. E. Hass, S. D. Spencer et al., "Stimulation of megakaryocytopoiesis and thrombopoiesis by the c-Mpl ligand," *Nature*, vol. 369, no. 6481, pp. 533–538, 1994.

[11] T. Temel, D. U. Cansu, H. E. Temel, and A. H. Ozakyol, "Serum thrombopoietin levels and its relationship with thrombocytopenia in patients with cirrhosis," *Hepatitis Monthly*, vol. 14, no. 5, Article ID e18556, 2014.

[12] S. J. Slichter, "Relationship between platelet count and bleeding risk in thrombocytopenic patients," *Transfusion Medicine Reviews*, vol. 18, no. 3, pp. 153–167, 2004.

[13] A. Tripodi and P. M. Mannucci, "The coagulopathy of chronic liver disease," *The New England Journal of Medicine*, vol. 365, no. 2, pp. 147–156, 2011.

[14] A. Tripodi, M. Primignani, V. Chantarangkul et al., "Thrombin generation in patients with cirrhosis: the role of platelets," *Hepatology*, vol. 44, no. 2, pp. 440–445, 2006.

[15] L. B. Seeff, G. T. Everson, T. R. Morgan et al., "Complication rate of percutaneous liver biopsies among persons with advanced chronic liver disease in the HALT-C trial," *Clinical Gastroenterology and Hepatology*, vol. 8, no. 10, pp. 877–883, 2010.

[16] G. D. Demetri, "Targeted approaches for the treatment of thrombocytopenia," *Oncologist*, vol. 6, supplement 5, pp. 15–23, 2001.

[17] T. A. Hadduck and J. P. McWilliams, "Partial splenic artery embolization in cirrhotic patients," *World Journal of Radiology*, vol. 6, no. 5, pp. 160–168, 2014.

[18] F. Rodeghiero and M. Ruggeri, "Short- and long-term risks of splenectomy for benign haematological disorders: should we revisit the indications?" *British Journal of Haematology*, vol. 158, no. 1, pp. 16–29, 2012.

[19] N. Jabbour, A. Zajko, P. Orons, W. Irish, J. J. Fung, and R. R. Selby, "Does transjugular intrahepatic portosystemic shunt (TIPS) resolve thrombocytopenia associated with cirrhosis?" *Digestive Diseases and Sciences*, vol. 43, no. 11, pp. 2459–2462, 1998.

[20] L. A. Solberg Jr., "Biologic aspects of thrombopoietins and the development of therapeutic agents," *Current Hematology Reports*, vol. 4, no. 6, pp. 423–428, 2005.

[21] M. Koruk, M. D. Onuk, F. Akçay, and M. C. Savas, "Serum thrombopoietin levels in patients with chronic hepatitis and liver cirrhosis, and its relationship with circulating thrombocyte counts," *Hepato-Gastroenterology*, vol. 49, no. 48, pp. 1645–1648, 2002.

[22] H. Miyazaki, "Update on thrombopoietin in preclinical and clinical trials," *Current Opinion in Hematology*, vol. 5, no. 3, pp. 197–202, 1998.

[23] C. Aguilar, "Potential usefulness of thrombopoietin receptor agonists in haemophiliacs with thrombocytopaenia due to chronic liver disease," *Blood Coagulation and Fibrinolysis*, vol. 24, no. 3, pp. 231–236, 2013.

[24] N. H. Afdhal, E. G. Giannini, G. Tayyab et al., "Eltrombopag before procedures in patients with cirrhosis and thrombocytopenia," *The New England Journal of Medicine*, vol. 367, no. 8, pp. 716–724, 2012.

[25] M. M. Moussa and N. Mowafy, "Preoperative use of romiplostim in thrombocytopenic patients with chronic hepatitis C and liver cirrhosis," *Journal of Gastroenterology and Hepatology*, vol. 28, no. 2, pp. 335–341, 2013.

[26] P. Basu, T. Nair, S. Farhat, N. Shah, M. Jafri, and S. Fousin, "Single use of romiplostim thrombopoietin analogue in severe thrombocytopenia for outpatient percutaneous liver biopsy in patients with chronic liver disease—a randomized double blinded prospective trial," *Journal of Hepatology*, vol. 56, supplement 2, p. S38, 2012.

[27] N. A. Terrault, T. Hassanein, C. D. Howell et al., "Phase II study of avatrombopag in thrombocytopenic patients with cirrhosis undergoing an elective procedure," *Journal of Hepatology*, vol. 61, no. 6, pp. 1253–1259, 2014.

[28] J. B. Bussel, G. Cheng, M. N. Saleh et al., "Eltrombopag for the treatment of chronic idiopathic thrombocytopenic purpura," *The New England Journal of Medicine*, vol. 357, no. 22, pp. 2237–2247, 2007.

[29] N. H. Afdhal, G. M. Dusheiko, E. G. Giannini et al., "Eltrombopag increases platelet numbers in thrombocytopenic patients with hcv infection and cirrhosis, allowing for effective antiviral therapy," *Gastroenterology*, vol. 146, no. 2, pp. 442.el–452.el, 2014.

[30] D. J. Kuter, J. B. Bussel, R. M. Lyons et al., "Efficacy of romiplostim in patients with chronic immune thrombocytopenic purpura: a double-blind randomised controlled trial," *The Lancet*, vol. 371, no. 9610, pp. 395–403, 2008.

[31] G. Buccoliero, T. Urbano, P. Mazza, F. Resta, and S. Pisconti, "Romiplostim for severe thrombocytopenia in the treatment of chronic hepatitis C virus infection: a new option for clinicians?" *New Microbiologica*, vol. 37, no. 1, pp. 97–101, 2014.

[32] M. Fukushima-Shintani, K.-I. Suzuki, Y. Iwatsuki et al., "AKR-501 (YM477) a novel orally-active thrombopoietin receptor agonist," *European Journal of Haematology*, vol. 82, no. 4, pp. 247–254, 2009.

[33] J. B. Bussel, D. J. Kuter, L. M. Aledort et al., "A randomized trial of avatrombopag, an investigational thrombopoietin-receptor agonist, in persistent and chronic immune thrombocytopenia," *Blood*, vol. 123, no. 25, pp. 3887–3894, 2014.

[34] R. Maan, R. J. de Knegt, and B. J. Veldt, "Management of thrombocytopenia in chronic liver disease: focus on pharmacotherapeutic strategies," *Drugs*, vol. 75, no. 17, pp. 1981–1992, 2015.

[35] J. G. McHutchison, G. Dusheiko, M. L. Shiffman et al., "Eltrombopag for thrombocytopenia in patients with cirrhosis associated with hepatitis C," *The New England Journal of Medicine*, vol. 357, no. 22, pp. 2227–2236, 2007.

[36] E. G. Giannini, A. Greco, S. Marenco, E. Andorno, U. Valente, and V. Savarino, "Incidence of bleeding following invasive procedures in patients with thrombocytopenia and advanced liver disease," *Clinical Gastroenterology and Hepatology*, vol. 8, no. 10, pp. 899–902, 2010.

# 23

# Randomized Controlled Study Comparing Use of Propofol Plus Fentanyl versus Midazolam Plus Fentanyl as Sedation in Diagnostic Endoscopy in Patients with Advanced Liver Disease

**Sameh Abdelkhalik Ahmed,[1] Amal Selim,[2] Nehad Hawash,[3] Ahmed Khaled Tawfik,[3] Mohamed Yousef,[3] Abdelrahman Kobtan,[3] Rehab Badawi,[3] Sally Elnawasany,[3] Reham Abdelkader Elkhouly,[3] Amr Shaaban Hanafy,[4] Fatma H. Rizk,[5] Loai Mansour,[3] and Sherief Abd-Elsalam[3]**

[1] *Department of Anesthesia, Tanta University, Tanta, Egypt*
[2] *Internal Medicine Department, Tanta University, Tanta, Egypt*
[3] *Tropical Medicine Department, Tanta University, Tanta, Egypt*
[4] *Internal Medicine Department, Zagazig University, Zagazig, Egypt*
[5] *Department of Physiology, Tanta University, Tanta, Egypt*

Correspondence should be addressed to Sherief Abd-Elsalam; sherif_tropical@yahoo.com

Academic Editor: Simon Bramhall

*Objectives.* We aimed to investigate the safety and efficacy of propofol plus fentanyl versus midazolam plus fentanyl as sedative for patients with advanced liver disease presented for gastrointestinal endoscopy. *Methods.* A total of 100 patients with liver cirrhosis referred for upper endoscopy were enrolled and divided equally in two groups, midazolam plus fentanyl group and propofol plus fentanyl group. All patients were subjected to history taking, estimation of level of sedation, endoscopist rating, and hemodynamic parameters including oxygen saturation, heart rate, mean arterial pressure, incidence of side effect as (bradycardia, hypotension, hypoxia, nausea and vomiting, cough, shivering, or diplopia), time needed for complete recovery, and time needed for discharge. *Results.* There was no statistical significant difference between the studied groups regarding age, sex, weight, Child–Pugh classification score, type and duration of endoscopic intervention, time needed for complete recovery, or time needed for discharge. Complication rates were similar in both groups except for mean arterial blood pressure which was significantly lower in group of patients receiving propofol and fentanyl ($P = 0.001$). *Conclusion.* The use of either propofol or midazolam in combination to fentanyl is effective in sedation of patients with advanced liver diseases presented for upper GIT endoscope. The trial is registered with ClinicalTrials.gov Identifier: NCT03063866.

## 1. Introduction

Gastrointestinal endoscopy is a common procedure in the patients with advanced liver disease. It requires variable level of sedation ranging from minimal sedation to standard general anesthesia aiming for alleviating pain, anxiety, tension, and awful memories of the procedure [1].

In conscious sedation, patients are capable of making purposeful responses to auditory and tactile clues, with maintenance of ventilatory and circulatory stability. Certainly, even as, in deep sedation, patients react only to painful stimuli, they regularly require airway support. At the level of general anesthesia, patients are unresponsive, and airway support is obligatory [2, 3].

The use of general anesthesia or deep sedation in patients with advanced liver disease carries an increased risk of perioperative morbidity and mortality, even with minor procedures. Thus, the use of conscious sedation for endoscopy in hepatic patients remains as the classical method [4, 5].

The level of sedation may require changing throughout the same procedure. Generally, diagnostic procedure usually can be managed by conscious sedation, while therapeutic interventions need more deep level of sedation [6, 7].

Propofol, the short acting intravenous anesthetic agent, is used to achieve a different level of sedation nowadays. Some authors recommend the use of propofol as a sedative agent in short procedure [8].

Midazolam, the short acting barbiturate, is a sedative drug that exerts its action through the effect on GABA receptor in the brain, thus relieving anxiety. It has sedative, amnesic, and anticonvulsant effect [9]. However, midazolam shows extensive hepatic metabolism that increases the risk of complications in patients with advanced liver disease especially with prolonged sedation [10].

Fentanyl, the short acting opioid, is commonly used as an additive to the sedative agents to improve the sedation level, analgesia, and amnesia and to allow the decrease in the used dose of the sedative [11].

The aim of this study is to compare the use of propofol plus fentanyl versus midazolam plus fentanyl as sedative for patients with advanced liver disease presented for gastrointestinal endoscopy. Our primary outcome is the safety and efficacy of the drugs.

## 2. Patients and Method

This randomized, double-blind prospective study was carried out on 100 adult patients admitted to Department of Gastroenterology, Tanta University Hospital, who presented for elective endoscopy.

The duration of study was 6 months starting immediately after obtaining ethical committee approval. An informed written consent was taken from each patient and the study was registered on clinicaltrials.gov (ClinicalTrials.gov Identifier: NCT03063866). All patients' data were confidential with secret codes and will be used for the current study only.

Any unexpected risk appearing during the course of the research was cleared to the participants and ethical committee on time and proper measures were taken to overcome or minimize these risks.

*Risk to the Patients.* Patients included in the study who had potential risk of airway obstruction were managed with adequate monitoring, anesthetist attendance, and available airway management devices.

There was adequate provisions to maintain privacy of participants and confidentiality of the data.

There were no conflicts of interest, or conflicts with religion, law, or social obligations.

The research was useful for society and carried no risk for environmental pollution.

Patients included in this study were aged 40–60 years old, with CTP score B or C presented for elective gastrointestinal endoscopy.

Patients were excluded from the study in the following cases: if they refused to participate in the study and patients with emergent condition like hematemesis, patients with any grade of hepatic encephalopathy, patients with hepatopulmonary syndrome, or patients with known or suspected hypersensitivity to the used medication.

All the maneuvers were performed in the operating theatre with attendance of anesthesiologist throughout the whole procedure for initiation and maintenance of patients sedation with monitoring of the patients' vital parameters. After preoperative evaluation of the patients through history, examination, and investigations, patients were counseled, reassured, and, then, transported to the operating theatre. Then, intravenous 22 gauge peripheral cannula was inserted. The patient was monitored with three leads, electrocardiogram, pulse oximetry, and noninvasive blood pressure. Supplemental oxygen (3-4 L/min) was given via a nasal cannula in all cases during the procedure with administration of 10 ml/kg of lactated ringer solution by i.v. infusion.

The patients were randomly allocated (using closed envelop method) into two groups, 50 patients in each group.

*2.1. Group I (M Group).* Patients in this group received sedation in the form of midazolam 3 mg i.v. added to fentanyl 0.5 ug/kg till reaching a satisfactory level of sedation. Supplementary dose of midazolam of 1 mg was given if the level of sedation reached was unsatisfactory.

*2.2. Group II (P Group).* Patients in this group received sedation in the form of propofol 1 mg/kg i.v. added to fentanyl 0.5 ug/kg i.v till reaching a satisfactory level of sedation. If the level of sedation was not satisfactory, an additional dose of propofol 0.2 mg/kg will be given.

After adequate sedation of the patient, all patients received lidocaine spray 10% applied to the posterior pharynx for minimizing gag reflex followed by application of mouth piece. All the endoscopic maneuvers were performed in left lateral position with continuous monitoring by anesthesiologist till the end of the procedure and recovery of patients to the fully conscious level. All resuscitation equipment and medications were available.

All the following data were assessed including demographic data including age, sex, CTP class, body weight (BWT), type of endoscopic intervention, duration of endoscopy, time for complete recovery, and time for discharge. Additionally, time for complete recovery is the time elapsed between the end of endoscopy and the complete return of conscious level and time to discharge is the time elapsed between regaining conscious level and complete hospital discharge. The level of sedation using Ramsay sedation agitation score before induction of sedation (T0), 5 min after sedation (T1), 10 min after sedation (T2), and then every 30 min till complete recovery (T3, T4, and T5) was also assessed. Moreover, Endoscopist rating (easy or difficult endoscope) was recorded.

Hemodynamic parameters including oxygen saturation (Spo2), heart rate (HR), and mean arterial pressure (MAP) before induction (T0), 5 min after sedation (T1), 10 min after sedation (T2), and then every 15 min till complete recovery (T3, T4, T5, T6, T7, and T8) were monitored and incidence of side effects (bradycardia, hypotension, nausea and vomiting, shivering, diplopia, or hypoxia) was recorded.

TABLE 1: Patient characteristics of two groups.

| | M group | P group | $P$ |
|---|---|---|---|
| Age (year) mean ± SD | 51.24 ± 5.80 | 49.94 ± 5.53 | 0.25 |
| Gender | | | 0.47 |
| Male NO. (%) | 28 (56%) | 29.0 (58%) | |
| Female NO. (%) | 22 (44%) | 21.0 (42%) | |
| CTP class | | | 0.34 |
| B NO. (%) | 31.00 (62%) | 30.0 (60%) | |
| C NO. (%) | 19.00 (38%) | 20.0 (40%) | |
| Weight (kg) mean ± SD | 73.02 ± 9.41 | 72.92 ± 8.88 | 0.96 |
| Type of endoscopic intervention | | | 0.22 |
| Diagnostic NO. (%) | 26 (52%) | 25 (50%) | |
| Sclerotherapy NO. (%) | 14 (28%) | 17 (34%) | |
| Band ligation NO. (%) | 10 (20%) | 8 (16%) | |
| Duration of endoscope (min) mean ± SD | 20.00 ± 5.80 | 20.90 ± 6.68 | 0.47 |
| Time for complete recovery (min) mean ± SD | 40.90 ± 11.90 | 36.60 ± 12.43 | 0.08 |
| Time for discharge (min) mean ± SD | 64.00 ± 14.98 | 61.80 ± 17.37 | 0.50 |

Bradycardia is a decrease in HR less than 50 B/min, while hypotension is a decrease in mean arterial pressure by more than 20 mmHg. Hypoxia is a decrease in Spo2 less than 90%.

Bradycardia was managed by 0.3 mg i.v. atropine, while hypotension was managed by ephedrine 10 mg i.v. and ringer lactate 5 ml/kg. Hypoxia was managed by adequate airway management and oxygenation.

*2.3. Statistical Analysis.* The statistical differences between the studied groups were tested using unpaired $t$-test for parametric variables and chi-square test for nonparametric variables. The sedation score was analyzed with Wilcoxon test. Statistical tests were performed with SPSS (Version 23). $P$ values < 0.05 were considered statistically significant.

## 3. Results

As regards patient characteristics of the two groups, there were no statistically significant differences between the studied groups regarding age, sex, CTP class, body weight, type of endoscopic intervention, duration of endoscopy, time for complete recovery, and time for discharge (Table 1).

Regarding sedation scores during the procedure, there were significant increases in sedation scores between T1, 2, 3, and 4 and baseline values in each group. However, there was no significant difference between T5 and baseline value in each group. In addition, there was no significant difference between groups in sedation scores (Table 2).

Considering endoscopist's rating, the rating was easy in 38% and 52% in M and P group, respectively. Moreover, the rating was difficult in 62% and 48% in M and P group, respectively. However, there were no significant differences in endoscopist's rating between both groups (Table 3).

Concerning side effects in studied groups, Hypotension was significantly more frequent in P group compared with M group, while there were no significant differences in frequency of bradycardia, nausea and vomiting, shivering, diplopia, or hypoxia between both groups (Table 4).

Regarding the changes in oxygen saturation (Spo2), heart rate (HR) and mean arterial pressure (MAP) in both studied groups concerned with the Spo2 levels. As regards the Spo2 levels, P group showed significant increases at T0, T6, T7, and T8 when compared with M group. In addition, HR levels showed significant increases in P group at T0 only when compared with M group. Moreover, MAP showed significant increases in P group at T4, T5, and T8 when compared with M group (Figure 1).

TABLE 2: Sedation scores during the procedure.

| | M group ($n$ = 50) Median (Minimum–maximum) | P group ($n$ = 50) Median (Minimum–maximum) |
|---|---|---|
| T0 | 0 (0-1) | 0 (0-1) |
| T1 | 4 (2–6)* | 4 (2–6)* |
| T2 | 4 (3–6)* | 4 (3–6)* |
| T3 | 4 (2–6)* | 4 (2–6)* |
| T4 | 2 (1–5)* | 2 (1–5)* |
| T5 | 0 (0-1) | 0 (0-1) |

* $P < 0.05$ compared with T0.

TABLE 3: Endoscopist's rating.

| | M group | P group | $P$ |
|---|---|---|---|
| Rating | | | |
| Easy NO. (%) | 19 (38%) | 26 (52%) | 0.22 |
| Difficult NO. (%) | 31 (62%) | 24 (48%) | |

TABLE 4: Side effects in the studied groups.

| | M group | P group | $P$ |
|---|---|---|---|
| Bradycardia | 9 (18%) | 14 (28%) | 0.67 |
| Hypotension | 1 (2%) | 4 (8%) | 0.001* |
| Nausea and vomiting | 30 (60%) | 24 (48%) | 0.13 |
| Shivering | 25 (50%) | 23 (46%) | 0.16 |
| Diplopia | 21 (42%) | 19 (38%) | 0.24 |
| Hypoxia | 14 (28%) | 12 (24%) | 0.64 |

* $P < 0.05$ (indicates significant difference between the studied groups). Bradycardia is a decrease in HR less than 50 B/min; hypotension is a decrease in mean arterial pressure by more than 20 mmHg.

## 4. Discussion

Patients with liver cirrhosis are commonly referred for upper gastrointestinal (GI) endoscopy for the screening and treatment of complications of portal hypertension, such as esophagogastric varices and portal hypertensive gastropathy [12].

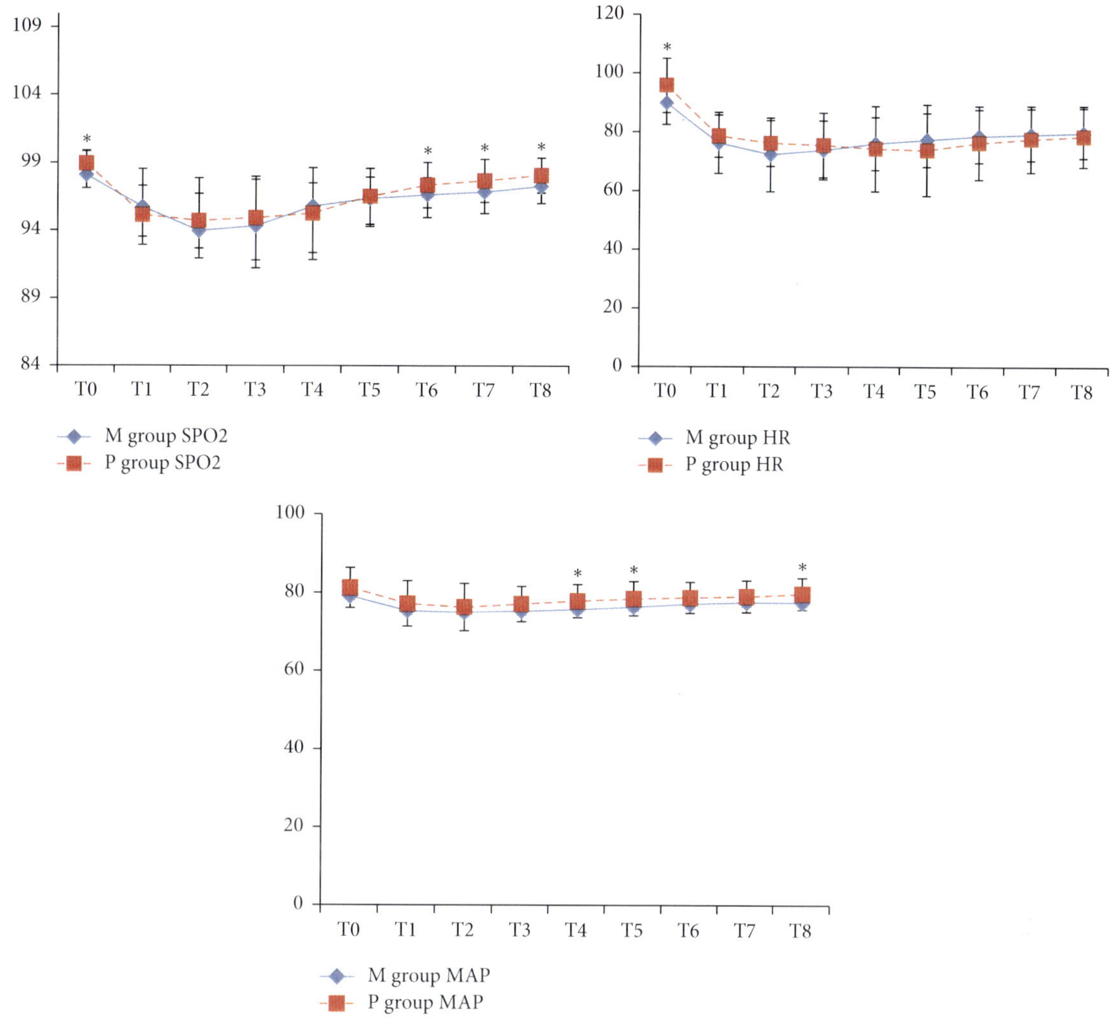


FIGURE 1: The changes in oxygen saturation (Spo2), heart rate (HR), and mean arterial pressure (MAP) in both studied groups. $^{*}P < 0.05$ between the two groups.

The main goals of sedation in GI endoscopy are rapid onset of hypnosis, anxiolysis, analgesia, amnesia, cooperation to complete the procedure, and rapid recovery of consciousness [13, 14].

The aim of our randomized study was to assess the safety and efficacy of the use of propofol plus fentanyl versus midazolam plus fentanyl as sedatives for patients with advanced liver disease presented for gastrointestinal endoscopy.

There was no statistically significant difference between the studied groups regarding age, sex, weight, Child-Pugh classification score, and type and duration of endoscopic intervention, as some of these factors may affect the dose of the sedating drug or its related complications [15]. Also there was no significant difference regarding endoscopist's rating.

There was no statistical difference in time needed for complete recovery or time needed for discharging between two studied groups. In contrast to our results, Correia et al. 2011 [16] studied 200 cirrhotic patients and compared propofol and fentanyl with midazolam and fentanyl and found that sedation with propofol plus fentanyl was more efficacious with a shorter recovery time compared with midazolam plus fentanyl; also Seleem et al. 2014 [17] who studied 99 cirrhotic patients and divided them into three groups, midazolam plus fentanyl group, propofol plus fentanyl group, and Ketamine group, found that there was a high statistically significant difference among the studied groups with the shortest recovery time which was observed in propofol plus fentanyl group followed by midazolam plus fentanyl and Ketamine groups; also Poulos et al. 2013 [18] reported that the use of propofol plus fentanyl resulted in less time in the endoscopy unit, quicker recovery, and faster discharge than regimen using midazolam plus fentanyl, and Tsai et al. 2015 [19] who performed meta-analysis included five studies between 2003 and 2012, including 433 patients, and concluded that propofol provided a shorter time to sedation (weight mean difference: −2.76 min, 95% confidence interval: −3.00 to −2.51) and a shorter recovery time (weight mean difference −6.17 min, 95% confidence interval: −6.81 to −5.54) than midazolam did.

We also did not find statistical difference regarding side effects including nausea, vomiting, shivering, and diplopia. Also, heart rate and hypoxia among our patients groups showed no significant differences as we recorded 9 patients had bradycardia and 14 patients had hypoxia in M group while 14 patients had bradycardia and 12 patients had hypoxia in P group. On the other hand, there was a significant difference between the studied two groups regarding hypotension. As 4 patients in P group and only 1 patient in M group suffered from hypotension, the mechanisms by which midazolam causes hypotension was attributed to reduction in systematic vascular resistance and myocardial contractility [20, 21]; fentanyl causes hypotension due to a centrally mediated decrease in sympathetic tone as declared by Laubie et al., 1974 [22], while propofol causes hypotension by decreasing preload, cardiac output, and contractility [23, 24] or decreasing systemic vascular resistance [25].

This was in agreement with Seleem et al., 2014 [17] who found no significant difference in heart rate among two groups receiving propofol-fentanyl and midazolam-fentanyl; our results were in partial agreement with results of Correia et al., 2011 [16] who concluded that complications rates were similar in both groups, which was similar to our results except for hypotension. While Tsai et al. 2015 [19] recorded no intergroup difference regarding incidence of hypotension, bradycardia, or hypoxemia.

Similar to our results dos Santos et al., 2013 [26] who studied 200 patients (divided into two groups who received propofol-fentanyl or midazolam-fentanyl) concluded that there were significant differences between two studied groups regarding oxygen saturation as oxygen supplementation was required in 42% of the propofol-fentanyl group and 26% of the midazolam-fentanyl group.

Moerman et al., 2004 [27], who used the same dose of propofol (1 mg/kg) as our study recorded that patients received propofol plus fentanyl had serious hypotension, bradycardia, and hypoxemia in 14% out of 50 patients.

In contrast to our results Seleem et al. 2014 [17] found no significant difference in mean arterial pressure among studied groups. Also, Suh et al., 2014 [28] who performed upper gastrointestinal endoscopy under sedation with propofol along with careful monitoring in 20 patients with liver cirrhosis and 20 control subjects and found that there were neither respiratory depression nor clinically significant hypotension observed among cirrhotic patients.

On the other hand Barriga et al., 2008 [29] reported serious hypotension in 16 patients out of 480 patients who received midazolam plus fentanyl; also serious hypoxemia occurred in one patient and this may be attributed to their use of a higher dose of midazolam (0.1 mg/kg) than the dose we used in our study (3 mg) and higher number of patients included in their study.

Finally, we can conclude that the use of either propofol or midazolam in combination to fentanyl is effective in the sedation of patients with advanced liver diseases who presented for upper GIT endoscope with indifference between the two drugs as regarding level of sedation, difficulty of technique, duration of recovery or discharge, and incidence of complication. However, the risk of hypotension seems to be increased with use of propofol.

## References

[1] D. S. Early, T. Ben-Menachem, G. A. Decker et al., "Appropriate use of GI endoscopy," *Gastrointestinal Endoscopy*, vol. 75, no. 6, pp. 1127–1131, 2012.

[2] D. O. Faigel, T. H. Baron, J. L. Goldstein et al., "Guidelines for the use of deep sedation and anesthesia for GI endoscopy," *Gastrointestinal Endoscopy*, vol. 56, no. 5, pp. 613–617, 2002.

[3] D. O. Faigel, G. M. Eisen, T. H. Baron et al., "Preparation of patients for GI endoscopy," *Gastrointestinal Endoscopy*, vol. 57, no. 4, pp. 446–450, 2003.

[4] J. Montomoli, R. Erichsen, C. F. Christiansen et al., "Liver disease and 30-day mortality after colorectal cancer surgery: a Danish population-based cohort study," *BMC Gastroenterology*, vol. 13, no. 1, article 66, 2013.

[5] L. S. Friedman, "Preoperative evaluation of the patient with liver disease," in *Schiff's Diseases of the Liver*, pp. 316–325, 11th edition, 2012.

[6] J. J. Vargo, G. Zuccaro, J. A. Dumot et al., "Gastroenterologist-administered propofol versus meperidine and midazolam for advanced upper endoscopy: a prospective, randomized trial," *Gastroenterology*, vol. 123, no. 1, pp. 8–16, 2002.

[7] M. Jung, C. Hofmann, R. Kiesslich, and A. Brackertz, "Improved sedation in diagnostic and therapeutic ERCP: propofol is an alternative to midazolam," *Endoscopy*, vol. 32, no. 3, pp. 233–238, 2000.

[8] H. Seifert, T. Schmitt, T. Gültekin, W. Caspary, and T. Wehrmann, "Sedation with propofol plus midazolam versus propofol alone for interventional endoscopic procedures: a prospective, randomized study," *Alimentary Pharmacology and Therapeutics*, vol. 14, no. 9, pp. 1207–1214, 2000.

[9] K. D. Mullen and E. A. Jones, *Natural Benzodiazepines and Hepatic Encephalopathy*, Seminars in liver disease, Thieme Medical Publishers, Inc., 1996.

[10] S. P. Wilkinson, "GABA, benzodiazepines and hepatic encephalopathy," *European Journal of Gastroenterology and Hepatology*, vol. 7, no. 4, pp. 323-324, 1995.

[11] N. Disma, M. Astuto, G. Rizzo et al., "Propofol sedation with fentanyl or midazolam during oesophagogastroduodenoscopy in children," *European Journal of Anaesthesiology*, vol. 22, no. 11, pp. 848–852, 2005.

[12] R. C. Cheung, S. Cooper, and E. B. Keeffe, "Endoscopic gastrointestinal manifestations of liver disease," *Gastrointestinal Endoscopy Clinics of North America*, vol. 11, pp. 15–44, 2001.

[13] D. Wang, C. Chen, J. Chen et al., "The use of propofol as a sedative agent in gastrointestinal endoscopy: a meta-analysis," *PLoS ONE*, vol. 8, no. 1, Article ID e53311, 2013.

[14] W.-H. Hsu, S. S. Wang, H.-Y. Shih et al., "Low effect-site concentration of propofol target-controlled infusion reduces the risk of hypotension during endoscopy in a Taiwanese population," *Journal of Digestive Diseases*, vol. 14, no. 3, pp. 147–152, 2013.

[15] S.-Y. Lee, J. S. Hee, M. L. Ji et al., "Identification of factors that influence conscious sedation in gastrointestinal endoscopy,"

*Journal of Korean Medical Science*, vol. 19, no. 4, pp. 536–540, 2004.

[16] L. M. Correia, D. Q. Bonilha, G. F. Gomes et al., "Sedation during upper GI endoscopy in cirrhotic outpatients: a randomized, controlled trial comparing propofol and fentanyl with midazolam and fentanyl," *Gastrointestinal Endoscopy*, vol. 73, no. 1, pp. 45–51, 2011.

[17] W. Seleem, M. Semary, K. El Hossieny, and A. Metwally, "Evaluation of different sedative approaches for cirrhotic patients during upper gastrointestinal endoscopy," *International Journal of Advanced Research*, vol. 2, no. 10, pp. 925–933, 2014.

[18] J. Poulos, P. Kalogerinis, and J. Caudle, "Propofol plus fentanyl compared with combination of midazolam plus fentanyl for endoscopy in a community setting," *AANA Journal*, vol. 81, no. 1, pp. 31–36, 2013.

[19] H.-C. Tsai, Y.-C. Lin, C.-L. Ko et al., "Propofol versus midazolam for upper gastrointestinal endoscopy in cirrhotic patients: a meta-analysis of randomized controlled trials," *PLoS ONE*, vol. 10, no. 2, Article ID e0117585, 2015.

[20] J. G. Reves, P. N. Samuelson, and S. Lewis, "Midazolam maleate induction in patients with ischaemic heart disease: Haemodynamic observations," *Canadian Anaesthetists' Society Journal*, vol. 26, no. 5, pp. 402–409, 1979.

[21] P. N. Samuelson, J. G. Reves, N. T. Kouchoukos, L. R. Smith, and K. M. Dole, "Hemodynamic responses to anesthetic induction with midazolam or diazepamin patients with ischemic heart disease," *Anesthesia & Analgesia*, vol. 60, no. 11, pp. 802–809, 1981.

[22] M. Laubie, H. Schmitt, J. Canellas, J. Roquebert, and P. Demichel, "Centrally mediated bradycardia and hypotension induced by narcotic analgesics: dextromoramide and fentanyl," *European Journal of Pharmacology*, vol. 28, no. 1, pp. 66–75, 1974.

[23] J.-Y. M. Lepage, M. L. Pinaud, J. H. Helias, A. Y. Cozian, Y. Le Normand, and R. J. Souron, "Left ventricular performance during propofol or methohexital anesthesia: isotopic and invasive cardiac monitoring," *Anesthesia and Analgesia*, vol. 73, no. 1, pp. 3–9, 1991.

[24] A. Gauss, H. Heinrich, and O. H. G. Wilder-smith, "Echocardiographic assessment of the haemodynamic effects of propofol: a comparison with etomidate and thiopentone," *Anaesthesia*, vol. 46, no. 2, pp. 99–105, 1991.

[25] D. P. Coates, C. R. Monk, C. Prys-Roberts, and M. Turtle, "Hemodynamic effects of infusions of the emulsion formulation of propofol during nitrous oxide anesthesia in humans," *Anesthesia and Analgesia*, vol. 66, no. 1, pp. 64–70, 1987.

[26] M. E. L. dos Santos, F. Maluf-Filho, D. M. Chaves et al., "Deep sedation during gastrointestinal endoscopy: propofol-fentanyl and midazolam-fentanyl regimens," *World Journal of Gastroenterology*, vol. 19, no. 22, pp. 3439–3446, 2013.

[27] A. T. Moerman, M. M. R. F. Struys, H. E. Vereecke, L. L. Herregods, M. M. De Vos, and E. P. Mortier, "Remifentanil used to supplement propofol does not improve quality of sedation during spontaneous respiration," *Journal of Clinical Anesthesia*, vol. 16, no. 4, pp. 237–243, 2004.

[28] S. J. Suh, H. J. Yim, E. L. Yoon et al., "Is propofol safe when administered to cirrhotic patients during sedative endoscopy?" *Korean Journal of Internal Medicine*, vol. 29, no. 1, pp. 57–65, 2014.

[29] J. Barriga, M. S. Sachdev, L. Royall, G. Brown, and C. R. Tombazzi, "Sedation for upper endoscopy: Comparison of midazolam versus fentanyl plus midazolam," *Southern Medical Journal*, vol. 101, no. 4, pp. 362–366, 2008.

# Cardiovascular Autonomic Dysfunction in Patients of Nonalcoholic Fatty Liver Disease

**Mavidi Sunil Kumar,[1] Akanksha Singh,[2] Ashok Kumar Jaryal,[2] Piyush Ranjan,[1] K. K. Deepak,[2] Sanjay Sharma,[3] R. Lakshmy,[4] R. M. Pandey,[5] and Naval K. Vikram[1]**

[1]*Department of Internal Medicine, All India Institute of Medical Sciences, New Delhi 110029, India*
[2]*Department of Physiology, All India Institute of Medical Sciences, New Delhi 110029, India*
[3]*Department of Radiodiagnosis, All India Institute of Medical Sciences, New Delhi 110029, India*
[4]*Department of Cardiac Biochemistry, All India Institute of Medical Sciences, New Delhi 110029, India*
[5]*Department of Biostatistics, All India Institute of Medical Sciences, New Delhi 110029, India*

Correspondence should be addressed to Naval K. Vikram; navalvikram@gmail.com

Academic Editor: Daisuke Morioka

*Aim.* The present study was designed to evaluate the heart rate variability (HRV) in nonalcoholic fatty liver disease (NAFLD) and to assess the effect of grade of NAFLD and diabetic status on HRV. *Methods.* This cross-sectional study included 75 subjects (25 NAFLD without diabetes, 25 NAFLD with diabetes, and 25 controls). Measurements included anthropometry, body composition analysis, estimation of plasma glucose, serum lipids, hsCRP, and serum insulin. HRV analysis was performed in both time and frequency domains. *Results.* The time and frequency domain indices of overall variability (SDNN, total power) were significantly lower in NAFLD with diabetes as compared to the controls. However, the LF : HF ratio did not differ among the three groups. The variables related to obesity, lipid profile, and glucose metabolism were also higher in NAFLD with diabetes and those with Grade II NAFLD without diabetes, as compared to controls. Multivariate stepwise regression analysis showed a negative correlation between HRV and total cholesterol and fat percentage. *Conclusion.* The grade of NAFLD as well as diabetic status contributes to the decrease in the cardiovascular autonomic function, with diabetic status rather than grade of NAFLD playing a critical role. Serum lipids and adiposity may also contribute to cardiac autonomic dysfunction.

## 1. Introduction

Nonalcoholic fatty liver disease (NAFLD) is a clinicopathological condition characterised by lipid deposition in the liver and is a common cause of liver dysfunction. The prevalence of NAFLD in Asian population ranges from 9% to 45% [1] and is estimated to be about 30% in western population [2]. Apart from an increased risk of liver-related morbidity and mortality, patients of NAFLD also have higher cardiovascular risk [3, 4] especially when present along with type 2 diabetes (T2DM) [4, 5].

A balanced autonomic output to liver is important for maintenance of circadian rhythms of liver metabolic enzymes and glucose level [6]. Imbalance in autonomic function has been proposed as a component in pathogenesis of NAFLD [7]. The autonomic dysfunction has been shown to be higher in the NAFLD. The autonomic symptom burden assessed by orthostatic grading scale was higher in nondiabetic NAFLD [8] and the sudomotor dysfunction was also higher in the NAFLD after accounting for all confounders [9].

A recent systematic review of 27 studies showed an association of NAFLD with subclinical atherosclerosis independent of traditional risk factors and metabolic syndrome [10]. Similar independent association of NAFLD with subclinical atherosclerosis has been observed in Asian Indians also [11]. In other clinical settings, it has been shown that arterial stiffness is inversely related to heart rate variability [12, 13]. However, there are only a few studies in which heart rate variability has been evaluated in NAFLD [9, 14, 15]. Decrease in indices of HRV has been reported by Liu et al. with decrease in parasympathetic component after adjustment of covariates [14]. A higher LF : HF ratio (low frequency : high frequency) of HRV was reported in patients ($n = 18$) with NAFLD along with a lower baroreflex sensitivity [15].

Cardiovascular autonomic neuropathy is a common complication of diabetes [16]. NAFLD commonly coexists with diabetes. Both may act synergistically leading to varied clinical outcomes [17]. The independent contribution of diabetes and grade of NAFLD in development of autonomic dysfunction is not known. The present study was designed to evaluate cardiovascular autonomic status in the patients of NAFLD with or without diabetes as compared to control population of individuals without either diabetes or NAFLD. In the present study we evaluated the association of indices of HRV with anthropometric variables, lipid profile, and diabetic status in patients with and without NAFLD.

## 2. Methods

This was a cross-sectional study approved by the Institute Ethics Committee of the All India Institute of Medical Sciences (AIIMS), New Delhi. The subjects were recruited from the medicine outpatient department. Informed written consent was obtained after explanation of the purpose, type, and duration of the study.

*2.1. Study Subjects.* A total of 75 subjects were recruited for the study. The subjects were grouped into NAFLD patients without diabetes ($n = 25$, 13 females and 12 males), NAFLD patients with diabetes of <5 years of duration ($n = 25$, 17 females and 8 males), and healthy controls with similar age distribution ($n = 25$, 9 females and 16 males). Subjects with alcohol consumption >140 gm/week, any secondary cause of fatty liver, hereditary disorders, any severe acute or chronic illness, seropositivity for hepatitis B, hepatitis C, and HIV, established coronary heart disease, pregnancy, and lactation were excluded. Diagnosis of NAFLD was made using ultrasonography performed by an experienced sonologist who was blinded to the clinical data of the patients, using a 3.5 MHz convex transducer by subcostal and intercostal approach (Volusion, GE).

*2.2. Measurements*

*2.2.1. Anthropometry and Body Composition.* A detailed clinical history and clinical examination was done. All the subjects underwent anthropometric measurements and body composition analysis by bioelectrical impedance method as described earlier [11]. Height and weight were recorded to the nearest 0.1 cm and nearest 0.1 kg with stadiometer and electronic scale. Body Mass Index (BMI) was calculated by weight (kg)/height ($m^2$). Waist circumference (WC) was measured midway between the iliac crest and the lower most margin of the ribs. Hip circumference (HC) was measured at the maximum circumference of buttocks. Body fat and percentage body fat were estimated by foot-to-foot bioelectrical impedance technique (TANITA, Japan).

*2.2.2. Biochemical Measurements.* Venous blood samples were obtained after an overnight fast of at least 10 hours. Biochemical measurements included liver function tests, fasting blood glucose (FBG) and postprandial blood glucose (PPBG) levels, and fasting lipid profile using standard methods as described earlier [11]. Serum levels of hsCRP were measured using a commercially available reagent kit based on the principle of solid phase enzyme-linked immune sorbent assay (Biocheck, Inc., Foster City, USA). Fasting insulin was measured using a commercially available reagent kit based on the principle of electrochemiluminescence (Liaison® Insulin, DiaSorin Inc., USA). The inter- and intra-assay coefficient of variation was <5%. The HOMA-IR was calculated by using the following formula: HOMA-IR = fasting insulin ($\mu$U/mL) $*$ fasting blood glucose (mmol/L)/22.5.

*2.2.3. Assessment of Heart Rate Variability.* The cardiovascular autonomic status was estimated in the Autonomic Function Testing Laboratory (AFT Lab), Department of Physiology, AIIMS, New Delhi. The subject was requested to lie down on the couch where electrodes for lead II ECG acquisition by Labchart Pro 7® (AD Instruments, Australia) were attached. The recording was performed in a controlled ambient temperature of 22 to 25°C. After an initial period of rest of 5 minutes, a 5-minute lead II ECG (sampling rate 1 KHz) was recorded for later offline analysis. The subject was instructed to avoid movement during data acquisition to prevent artefacts in the recording.

Offline analysis of ECG was done using Labchart Pro 7 (AD Instruments, Australia) and HRV was computed using Hemolab software (version 8.5, Harald Stauss Scientific, Iowa). For time domain analysis the beat-to-beat heart rate series was computed from ECG using Labchart Pro and was then exported as a $*$.txt file. The file format was converted to $*$.asc as required by the Hemolab software for batch processing. The time domain indices of HRV computed were SDNN (standard deviation of all NN intervals), SDSD (standard deviation of differences between adjacent NN intervals), and pNN50% (NN50 count divided by the total number of all NN intervals). For frequency domain analysis RR intervals were computed from ECG using Labchart Pro and were then exported as a.txt file. The file format was converted to $*$.asc and then to $*$.tsa for batch processing. This was followed by spline interpolation at sampling frequency of 5 Hz followed by the power spectral density (PSD) calculation using Fast Fourier Transformation (FFT). The measurement of low frequency (LF: 0.04–0.15 Hz) and high frequency (HF: 0.15–0.40 Hz) power components was made in absolute values of power ($ms^2$). The powers were further normalized to account for changes in the total power of the HRV.

*2.3. Statistical Analysis.* The data was analysed using SPSS software (Version 22, IBM). The normality of distribution was estimated with Shapiro-Wilk test. Quantitative data is expressed as mean ± SD for normally distributed data, and median with interquartile range (IQR) is used to express skewed data. For parametric data, one-way ANOVA followed by Tukey's test was used and for nonparametric data Kruskal Wallis H test followed by Dunn's comparison was done. $p <$

0.05 was considered to be statistically significant. Two-way ANOVA was employed to evaluate the relative contribution of the diabetic status and grade of NAFLD. Correlation analysis was done with Spearman's test followed by stepwise multivariate analysis.

## 3. Results

The anthropometric measures, biochemical investigation, and lead II ECG recordings were measured in all the subjects. The data of 7 subjects in the NAFLD without diabetes group was excluded from HRV due to presence of artefacts that prevented computation.

*3.1. Anthropometric Features and Biochemical Profile.* Table 1 shows the general, anthropometric, and biochemical parameters of the subjects. Patients with NAFLD and diabetes were older (42.9 ± 7.6 yrs) than patients with NAFLD without diabetes (41.8 ± 7.3 yrs) and controls (37.9 ± 8.4 yrs). The BMI, fat mass, and fat percentage were higher in NAFLD with diabetes group as well as NAFLD without diabetes group as compared to the controls but there was no difference between NAFLD with and without diabetes. Value of WHR was higher only in NAFLD without diabetes as compared to the controls. The fat percentage was the only measure that was higher in the NAFLD with diabetes as compared to the NAFLD without diabetes.

The ESR was higher in NAFLD with diabetes while hsCRP was higher in NAFLD without diabetes as compared to controls. All the indices of liver function (bilirubin, SGOT, SGPT, and ALP) were not significantly different among the three groups. As expected, the values of FBG, PPBG, and HOMA-IR were significantly higher in NAFLD with diabetes group as compared to the other two groups. Serum levels of TC and LDL were higher in NAFLD with diabetes group as compared to the control group.

*3.2. Heart Rate Variability (HRV).* The time and frequency domain indices of HRV are shown in Table 2. The overall variability (time domain: SDNN and frequency domain: total power) was lower in NAFLD with diabetes group as compared to the control group. Even though median values of the overall variability of HRV were lower in NAFLD group without diabetes as compared to controls, the difference was not statistically significant. Similarly, the overall variability of NAFLD with diabetes was not statistically different from NAFLD without diabetes even though the median values were lower. The low frequency and high frequency component of HRV and the LF : HF ratio were similar in all three groups. In time domain analysis, the indices of parasympathetic component of HRV (SDSD and pNN50) were lower in NAFLD with diabetes group as compared to controls as well as NAFLD without diabetes.

The proportional distribution of Grade I and Grade II was not different in the NAFLD groups with or without diabetes. The subjects were regrouped depending upon the grades of NAFLD irrespective of their diabetic status and statistical analysis was done (Table 3). The distribution of diabetics in NAFLD Grade I and Grade II was not statistically different. The indices of overall variability (SDNN and total power) and parasympathetic component (SDSD, pNN50) were lower in Grade II as compared to controls. Even though the median values of the same parameters were lower in Grade I when compared with controls, it was not statistically significant.

In order to delineate the relative contribution of the diabetic status and grade of NAFLD, two-way ANOVA was done on all the NAFLD subjects. The presence of diabetes was found to be significantly associated with decrease in SDSD and total power (Table 4).

*3.3. Association between Indices of HRV and Anthropometric and Biochemical Parameters.* The result of Spearman's correlation performed between the selected indices of HRV (SDNN, SDSD, and total power) and anthropometric and biochemical parameters is shown in Table 5. No significant association was found between indices of HRV, parameters of inflammation (ESR, hsCRP), liver function (serum bilirubin, SGOT, SGPT, and ALP), or insulin resistance (HOMA-IR, fasting insulin). The rest of the parameters were negatively correlated with the indices of HRV.

A further multivariate stepwise regression analysis was performed between indices of HRV as dependent variable and selected independent variables (with significant association in univariate analysis). Table 6 shows the two models. Of all the parameters that were negatively associated with HRV, only total cholesterol (TC) and fat percentage significantly associated with SDNN and total power after multivariate analysis.

## 4. Discussion

The study was done to assess the heart rate variability in patients of NAFLD with or without diabetes. Since diabetes is known to independently cause autonomic dysfunction, the patients of nonalcoholic fatty liver disease were grouped into NAFLD without diabetes and NAFLD with diabetes.

*4.1. Anthropometric Features and Biochemical Profile.* As expected, the variables related to obesity, lipid profile, and glucose metabolism were higher in NAFLD with diabetes and those with Grade II NAFLD as compared to controls [18–20]. A higher ESR in NAFLD with diabetes and higher hsCRP in NAFLD without diabetes indicate ongoing inflammatory process. Similar high hsCRP was reported by Nigam et al. [21] and Ajmal et al. [22], even after adjusting for covariates.

*4.2. Heart Rate Variability (HRV).* The time domain and frequency domain indices of overall variability of HRV were lower in the NAFLD with diabetes group as compared to the control. Even though the median values of these parameters were lower in NAFLD without diabetes, the difference was not significant. The indices of parasympathetic component of HRV (SDNN, pNN50) were lower in NAFLD with diabetes as compared to controls as well as NAFLD without diabetes. When the analysis was done on the basis of grades of NAFLD irrespective of the diabetic status, the indices of overall HRV were found to be lower in Grade II NAFLD as compared to controls. Though the median values of the theses indices

TABLE 1: General, anthropometric, and biochemical parameters of the subjects.

| | Controls | NAFLD without diabetes | NAFLD with diabetes | $p$ value |
|---|---|---|---|---|
| Age (years) | 37.9 ± 8.4 | 41.8 ± 7.3 | 42.9 ± 7.6 | 0.04 |
| NAFLD Grades I, II, and III ($n$) | — | 15, 10, 0 | 16, 8, 1 | 0.62 |
| *Variables related to whole body fat* | | | | |
| BMI ($kg/m^2$) | 24.2 (21.7–26.6) | 27.8* (24.8–31.2) | 27.9* (25.7–30.1) | 0.0001 |
| WHR | 0.95 ± 0.1 | 1.0 ± 0.1* | 1.0 ± 0.1 | 0.052 |
| Fat percentage (%) | 24.0 ± 6.7 | 26.6 ± 7.0 | 31.4 ± 6.2*# | 0.001 |
| Fat mass (kg) | 15.4 ± 5.6 | 20.2 ± 7.5* | 21.7 ± 5.2* | 0.002 |
| *Variables related to inflammation* | | | | |
| ESR (mm/hr) | 12.0 (8.5–19.0) | 18.0 (12.0–28.5) | 20.0* (10.5–33.5) | 0.020 |
| hsCRP (mg/L) | 6.7 (1.5–12.3) | 11.3* (9.6–13.0) | 8.0 (4.0–12.0) | 0.007 |
| *Variables related to liver function* | | | | |
| Bilirubin (mg/dL) | 0.6 (0.4–0.8) | 0.5 (0.4–0.8) | 0.5 (0.3–0.8) | 0.916 |
| SGOT (AST) (IU/L) | 25.0 (21.5–31.0) | 30.0 (22.0–44.5) | 27.0 (22.0–44.5) | 0.354 |
| SGPT (ALT) (IU/L) | 25.0 (18.5–36.0) | 36.0 (23.0–57.0) | 36.0 (23.0–51.5) | 0.111 |
| ALP (IU/L) | 180.0 (158.5–213.5) | 204.0 (165.0–250.0) | 189.0 (154.0–229.5) | 0.545 |
| *Variables related to lipid profile* | | | | |
| TG (mg/dL) | 132.0 (81.0–173.5) | 140.0 (98.5–222.0) | 161.0 (115.5–201.5) | 0.228 |
| TC (mg/dL) | 168.0 (144.0–196.5) | 191.0 (162.5–235.5) | 218.0* (171.5–230.0) | 0.005 |
| LDL (mg/dL) | 100.0 (82.5–126.0) | 117.0 (99.0–138.0) | 134.00* (102.0–148.5) | 0.009 |
| HDL (mg/dL) | 44.0 (40.5–49.5) | 45.0 (40.5–47.5) | 46.0 (41.0–53.5) | 0.423 |
| VLDL (mg/dL) | 20.0 (16.0–26.5) | 30.0* (19.5–42.0) | 32.0* (23.5–43.5) | 0.003 |
| *Variables related to diabetic status* | | | | |
| FBG (mg/dL) | 89.0 (86.0–95.0) | 97.0 (90.5–101.0) | 118.0*# (109.5–164.0) | 0.0001 |
| PPBG (mg/dL) | 119.0 (104.0–128.0) | 129.0 (118.5–142.0) | 179.0*# (154.5–218.5) | 0.0001 |
| Fasting insulin ($\mu$IU/mL) | 10.5 (5.9–17.2) | 15.6 (5.4–20.7) | 11.4 (10.0–17.2) | 0.323 |
| HOMA-IR | 2.0 (1.3–4.0) | 3.8 (1.3–5.1) | 3.8*# (2.6–5.5) | 0.0001 |

Values are expressed as median (IQR) or mean ± SD; *significant versus control; #significant versus NAFLD without diabetes.
BMI: Body Mass Index; WHR: Waist Hip Ratio; ESR: Erythrocyte Sedimentation Rate; hsCRP: High-Sensitivity C Reactive Protein; SGOT: Serum Glutamic Oxaloacetic Transaminase; AST: Aspartate Transaminase; SGPT: Serum Glutamate Pyruvate Transaminase; ALT: Alanine Transaminase; ALP: Alkaline Phosphatase; IU: International Unit; TG: Triglycerides; TC: total cholesterol; LDL: Low Density Lipoprotein; HDL: High Density Lipoprotein; VLDL: Very Low Density Lipoprotein; FBG: fasting blood glucose; PPBG: postprandial blood glucose; HOMA-IR: Homeostatic Model Assessment for Insulin Resistance.

Table 2: Time domain and frequency domain indices of HRV in the study population.

| | Controls | NAFLD without diabetes | NAFLD with diabetes | $p$ value |
|---|---|---|---|---|
| *Time domain indices* | | | | |
| SDNN (ms) | 40.7 (24.6–61.5) | 30.2 (15.5–47.8) | 22.2* (17.59–28.2) | 0.006 |
| SDSD (ms) | 24.2 (17.3–43.2) | 25.9 (8.8–36.8) | 13.5*# (9.36–19.6) | 0.009 |
| pNN50 (%) | 0.04 (0.00–0.22) | 0.04 (0.00–0.16) | 0.00*# (0.00–0.01) | 0.008 |
| *Frequency domain indices* | | | | |
| LF nu | 40.2 (33.4–53.6) | 41.9 (27.1–52.3) | 37.8 (23.9–53.2) | 0.855 |
| HF nu | 29.2 (18.4–43.9) | 26.8 (15.6–36.3) | 19.7 (15.5–38.9) | 0.575 |
| LF : HF ratio | 1.5 (1.0–2.6) | 1.6 (1.0–2.2) | 1.6 (0.9–2.9) | 0.843 |
| Total power ($ms^2$) | 1166.5 (383.5–2312.6) | 658.4 (202.9–1379.2) | 310.6* (173.3–545.4) | 0.005 |

Values are expressed as median (IQR); *significant versus control; #significant versus NAFLD without diabetes.
SDNN: standard deviation of all NN intervals; SDSD: standard deviation of differences between adjacent NN intervals; pNN50%: NN50 count divided by the total number of all NN intervals; LF: low frequency (0.04–0.15 Hz); HF: high frequency (0.15–0.40 Hz); nu: normalized unit.

Table 3: Time domain and frequency domain indices of HRV in controls, Grade I and Grade II NAFLD.

| | Controls ($n = 25$) | Grade I ($n = 31$) | Grade II ($n = 18$) | $p$ value |
|---|---|---|---|---|
| Diabetics ($n$, %) | — | 16, 51.6% | 8, 44.4% | 0.62 |
| *Time domain indices* | | | | |
| SDNN (ms) | 40.7 (24.6–61.5) | 28.3 (19.5–46.3) | 21.2* (14.7–26.0) | 0.010 |
| SDSD (ms) | 24.2 (17.3–43.2) | 18.8 (12.4–29.8) | 12.2* (9.1–28.4) | 0.026 |
| pNN50 (%) | 0.04 (0.00–0.22) | 0.01 (0.00–0.07) | 0.00* (0.00–0.01) | 0.016 |
| *Frequency domain indices* | | | | |
| LF nu | 40.2 (33.4–53.6) | 37.8 (27.1–53.3) | 44.5 (20.1–50.0) | 0.435 |
| HF nu | 29.2 (18.4–43.9) | 19.7 (14.9–37.9) | 23.1 (19.3–35.8) | 0.650 |
| LF : HF ratio | 1.5 (0.9–3.0) | 1.6 (0.9–3.4) | 1.4 (0.8–2.7) | 0.804 |
| Total power ($ms^2$) | 1166.5 (383.5–2312.6) | 515.0 (271.1–1374.3) | 255.1* (157.5–382.6) | 0.006 |

Values are expressed as median (IQR); *significant versus control.
SDNN: standard deviation of all NN intervals; SDSD: standard deviation of differences between adjacent NN intervals; pNN50%: NN50 count divided by the total number of all NN intervals; LF: low frequency (0.04–0.15 Hz); HF: high frequency (0.15–0.40 Hz); nu: normalized unit.

were lower in Grade I NAFLD they were not statistically significant. This indicates an independent contribution of diabetic status as well as grade of NAFLD in development of autonomic dysfunction. Within the patients of NAFLD, the diabetic status had significant main effect in decreasing HRV rather than the grade.

Similar decrease in indices of overall HRV (Ln SDNN) and parasympathetic components (Ln RMSSD) was noted by Liu et al. [23]. In the present study, no change in normalized low frequency, high frequency, or their ratio was found. Liu et al., however, have reported lower low frequency and high frequency components of HRV [14, 23]. This difference is

TABLE 4: Two-way ANOVA for determination of main effect of diabetic status, NAFLD grade, and their interaction.

| | Presence of diabetes | NAFLD grade | Interaction between diabetes and NAFLD grade |
|---|---|---|---|
| SDNN | 0.054 | 0.140 | 0.461 |
| SDSD | 0.009* | 0.817 | 0.201 |
| Total power | 0.001* | 0.903 | 0.902 |

*Significant.

likely due to reporting absolute values rather than normalizing the values to total power of the HRV as was done in the present study. The data of the present study suggests that decrease in total power of HRV results from a decrease in both sympathetic and parasympathetic components. In the presence of diabetes, the decrease in the parasympathetic component is more [24]. Jakovljevic et al. had reported higher values of LF : HF ratio though it had not been compared with any control group. In the present study LF : HF ratio was similar in NAFLD with or without diabetes as compared to controls. This difference could be due to inclusion of diabetics with less 5 years of history as well as lower BMI of the study subjects in the present study as compared to the report by Jakovljevic et al. [15].

In univariate analysis, the decrease in indices of HRV was significantly and negatively correlated with variables of lipid profile, obesity, and diabetic status. Interestingly, the decrease in HRV was not associated either with HOMA-IR or with fasting insulin but with fasting blood and post-prandial glucose level. These observations are in tune with the known role blood glucose level and glycation play in the pathogenesis of diabetic autonomic neuropathy [25]. However, in multivariate stepwise regression analysis, indices of HRV were negatively associated with total cholesterol and fat percentage only. The importance of total serum cholesterol in the development of diabetic autonomic neuropathy has also been reported earlier [26]. These observations are similar to a report by Pimenta et al. where the autonomic control in NAFLD (measured by heart rate recovery after maximum graded exercise test) correlated with body composition and body fat [27]. In a recent review, importance of hepatic accumulation of fat in a setting of obesity for the development of hepatic/peripheral insulin resistance has been proposed [20]. NAFLD and diabetes then independently lead to the development of cardiac autonomic dysfunction.

The observation of importance of diabetic status in decrease in overall HRV is in line with observations of increase prevalence of cardiovascular disease in NAFLD with diabetes [28–30]. A recent systematic review of 27 studies showed an association of NAFLD with subclinical atherosclerosis independent of traditional risk factors and metabolic syndrome [10]. In other clinical settings, it has been shown that arterial stiffness is inversely related to heart rate variability [12, 13]. It is probable that increase in stiffness of arteries due to subclinical atherosclerosis leads to decrease in the transducer function of the baroreceptors. A lower baroreflex sensitivity in NAFLD has been reported in a single study [15]. A decrease in baroreflex function will decrease the heart rate variability of both sympathetic and parasympathetic components.

## 5. Conclusion

The result of the present study indicates that the grade of NAFLD as well as diabetic status contributes to the decrease in the cardiovascular autonomic function with a decrease in overall variability but an unchanged sympathovagal balance. It also shows that once NAFLD is developed a further decrease is more likely due to diabetes rather than further increase in the grade of NAFLD and the important role of dyslipidemia and obesity in the cardiac autonomic dysfunction represented by heart rate variability.

## Abbreviations

ANOVA: Analysis of variance
ALP: Alkaline Phosphatase
ALT: Alanine Transaminase
AST: Aspartate Transaminase
BMI: Body Mass Index
ESR: Erythrocyte Sedimentation Rate
FBG: Fasting blood glucose
FFT: Fast Fourier Transformation
HC: Hip circumference
HDL: High Density Lipoprotein
HF: High frequency (0.15–0.40 Hz)
HOMA-IR: Homeostatic Model Assessment for Insulin Resistance
HRV Heart rate variability
hsCRP: High-Sensitivity C Reactive Protein
IQR: Interquartile range.

*Reactive Protein*

IU: International Unit
LDL: Low Density Lipoprotein
LF: Low frequency (0.04–0.15 Hz)
NAFLD: Nonalcoholic fatty liver disease
nu: Normalized unit
pNN50%: NN50 count divided by the total number of all NN intervals
PPBG: Postprandial blood glucose
PSD: Power spectral density
SDNN: Standard deviation of all NN intervals
SDSD: Standard deviation of differences between adjacent NN intervals
SGOT: Serum Glutamic Oxaloacetic Transaminase
SGPT: Serum Glutamate Pyruvate Transaminase
T2DM: Type 2 diabetes mellitus
TC: Total cholesterol
TG: Triglycerides
VLDL: Very Low Density Lipoprotein
WC: Waist circumference
WHR: Waist Hip Ratio.

TABLE 5: Linear correlation analysis between the indices of HRV (dependent) and independent variables.

| | SDNN | | SDSD | | Total power | |
|---|---|---|---|---|---|---|
| | $R$ | $p$ value | $R$ | $p$ value | $R$ | $p$ value |
| Age (yr) | −0.242* | 0.046 | −0.301* | 0.013 | −0.212 | 0.083 |
| *Variable related to whole body fat* | | | | | | |
| BMI (kg/m$^2$) | −0.391* | 0.001 | −0.255* | 0.036 | −0.401* | 0.001 |
| WHR | −0.071 | 0.563 | 0.004 | 0.976 | −0.106 | 0.391 |
| Fat percentage (%) | −0.302* | 0.012 | −0.204 | 0.095 | −0.309* | 0.010 |
| Fat Mass (kg) | −0.319* | 0.008 | −0.220 | 0.071 | −0.333* | 0.006 |
| *Variable related to inflammation* | | | | | | |
| ESR (mm/hr) | −0.085 | 0.493 | −0.002 | 0.986 | −0.083 | 0.501 |
| hsCRP (mg/L) | −0.139 | 0.258 | −0.130 | 0.292 | −0.149 | 0.226 |
| *Variable related to liver function* | | | | | | |
| Bilirubin (mg/dL) | −0.033 | 0.788 | −0.067 | 0.590 | −0.026 | 0.833 |
| SGOT (AST) (IU/L) | 0.117 | 0.344 | 0.137 | 0.265 | 0.062 | 0.615 |
| SGPT (ALT) (IU/L) | 0.007 | 0.955 | 0.035 | 0.779 | −0.041 | 0.739 |
| ALP (IU/L) | −0.137 | 0.266 | −0.103 | 0.405 | −0.137 | 0.266 |
| *Variable related to lipid profile* | | | | | | |
| TG (mg/dL) | −0.240* | 0.048 | −0.178 | 0.147 | −0.281* | 0.020 |
| TC (mg/dL) | −0.405* | 0.001 | −0.301* | 0.013 | −0.390* | 0.001 |
| LDL (mg/dL) | −0.359* | 0.003 | −0.286* | 0.018 | −0.333* | 0.006 |
| HDL (mg/dL) | −0.081 | 0.512 | 0.001 | 0.995 | −0.051 | 0.678 |
| VLDL (mg/dL) | −0.368* | 0.002 | −0.270* | 0.026 | −0.401* | 0.001 |
| *Variables related to diabetic status* | | | | | | |
| FBG (mg/dL) | −0.493* | 0.000 | −0.414* | 0.000 | −0.442* | 0.000 |
| PPBG (mg/dL) | −0.474* | 0.000 | −0.451* | 0.000 | −0.511* | 0.000 |
| Fasting insulin ($\mu$IU/mL) | −0.097 | 0.431 | −0.020 | 0.873 | −0.088 | 0.475 |
| HOMA-IR score | −0.225 | 0.065 | −0.150 | 0.223 | −0.200 | 0.102 |

*Significant.
BMI: Body Mass Index; WHR: Waist Hip Ratio; ESR: Erythrocyte Sedimentation Rate; hsCRP: High-Sensitivity C Reactive Protein; SGOT: Serum Glutamic Oxaloacetic Transaminase; AST: Aspartate Transaminase; SGPT: Serum Glutamate Pyruvate Transaminase; ALT: Alanine Transaminase; ALP: Alkaline Phosphatase; IU: International Unit; TG: Triglycerides; TC: total cholesterol; LDL: Low Density Lipoprotein; HDL: High Density Lipoprotein; VLDL: Very Low Density Lipoprotein; FBG: fasting blood glucose; PPBG: postprandial blood glucose; HOMA-IR: Homeostatic Model Assessment for Insulin Resistance.

TABLE 6: Stepwise multivariate regression analysis of the indices of HRV with independent variables.

| | SDNN | | SDSD | | Total power | |
|---|---|---|---|---|---|---|
| | Beta | $p$ value | Beta | $p$ value | Beta | $p$ value |
| Model 1 | | | | | | |
| TC | −0.482 | 0.0001 | −0.329 | 0.006 | −0.422 | 0.0001 |
| Model 2 | | | | | | |
| TC | −0.428 | 0.0001 | | | −0.369 | 0.001 |
| Fat% | −0.268 | 0.014 | | | −0.262 | 0.020 |

TC: total cholesterol.

## Additional Points

*Strengths and Limitations.* The present study is first study on effect of grade and diabetic status of NAFLD on heart rate variability. The exclusion of subjects with duration longer than 5 years of diabetes provides a suitable group to elucidate the contribution of diabetic status. A limitation of the study is that it is cross-sectional in design with number not sufficient to have subgroup analysis based on Grade I with or without diabetes and Grade II with or without diabetes. A prospective design with long term follow-up can further establish the observation of the present study.

## Competing Interests

Authors declare no conflict of interests.

## Acknowledgments

The authors are thankful to Dr. Surya Prakash for his assistance in performing anthropometric and biochemical measurements. The cooperation of subjects who agreed to participate in this study is highly appreciated.

## References

[1] G. C. Farrell, V. W.-S. Wong, and S. Chitturi, "NAFLD in Asia—as common and important as in the West," *Nature Reviews*

*Gastroenterology and Hepatology*, vol. 10, no. 5, pp. 307–318, 2013.

[2] S. A. Harrison and C. P. Day, "Benefits of lifestyle modification in NAFLD," *Gut*, vol. 56, no. 12, pp. 1760–1790, 2007.

[3] M. Stepanova and Z. M. Younossi, "Independent association between nonalcoholic fatty liver disease and cardiovascular disease in the us population," *Clinical Gastroenterology and Hepatology*, vol. 10, no. 6, pp. 646–650, 2012.

[4] M. Hamaguchi, T. Kojima, N. Takeda et al., "Nonalcoholic fatty liver disease is a novel predictor of cardiovascular disease," *World Journal of Gastroenterology*, vol. 13, no. 10, pp. 1579–1584, 2007.

[5] H. Lu, L. Zeng, B. Liang, X. Shu, and D. Xie, "High prevalence of coronary heart disease in type 2 diabetic patients with non-alcoholic fatty liver disease," *Archives of Medical Research*, vol. 40, no. 7, pp. 571–575, 2009.

[6] C. Cailotto, C. Van Heijningen, J. Van Der Vliet et al., "Daily rhythms in metabolic liver enzymes and plasma glucose require a balance in the autonomic output to the liver," *Endocrinology*, vol. 149, no. 4, pp. 1914–1925, 2008.

[7] E. Sabath, A. Báez-Ruiz, and R. M. Buijs, "Non-alcoholic fatty liver disease as a consequence of autonomic imbalance and circadian desynchronization," *Obesity Reviews*, vol. 16, no. 10, pp. 871–882, 2015.

[8] J. L. Newton, J. Pairman, K. Wilton, D. E. J. Jones, and C. Day, "Fatigue and autonomic dysfunction in non-alcoholic fatty liver disease," *Clinical Autonomic Research*, vol. 19, no. 6, pp. 319–326, 2009.

[9] W. Sun, D. Zhang, J. Sun et al., "Association between non-alcoholic fatty liver disease and autonomic dysfunction in a Chinese population," *QJM*, vol. 108, no. 8, pp. 617–624, 2015.

[10] E. T. Oni, A. S. Agatston, M. J. Blaha et al., "A systematic review: burden and severity of subclinical cardiovascular disease among those with nonalcoholic fatty liver; Should we care?" *Atherosclerosis*, vol. 230, no. 2, pp. 258–267, 2013.

[11] M. L. Thakur, S. Sharma, A. Kumar et al., "Nonalcoholic fatty liver disease is associated with subclinical atherosclerosis independent of obesity and metabolic syndrome in Asian Indians," *Atherosclerosis*, vol. 223, no. 2, pp. 507–511, 2012.

[12] M. Kaur, D. Chandran, C. Lal et al., "Renal transplantation normalizes baroreflex sensitivity through improvement in central arterial stiffness," *Nephrology Dialysis Transplantation*, vol. 28, no. 10, pp. 2645–2655, 2013.

[13] E. R. Carthy, "Autonomic dysfunction in essential hypertension: a systematic review," *Annals of Medicine and Surgery*, vol. 3, no. 1, pp. 2–7, 2014.

[14] Y.-C. Liu, C.-S. Hung, Y.-W. Wu et al., "Influence of non-alcoholic fatty liver disease on autonomic changes evaluated by the time domain, frequency domain, and symbolic dynamics of heart rate variability," *PLoS ONE*, vol. 8, no. 4, article e61803, 2013.

[15] D. G. Jakovljevic, K. Hallsworth, P. Zalewski et al., "Resistance exercise improves autonomic regulation at rest and haemodynamic response to exercise in non-alcoholic fatty liver disease," *Clinical Science*, vol. 125, no. 3, pp. 143–149, 2013.

[16] M. Kuehl and M. J. Stevens, "Cardiovascular autonomic neuropathies as complications of diabetes mellitus," *Nature Reviews Endocrinology*, vol. 8, no. 7, pp. 405–416, 2012.

[17] J. M. Hazlehurst, C. Woods, T. Marjot, J. F. Cobbold, and J. W. Tomlinson, "Non-alcoholic fatty liver disease and diabetes," *Metabolism*, vol. 65, no. 8, pp. 1096–1108, 2016.

[18] M. R. Souza, M. D. Diniz, J. E. Medeiros-Filho, and M. S. Araújo, "Metabolic syndrome and risk factors for non-alcoholic fatty liver disease," *Arquivos de Gastroenterologia*, vol. 49, no. 1, pp. 89–96, 2012.

[19] M. Gaggini, M. Morelli, E. Buzzigoli, R. A. DeFronzo, E. Bugianesi, and A. Gastaldelli, "Non-alcoholic fatty liver disease (NAFLD) and its connection with insulin resistance, dyslipidemia, atherosclerosis and coronary heart disease," *Nutrients*, vol. 5, no. 5, pp. 1544–1560, 2013.

[20] C. D. Byrne and G. Targher, "NAFLD: a multisystem disease," *Journal of Hepatology*, vol. 62, no. 1, pp. S47–S64, 2015.

[21] P. Nigam, S. P. Bhatt, A. Misra, M. Vaidya, J. Dasgupta, and D. S. Chadha, "Non-alcoholic fatty liver disease is closely associated with sub-clinical inflammation: a case-control study on Asian Indians in North India," *PLoS ONE*, vol. 8, no. 1, Article ID e49286, 2013.

[22] M. R. Ajmal, M. Yaccha, M. A. Malik et al., "Prevalence of nonalcoholic fatty liver disease (NAFLD) in patients of cardiovascular diseases and its association with hs-CRP and TNF-$\alpha$," *Indian Heart Journal*, vol. 66, no. 6, pp. 574–579, 2014.

[23] Y. Liu, M. Dai, Y. Bi et al., "Active smoking, passive smoking, and risk of nonalcoholic fatty liver disease (NAFLD): A Population-Based Study in China," *Journal of Epidemiology*, vol. 23, no. 2, pp. 115–121, 2013.

[24] N. Oikawa, M. Umetsu, T. Toyota, and Y. Goto, "Quantitative evaluation of diabetic autonomic neuropathy by using heart rate variations: relationship between cardiac parasympathetic or sympathetic damage and clinical conditions," *Tohoku Journal of Experimental Medicine*, vol. 148, no. 2, pp. 125–133, 1986.

[25] A. Verrotti, G. Loiacono, A. Mohn, and F. Chiarelli, "New insights in diabetic autonomic neuropathy in children and adolescents," *European Journal of Endocrinology*, vol. 161, no. 6, pp. 811–818, 2009.

[26] H. Ueda, N. Kuroda, M. Ogura et al., "Importance of serum cholesterol level in development of diabetic autonomic neuropathy," *Diabetes Research and Clinical Practice*, vol. 21, no. 2-3, pp. 123–126, 1993.

[27] N. M. Pimenta, H. Santa-Clara, H. Cortez-Pinto et al., "Body composition and body fat distribution are related to cardiac autonomic control in non-alcoholic fatty liver disease patients," *European Journal of Clinical Nutrition*, vol. 68, no. 2, pp. 241–246, 2014.

[28] G. Targher, I. Pichiri, G. Zoppini, M. Trombetta, and E. Bonora, "Increased prevalence of cardiovascular disease in type 1 diabetic patients with non-alcoholic fatty liver disease," *Journal of Endocrinological Investigation*, vol. 35, no. 5, pp. 535–540, 2012.

[29] L. H. Yan, B. Mu, Y. Guan et al., "Assessment of the relationship between non-alcoholic fatty liver disease and diabetic complications," *Journal of Diabetes Investigation*, vol. 7, no. 6, pp. 889–894, 2016.

[30] I. S. Idilman, D. Akata, T. Hazirolan, B. Doganay Erdogan, K. Aytemir, and M. Karcaaltincaba, "Nonalcoholic fatty liver disease is associated with significant coronary artery disease in type 2 diabetic patients: A Computed Tomography Angiography Study," *Journal of Diabetes*, vol. 7, no. 2, pp. 279–286, 2015.

# 25

# Relationship between Experimental Diet in Rats and Nonalcoholic Hepatic Disease: Review of Literature

**Ayane A. Rodrigues,[1] Raíssa S. B. Andrade,[2] and Daniel F. P. Vasconcelos[1,2,3]**

[1] *Postgraduate Program in Biomedical Sciences, Federal University of Piaui, Parnaiba, PI, Brazil*
[2] *Postgraduate Program in Biotechnology, Federal University of Piaui, Parniba, PI, Brazil*
[3] *Department of Biomedicine, Federal University of Piaui, Parnaiba, PI, Brazil*

Correspondence should be addressed to Daniel F. P. Vasconcelos; vasconcelos@ufpi.edu.br

Academic Editor: Heather Francis

*Background.* The pathophysiology of nonalcoholic fatty liver disease (NAFLD) is related to unhealthy lifestyles that combine sedentary lifestyle, hypercaloric diets, excessive saturated fats, refined carbohydrates, and high intake of fructose as a food additive to various processed products. Both the broader recognition of the disease and the additional efforts to elucidate the NAFLD pathogenesis have led to an increase in animal models in recent years. *Objective.* This review was performed to provide better understanding of the association between the NAFLD and animal models. *Methods.* The search in the literature occurred before May of 2018 in the PUBMED database. *Results.* Most studies investigating the influence of diet on liver fat content have been performed using a high-calorie diet that leads to a significant increase in fat content in the liver. *Conclusion.* The findings of this review show that diet is one of the factors that predisposes to the appearance of NAFLD and that the studies presented a wide variety of designs.

## 1. Introduction

The prevalence of predictive metabolic diseases, especially dyslipidemias and nonalcoholic fatty liver disease (NAFLD), has increased worldwide [1, 2]. NAFLD and metabolic diseases associated with obesity, diabetes mellitus, and dyslipidemia are a growing public health problem both in the United States and worldwide [3]. The global population is affected by NAFLD with rates between 25% and 30% with higher prevalence in the Middle East and South America. In North America and Europe, a quarter of the adult population is affected by NAFLD [4]. It is a leading cause of liver transplantation and, by 2030, it is predicted to become one of the most common reasons for transplantation in the United States [5].

This pathology has drawn attention in recent years. Diagnosis and assessment of NAFLD can be performed based on physical examination, history of the disease, ultrasound examination, and hepatic imaging [6]. Although other noninvasive tests have been suggested, they must still be validated in large scales [1]. NAFLD presents an episode of variable hepatopathy of simple steatosis to nonalcoholic hepatitis (NASH), which is localized in the presence of hepatitis and inflammation, related to the death of hepatocytes; many patients progress to insufficient fibrosis/cirrhosis and hepatic failure [7]. The NAFLD is diagnosed histologically when > 5% of hepatocytes/field present lipid accumulation. That is the gold standard mean of diagnosis and should be considered in patients with NAFLD who present high risk to have fibrosis and steatohepatitis [8, 9].

The pathophysiology of NAFLD is associated with unhealthy lifestyles, which combine sedentary lifestyle, hypercaloric diets, excessive saturated fat, refined carbohydrates, and high fructose intake as a food additive to various processed products [10, 11].

Although the etiologies of dyslipidemias and NAFLD are complex and multifactorial, these diseases contain an important genetic component that is influenced by environmental factors and life habits, especially the food consumption profile [2, 12].

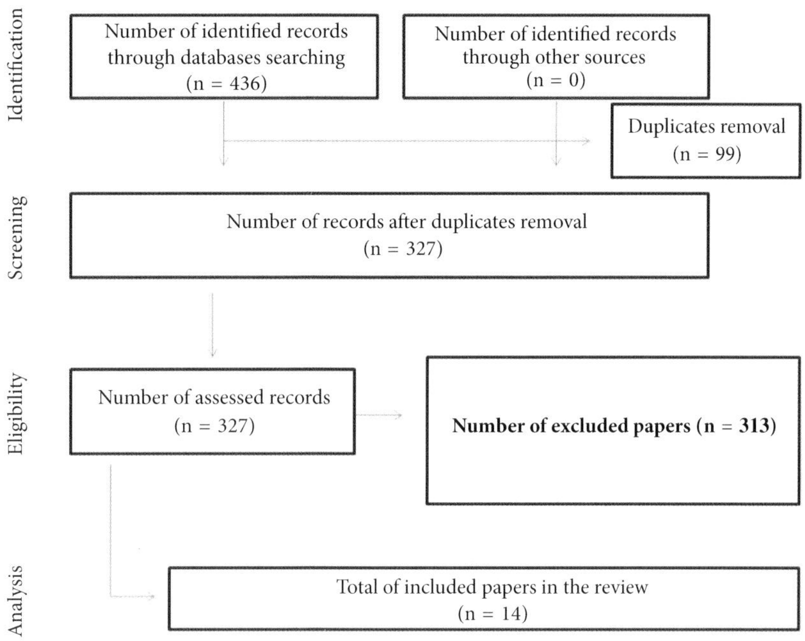


FIGURE 1: Flow diagram for identification, screening, eligibility, and analysis of studies included in the review.

Improved knowledge of the disease and its complementary data to elucidate the NAFLD pathogenesis have led to an increase in the animal models in recent years [13, 14].

Taking into account the increase in studies with NAFLD, the objective of this study was to investigate the different study designs that targeted the diet relationship with the appearance of NAFLD experimentally in rats.

## 2. Materials and Methods

This review was performed according to the PRISMA (Preferred Reporting Items for Systematic Reviews and Meta-Analyses) statement according to Moher et al., 2009 [15].

*2.1. Eligibility Criteria.* For the eligibility of publications, each title and abstract was read exhaustively to confirm whether they addressed the guiding question of this research and whether it would meet the inclusion and exclusion criteria established. Then, the same happened to the stage of inclusion of the articles. The selection of studies is shown in Figure 1. In the identification and screening, the following inclusion criteria were adopted: be available on the electronic address, be free of charge, be fully presented, and be disclosed in English, Portuguese, or Spanish. Investigations that did not present enough information about NAFLD were excluded. In addition, dissertations, theses, reports, news, letters to the editor, and scientific articles not fully available online and those that were repeated in the databases were excluded. Studies that used diet inducing alcoholic liver disease (ALD) were also excluded.

*2.2. Search Strategy.* The following keywords or descriptors were used in the Health Sciences Descriptors (DeCS) of the Virtual Health Library: "NAFLD", "diet", and "rat model".

The search in literature was executed by two investigators in the databases: Cochrane Library, Google Scholar, and PubMed for studies published before 28 Mai 2018 and addressing the NAFLD associated with rat model. The following combined keywords were used to search the literature: ("NAFLD", "diet", and "rat model"). Figure 1 demonstrates the search strategy and details from the review.

## 3. Results

Through the search carried out in PUBMED, 436 articles were found, of which 89 articles were not related to the theme, 8 articles were repeated, 2 articles were not available, 2 articles were excluded due to the used diet, which induces alcoholic liver disease (ALD) and thus was not the focus of this review, and 313 were related to the subject, but they were testing other compounds. This way, 14 articles were analyzed (Figure 1). Regarding the periodical and language, they were all published in international journals with English language.

As for the articles discussing diet and the onset of NAFLD, 1 used the iron-fructose-enriched diet (Ackerman et al., 2005) [15]; 2 induced steatohepatitis through the diet deficient in methionine-choline (Kirsch et al., 2003; Wu et al., 2011) [16, 21]; 1 used the high-fat diet associated with sucrose (Torres-Vilalobos et al., 2015) [23]; 1 used the high-fat, fructose, and high-fat diets associated with fructose (Lee et al., 2015) [24]; 2 used the high-fat diet (Zou et al., 2006; McDonald, 2011) [17, 20]; 2 used a high-fat and a methionine-deficient diet (Xu et al., 2010; De Lima, 2008) [18, 19]; 1 used rich diet and fat and diet deficient in methionine and choline (Han et al., 2017) [28]; 4 reviewed experimental models that induce NAFLD (Kucera, Cervinkova, 2014; Eslamparast et al., 2017; Goossens, 2017; Mikhail et al., 2017) [22, 25–27]. The respective data are presented in Table 1.

Table 1: Characteristics of the studies included in this study.

| Authors and year of publication | Title of the article | Objective | Diet model | Results |
|---|---|---|---|---|
| Kirsch et al., 2003 [16] | Nutritional model of non-alcoholic steatohepatitis: species studies, strains and sex differences | To investigate the differences between species, lineages, and sex in the nutritional model of diet deficient in methionine choline to induce nonalcoholic steatohepatitis (NASH). | They were fed with a diet deficient in methionine and choline; the control group received an identical diet to which choline bitartrate (2 g / kg) and DL-methionine (3 g / kg) were added. | The present study has demonstrated profound species, strain, and sex differences in the MCD nutritional model of NASH. |
| Ackerman et al., 2005 [15] | Hepatic Effects of Blood Pressure and Reduction of Plasma Triglycerides | To characterize hepatic pathology and function, hepatic lipid composition and hepatic iron concentration, and fasting plasma insulin changes occurring in rats as a result of the fructose-enriched diet, with and without therapeutic maneuvers to reduce blood pressure and plasma triglycerides. | Diet enriched with fructose (as supplied by Harlan Teklad) 20.7% (by weight basis) of protein (as casein), 5% fat (as lard), 60% carbohydrates (as fructose), 8% cellulose, 5% mineral blend, and 1% blend of vitamins. This diet contains 50 mg of iron in 1 kg of diet. For 5 weeks. | This study demonstrates that the model of fructose-treated rats can be a suitable model for studying various aspects of human NAFLD. |
| Zou. et al., 2006 [17] | High-fat emulsion-induced rat model of non-alcoholic steatohepatitis | The objective of the present study is to produce a practical and repetitive experimental rat model for steatohepatitis by designing a high-fat emulsion containing high fat, sucrose, and protein. | The rats were divided into normal control group (NC group) and hyperlipid emulsion model group (HF group). All rats received standard ration and water. In addition, they had free access to a sucrose solution (18%). Model mice were orally treated with the high-fat emulsion (10 ml / kg) once daily. For 6 weeks. | A new rat model of steatohepatitis was established. This model provides new opportunities to study the pathogenesis and treatment. |
| De Lima et al., 2008 [18] | A model of NASH rodents with cirrhosis, oval cell proliferation and hepatocellular carcinoma | Produce a mouse model of NASH, cirrhosis, and HCC. | Diet rich in fat (35% total fat, 54% trans fatty acid) and choline-deficient for 16 weeks | Our initial experience with this model demonstrates the development of histological NASH with cirrhosis, oval cell proliferation, and CK 19 positive hepatocellular carcinoma. |
| Xu et al., 2009 [19] | Characterization of High-Fat, Diet-Induced, Non-alcoholic Steatohepatitis with Fibrosis in Rats | Create a new NASH model by feeding animals on a high-fat diet (DHC), with a hope of reproduction as key features of human NASH for future research. | DHC was composed of the following energy sources: 52% were provided by carbohydrates, 30% by fat, and 18% by protein (total calories: 4.8 kcal/g). Comparison with the diet deficient in methionine-choline. | In conclusion, we created a practically simple but accurate rat NASH model. It reproduced the pathological sequence of events typical of human NASH. |

Table 1: Continued.

| Authors and year of publication | Title of the article | Objective | Diet model | Results |
|---|---|---|---|---|
| McDonald et al., 2011 [20] | Adverse metabolic effects of a high-calorie, high-fat diet (HFD) in rodents precede observable changes in body weight | The specific objective was to determine the impact of a lifetime exposure to a hypercaloric, DH on adiposity, its distribution, and its glycemic control markers | Hyperlipid diet with 5% fat energy in the control group and a hypercaloric diet, rich in 41% fat, for 39 weeks. | In conclusion, after only 4 weeks, animals fed on a HFD from weaning had increased intra-abdominal fat, which preceded an increase in overall body weight and was accompanied by metabolic abnormalities including high TG and hyperglycemia in response to a glucose challenge. |
| Wu et al., 2011[21] | Hepatic steatosis: an experimental model for quantification | Introduce an experimental method to quantify hepatic steatosis in rats and provide an alternative experimental model in the following studies. | Two groups fed with commercial diet and choline/methionine deficient-diet (DMC) for two weeks. | By this model, researchers can directly measure the degree of steatosis with a lesser concern about heterogeneous fatty infiltration and provide a continuous but not categorical measurement of hepatic steatosis. |
| Kucera, Cervinkova, 2014 [22] | Experimental models of non-alcoholic fatty liver disease in rats | This article reviews the widely used experimental models of NAFLD in rats. We discuss the nutritional, genetic, and combined models of NAFLD and its pros and cons. | Diets high in fat; diet rich in fructose/sucrose; diet deficient in methionine and choline; atherogenic diets; genetic and combined models. | Although there is no ideal model for human nonalcoholic fatty liver disease that reflects all the clinical aspects of human disease, choosing an appropriate model for studying particular events of NAFLD while respecting its limitations has contributed greatly to the understanding of this disease and its progression and treatment. |
| Torres-Vilalobos G, et al., 2015[23] | High-fat combined diet and sustained high sucrose consumption promotes NAFLD | To evaluate the impact of 4 different diets on the production of NAFLD with emphasis on a high combined consumption of high fat and sustained sucrose. | (1) Control diet. (2) High fat and cholesterol + 5% sucrose diet in drinking water. (3) High-fat corn starch diet + 5% sucrose in drinking water. (4) Food diet + 20% sucrose in drinking water for 90 days. | The HFC diet with combination of high fat and high sucrose is more effective in producing NAFLD compared with a high-sucrose diet only. |
| Lee et al., 2015 [24] | Histological and Metabolic Breakdown in high-fat, high-fructose and combined dietary animal models | To evaluate and compare the differences in the induction of histological and metabolic characteristics induced by the combined diets to characterize the resulting NAFLD and NASH mouse models. | G1: normal ration, G2: hyperlipid diet fed on high-fat diet (60% total calories), G3: high fructose (30% fructose in drinking water), G4: high fat + high fructose combination (60% fat + 20% fructose) for 20 weeks. | Intrahepatic inflammation and metabolic derangements were more prominent in the HF and HFr combination model than in the HF monodiet model. |

Table 1: Continued.

| Authors and year of publication | Title of the article | Objective | Diet model | Results |
|---|---|---|---|---|
| Mikhail et al., 2017 [25] | Animal Models of Non-Alcoholic Fatty Liver Disease - A Beginner's Guide | This review provides a brief overview of the most commonly used animal models in NDFL research and maternal health care, following the broader maritime guidance model, focusing on the key phenotypic characteristics of each model. | Diet deficient in methionine and choline; diet deficient in hill-deficient L-amino acids; atherogenic diet; fructose; high-fat diet, variations in high-fat diet. | This review presents a brief overview of these models with a particular focus on the basic mechanisms and physical, biochemical, and histological phenotypes. |
| Eslamparast et al., 2017 [26] | Independent dietary weight loss composition in the treatment of non-alcoholic fatty liver disease | Literature review evaluating the evidence behind dietary components, including meat, omega-3-rich diets, and depending on more evidence, we agree with the EASL-EASO Clinical Guidelines recommendation of the Mediterranean diet as the diet of choice in these patients. | Dietary Approach to Stop Hypertension (DASH) is a plant-rich dietary standard, Fiber Intervention (Soluble, Prebiotic), Omega-3 Intervention, Low Fat Interventions vs. Low-CHO, probiotics. | At this time, we do not have a definitive answer for the optimal proportions of total macronutrients (CHO, fat, and protein) in the diet of NAFLD patients. |
| Goossens, Jornayvaz, 2017 [27] | Translational aspects of diet and non-alcoholic fatty liver disease | Discuss some key questions of the translational aspects of NAFLD research from the perspective of nutrition and dietary interventions, literature review. | High-fat, methionine-deficient diet; high cholesterol; high fructose and ketogenic content. | NAFLD is a complex disease with an increasing epidemiology. Currently, no specific therapeutic alternative has been developed, partly due to the lack of robust reproducible dietary animal models of the disease. |
| Han et al., 2017 [28] | Distinction of the Metabolic Profile of the Progression of Non-Alcoholic Fatty Liver Disease from a Common Mouse Model | Perform complete metabolomic analyses on liver samples to determine which pathways are more markedly altered in the human condition and compare these changes with nonalcoholic fatty liver (NAFLD) models. | Alternately, the rats were fed on high-fat diet (high cholesterol, 18% butterfat) or methionine-choline deficient diet for eight weeks. | These results indicate that metabolites of specific pathways may be useful biomarkers for NASH progression, although these markers may not correspond to rodents. |

Dietary models are considered more similar to human metabolic diseases, but there are no standard composition and duration for these diets today: high-fat diets range from 30% to 60% fat content, including saturated fat, monounsaturated fatty acids, and polyunsaturated fatty acids, and last from a few days (short term) to more than a week (long term) [29]. In addition, theoretically composed diets of identical fat types can produce different results and data are often difficult to compare due to uncontrollable differences between primary fat sources and diet preparation [30].

It was observed that most articles found in the literature were related to the subject, but the studies used animal diet models to induce NAFLD in order to test compounds that interfere in the progression of the disease.

Ackerman et al. (2005) [15] demonstrated that the model of fructose-treated rats may be a suitable model for studying various aspects of human NAFLD, especially if it is associated with iron, since it generates an increase in liver fibrosis. This model contained 20.7% protein, 5% fat, 60% carbohydrate (fructose), 8% cellulose, 5% mineral blend, and 1% vitamin blend, combined with 50 mg of iron for each 1 kg diet during 5-week period. The model of fructose-iron showed evidence of mild to moderate deposition of macrovesicular and microvesicular fat with minimal signs of perisinusoidal fibrosis in 3 of 12 rats.

De Lima et al. (2008) [18] proposed a diet rich in fat (35% total fat, 54% transfatty acid) and choline-deficient for 16 weeks. This model demonstrated the development of histological NASH with cirrhosis, oval cell proliferation, and CK 19 positive hepatocellular carcinoma. In 2009, Xu et al. [19] tested a high-fat diet in rats and serum levels of glucose, triglyceride, cholesterol, alanine aminotransferase (ALT), free fatty acids (FFA), insulin, and tumor necrosis factor-alpha (TNF-alpha) were determined. Hepatic histology was also examined by H&E stain. The liver weight and liver index increased within one month, when hepatic steatosis was also observed. By month 2, the body weight and epididymal fat weight started increasing, which was associated with increased serum levels of FFA, cholesterol, and TNF-alpha, as well as development of fatty liver. The serum ALT level increased from month 3 on. Steatohepatitis occurred after three months. Thus, this model is recommended for the study of NASH and its implications.

The study by Wu et al. (2011) [21] and later Han et al. (2017) [28] used a diet deficient in choline/methionine (methionine 0.15%, choline 20 ppm, and 12% lipid component) for 2 weeks and concluded that researchers can directly measure the degree of steatosis with less concern about heterogeneous fatty infiltration and, moreover, provide a continuous, but not categorical, measure of hepatic steatosis.

The diet deficient in methionine and choline (MCD) in the study by Kirsch et al. (2003) [16] was composed of 2 g/kg of choline and 3 g/kg of methionine for 4 weeks. The research demonstrated profound differences between species, lineages, and sex in the nutritional model of MCD of NASH. From the groups studied, C57/BL6 male mice developed the histological characteristics that most resemble those observed in human NASH.

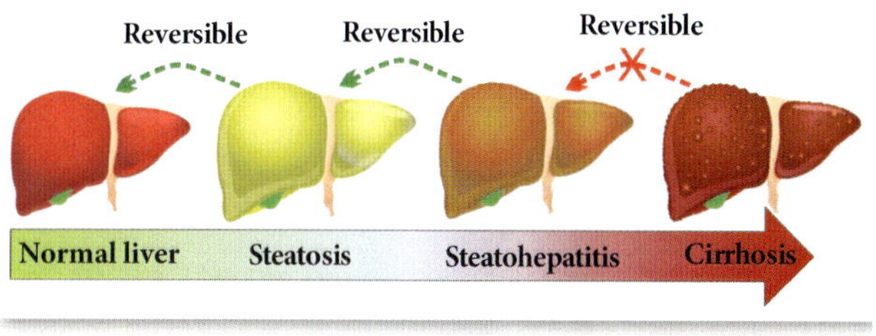


Figure 2: The progression of nonalcoholic fatty liver disease (NAFLD).

According to McDonald et al. (2011) [20], the high-calorie, high-fat diet with 41% fat energy was able to increase intra-abdominal fat, which preceded an increase in total body weight and was accompanied by metabolic abnormalities, including elevated triglyceride level and hyperglycemia in response to a glucose challenge.

Zou et al. (2006) [17] also stated that the hypercaloric diet model (77% of fat energy, 14% of total milk powder, and 9% of carbohydrates) provides new opportunities to study the pathogenesis and treatment of the metabolic syndrome associated with steatohepatitis, such as obesity, abnormal aminotransferase, hyperlipidemia, hyperinsulinemia, hyperglycemia, and insulin resistance. The progression of NAFLD also must be highlighted, which has potential to advance to steatohepatitis or even cirrhosis, as seen in Figure 2. It was demonstrated that the hypercaloric diet models showed the same metabolic profile observed in humans, such as increased levels of insulin, insulin resistance, hyperglycemia, hyperleptinemia, glucose intolerance, and increased levels of visceral white adipose tissue [17, 31].

The study by Kucera and Cervinkova [22] aimed to review several diets used to develop NAFLD and discuss nutritional, genetic, and combined models of NAFLD, as well as pros and cons. The choice of a suitable animal model for this disease, while respecting its limitations, may help to understand its complex pathogenesis and discover new therapeutic strategies.

In 2015, Torres-Vilalobos et al. [23] aimed to evaluate the impact of four different diets on the production of NAFLD with emphasis on high combined consumption of high fat and sustained sucrose. Their methodology used the following diets: control diet, high-fat, and cholesterol + 5% sucrose diet in drinking water, high-fat corn starch diet + 5% sucrose in drinking water, and food diet + 20% sucrose in drinking water for 90 days. They concluded that the high-fat + cholesterol diet with combination of high fat and high sucrose is more effective in producing NAFLD compared with a high-sucrose diet only.

Lee et al. (2015) [24] observed consequences of high-fat (HF) and high-fructose (HFr) diets in rats. Intrahepatic inflammation and metabolic derangements were more prominent in the HF and HFr combination model than in the HF monodiet model, which shows that a type of sugar aggravates the liver disease when associated with fat.

Eslamparast et al. (2017) [26] proposed in a review that poor dietary composition is an important factor in the progression of NAFLD and proposed that "high-quality healthy diet" improves hepatic steatosis and metabolic dysfunction in patients with NAFLD. They highlighted that most patients with NAFLD follow diets with overconsumption of simple carbohydrates and total and saturated fat, with reduced intake of dietary fiber and omega 3-rich foods.

Studies investigating the influence of diet on liver fat content were performed using a high-calorie diet that leads to a significant increase in liver fat content. DHC is well known to induce some metabolic disorders, and the consequences are completely dependent on the composition and duration of the diet [32, 33].

A broad view of the publications that study the diets used to simulate NAFLD in animals shows a break in nutritional, genetic, and combined diets. Goossens and Jornayvaz [27] describe the nutritional models of NAFLD that tried to mimic the metabolic disorders observed in the disease, as well as the histological alterations in the liver: hyperlipid diet, diet deficient in methionine and choline, high-cholesterol diet, high-fructose diet, ketogenic diet, and other models. Among these diets, Goossens and Jornayvaz [27] described the fat-rich diet model mentioned, tested in male Sprague-Dawley rats by Lieber et al. [34] (71% fat energy, 11% carbohydrate, and 18% protein). They demonstrated the development of steatosis in three weeks associated with insulin resistance and increased fibrogenesis markers. This same study also suggests that the fructose-rich diet model associated or not with the high-fat model induces steatosis over a period of four to eight weeks. DHC is well known to induce some metabolic disorders and the consequences are completely dependent on the composition and duration of the diet [29].

According to Mikhail et al. [25], the chemical models are divided into streptozotocin, carbon tetrachloride, and diethylnitrosamine, while the genetic models are models of diabetes mellitus type 2 and models of atherosclerosis and hepatocellular carcinoma.

These models allow researchers to control, *in vivo*, genetic and environmental factors that may influence the development of the disease and its secondary complications [29], thus obtaining useful information about its management and treatment in humans.

## 4. Conclusion

In conclusion, the findings of this review show that the diet is one of the factors that predisposes to the appearance of NAFLD and that the studies presented a wide variety of designs, with the DHC being the most frequent diets in studies with experimental models of NAFLD. These reinforce that animal diet models are able to mimic the pathophysiological characteristics of NAFLD and are still widely used in research, mainly related to the testing of compounds that interfere with the progression of the disease.

## References

[1] A. R. Araújo, N. Rosso, G. Bedogni, C. Tiribelli, and S. Bellentani, "Global epidemiology of non-alcoholic fatty liver disease/non-alcoholic steatohepatitis: What we need in the future," *Liver International*, vol. 38, pp. 47–51, 2018.

[2] R. W. Schwenk, H. Vogel, and A. Schürmann, "Genetic and epigenetic control of metabolic health," *Molecular Metabolism*, vol. 2, no. 4, pp. 337–347, 2013.

[3] T. Deng, C. J. Lyon, S. Bergin, M. A. Caligiuri, and W. A. Hsueh, "Obesity, inflammation, and cancer," *Annual Review of Pathology: Mechanisms of Disease*, vol. 11, pp. 421–449, 2016.

[4] Y. Fazel, A. B. Koenig, M. Sayiner, Z. D. Goodman, and Z. M. Younossi, "Epidemiology and natural history of non-alcoholic fatty liver disease," *Metabolism - Clinical and Experimental*, vol. 65, no. 8, pp. 1017–1025, 2016.

[5] J. Vizuete, A. Camero, M. Malakouti, K. Garapati, and J. Gutierrez, "Perspectives on Nonalcoholic Fatty Liver Disease: An Overview of Present and Future Therapies," *Journal of Clinical and Translational Hepatology*, vol. 5, no. 1, pp. 67–75, 2017.

[6] J. F. Cobbold, D. Patel, and S. D. Taylor-Robinson, "Assessment of inflammation and fibrosis in non-alcoholic fatty liver disease by imaging-based techniques," *Journal of Gastroenterology and Hepatology*, vol. 27, no. 8, pp. 1281–1292, 2012.

[7] X. Dou, S. Li, and L. Hu, "Glutathione disulfide sensitizes hepatocytes to TNFa-mediated cytotoxicity via IKK-$\beta$ S-glutathionylation: a potential mechanism underlying non-alcoholic fatty liver disease," *Experimental & Molecular Medicine*, vol. 50, no. 7, 2018.

[8] S. Tandra, M. M. Yeh, E. M. Brunt et al., "Presence and significance of microvesicular steatosis in nonalcoholic fatty liver disease," *Journal of Hepatology*, vol. 55, no. 3, pp. 654–659, 2011.

[9] N. Chalasani, Z. Younossi, and J. E. Lavine, "The diagnosis and management of non-alcoholic fatty liver disease: practice guideline by the American Association for the Study of Liver Diseases, American College of Gastroenterology, and the American Gastroenterological Association," *Hepatology*, vol. 55, no. 6, pp. 2005–2023, 2012.

[10] L. Gerber, M. Otgonsuren, A. Mishra et al., "Non-alcoholic fatty liver disease (NAFLD) is associated with low level of physical activity: a population-based study," *Alimentary Pharmacology & Therapeutics*, vol. 36, no. 8, pp. 772–781, 2012.

[11] B. A. Neuschwander-Tetri, "Non-alcoholic fatty liver disease," *BMC Medicine*, vol. 15, no. 1, article 45, 2017.

[12] J. K. C. Lau, X. Zhang, and J. Yu, "Animal models of non-alcoholic fatty liver disease: current perspectives and recent advances," *The Journal of Pathology*, vol. 241, no. 1, pp. 36–44, 2017.

[13] S. H. Ibrahim, P. Hirsova, H. Malhi, and G. J. Gores, "Animal models of nonalcoholic steatohepatitis: eat, delete, and inflame," *Digestive Diseases and Sciences*, vol. 61, no. 5, pp. 1325–1336, 2016.

[14] D. Moher, A. Liberati, J. Tetzlaff, and D. G. Altman, "Reprint-Preferred Reporting items for systematic reviews and meta-analyses: the PRISMA statement," *Physical Therapy in Sport*, vol. 89, no. 9, pp. 873–880, 2009.

[15] Z. Ackerman, M. Oron-Herman, M. Grozovski et al., "Fructose-induced fatty liver disease: hepatic effects of blood pressure and plasma triglyceride reduction," *Hypertension*, vol. 45, no. 5, pp. 1012–1018, 2005.

[16] R. Kirsch, V. Clarkson, E. G. Shephard et al., "Rodent nutritional model of non-alcoholic steatohepatitis: Species, strain and sex difference studies," *Journal of Gastroenterology and Hepatology*, vol. 18, no. 11, pp. 1272–1282, 2003.

[17] Y. Zou, J. Li, C. Lu et al., "High-fat emulsion-induced rat model of nonalcoholic steatohepatitis," *Life Sciences*, vol. 79, no. 11, pp. 1100–1107, 2006.

[18] V. M. R. de Lima, C. P. M. S. Oliveira, V. A. F. Alves et al., "A rodent model of NASH with cirrhosis, oval cell proliferation and hepatocellular carcinoma," *Journal of Hepatology*, vol. 49, no. 6, pp. 1055–1061, 2008.

[19] Z. J. Xu, J. G. Fan, X. D. Ding, L. Qiao, and G. L. Wang, "Characterization of high-fat, diet-induced, non-alcoholic steatohepatitis with fibrosis in rats," *Digestive Diseases and Sciences*, vol. 55, no. 4, pp. 931–940, 2010.

[20] S. D. McDonald, E. Pesarchuk, A. Don-Wauchope, H. El Zimaity, and A. C. Holloway, "Adverse metabolic effects of a hypercaloric, high-fat diet in rodents precede observable changes in body weight," *Nutrition Research*, vol. 31, no. 9, pp. 707–714, 2011.

[21] T. Wu, L. Chen, S. Tsai, Y. Liaw, and B. Hwang, "Hepatic steatosis: An experimental model for quantification," *Archives of Gerontology and Geriatrics*, vol. 52, no. 2, pp. 164–166, 2011.

[22] O. Kucera and Z. Cervinkova, "Experimental models of nonalcoholic fatty liver disease in rats," *World Journal of Gastroenterology*, vol. 20, no. 26, pp. 8364–8376, 2014.

[23] G. Torres-Villalobos, N. Hamdan-Pérez, A. R. Tovar et al., "Combined high-fat diet and sustained high sucrose consumption promotes NAFLD in a murine model," *Annals of Hepatology*, vol. 14, no. 4, pp. 540–546, 2015.

[24] J. S. Lee, D. W. Jun, E. K. Kim, H. J. Jeon, H. H. Nam, and W. K. Saeed, "Histologic and Metabolic Derangement in High-Fat, High-Fructose, and Combination Diet Animal Models," *The Scientific World Journal*, vol. 2015, Article ID 306326, 9 pages, 2015.

[25] M. A. Van Herck, L. Vonghia, and S. M. Francque, "Animal Models of Nonalcoholic Fatty Liver Disease- A Starter's Guide," *Nutrients*, vol. 9, no. 10, 2017.

[26] T. Eslamparast, P. Tandon, and M. Raman, "Dietary composition independent of weight loss in the management of nonalcoholic fatty liver disease," *Nutrients*, vol. 9, no. 8, 2017.

[27] N. Goossens and F. R. Jornayvaz, "Translational aspects of diet and non-alcoholic fatty liver disease," *Nutrients*, vol. 9, no. 10, 2017.

[28] J. H. Han, A. L. Dzierlenga, Z. Lu et al., "Distinction of the metabolic profile of the progression of non-alcoholic fatty liver disease from a common mouse model," *Obesity*, vol. 6, pp. 1069–1076, 25.

[29] I. Lozano, R. V. der Werf, and W. Bietiger, "High-fructose and high-fat diet-induced disorders in rats: impact on diabetes risk, hepatic and vascular complications," *Nutrition & Metabolism*, vol. 13, no. 15, 2016.

[30] R. Buettner, K. G. Parhofer, M. Woenckhaus et al., "Defining high-fat-diet rat models: metabolic and molecular effects of different fat types," *Molecular Endocrinology*, vol. 36, no. 3, pp. 485–501, 2006.

[31] L. Ghibaudi, J. Cook, C. Farley, M. van Heek, and J. J. Hwa, "Fat intake affects adiposity, comorbidity factors, and energy metabolism of Sprague-Dawley rats," *Obesity Research*, vol. 10, no. 9, pp. 956–963, 2002.

[32] A. Pocai, K. Morgan, C. Buettner, R. Gutierrez-Juarez, S. Obici, and L. Rossetti, "Central leptin acutely reverses diet-induced hepatic insulin resistance," *Diabetes*, vol. 54, no. 11, pp. 3182–3189, 2005.

[33] R. Buettner, J. Schölmerich, and L. C. Bollheimer, "High-fat diets: modeling the metabolic disorders of human obesity in rodents," *Obesity*, vol. 15, no. 4, pp. 798–808, 2007.

[34] C. S. Lieber, M. A. Leo, K. M. Mak et al., "Model of nonalcoholic steatohepatitis," *American Journal of Clinical Nutrition*, vol. 79, no. 3, pp. 502–509, 2004.

# 26

# Prevalence and Determinants of Significant Liver Fibrosis by Vibration-Controlled Transient Elastography in Thai Chronic Hepatitis B Patients

**Apichet Sirinawasatien, Thanaya Techasirioangkun, and Siriporn Thongsri**

*Division of Gastroenterology, Department of Medicine, Rajavithi Hospital, College of Medicine, Rangsit University, Bangkok, Thailand*

Correspondence should be addressed to Apichet Sirinawasatien; sui-apichet@hotmail.com

Academic Editor: Dirk Uhlmann

*Aims.* To describe the prevalence of significant liver fibrosis by ultrasound-based vibration-controlled transient elastography (VCTE; FibroScan®) and to identify the determinants of significant liver fibrosis in Thai chronic hepatitis B patients. *Methods.* A cross-sectional study of consecutive chronic hepatitis B patients performed VCTE and followed up at Rajavithi Hospital, Bangkok, Thailand, was conducted between 1 January, 2013, and 31 December, 2016. Liver fibrosis was defined as minimal (METAVIR F0-1) by VCTE < 7.2 kPa and significant (METAVIR F2-4) by VCTE ≥ 7.2 kPa. VCTE assessments and medical records were retrospectively reviewed. The prevalence and determinants of significant liver fibrosis were analyzed. *Results.* A total of 206 eligible patients were included; 120 patients (58.3%) were female. The mean age was 50 years (SD 12.4 years), and 32.5% had a body mass index ≥ 25. The prevalences of minimal (F 0-1) and significant fibrosis (F2-4) were 74.3% and 25.7%, respectively. The prevalence of hepatitis B e antigen negative (HBeAg -ve) was 83%. The median serum hepatitis B virus viral load was 4,340 IU/mL (range 20-271,883,036). Significant determinants of significant fibrosis (F2-4) were male gender (aOR 3.24 [95%CI: 1.36-7.72]) and high aspartate transaminase (AST) level (aOR 5.71 [95%CI: 2.03-16.04]). *Conclusion.* Around one-quarter of the Thai patients with chronic viral hepatitis B had significant liver disease defined by VCTE, requiring further evaluation for specific treatment for hepatitis B virus. Determinants of significant liver fibrosis were male gender and high AST level.

## 1. Introduction

Hepatitis B virus (HBV) is among the common causes of cirrhosis and hepatocellular carcinoma worldwide, especially in the Asia-Pacific region, including Thailand [1]. Patients have a wide range of clinical manifestations from inactive hepatitis B surface antigen carriers with normal histology to advanced liver fibrosis. The management of chronic hepatitis B infection is thus complex and based upon multiple factors, e.g., HBV viral load, hepatitis B e antigen (HBeAg) status, the presence or absence of liver inflammation, fibrosis, and cirrhosis. Patients with persistently high viremia with moderate to severe fibrosis (i.e. a METAVIR score ≥ F2) or cirrhosis should have antiviral treatment initiated with either a finite duration of pegylated interferon or long-term treatment with nucleos(t)ide analogues [2–4].

Liver biopsy remains the gold standard for evaluating the degree of liver fibrosis. It has, however, several disadvantages, including invasiveness, associations with rare serious complications, and susceptibility to sampling variation due to sampling only a small portion of the liver parenchyma. Many radiologic methods for staging liver fibrosis, including ultrasound-based and vibration-controlled transient elastography (VCTE), have recently been increasingly used in clinical practice instead of liver biopsy. VCTE is quick, reproducible, and painless, and it examines a large portion of liver parenchyma, thereby reducing sampling error. VCTE is the most studied radiologic method and is reliable for staging liver fibrosis in HBV- or hepatitis C virus (HCV)-infected patients, and other liver diseases [5–11]. Recent guidelines from the European Association for the Study of Liver Diseases and the Latin American Association for the Study of the Liver recommends VCTE as a valid noninvasive test for assessing liver fibrosis in HBV- and HCV-infected patients with a >90% negative predictive value for ruling out cirrhosis [12].

There have been few studies about the prevalence of significant liver fibrosis in chronic viral hepatitis B patients in Thailand. It is also important to identify the predictors of underlying significant liver fibrosis to select the patients who may benefit from early initiation of antiviral treatment. We thus aimed to describe the prevalence of significant liver fibrosis by noninvasive test (VCTE) in Thai chronic viral hepatitis B patients and also to identify the determinants of significant liver fibrosis.

## 2. Materials and Methods

*2.1. Patients.* This cross-sectional study was conducted by reviewing the medical records of all chronic hepatitis B patients who has VCTE performed from 1 January, 2013, to 31 December, 2016, at the outpatient clinic of the Department of Medicine at Rajavithi Hospital, a tertiary referral center in Bangkok, Thailand. Patients older than 18 years with chronic hepatitis B infection defined as having a positive HBs antigen for 6 months or more were included. None received antiviral treatment, namely nucleos(t)ide analogues or pegylated interferon, before VCTE was performed.

The exclusion criteria were (1) the presence of HCV or human immunodeficiency virus coinfection, (2) a positive test for anti-nuclear antibody, anti-smooth muscle antibody or anti-mitochondrial antibody, (3) a significant elevation of liver enzymes (aminotransferases > 5-fold the upper limit of normal [ULN]), and (4) an invalid VCTE result. The study protocol was reviewed and approved by the ethics committee of Rajavithi Hospital (No. 110/2560).

*2.2. Vibration-Controlled Transient Elastography.* VCTE were performed by one experienced operator (Thanaya Techasirioangkun, RN), using a Fibroscan® device (Echosens, France). This device sends a shear wave through the liver. The velocity of the propagation of this wave is assessed as a measure of the elasticity, or the stiffness, of the liver. Higher liver stiffness causes the shear wave to move faster, and higher liver stiffness indicates the presence of fibrosis. The VCTE measurement technique used involves a piston vibrator placed in the 9th-11th intercostal space on the right lobe of the liver with the patient positioned supine with the right arm at maximal abduction. The velocity is measured in a region 25-65 mm below the skin surface with the standard adult M probe. The unit of measurement is kPa with a range from 2.5 to 75 kPa. A valid VCTE result requires at least 10 successful measurements and an interquartile range (reflects variations among measurements) <30% of the median value [13, 14].

Factors influencing viscoelasticity of the liver may also contribute to increased liver stiffness such as the presence of severe hepatic inflammation [15] and nonfasting state [16]. Patients with significant elevation in liver enzymes (aminotransferases >5-fold the ULN) were thus excluded from the study, and VCTE was performed after the patient had fasted for at least 2 hours.

Stages of liver fibrosis were categorized according to the previous study by Marcellin et al. [8]. Liver stiffness scores of <7.2 kPa, ≥7.2 kPa, ≥8.1 kPa, and ≥11 kPa were used as cutoffs for the presence of minimal fibrosis (F0-1), significant fibrosis (F≥2), advanced fibrosis (F≥3), and cirrhosis (F=4), respectively. We classified the patients into two groups, namely, a minimal fibrosis group (F0-1) and a significant fibrosis group (F2-4), based on the different treatment strategies for these patients.

*2.3. Clinical and Laboratory Data.* Patient data collected retrospectively from medical records for description as well as comparison between VCTE-classified groups of severities of liver fibrosis were patient demographics and baseline characteristics including body mass index (BMI), serum albumin (g/dL), total bilirubin (mg/dL), serum creatinine (mg/dL), HBeAg serostatus, HBV DNA level (IU/mL), aspartate transaminase (AST) level (U/L), alanine transaminase (ALT) level (U/L), alkaline phosphatase (ALP) level (U/L), international normalized ratio (INR), white blood cell count (WBC) (/mm3), hemoglobin (g/dL), and platelet (x109/L). Determinants of significant liver fibrosis in chronic hepatitis B patients for multivariable logistic regression analysis were gender (reference, female gender), BMI, comorbidity of diabetes mellitus, AST (reference, ULN and unit of AST independent variable, n-fold ULN), ALT (reference, ULN and unit of ALT independent variable, n-fold ULN), ALP (U/L), and hemoglobin (g/dL). BMI was categorized as normal (BMI <23 kg/m2), overweight (BMI ≥23 kg/m2 and <25 kg/m2), or obese (BMI ≥25 kg/m2) according to the World Health Organization guidelines for adult Asian population [17]. The ULN for AST and ALT were both defined as 40 U/L, and a normal range of INR was defined as 0.80-1.10. Serum samples were tested for the presence of hepatitis B surface antigen (HBsAg), HBeAg, and anti-HBeAg antibody using radioimmunoassay (Abbott Laboratories, Irving, TX). Serum HBV viral load was measured using real-time HBV assays by polymerase chain reaction using the COBAS® AmpliPrep/COBAS® TaqMan® HBV Test, (Roche Molecular Diagnostics, Indianapolis, IN) with the range from 20 - 1.7 x 108 IU/mL.

*2.4. Statistical Analysis.* Data analysis was performed using SPSS software version 17.0 (SPSS Inc., Chicago, IL). Descriptive statistics were presented a mean (SD) or median (range and IQR) as appropriate for continuous data as well as numbers and prevalences for categorical data. Categorical variables were compared using the Chi-square test or Fisher exact test as appropriate. Continuous variables were compared for significant differences between multiple groups using one-way ANOVA test or Kruskal-Wallis test as appropriate. Multivariable logistic regression analysis was used to identify the determinants of liver fibrosis and cirrhosis, and results were presented as adjusted odds ratios (aOR) with 95% confidence intervals. A p-value <0.05 was considered statistically significant.

## 3. Results

Two hundred twenty-nine Thai chronic hepatitis B patients were identified and assessed for eligibility. Three patients

(1.3%) with invalid VCTE results and 20 patients (9.6%) with missing laboratory data were excluded. The remaining 206 patients were included, and none of them had received any antiviral therapy. The median liver stiffness was 5.50 kPa (range 2.50-63.90; IQR 1.40-24.60). Of the 206 included patients, 120 patients (58.3%) were female, and 86 patients (41.7%) were male. The mean age of patients was 50 years (SD 12.4), and 32.5% were obese (BMI ≥25 kg/m2). The prevalence of hepatitis B e antigen negative (HBeAg -ve) was 83%. The median serum HBV viral load was 4340 IU/mL (range 20 - 271883036). VCTE results, demographics, and laboratory data of the patients are summarized in Table 1.

The prevalences of liver fibrosis defined by VCTE were minimal fibrosis (F 0-1) in 74.3%, significant fibrosis (F2) in 5.34%, advanced fibrosis (F3) in 11.7%, and cirrhosis (F4) in 8.74% (Table 2).

Comparison of the baseline characteristics of the patients with minimal fibrosis (F0-1) and significant fibrosis (F2-4) are shown in Table 3. A higher proportion of male patients had significant fibrosis compared with minimal fibrosis (64.2 versus 34.0%, P <0.001). BMI was significantly higher in patients with significant fibrosis than minimal fibrosis (25.30 [SD 4.64] versus 23.50 [SD 3.49] kg/m$^2$, P = 0.004). Diabetes mellitus was observed significantly less frequently in patients with minimal fibrosis than significant fibrosis (5.23 versus 17.0%, P = 0.007). Both HBeAg status and serum HBV viral load were not significantly different among patients with different stages of liver fibrosis. Laboratory data showed significantly higher levels of ALP, WBC, hemoglobin, and higher prevalences of AST and ALT level >1 x ULN in the significant fibrosis group than the minimal fibrosis group (P <0.05).

Univariate analysis showed determinants for significant liver fibrosis (F2-4) were male gender, BMI, comorbidity with diabetes mellitus, hemoglobin, ALP, and high AST and ALT levels (>1 x ULN). Multivariable logistic regression analysis, however, showed that only male gender and a high AST level (>1 x ULN) were significant determinants of significant liver fibrosis (F2-4) with an aOR of 3.24 (95%CI: 1.36-7.72) and 5.71 (95%CI: 2.03-16.04), respectively (Table 4).

## 4. Discussion

The present study demonstrated a prevalence of liver fibrosis in Thai chronic hepatitis B patients defined by VCTE, a validated noninvasive test for assessment of liver fibrosis. The prevalences were minimal fibrosis (F0-1) in 74.3%, significant fibrosis (F2) in 5.34%, advanced fibrosis (F3) in 11.7%, and cirrhosis (F4) in 8.74%. Around one-quarter of these patients thus had significant liver disease (F2-4), requiring further evaluation for specific treatment for hepatitis B virus infection.

Male gender appears to hasten the progression in HBV-related liver disease. The male-to-female ratio increased from 1.2 in asymptomatic carriers to 6.3 in chronic liver disease and finally to 9.8 in hepatocellular carcinoma [18]. This gender disparity was experimentally confirmed in a HBV-transgenic-mice model. Wang et al. study demonstrated the androgen hormone could increase the transcription of HBV through direct binding to the androgen-responsive element sites in viral enhancer I. The adult male mice consequently showed higher serum titers of both viral DNA and HBsAg than the female mice [19]. This may explain the increased risk of liver-related disease in human males compared with females. We found similar results in the present study from multivariate analysis, in which male gender was a significant determinant of significant liver fibrosis (F2-4) with an aOR of 3.24 (95%CI: 1.36-7.72).

Obesity leads to adverse health consequences, including diabetes mellitus and atherosclerosis, and it contributes to the development of hepatic steatosis, nonalcoholic fatty liver disease and nonalcoholic steatohepatitis [20]. Lee et al. studied the impact of BMI on liver histology in chronic HBeAg -ve patients, and they found that overweight (BMI ≥23 kg/m$^2$) contributed to hepatic necroinflammation and obesity (BMI ≥25 kg/m$^2$) led to hepatic fibrosis [21]. Diabetes mellitus has also been reported to be associated with more severe liver fibrosis and cirrhosis in chronic hepatitis B patients [22]. From our data, both factors seemed to be associated with significant liver fibrosis in the univariate analysis, but were not significant in the multivariable analysis. These results might be explained by the difference of patient characteristics between the present study and Lee et al.'s study. That study had a higher HBV DNA viral load compared with our study (1.09 x $10^6$ versus 4.34 x $10^3$ IU/mL, respectively), and this factor potentiates more severe liver disease. The lower prevalence of diabetes mellitus in the present study (8.3%) compared with that of Papatheodoridis et al.'s study (14.4%)[22] might explain our the lack of significant association of diabetes mellitus with significant liver disease in multivariable analysis.

Elevations in AST level greater than ALT have been associated with more advanced fibrosis [23, 24] and are partially related to delayed clearance of AST relative to ALT [25] or to mitochondrial injury associated with more advanced fibrosis [26]. Our finding that a high AST level was, therefore, associated with more advanced fibrosis, is consistent with previous studies [27, 28]. The present study showed that patients with an AST levels of >1 x ULN have a higher rate of significant fibrosis compared with minimal fibrosis (45.3 versus 7.2%, respectively; p <0.001). From the multivariable analysis, a high AST level of >1 x ULN was associated with significant fibrosis with an aOR of 5.71 (95%CI: 2.03-16.04). This simple surrogate biomarker of liver disease, which is routinely collected in the follow-up visits by our chronic hepatitis B patients, is thus valuable because it is strongly suggestive of high risk for significant liver disease. This positive finding should cause the doctor to have a low threshold for further evaluation by either VCTE or liver biopsy to define the underlying liver fibrosis status.

Our study had several limitations including the retrospective study design, the limited number of patients, the diagnosis of liver fibrosis, and cirrhosis not based on liver biopsy, which is still the gold standard. There was also a rather low prevalence of significant fibrosis in the present study compared with a previous study [8] (25.7 versus 50.3%). This might be explained by selection bias. This is because some patients who already were diagnosed as cirrhosis by ultrasonography may not have had VCTE performed and

Table 1: Demographic and laboratory data of patients.

| Variable | Value |
|---|---|
| Total patients with a valid transient elastography scan, n | 206 |
| Liver stiffness, median (range), kPa | 5.50 (2.50-63.90) |
| Interquartile range, median (range) | 11.00 (1.40-24.60) |
| Failed scan, n (%) | 3 (1.3) |
| Success rate, % | 98.7 |
| Treatment naïve patients, n (%) | 206 (100.0) |
| Age, mean (SD), y | 50.01 (12.39) |
| Gender, n (%) | |
| Female | 120 (58.3) |
| Male | 86 (41.7) |
| BMI, mean (SD), kg/m$^2$ | 23.95 (3.88) |
| <23, n (%) | 94 (45.6) |
| ≥23, n (%) | 45 (21.9) |
| ≥25, n (%) | 67 (32.5) |
| Diabetes mellitus, n (%) | 17 (8.3) |
| HBeAg, n (%) | |
| Positive | 35 (17.0) |
| Negative | 171 (83.0) |
| HBV DNA, median (range), IU/mL | 4340 (20-271883036) |
| Biochemical markers | |
| Total bilirubin, median (range), mg/dL | 0.58 (0.19-3.53) |
| AST, median (range), U/L | 26 (8-199) |
| ≤1 x ULN, n (%) | 171 (83.0) |
| >1 x ULN, n (%) | 35 (17.0) |
| ALT, median (range), U/L | 25 (5-166) |
| ≤1 x ULN, n (%) | 155 (75.2) |
| >1 x ULN, n (%) | 51 (24.8) |
| ALP, median (range), U/L | 65 (29-511) |
| Albumin, median (range), g/dL | 4.40 (2.20-5.40) |
| INR, median (range) | 1.00 (0.90-2.40) |
| WBC, median (range), /mm$^3$ | 6500 (2700-18900) |
| Hemoglobin, mean (SD), g/dL | 13.13 (1.58) |
| Platelet, mean (SD), x10$^9$/L | 220.00 (63.60) |
| Creatinine, mean (SD), mg/dL | 1.14 (1.61) |

kPa: Kilopascal; BMI: Body mass index; HBeAg: Hepatitis B e antigen;
AST: Aspartate aminotransferase; ALT: Alanine aminotransferase; ULN: Upper limit of normal;
ALP: Alkaline phosphatase; INR: International normalized ratio.

Table 2: Prevalence of liver fibrosis by vibration-controlled transient elastography in chronic hepatitis B patients.

| Liver fibrosis stage | Overall n (%) |
|---|---|
| F0-1 | 153 (74.3) |
| F2 | 11 (5.3) |
| F3 | 24 (11.7) |
| F4 | 18 (8.7) |

were thus not included. Finally, as this study represents patients already referred to a tertiary care center, referral bias was always a possibility, by which patients with persistently normal ALT and low viremia are less likely to be referred.

In conclusion, our study demonstrated that a small but significant proportion of Thai chronic hepatitis B patients (about 25%) had significant liver fibrosis (F2-4). Male patients with an AST level >1 x ULN were especially at high risk of significant liver disease. VCTE or liver biopsy should therefore be performed in these patients to evaluate the status of liver fibrosis and provide an indication for antiviral treatment to prevent the development of end-stage liver disease.

Table 3: Comparison of the baseline characteristics of patients with minimal fibrosis (F0-1) and significant fibrosis (F2-4).

| Variable | F0-1 (n = 153) | F2-4 (n = 53) | P-value |
|---|---|---|---|
| Age, mean (SD), y | 49.60 (12.73) | 51.21 (11.39) | 0.417 |
| Male gender, n (%) | 52 (34.0) | 34 (64.2) | <0.001 |
| BMI, mean (SD), kg/m$^2$ | 23.50 (3.49) | 25.30 (4.64) | 0.004 |
| <23, n (%) | 75 (49.0) | 19 (35.8) | |
| ≥23, n (%) | 34 (22.2) | 11 (20.8) | |
| ≥25, n (%) | 44 (28.8) | 23 (43.4) | |
| Diabetes mellitus, n (%) | 8 (5.2) | 9 (17.0) | 0.007 |
| HBeAg, n (%) | | | 0.998 |
| Positive | 26 (17.0) | 9 (17.0) | |
| Negative | 127 (83.0) | 44 (83.0) | |
| HBV DNA level, n (%) | | | 0.395 |
| <2000 IU/mL | 68 (44.4) | 20 (37.7) | |
| ≥2000 IU/mL | 85 (55.6) | 33 (62.3) | |
| Total bilirubin, mean (SD), mg/dL | 0.60 (0.25) | 0.75 (0.54) | 0.053 |
| AST level, n (%) | | | <0.001 |
| ≤1 x ULN | 142 (92.8) | 29 (54.7) | |
| >1 x ULN | 11 (7.2) | 24 (45.3) | |
| ALT level, n (%) | | | <0.001 |
| ≤1 x ULN | 130 (85.0) | 25 (47.2) | |
| >1 x ULN | 23 (15.0) | 28 (52.8) | |
| ALP, median (range), U/L | 63 (29-280) | 73 (32-511) | 0.011 |
| Albumin, mean (SD), g/dL | 4.40 (0.40) | 4.30 (0.40) | 0.134 |
| INR, mean (SD) | 1.00 (0.10) | 1.10 (0.20) | 0.051 |
| WBC, median (range), /mm$^3$ | 6800 (2700-18900) | 8200 (3800-11100) | 0.036 |
| Hemoglobin, mean (SD), g/dL | 13.00 (1.54) | 13.50 (1.63) | 0.044 |
| Platelet, mean (SD), x10$^9$/L | 239.00 (60.50) | 221.00 (70.90) | 0.082 |

BMI: Body mass index; HBeAg: Hepatitis B e antigen;
AST: Aspartate aminotransferase; ALT: Alanine aminotransferase; ULN: Upper limit of normal;
ALP: Alkaline phosphatase; INR: International normalized ratio.

Table 4: Multivariable logistic regression analysis on factors associated with significant fibrosis (F2-4).

| Variable | Crude OR (95%CI) | P-value | Adjusted OR (95%CI) | P-value |
|---|---|---|---|---|
| Gender (Ref=female) | 3.48(1.81-6.68) | <0.001 | 3.24(1.36-7.72) | 0.008 |
| Body mass index (kg/m$^2$) | 1.12(1.03-1.21) | 0.006 | 1.03(0.92-1.14) | 0.650 |
| Diabetes mellitus | 3.71(1.35-10.18) | 0.011 | 2.32(0.72-7.49) | 0.160 |
| AST (Ref=≤1 x ULN) | 10.68(4.72-24.20) | <0.001 | 5.71(2.03-16.04) | 0.001 |
| ALT (Ref=≤1 x ULN) | 6.33(3.15-12.72) | <0.001 | 1.90(0.75-4.84) | 0.178 |
| ALP (U/L) | 1.02(1.01-1.03) | 0.004 | 1.01(1.00-1.02) | 0.520 |
| Hemoglobin (g/dL) | 1.24(1.00-1.54) | 0.046 | 0.97(0.72-1.29) | 0.825 |

AST: Aspartate aminotransferase; ALT: Alanine aminotransferase; ULN: Upper limit of normal;
ALP: Alkaline phosphatase; OR: Odds ratio; 95%CI: Confidence interval 95%.

## Additional Points

*Study Highlights.* VCTE have recently been increasingly used in clinical practice to evaluate liver fibrosis stage instead of liver biopsy. Recent guidelines from the EASL-ALEH recommends VCTE as a valid noninvasive test for assessing liver fibrosis in HBV-infected patients. By VCTE we demonstrated that the prevalence of significant liver fibrosis in Thai chronic hepatitis B patients was 25.7% and determinants of significant liver fibrosis were male gender and high AST level.

## Authors' Contributions

Apichet Sirinawasatien conceived the project, analyzed, and interpreted the data and drafted the manuscript. Thanaya Techasirioangkun and Siriporn Thongsri collected the data.

## Acknowledgments

The authors are thankful to all gastrointestinal (GI) specialty staff (Dr. Piyathida Hansomburana, Dr. Siam Sirinthornpunya, Dr. Kitti Chuengyong, Dr. Chalermrat Bunchorntavakul and Dr. Kanokpoj Chanpiwat), the GI fellows, and Mrs. Thanaya Techasirioangkun, Hepatology Nurse at the GI Clinic, Division of Gastroenterology, Department of Medicine, Rajavithi Hospital, for their contributions to the care of chronic hepatitis B patients included in the present study.

## References

[1] L. A. Torre, F. Bray, R. L. Siegel, J. Ferlay, and J. Lortet-Tieulent, "Global cancer statistics, 2012," *CA: A Cancer Journal for Clinicians*, vol. 65, no. 2, pp. 87–108, 2015.

[2] N. A. Terrault, N. H. Bzowej, K.-M. Chang, J. P. Hwang, M. M. Jonas, and M. H. Murad, "AASLD guidelines for treatment of chronic hepatitis B," *Hepatology*, vol. 63, no. 1, pp. 261–283, 2016.

[3] G. Papatheodoridis, M. Buti, M. Cornberg, H. L. Janssen, D. Mutimer, S. Pol et al., "EASL clinical practice guidelines: management of chronic hepatitis B virus infection," *Journal of Hepatology*, vol. 57, no. 1, pp. 167–185, 2013.

[4] S. K. Sarin, M. Kumar, G. K. Lau et al., "Asian-Pacific clinical practice guidelines on the management of hepatitis B: a 2015 update," *Hepatology International*, vol. 10, no. 1, pp. 1–98, 2016.

[5] M. Ziol, A. Handra-Luca, A. Kettaneh et al., "Noninvasive assessment of liver fibrosis by measurement of stiffness in patients with chronic hepatitis C," *Hepatology*, vol. 41, no. 1, pp. 48–54, 2005.

[6] M. Friedrich-Rust, M.-F. Ong, S. Martens et al., "Performance of transient elastography for the staging of liver fibrosis: a meta analysis," *Gastroenterology*, vol. 134, no. 4, pp. 960.e8–974.e8, 2008.

[7] L. Castera, X. Forns, and A. Alberti, "Non-invasive evaluation of liver fibrosis using transient elastography," *Journal of Hepatology*, vol. 48, no. 5, pp. 835–847, 2008.

[8] P. Marcellin, M. Ziol, P. Bedossa et al., "Non-invasive assessment of liver fibrosis by stiffness measurement in patients with chronic hepatitis B," *Liver International*, vol. 29, no. 2, pp. 242–247, 2009.

[9] Y. S. Seo, M. Y. Kim, S. U. Kim et al., "Accuracy of transient elastography in assessing liver fibrosis in chronic viral hepatitis: A multicentre, retrospective study," *Liver International*, vol. 35, no. 10, pp. 2246–2255, 2015.

[10] W. Kemp, M. Levy, M. Weltman, and J. Lubel, "Australian Liver Association (ALA) expert consensus recommendations for the use of transient elastography in chronic viral hepatitis," *Journal of Gastroenterology and Hepatology*, vol. 30, no. 3, pp. 453–462, 2015.

[11] Y. Li, Y.-S. Huang, Z.-Z. Wang et al., "Systematic review with meta-analysis: The diagnostic accuracy of transient elastography for the staging of liver fibrosis in patients with chronic hepatitis B," *Alimentary Pharmacology & Therapeutics*, vol. 43, no. 4, pp. 458–469, 2016.

[12] European Association for Study of Liver and Asociacion Latinoamericana para el Estudio del Higado, "EASL-ALEH Clinical Practice Guidelines: non-invasive tests for evaluation of liver disease severity and prognosis," *Journal of Hepatology*, vol. 63, no. 1, pp. 237–264, 2015.

[13] L. Castera, "Noninvasive methods to assess liver disease in patients with hepatitis B or C," *Gastroenterology*, vol. 142, no. 6, pp. 1293–1302, 2012.

[14] E. B. Tapper, L. Castera, and N. H. Afdhal, "FibroScan (vibration-controlled transient elastography): Where does it stand in the United States practice," *Clinical Gastroenterology and Hepatology*, vol. 13, no. 1, pp. 27–36, 2015.

[15] U. Arena, F. Vizzutti, G. Corti et al., "Acute viral hepatitis increases liver stiffness values measured by transient elastography," *Hepatology*, vol. 47, no. 2, pp. 380–384, 2008.

[16] U. Arena, M. L. Platon, C. Stasi et al., "Liver stiffness is influenced by a standardized meal in patients with chronic hepatitis C virus at different stages of fibrotic evolution," *Hepatology*, vol. 58, no. 1, pp. 65–72, 2013.

[17] WHO Expert Consultation, "Appropriate body-mass index for Asian populations and its implications for policy and intervention strategies," *The Lancet*, vol. 363, no. 9403, pp. 157–163, 2004.

[18] C. Chu, Y. Liaw, I. Sheen, D. Lin, and M. Huang, "Sex Difference in Chronic Hepatitis B Virus Infection: An Appraisal Based on the Status of Hepatitis B e Antigen and Antibody," *Hepatology*, vol. 3, no. 6, pp. 947–950, 1983.

[19] S.-H. Wang, S.-H. Yeh, W.-H. Lin, H.-Y. Wang, D.-S. Chen, and P.-J. Chen, "Identification of androgen response elements in the enhancer I of hepatitis B virus: a mechanism for sex disparity in chronic hepatitis B," *Hepatology*, vol. 50, no. 5, pp. 1392–1402, 2009.

[20] S. E. Shoelson, L. Herrero, and A. Naaz, "Obesity, inflammation, and insulin resistance," *Gastroenterology*, vol. 132, no. 6, pp. 2169–2180, 2007.

[21] I.-C. Lee, Y.-H. Huang, C.-C. Chan et al., "Impact of body mass index and viral load on liver histology in hepatitis B e antigen-negative chronic hepatitis B," *Clinical Nutrition*, vol. 30, no. 5, pp. 647–652, 2011.

[22] G. V. Papatheodoridis, N. Chrysanthos, S. Savvas et al., "Diabetes mellitus in chronic hepatitis B and C: prevalence and potential association with the extent of liver fibrosis," *Journal of Viral Hepatitis*, vol. 13, no. 5, pp. 303–310, 2006.

[23] S. G. Sheth, S. L. Flamm, F. D. Gordon, and S. Chopra, "AST/ALT ratio predicts cirrhosis in patients with chronic hepatitis C virus infection," *American Journal of Gastroenterology*, vol. 93, no. 1, pp. 44–48, 1998.

[24] A. Pohl, C. Behling, D. Oliver, M. Kilani, P. Monson, and T. Hassanein, "Serum aminotransferase levels and platelet counts as predictors of degree of fibrosis in chronic hepatitis C virus infection," *American Journal of Gastroenterology*, vol. 96, no. 11, pp. 3142–3146, 2001.

[25] Y. Kamimoto, S. Horiuchi, S. Tanase, and Y. Morino, "Plasma clearance of intravenously injected aspartate aminotransferase isozymes: Evidence for preferential uptake by sinusoidal liver cells," *Hepatology*, vol. 5, no. 3, pp. 367–375, 1985.

[26] B. Nalpas, A. Vassault, A. L. Guillou et al., "Serum Activity of Mitochondrial Aspartate Aminotransferase: A Sensitive Marker of Alcoholism With or Without Alcoholic Hepatitis," *Hepatology*, vol. 4, no. 5, pp. 893–896, 1984.

# 27

# Chronic Hepatitis C: An Overview of Evidence on Epidemiology and Management from a Brazilian Perspective

**Rodolfo Castro,[1] Hugo Perazzo,[1] Beatriz Grinsztejn,[1] Valdilea G. Veloso,[1] and Chris Hyde[2]**

[1]*Evandro Chagas National Institute of Infectious Diseases, Oswaldo Cruz Foundation, Laboratory of Clinical Research on STD/AIDS, Avenida Brasil 4365, 21040-900 Manguinhos, RJ, Brazil*
[2]*Institute of Health Research, Peninsula Technology Assessment Group (PenTAG), Evidence Synthesis and Modelling for Health Improvement (ESMI), University of Exeter Medical School, University of Exeter, St Luke's Campus, South Cloisters, Exeter EX1 2LU, UK*

Correspondence should be addressed to Rodolfo Castro; rodolfoalcastro@gmail.com

Academic Editor: Maria Buti

Chronic hepatitis C remains one of the main causes of chronic liver disease worldwide and presents a variable natural history ranging from minimal changes to advanced fibrosis and cirrhosis and its complications, such as development of hepatocellular carcinoma. Approximately, 1.45 million people are estimated to be infected by HCV in Brazil representing a major public health issue. The aim of this paper was to review the epidemiology and management of chronic hepatitis C from a Brazilian perspective. The management of chronic hepatitis C has been challenged by the use of noninvasive methods to stage liver fibrosis as an alternative to liver biopsy and the high cost of new interferon-free antiviral treatments. Moreover, the need of cost-effectiveness analysis in hepatitis C and the recent changes in treatment protocols were discussed.

## 1. Introduction

Hepatitis C virus (HCV) was first described as non-A, non-B hepatitis in the 1990s in patients who presented with acute hepatitis after transfusion of blood products [1]. HCV is an enveloped RNA virus with 10 protein coding genes and a member of the family Flaviviridae, which targets hepatocytes leading to liver damage [2]. Parenteral transmission due to intravenous drug use, followed by transfusion of blood products before HCV screening, has been described as the most frequent route of infection. However, HCV can also be transmitted sexually or vertically [3]. Among patients exposed to HCV, a minority can spontaneously clear the virus [1] and around 85% of patients who still have detectable serum HCV RNA after 6 months should be considered as chronically infected [4].

Chronic hepatitis C (CHC) remains one of the main causes of chronic liver disease worldwide and presents a variable natural history ranging from minimal changes to extensive fibrosis and cirrhosis and its complications, such as development of hepatocellular carcinoma [5]. The correct determination of liver fibrosis stage has important implications for prognostic, therapeutic, and monitoring purposes [6]. Considerable progress in research and clinical practice has been made on hepatitis C infection since its discovery. Diagnosis and monitoring of infected patients were improved by molecular virological techniques and fibrosis staging using noninvasive methods. In addition, a promising new era in CHC treatment has been heralded by the recent approval of new drugs by licensing authorities around the world.

## 2. Diagnosis

Screening for HCV infection is performed by measuring anti-HCV antibody by serological enzyme immunoassay (EIA) that has been used as an indicator of past or present infection. The current third- and fourth-generation screening tests contain multiple recombinant antigens from HCV core and viral nonstructural proteins, such as NS3, NS4, and NS5, providing high accuracy for detection of exposure to HCV [7]. HCV antibodies can be detected by rapid diagnostic tests that use finger-stick whole-blood samples. These tests do not require complex instruments, yield the result in 20 minutes, and might be used in high burden HCV and low resources countries [8]. According to the recommendations from the US Center for Disease Control and Prevention (CDC) [9], all persons born between 1945 and 1965 or individuals presenting at least one of the following risk factors should be screened for HCV infection: patients who (i) have ever injected themselves with illegal drugs; (ii) received blood transfusion or organs transplant before the 1990s; (iii) have ever been in hemodialysis; (iv) have a persistently abnormal alanine aminotransferase (ALT) level; (v) were born to an HCV-positive mother; (vi) have human immunodeficiency virus (HIV) infection; and (vii) had a needle-stick injury or mucosal exposure to HCV-positive blood.

Patients with a positive anti-HCV should be tested for serum HCV RNA that quantifies the amount of RNA in serum and indicates ongoing HCV infection. Usually, HCV RNA is extracted from serum or plasma and amplified by polymerase chain reaction (PCR) [10]. Individuals with a positive HCV RNA should undergo disease staging to assess the extent of fibrosis by liver biopsy or noninvasive methods. In addition, the HCV genotype should be established in patients with CHC. Genotypes 1 to 6 are the most common in chronic viral infection, further divided into subtypes and strains. HCV genotyping is usually performed by direct sequencing of specific regions within the viral genome, followed by alignment to reference sequences and phylogenic analysis [11]. Genotype distribution varies according to geographic localization: HCV genotype 1 is the most frequent in the United States [12] and in Brazil [13, 14] and genotype 3 in India [15]. The definition of HCV genotype might guide the drug selection, dosage, and overall treatment duration.

## 3. Epidemiology of Chronic Hepatitis C

CHC is a disease that has global importance, since it was estimated to affect 2 to 3% of the world population, with 130–170 million people infected. The prevalence of HCV has a high variability between countries, with developed nations characterized by lower prevalence. A higher endemicity is present in countries of the African and the Eastern Mediterranean region [17, 18].

The Brazilian epidemiologic surveillance system uses a positive serum HCV RNA to define a confirmed case of hepatitis C infection. The compulsory notification of viral hepatitis started in 1996 in Brazil: 82,041 cases of HCV were notified, 60.1% in males and 39.9% in female patients from 1999 to 2011 [19]. Including the cases registered from 2012 to 2015, more than 150,000 confirmed HCV-positive patients were identified by the Brazilian surveillance system [20]. However, a very recently published report from Brazilian Ministry of Health estimated using mathematic modelling that around 1,450,000 people are living with HCV in Brazil [21]. These data justify all investments on HCV screening programs, implemented in order to reduce the number of people unaware of their HCV-positive status, and improve access to HCV-care. The quality of information about the infected patients will be improved with these testing strategies, reinforcement of the surveillance system, and research budgets offered for epidemiologic studies on HCV-prevalence in Brazil. The scarce data on HCV epidemiology, considering the real number of patients infected, is a problem in Brazil as in most of the Latin American countries [22].

The last extensive epidemiologic study was conducted from 2005 to 2009 using data from all major Brazilian cities. This research reported a prevalence of 1.38% (95% CI: 1.12%–1.64%) in 10–69-year-old subjects [23]. The predictors of HCV infection were age (OR = 1.01, 95% CI: 1.01–1.04), injected drug use (OR = 6.65, 95% CI: 2.47–17.91), sniffed drug use (OR = 2.59, 95% CI: 1.34–5.01), hospitalization (OR = 1.90, 95% CI: 1.03–3.51), and groups socially deprived by the lack of sewage disposal (OR = 2.53, 95% CI: 1.38–4.65) [23]. Genotype 1 was the most prevalent (79%) in a Brazilian study that aimed to evaluate the presence of cognitive dysfunction in CHC patients [13]. The higher prevalence of genotype 1 in Brazil was confirmed in a study that evaluated 283 patients: genotype 1 was present in 57.6%, genotype 3 in 39.6%, genotype 2 in 2.5%, and genotype 4 in 0.35% patients [14].

## 4. Prevalence of Liver Fibrosis and Cirrhosis and Its Complications in Brazil

The prevalence of liver fibrosis stages and cirrhosis was reported in small sample studies in Brazil. Using liver biopsy as the reference, mild to moderate fibrosis (F0F1F2) was observed in up to 70% of patients [13]. Fibrosis stages estimated by transient elastography were reported in 120 CHC patients: 54%, 30%, 9%, and 7% for METAVIR stages F0F1, F2, F, and F4, respectively [24]. These results were confirmed in a more recent study [25]. Up to 8% of Brazilian patients with cirrhosis developed hepatocellular carcinoma (HCC) in a 10-year follow-up period [26].

End-stage cirrhosis due to HCV is the main indication for liver transplantation worldwide [27]. Up to 75% of patients submitted to liver transplantation in a Brazilian tertiary hospital had CHC [28]. The number of liver transplants has been growing in Latin America, especially in Brazil: this country has achieved the third largest volume of liver transplantation in the world with more than 1,600 liver transplantations performed in 2012 [29].

## 5. Natural History

Most patients exposed to HCV cannot clear the virus spontaneously and develop chronic infection. The host's age, gender, and other comorbidities, such as body weight, hepatic steatosis, alcohol abuse, and coinfection with hepatitis B virus and/or HIV, might play a crucial role in the ability to spontaneously clear the virus [30]. The natural history of CHC is extremely variable ranging from minimal changes to extensive fibrosis, cirrhosis, and development of severe complications, such as end-stage liver disease, portal hypertension, and hepatocellular carcinoma [5]. The chronic disease is generally slowly progressive and cirrhosis develops within 20 years in about 10–20% of patients chronically infected [31]. The prevalence of cirrhosis after 20 years of HCV infection was estimated at 16% (95% CI 14–90%) in a systematic review that included 111 studies [32]. Similar results were reported in studies in France [33]. Several factors might influence the progression of liver disease, such as the age of acquisition, gender, coexisting viral disease particularly HBV or HIV coinfection, concomitant alcohol abuse, and the host immune response [34].

HCV infection might be associated with extrahepatic manifestations such as cryoglobulinaemia, vasculitis, lichen planus, porphyria cutanea tarda, lymphocytic sialoadenitis, and membranous glomerulonephritis [35]. In addition, CHC might be associated with non-Hodgkin's lymphoma [36]. The development of cirrhosis might be associated with major complications such as ascites, gastrointestinal bleeding, severe bacterial infection, and encephalopathy [37]. Cirrhotic patients with compensated disease have a risk of 1–4% per year of developing hepatocellular carcinoma and a risk of 4% per year of developing hepatic decompensation. Those with decompensated cirrhosis have a survival rate of 50% at 5 years [38].

## 6. Staging Liver Fibrosis

Accurate assessment of the fibrosis stage and the grade of necroinflammatory activity are essential for the management of patients with CHC. Historically, the severity of liver disease has been measured by liver biopsy using semiquantitative histological scoring systems, such as METAVIR [39] and Ishak score [40]. However, liver biopsy is a painful invasive method and might be associated with potential complications that range from local pain to intraperitoneal bleeding, associated in turn with transfusion of blood products, surgery, or death [41]. In Brazil, Bergesch D'Incao et al. reported 0.3% of severe complications in a study that evaluated 1955 liver biopsies in patients with chronic liver disease, most infected by viral hepatitis. In this study, the majority of severe complications were gallbladder perforation and all patients with complications were submitted to surgery after liver biopsy [42]. In addition, the usefulness of liver biopsy has been challenged by limited feasibility, adverse effects, sampling error, and interobserver variability [43–45].

Several noninvasive methods have been proposed to assess liver fibrosis in patients with chronic viral hepatitis as an alternative to liver biopsy: serological biomarkers and imaging techniques [46]. Few biomarkers, such as aspartate-to-platelet ratio index (APRI) or Fibrosis-4 score (FIB-4) are nonpatented tests that use simple and worldwide available parameters in their formula. Other biomarkers are patented and involve the combination of more complex biological parameters, such as hyaluronic acid, alpha-2-macroglobulin, or serum markers involved in the synthesis and breakdown of the extracellular matrix [47]. Transient elastography by FibroScan (EchoSens, Paris, France) is one of the most validated noninvasive methods based on imaging techniques [48]. Table 1 summarizes the several noninvasive methods currently available for estimation of liver fibrosis in chronic viral hepatitis.

Liver fibrosis can be estimated by APRI using simple and worldwide available serological parameters such as AST and platelet count. This biomarker can be calculated according to the following formula: AST level (/ULN)/Platelets count ($10^9$/L) $*$ 100. Liver fibrosis, estimated by APRI, can be converted to the METAVIR scoring system [39] as proposed by Wai et al. [49] using dual cut-offs: >0.5 and >1.5 for fibrosis stage $F \geq 2$ and >1.0 and >2.0 for cirrhosis ($F = 4$). In this first study, APRI yielded 0.91 of sensitivity and 0.47 of specificity for fibrosis stage $F \geq 2$ and 0.89 of sensitivity and 0.75 of specificity for cirrhosis when the lower set of cut-offs >0.5 for $F \geq 2$ and >1.0 for $F = 4$. In addition, this test yielded 0.41 of sensitivity and 0.95 of specificity for fibrosis stage $F \geq 2$ and 0.57 of sensitivity and 0.93 of specificity considering the higher set of cut-off (>1.5 for $F \geq 2$ and >2.0 for $F = 4$).

A potential criticism to this test could be the impact of necroinflammatory activity in the estimation of liver fibrosis due to the use of transaminases in its formula and the fact that upper limit of normal for AST is extremely variable from a laboratory to another depending on the control group used. This variability induces a spectrum effect, which could cause misleading interpretations of APRI performance for the staging of fibrosis [50].

The performance of APRI to stage liver fibrosis was validated in a systematic review yielding an area under the receiver-operating characteristic curve [AUROC (95% CI)] of 0.77 (0.58–0.95) for fibrosis stage $F \geq 2$ and 0.84 (0.54–0.97) for cirrhosis ($F = 4$) [51]. APRI has also been reported to be predictive of mortality in CHC [52–54]. Few studies have been published regarding the diagnostic performance of APRI with data from Brazilian centers. Initially, Parise et al. reported the diagnostic performance of APRI in 206 patients with HCV infection: AUROC = 0.824 (0.772–0.903) for fibrosis stage $F \geq 2$ [55]. In addition, da Silva Jr. et al. described AUROC of 0.92 (0.83–1.00) and 0.92 (0.85–1.00) for diagnosis of fibrosis stage $F \geq 2$ and cirrhosis, respectively, using liver biopsy as the reference in a small sample ($n$ = 41) of patients with CHC [56]. Following the same trend, Amorim et al. reported an AUROC of 0.793 ± 0.047 for APRI to estimate fibrosis stage $F \geq 2$ in 119 HCV-infected patients [57] and, more recently, Silva Junior et al. reported AUROC of 0.82 for both diagnosis of fibrosis stage $F \geq 2$ and cirrhosis [58].

Transient elastography (TE), assessed by FibroScan (EchoSens, Paris, France), is an imaging method that estimates liver fibrosis based on liver stiffness measurement (LSM) [59]. The examination is very well accepted by patients, is painless and fast (<10 minutes), and can be easily performed at bedside or in the outpatient clinic without potential complications. The performance of 100 exams can be used to define an experimented operator [60]. However, TE requires an expensive medical device operated by an experienced operator and this method has been challenged concerning its reproducibility and overestimation of fibrosis in special situations.

The performance of TE, expressed as AUROC, for diagnosis of fibrosis stage $F \geq 2$ and cirrhosis ($F = 4$) varies from 0.79 to 0.83 and from 0.95 to 0.97 in HCV-infected patients.

TABLE 1: Noninvasive methods for staging fibrosis in chronic hepatitis C.

| Noninvasive method for estimation of liver fibrosis | Parameters |
|---|---|
| Biomarkers | |
| APRI | AST and platelet count |
| ELF | PIIINP, TIMP-1, and hyaluronic acid |
| FIB-4 | Platelet count, ALT and AST adjusted for age |
| FibroIndex | platelet count, AST, and gamma-globulin |
| FibroMeter | Alpha-2-macroglobulin, hyaluronic acid, platelet count, AST, prothrombin time, and urea adjusted for age |
| FibroSpect II | Hyaluronic acid, TIMP-1, and alpha-2-macroglobulin |
| FibroTest | Apolipoprotein A1, haptoglobin, alpha-2-macroglobulin, GGT, and total bilirubin adjusted for age and gender |
| Forns index | Platelet count, GGT, and total cholesterol adjusted for age and gender |
| HepaScore | Alpha-2-macroglobulin, GGT, total bilirubin, and hyaluronic acid adjusted for age and gender |
| Imaging techniques | |
| AixPlorer | Real-time shear wave elastography |
| ARFI | Elastography |
| Fibroscan | Transient elastography |
| Magnetic Resonance Imaging | Elastography and water-diffusion abnormalities |

ALT, alanine aminotransferase; AST, aspartate aminotransferase; ARFI, Acoustic Radiation Force Impulse; ELF, enhanced liver fibrosis; GGT, gamma-glutamyl transferase; PIIINP, serum amino-terminal propeptide of type III procollagen; TIMP-1, tissue inhibitors of matrix metalloproteinase.

A cut-off value of 12.5 kPa yielded sensitivity, specificity, and AUROC values of 0.87, 0.91, and 0.95, respectively, for the diagnosis of cirrhosis [61], whereas a cut-off of 14.6 kPa yielded sensitivity, specificity, and AUROC values of 0.86, 0.96, and 0.97, respectively [62]. A meta-analysis validated the diagnostic performance of TE: for detection of cirrhosis, the summary sensitivity was 0.92 (95% CI: 0.78–0.97) and the summary specificity was 0.86 (95% CI: 0.82–0.90). TE has a prognostic value for 5-year prediction of overall mortality [53] and severe outcomes in CHC patients [63]. In Brazil, a single study has reported the diagnostic accuracy of TE: AUROC ranged from 0.87 to 0.94 for diagnosis of fibrosis stage $F \geq 2$ and cirrhosis, respectively, in 120 patients with CHC, mostly with mild fibrosis (F0 or F1) [24]. Another two studies have evaluated the intra- and interobserver agreement of this method in a Brazilian population [25, 60].

## 7. Health-Related Quality of Life and Cost-Effectiveness of Noninvasive Diagnostic Tests for Surveillance of Liver Disease in Brazil

Studies have reported worse health-related quality of life (HRQOL) for people living with HCV in Brazil [64–67]. These results demonstrate that CHC has impact on the quality of life, which might be due to the HCV itself according to a study with blood donors unaware of the HCV-positive diagnosis [66]. CHC was associated with depression [68] and sexual dysfunction [69] and the diagnosis of HCV was frequently considered a traumatic experience [70]. Few studies used quality-adjusted life years (QALY) as an outcome measure to estimate effects of interventions for Brazilian patients [71, 72]. However, both studies have used international data for utilities estimation due to local information unavailability. Few studies have used cost-effectiveness analysis to evaluate interventions for CHC from a Brazilian perspective: treatment with Peg-interferon and Ribavirin and hypothetical vaccine should be cost-effective [71–74]. Similar results were reported for HCV/HIV coinfected patients [74].

Since CHC is a major public health issue with new costly drugs for treatment, leading to an economic impact on the healthcare systems [75], more health technology assessments for treating and preventing CHC in Brazil are urgently needed to tackle this public health issue. Moreover, cost-effectiveness analysis of noninvasive methods for staging liver fibrosis in CHC patients must be conducted to establish evidence-based criteria for treatment decisions.

## 8. Evidences on HCV-Treatment and the Promising New Brazilian Guidelines

The main objective of treatment of CHC remains eradication of HCV represented as sustained virological response (SVR) that has been associated with lower overall and liver-related mortality [76]. Several factors can influence the response rate, such as HCV genotype, stage of fibrosis, or results of previous HCV-treatment [77]. Treatment using Peg-interferon has been challenged by low response rates, especially in genotypes 1 and 4 and significant side effects [78].

Considering the effectiveness of retreatment, results from a Brazilian cohort of patients with HCV genotypes 2 and 3 showed 34.4% of SVR rate for nonresponders to previous treatment and 50% for relapsers with Peg-interferon combined with Ribavirin [79]. Other Brazilian cohort studies obtained 79.3% (46/58) of SVR for patients with HCV genotypes 2 or 3 treated with Peg-interferon plus Ribavirin and 49.1% (56/114) among those treated with biosimilar standard interferon plus Ribavirin [80].

In recent years, the standard of care has been replaced by new direct-acting antiviral drugs (DAAs) that act by inhibiting protease or nonstructural proteins of HCV. Currently, these drugs are in various stages of preclinical and clinical development. The new treatment regimens has been based on the combination of DAA that can be classified as protease inhibitor (first-generation: Boceprevir and Telaprevir; second-generation: Simeprevir, Paritaprevir), NS5A inhibitor (Ledipasvir, Daclatasvir, and Ombitasvir), or NS5B inhibitor (Sofosbuvir, Dasabuvir, and Beclabuvir) [81].

In 2011, the first-generation protease inhibitors were approved for clinical use. Patients with genotype 1 treated by a combination of Boceprevir or Telaprevir plus Peg-interferon and Ribavirin had a significantly higher SVR compared to those treated by the standard of care with Peg-interferon and Ribavirin [82, 83]. However, patients also suffered high rates of side effects [84] and several drug interactions [85] and viral resistance might occur and patients with cirrhosis need a longer duration treatment [86]. In 2014, new DAAs, such as Simeprevir (second-generation protease inhibitor), Daclatasvir (NS5A inhibitor), and Sofosbuvir (NS5B inhibitor), were licensed for treatment in combination with Peg-interferon and Ribavirin in genotype 1 patients. Peg-interferon plus Ribavirin in combination with Simeprevir [87] or Sofosbuvir [88] had a SVR in about 80% and 90% of patients, respectively. New interferon-free treatments will probably be the standard of care due to their high efficacy and low adverse events for untreated patients and previous interferon nonresponders. These regimens might comprise the following combinations: (i) protease or NS5A inhibitor plus a NS5B inhibitor with or without Ribavirin; (ii) a protease inhibitor plus a NS5A and a NS5B inhibitor with or without Ribavirin; or (iii) a protease inhibitor and a NS5A inhibitor with or without Ribavirin.

Several studies have evaluated the efficacy of interferon-free regimens in HCV genotype 1 patients. The combination of Sofosbuvir (NS5B inhibitor) with Ledipasvir (NS5A) in combined pill once daily without Ribavirin for 12 weeks is highly effective in untreated (SVR 97%) [89] and previously treatment-experienced patients (SVR 93%) [90]. In addition, the same regimen can achieve a 94% SVR in treatment-naive patients in 8-week treatment. The efficacy of Sofosbuvir/Ledipasvir with Ribavirin remains very high in patients with well-compensated cirrhosis (Child-Pugh-Turcotte class A) in a 12-week treatment (96% SVR) [90]. Other potentially effective oral combination regimens have been described. The combination of Paritaprevir (second generation protease inhibitor) boosted by Ritonavir with Ombitasvir (NS5A inhibitor) and Dasabuvir (NS5B inhibitor) in a combined pill twice daily with Ribavirin had a 96% SVR in treatment-naive genotype 1 patients and 96% of SVR in noncirrhotic nonresponders to Peg-interferon and Ribavirin [91]. Similar results were described in cirrhotic treatment-naive or treatment experimented patients treated for 12 (with 92% of SVR) or 24 weeks (96% SVR) [92]. In addition, the coformulation Sofosbuvir/Simeprevir had a 92–96% SVR depending on stage of fibrosis or previous treatment [93].

Similar results have been described in genotypes 2 and 3 patients. Sofosbuvir with Ribavirin is highly effective in 12-week treatment of genotype 2 (97%) but a longer treatment is needed in those with genotype 3. In addition, response rate is lower in those with cirrhosis [94, 95]. High rates of SVR (94–100%) have been reported in genotypes 2 and 3 patients treated with the combination Sofosbuvir/Daclatasvir [96]. Similar results were reported in a regimen combining Sofosbuvir and Ledipasvir for patients with genotype 3 [97]. Those combinations, Sofosbuvir/Daclatasvir and Sofosbuvir/Simeprevir or others such as Ritonavir boosted Paritaprevir/Ombitasvir, showed efficacy in patients with genotype 4 [98, 99].

The Brazilian Ministry of Health has recently approved guidelines for treatment of CHC with interferon-free regimens [16]. Sofosbuvir, Daclatasvir, and Simeprevir were included for interferon-free treatment. These drugs have been adopted by the Brazilian government and delivered free to patients with advanced fibrosis (stages $F \geq 3$) by the public health system (SUS; *Sistema Único de Saúde*). Liver biopsy, serological biomarkers (APRI and FIB-4), or elastography methods have been accepted to stage liver fibrosis. Special populations, such as HIV-HCV coinfected patients can be treated without need of fibrosis staging. Patients can be treated with a specific regimen during 12 or 24 weeks according to genotype, previous response, and presence of cirrhosis (Table 2). Due to the short period since implementation, the effectiveness of these new Brazilian guidelines was still not evaluated.

The access to DAAs is still incipient across Latin American countries. The process for introduction of DAAs in public health systems has just started in Mexico, Venezuela, Chile, and Argentina [22], Colombia has unofficial guideline from the local society of hepatology recommending the use of these drugs. Furthermore, Brazil is the first country where these innovative treatments could be recommended in officially published guidelines [16]. This situation is somewhat different from North America, where Canada and the United States of America already have interferon-free therapies in their national guidelines [100, 101].

Resistance to HCV treatment with Peg-interferon has been previously studied in Brazilian cohorts [102, 103]. The high specificity of DAAs against their viral targets might result in emergence of antiviral resistance and treatment failure in some patients. Resistance-associated mutants may arise prior to or during therapy and cross-resistance among DAAs is high, with resistance to one drug often conferring at least partial resistance to other drugs in the same class. Although methods for detecting resistance-associated variants (RAVs) have been described and commercial assays are available for certain variants (e.g., NS3 Q80K), there is no standard recommendation to evaluate patients for the presence of RAVs in clinical practice and there are few guidelines on their effective use [104]. Phase 3 studies and real-world experience have been showing that treatment

Table 2: Guidelines for CHC treatment according to Brazilian Ministry of Health.

| Conditions | Treatment | Duration |
|---|---|---|
| *Genotype 1* | | |
| HCV monoinfected | Sofosbuvir + Simeprevir<br>OR<br>Sofosbuvir + Daclatasvir | 12 weeks |
| HCV monoinfected with Child-Pugh B/C<br>OR<br>previously treated by Telaprevir/Boceprevir OR<br>HIV-HCV coinfection | Sofosbuvir + Daclatasvir | 24 weeks |
| *Genotype 2* | | |
| HCV monoinfected | Sofosbuvir + Ribavirin | 12 weeks |
| *Genotype 3* | | |
| No contraindication for Peg-interferon | Sofosbuvir + Peg-interferon + Ribavirin | 12 weeks |
| Contraindication for Peg-interferon | Sofosbuvir + Daclatasvir | 12 weeks |
| *Genotype 4* | | |
| No contraindication for Peg-interferon | Daclatasvir + Peg-interferon + Ribavirin | 24 weeks |
| Contraindication for Peg-interferon | Sofosbuvir + Daclatasvir | 12 weeks |

Source: Brazilian Ministry of Health [16].

using DAAs seems to be safe with very low rates of serious adverse effects [105].

The growing complexity of CHC treatment may reach a future point where a new specialty could emerge just to treat people living with HCV [106]. Due to this scenario, the effort to synthetize scientific knowledge into clear and evidence-based guidelines should be made [16, 100, 107].

New treatment regimens with DAAs are highly effective and safe, have short duration, and involve simple interferon-free oral coformulations, most of which without association of Ribavirin. However, these regimens are costly which might lead to a restricting societal benefit. Health policies might be implemented based on cost-effectiveness, stage of disease, and potential gain from treatment.

## 9. Conclusions

An estimated number of 1.45 million people are living with chronic hepatitis C in Brazil, representing a major public health issue. This liver disease presents a variable natural history ranging from minimal changes to advanced fibrosis and cirrhosis and its complications. Liver fibrosis might be accurately staged by noninvasive methods and new antiviral treatments might eradicate the virus in high rates. However, further research is needed to analyze the cost-effectiveness of noninvasive diagnostic strategies and prompt treatment with new antiviral drugs in the perspective of Brazilian universal health system.

## Acknowledgments

The authors would like to acknowledge the following research grants: Newton Fund RCUK-CONFAP Research Partnerships call, Project "Brazil-UK collaboration in Health Technology Assessment of diagnostic strategies for infectious diseases," Fundação Carlos Chagas Filho de Amparo à Pesquisa do Estado do Rio de Janeiro (FAPERJ) under Grant E-26/170.021/2015 (Brazil) and Medical Research Council (MRC) Grant Reference MR/M026515/1 (UK), and Conselho Nacional de Desenvolvimento Científico e Tecnológico (CNPq), Bolsa Jovem Talento (BJT), Programa Ciências Sem Fronteiras, Brazil, under Grant 301520/2014-3.

## References

[1] M. J. Alter, H. S. Margolis, K. Krawczynski et al., "The natural history of community-acquired hepatitis C in the United States," *The New England Journal of Medicine*, vol. 327, no. 27, pp. 1899–1905, 1992.

[2] J.-M. Pawlotsky, "Virology of hepatitis B and C viruses and antiviral targets," *Journal of Hepatology*, vol. 44, supplement 1, pp. S10–S13, 2006.

[3] N. A. Terrault, J. L. Dodge, E. L. Murphy et al., "Sexual transmission of hepatitis C virus among monogamous heterosexual couples: the HCV partners study," *Hepatology*, vol. 57, no. 3, pp. 881–889, 2013.

[4] National Institutes of Health, "National institutes of health consensus development conference statement: management of hepatitis C: 2002—June 10–12, 2002," *Hepatology*, vol. 36, supplement 1, pp. S3–S20, 2002.

[5] M. V. Reggiardo, F. Fay, M. Tanno et al., "Natural history of hepatitis c virus infection in a cohort of asymptomatic post-transfused subjects," *Annals of Hepatology*, vol. 11, no. 5, pp. 658–666, 2012.

[6] European Association for Study of the Liver, *EASL Recommendations on Treatment of Hepatitis C 2014*, EASL, Geneva, Switzerland, 2014.

[7] S. Maity, S. Nandi, S. Biswas, S. K. Sadhukhan, and M. K. Saha, "Performance and diagnostic usefulness of commercially available enzyme linked immunosorbent assay and rapid kits for detection of HIV, HBV and HCV in India," *Virology Journal*, vol. 9, no. 1, article 290, 2012.

[8] B. D. Smith, J. Drobeniuc, A. Jewett et al., "Evaluation of three rapid screening assays for detection of antibodies to hepatitis C virus," *Journal of Infectious Diseases*, vol. 204, no. 6, pp. 825–831, 2011.

[9] V. A. Moyer, "Screening for hepatitis C virus infection in adults: U.S. preventive services task force recommendation statement," *Annals of Internal Medicine*, vol. 159, no. 5, pp. 349–357, 2013.

[10] T. J. Liang and M. G. Ghany, "Current and future therapies for hepatitis C virus infection," *The New England Journal of Medicine*, vol. 368, no. 20, pp. 1907–1917, 2013.

[11] D. G. Murphy, B. Willems, M. Deschênes, N. Hilzenrat, R. Mousseau, and S. Sabbah, "Use of sequence analysis of the NS5B region for routine genotyping of hepatitis C virus with reference to C/E1 and 5′ untranslated region sequences," *Journal of Clinical Microbiology*, vol. 45, no. 4, pp. 1102–1112, 2007.

[12] T. Sy and M. M. Jamal, "Epidemiology of hepatitis C virus (HCV) infection," *International Journal of Medical Sciences*, vol. 3, no. 2, pp. 41–46, 2006.

[13] J. Abrantes, D. S. Torres, and C. E. B. de Mello, "Patients with hepatitis C infection and normal liver function: an evaluation of cognitive function," *Postgraduate Medical Journal*, vol. 89, no. 1054, pp. 433–439, 2013.

[14] A. G. Vigani, M. H. Pavan, R. Tozzo et al., "Comparative study of patients with chronic hepatitis C virus infection due to genotypes 1 and 3 referred for treatment in southeast Brazil," *BMC Infectious Diseases*, vol. 8, article 164, 2008.

[15] B. R. Das, B. Kundu, R. Khandapkar, and S. Sahni, "Geographical distribution of hepatitis C virus genotypes in India," *Indian Journal of Pathology and Microbiology*, vol. 45, no. 3, pp. 323–328, 2002.

[16] Ministério da Saúde. Secretaria de Vigilância em Saúde. Departamento de DST. Aids e Hepatites Virais, *Protocolo Clínico e Diretrizes Terapêuticas para Hepatite C e Coinfecções*, MS, Brasília, Brazil, 2015.

[17] F. Ansaldi, A. Orsi, L. Sticchi, B. Bruzzone, and G. Icardi, "Hepatitis C virus in the new era: perspectives in epidemiology, prevention, diagnostics and predictors of response to therapy," *World Journal of Gastroenterology*, vol. 20, no. 29, pp. 9633–9652, 2014.

[18] D. Lavanchy, "The global burden of hepatitis C," *Liver International*, vol. 29, no. 1, pp. 74–81, 2009.

[19] Brasil. Ministério da Saúde, Secretaria de Vigilância em Saúde, Departamento de DST, and Aids e Hepatites Virais, *Boletim Epidemiológico—Hepatites Virais*, Ministério da Saúde, Brasília, Brazil, 2012.

[20] Ministério da Saúde, Secretaria de Vigilância em Saúde, Sistema de Informação de Agravos de Notificação, and Sinan Net, *Hepatites Virais Casos Confirmados Notificados no Sistema de Informação de Agravos de Notificação por Ano de Diagnóstico/Sintomas*, Ministério da Saúde, Brasília, Brazil, 2015.

[21] Brasil. Ministério da Saúde, Secretaria de Vigilância em Saúde, Departamento de DST, and Aids e Hepatites Virais, *Boletim Epidemiológico—Hepatites Virais*, Ministério da Saúde, Brasília, Brazil, 2015.

[22] R. C. Botero and M. Tagle, "New therapies for hepatitis C: Latin American perspectives," *Clinical Liver Disease*, vol. 5, no. 1, pp. 8–10, 2015.

[23] L. M. M. B. Pereira, C. M. T. Martelli, R. C. Moreira et al., "Prevalence and risk factors of Hepatitis C virus infection in Brazil, 2005 through 2009: a Cross-Sectional Study," *BMC Infectious Diseases*, vol. 13, article 60, 2013.

[24] F. F. Fernandes, M. L. Ferraz, L. E. Andrade et al., "Enhanced liver fibrosis panel as a predictor of liver fibrosis in chronic hepatitis C patients," *Journal of Clinical Gastroenterology*, vol. 49, no. 3, pp. 235–241, 2015.

[25] H. Perazzo, F. F. Fernandes, A. Gomes, C. Terra, R. M. Perez, and F. A. F. Figueiredo, "Interobserver variability in transient elastography analysis of patients with chronic hepatitis C," *Liver International*, vol. 35, no. 5, pp. 1533–1539, 2015.

[26] D. C. Paranaguá-Vezozzo, S. K. Ono, M. V. Alvarado-Mora et al., "Epidemiology of HCC in Brazil: incidence and risk factors in a ten-year cohort," *Annals of Hepatology*, vol. 13, no. 4, pp. 386–393, 2014.

[27] N. Akamatsu and Y. Sugawara, "Liver transplantation and Hepatitis C," *International Journal of Hepatology*, vol. 2012, Article ID 686135, 22 pages, 2012.

[28] F. Klaus, C. Keitel da Silva, G. Meinerz et al., "Acute kidney injury after liver transplantation: incidence and mortality," *Transplantation Proceedings*, vol. 46, no. 6, pp. 1819–1821, 2014.

[29] P. R. Salvalaggio, J. C. Caicedo, L. C. de Albuquerque et al., "Liver transplantation in Latin America: the state-of-the-art and future trends," *Transplantation*, vol. 98, no. 3, pp. 241–246, 2014.

[30] J. M. Barrera, M. Bruguera, M. Guadalupe Ercilla et al., "Persistent hepatitis C viremia after acute self-limiting posttransfusion hepatitis C," *Hepatology*, vol. 21, no. 3, pp. 639–644, 1995.

[31] T. Poynard, V. Ratziu, Y. Benmanov, V. Di Martino, P. Bedossa, and P. Opolon, "Fibrosis in patients with chronic hepatitis C: detection and significance," *Seminars in Liver Disease*, vol. 20, no. 1, pp. 47–56, 2000.

[32] S. A. Villano, D. Vlahov, K. E. Nelson, S. Cohn, and D. L. Thomas, "Persistence of viremia and the importance of long-term follow-up after acute hepatitis C infection," *Hepatology*, vol. 29, no. 3, pp. 908–914, 1999.

[33] T. Poynard, P. Bedossa, and P. Opolon, "Natural history of liver fibrosis progression in patients with chronic hepatitis C," *The Lancet*, vol. 349, no. 9055, pp. 825–832, 1997.

[34] H. J. Alter and L. B. Seeff, "Recovery, persistence, and sequelae in hepatitis C virus infection: a perspective on long-term outcome," *Seminars in Liver Disease*, vol. 20, no. 1, pp. 17–35, 2000.

[35] P. Cohen, "Extrahepatic manifestations of the hepatitis C virus," *Presse Medicale*, vol. 29, no. 4, pp. 209–214, 2000.

[36] D. Prati, A. Zanella, C. De Mattei et al., "Chronic hepatitis C virus infection and primary cutaneous B-cell lymphoma," *British Journal of Haematology*, vol. 105, no. 3, p. 841, 1999.

[37] R. Planas, B. Ballesté, M. A. Álvarez et al., "Natural history of decompensated hepatitis C virus-related cirrhosis. A study of 200 patients," *Journal of Hepatology*, vol. 40, no. 5, pp. 823–830, 2004.

[38] S. L. Chen and T. R. Morgan, "The natural history of hepatitis C virus (HCV) infection," *International Journal of Medical Sciences*, vol. 3, no. 2, pp. 47–52, 2006.

[39] P. Bedossa, "Intraobserver and interobserver variations in liver biopsy interpretation in patients with chronic hepatitis C," *Hepatology*, vol. 20, no. 1, part 1, pp. 15–20, 1994.

[40] K. Ishak, A. Baptista, L. Bianchi et al., "Histological grading and staging of chronic hepatitis," *Journal of Hepatology*, vol. 22, no. 6, pp. 696–699, 1995.

[41] D. B. McGill, J. Rakela, A. R. Zinsmeister, and B. J. Ott, "A 21-year experience with major hemorrhage after percutaneous liver biopsy," *Gastroenterology*, vol. 99, no. 5, pp. 1396–1400, 1990.

[42] R. Bergesch D'Incao, M. C. A. da Silva, P. R. L. de Almeida, V. Plasse Renon, and C. V. Tovo, "Percutaneous liver biopsy—2 decades of experience in a public hospital in the South of Brazil," *Annals of Hepatology*, vol. 12, no. 6, pp. 876–880, 2013.

[43] A. A. Bravo, S. G. Sheth, and S. Chopra, "Liver biopsy," *The New England Journal of Medicine*, vol. 344, no. 7, pp. 495–500, 2001.

[44] P. Bedossa, D. Dargère, and V. Paradis, "Sampling variability of liver fibrosis in chronic hepatitis C," *Hepatology*, vol. 38, no. 6, pp. 1449–1457, 2003.

[45] M.-C. Rousselet, S. Michalak, F. Dupré et al., "Sources of variability in histological scoring of chronic viral hepatitis," *Hepatology*, vol. 41, no. 2, pp. 257–264, 2005.

[46] T. Poynard, R. Morra, P. Ingiliz et al., "Assessment of liver fibrosis: noninvasive means," *Saudi Journal of Gastroenterology*, vol. 14, no. 4, pp. 163–173, 2008.

[47] S. Sharma, K. Khalili, and G. C. Nguyen, "Non-invasive diagnosis of advanced fibrosis and cirrhosis," *World Journal of Gastroenterology*, vol. 20, no. 45, pp. 16820–16830, 2014.

[48] S. Bota, H. Herkner, I. Sporea et al., "Meta-analysis: ARFI elastography versus transient elastography for the evaluation of liver fibrosis," *Liver International*, vol. 33, no. 8, pp. 1138–1147, 2013.

[49] C.-T. Wai, J. K. Greenson, R. J. Fontana et al., "A simple noninvasive index can predict both significant fibrosis and cirrhosis in patients with chronic hepatitis C," *Hepatology*, vol. 38, no. 2, pp. 518–526, 2003.

[50] H. Perazzo, R. Pais, M. Munteanu et al., "Variability in definitions of transaminase upper limit of the normal impacts the APRI performance as a biomarker of fibrosis in patients with chronic hepatitis C: 'APRI c'est fini?'," *Clinics and Research in Hepatology and Gastroenterology*, vol. 38, no. 4, pp. 432–439, 2014.

[51] R. Chou and N. Wasson, "Blood tests to diagnose fibrosis or cirrhosis in patients with chronic hepatitis C virus infection: a systematic review," *Annals of Internal Medicine*, vol. 158, no. 11, pp. 807–820, 2013.

[52] D. Nunes, C. Fleming, G. Offner et al., "Noninvasive markers of liver fibrosis are highly predictive of liver-related death in a cohort of HCV-infected individuals with and without HIV infection," *American Journal of Gastroenterology*, vol. 105, no. 6, pp. 1346–1353, 2010.

[53] J. Vergniol, J. Foucher, E. Terrebonne et al., "Noninvasive tests for fibrosis and liver stiffness predict 5-year outcomes of patients with chronic hepatitis C," *Gastroenterology*, vol. 140, no. 7, pp. 1970–1979, 2011.

[54] T. Poynard, Y. Ngo, H. Perazzo et al., "Prognostic value of liver fibrosis biomarkers: a meta-analysis," *Gastroenterology & Hepatology*, vol. 7, no. 7, pp. 445–454, 2011.

[55] E. R. Parise, A. C. Oliveira, C. Figueiredo-Mendes et al., "Noninvasive serum markers in the diagnosis of structural liver damage in chronic hepatitis C virus infection," *Liver International*, vol. 26, no. 9, pp. 1095–1099, 2006.

[56] R. G. da Silva Jr., R. Fakhouri, T. V. B. do Nascimento, I. M. Santos, and L. M. M. Barbosa, "Aspartate aminotransferase-to-platelet ratio index for fibrosis and cirrhosis prediction in chronic hepatitis C patients," *Brazilian Journal of Infectious Diseases*, vol. 12, no. 1, pp. 15–19, 2008.

[57] T. G. F. Amorim, G. J. Staub, C. Lazzarotto et al., "Validation and comparison of simple noninvasive models for the prediction of liver fibrosis in chronic hepatitis C," *Annals of Hepatology*, vol. 11, no. 6, pp. 855–861, 2012.

[58] R. G. Silva Junior, J. Schmillevitch, M. D. F. A. Nascimento et al., "Acoustic radiation force impulse elastography and serum fibrosis markers in chronic hepatitis C," *Scandinavian Journal of Gastroenterology*, vol. 49, no. 8, pp. 986–992, 2014.

[59] V. de Lédinghen and J. Vergniol, "Transient elastography (FibroScan)," *Gastroenterologie Clinique et Biologique*, vol. 32, supplement 1, no. 6, pp. 58–67, 2008.

[60] H. Perazzo, F. F. Fernandes, J. C. Soares et al., "Learning curve and intra/interobserver agreement of transient elastography in chronic hepatitis C patients with or without HIV co-infection," *Clinics and Research in Hepatology and Gastroenterology*, 2015.

[61] L. Castéra, J. Vergniol, J. Foucher et al., "Prospective comparison of transient elastography, Fibrotest, APRI, and liver biopsy for the assessment of fibrosis in chronic hepatitis C," *Gastroenterology*, vol. 128, no. 2, pp. 343–350, 2005.

[62] M. Ziol, A. Handra-Luca, A. Kettaneh et al., "Noninvasive assessment of liver fibrosis by measurement of stiffness in patients with chronic hepatitis C," *Hepatology*, vol. 41, no. 1, pp. 48–54, 2005.

[63] T. Poynard, J. Vergniol, Y. Ngo et al., "Staging chronic hepatitis C in seven categories using fibrosis biomarker (FibroTest) and transient elastography (FibroScan)," *Journal of Hepatology*, vol. 60, no. 4, pp. 706–714, 2014.

[64] G. A. Alves, M. Z. Baldessar, G. W. Pereira, V. M. Kuehlkamp, C. Hilzendeger, and J. da Silva, "Quality of life of patients with hepatitis C," *Revista da Sociedade Brasileira de Medicina Tropical*, vol. 45, no. 5, pp. 553–557, 2012.

[65] A. C. El Khoury, J. Vietri, and G. Prajapati, "Health-related quality of life in patients with hepatitis C virus infection in Brazil," *Pan American Journal of Public Health*, vol. 35, no. 3, pp. 200–206, 2014.

[66] E. Strauss, F. A. Porto-Ferreira, C. de Almeida-Neto, and M. C. D. Teixeira, "Altered quality of life in the early stages of chronic hepatitis C is due to the virus itself," *Clinics and Research in Hepatology and Gastroenterology*, vol. 38, no. 1, pp. 40–45, 2014.

[67] M. C. D. Teixeira, M. D. F. G. S. Ribeiro, L. C. D. C. Gayotto, D. D. A. F. Chamone, and E. Strauss, "Worse quality of life in volunteer blood donors with hepatitis C," *Transfusion (Paris)*, vol. 46, no. 2, pp. 278–283, 2006.

[68] B. C. Fábregas, R. E. de Ávila, M. N. Faria, A. S. Moura, R. A. Carmo, and A. L. Teixeira, "Health related quality of life among patients with chronic hepatitis C: a cross-sectional study of sociodemographic, psychopathological and psychiatric determinants," *Brazilian Journal of Infectious Diseases*, vol. 17, no. 6, pp. 633–639, 2013.

[69] B. C. Fábregas, A. S. Moura, R. E. de Ávila, M. N. Faria, R. A. Carmo, and A. L. Teixeira, "Sexual dysfunction and dissatisfaction in chronic hepatitis C patients," *Revista da Sociedade Brasileira de Medicina Tropical*, vol. 47, no. 5, pp. 564–572, 2014.

[70] M. Morais-de-Jesus, R. Daltro-Oliveira, K. M. Pettersen et al., "Hepatitis C virus infection as a traumatic experience," *PLoS ONE*, vol. 9, no. 10, Article ID e110529, 2014.

[71] M. C. M. Fonseca, G. T. B. de Araújo, and D. V. Araújo, "Cost effectiveness of peginterferon alfa-2B combined with ribavirin for the treatment of chronic hepatitis C in Brazil," *Brazilian Journal of Infectious Diseases*, vol. 13, no. 3, pp. 191–199, 2009.

[72] F. M. R. Barros, H. Cheinquer, C. T. Tsuchiya, and E. A. V. Santos, "Cost-effectiveness analysis of treatment with peginterferon-alfa-2a versus peginterferon-alfa-2b for patients with chronic hepatitis C under the public payer perspective in Brazil," *Cost Effectiveness and Resource Allocation*, vol. 11, no. 1, article 25, 2013.

[73] E. Massad, F. A. B. Coutinho, E. Chaib, and M. N. Burattini, "Cost-effectiveness analysis of a hypothetical hepatitis C vaccine compared to antiviral therapy," *Epidemiology and Infection*, vol. 137, no. 2, pp. 241–249, 2009.

[74] M. P. da S. Rodrigues, C. M. de M. Vianna, G. B. G. Mosegui, F. V. Costa e Silva, A. A. de F. Peregrino, and F. N. Jardim, "Cost-effectiveness of hepatitis C treatment in slow virologic responders coinfected with HIV," *Cadernos de Saúde Pública*, vol. 29, supplement 1, pp. S146–S158, 2013.

[75] K. Bichoupan, V. Martel-Laferriere, D. Sachs et al., "Costs of telaprevir-based triple therapy for hepatitis C: $189,000 per sustained virological response," *Hepatology*, vol. 60, no. 4, pp. 1187–1195, 2014.

[76] A. J. van der Meer, B. J. Veldt, J. J. Feld et al., "Association between sustained virological response and all-cause mortality among patients with chronic hepatitis C and advanced hepatic fibrosis," *The Journal of the American Medical Association*, vol. 308, no. 24, pp. 2584–2593, 2012.

[77] M. Imran, S. Manzoor, J. Ashraf et al., "Role of viral and host factors in interferon based therapy of hepatitis C virus infection," *Virology Journal*, vol. 10, article 299, 2013.

[78] S. Chevaliez, "Antiviral activity of the new DAAs for the treatment of hepatitis C virus infection: virology and resistance," *Clinics and Research in Hepatology and Gastroenterology*, vol. 35, pp. S46–S51, 2011.

[79] S. Artico, K. M. Amaral, C. B. T. Gonçalves, and P. D. Picon, "The effectiveness of retreatment with peginterferon alfa and ribavirin in patients with chronic viral hepatitis C genotype 2 and 3: a prospective cohort study in Brazil," *BMC Infectious Diseases*, vol. 12, article 377, 2012.

[80] A. G. Vigani, E. S. Gonçales, M. H. P. Pavan et al., "Therapeutic effectiveness of biosimilar standard interferon versus pegylated interferon for chronic hepatitis C genotypes 2 or 3," *Brazilian Journal of Infectious Diseases*, vol. 16, no. 3, pp. 232–236, 2012.

[81] D. P. Webster, P. Klenerman, and G. M. Dusheiko, "Hepatitis C," *The Lancet*, vol. 385, no. 9973, pp. 1124–1135, 2015.

[82] F. Poordad, J. McCone Jr., B. R. Bacon et al., "Boceprevir for untreated chronic HCV genotype 1 infection," *The New England Journal of Medicine*, vol. 364, no. 13, pp. 1195–1206, 2011.

[83] I. M. Jacobson, J. G. McHutchison, G. Dusheiko et al., "Telaprevir for previously untreated chronic hepatitis C virus infection," *The New England Journal of Medicine*, vol. 364, no. 25, pp. 2405–2416, 2011.

[84] C. Hézode, H. Fontaine, C. Dorival et al., "Effectiveness of telaprevir or boceprevir in treatment-experienced patients with HCV genotype 1 infection and cirrhosis," *Gastroenterology*, vol. 147, no. 1, pp. 132–142.e4, 2014.

[85] J. J. Kiser, J. R. Burton, and G. T. Everson, "Drug-drug interactions during antiviral therapy for chronic hepatitis C," *Nature Reviews Gastroenterology and Hepatology*, vol. 10, no. 10, pp. 596–606, 2013.

[86] J.-M. Pawlotsky, "Treatment failure and resistance with direct-acting antiviral drugs against hepatitis C virus," *Hepatology*, vol. 53, no. 5, pp. 1742–1751, 2011.

[87] M. Manns, P. Marcellin, F. Poordad et al., "Simeprevir with pegylated interferon alfa 2a or 2b plus ribavirin in treatment-naive patients with chronic hepatitis C virus genotype 1 infection (QUEST-2): a randomised, double-blind, placebo-controlled phase 3 trial," *The Lancet*, vol. 384, no. 9941, pp. 414–426, 2014.

[88] K. V. Kowdley, E. Lawitz, I. Crespo et al., "Sofosbuvir with pegylated interferon alfa-2a and ribavirin for treatment-naive patients with hepatitis C genotype-1 infection (ATOMIC): an open-label, randomised, multicentre phase 2 trial," *The Lancet*, vol. 381, no. 9883, pp. 2100–2107, 2013.

[89] N. Afdhal, K. R. Reddy, D. R. Nelson et al., "Ledipasvir and sofosbuvir for previously treated HCV genotype 1 infection," *The New England Journal of Medicine*, vol. 370, no. 16, pp. 1483–1493, 2014.

[90] K. V. Kowdley, S. C. Gordon, K. R. Reddy et al., "Ledipasvir and sofosbuvir for 8 or 12 weeks for chronic HCV without cirrhosis," *The New England Journal of Medicine*, vol. 370, no. 20, pp. 1879–1888, 2014.

[91] S. Zeuzem, I. M. Jacobson, T. Baykal et al., "Retreatment of HCV with ABT-450/r—ombitasvir and dasabuvir with ribavirin," *The New England Journal of Medicine*, vol. 370, no. 17, pp. 1604–1614, 2014.

[92] F. Poordad, C. Hezode, R. Trinh et al., "ABT-450/r-ombitasvir and dasabuvir with ribavirin for hepatitis C with cirrhosis," *The New England Journal of Medicine*, vol. 370, no. 21, pp. 1973–1982, 2014.

[93] E. Lawitz, M. S. Sulkowski, R. Ghalib et al., "Simeprevir plus sofosbuvir, with or without ribavirin, to treat chronic infection with hepatitis C virus genotype 1 in non-responders to pegylated interferon and ribavirin and treatment-naive patients: the COSMOS randomised study," *The Lancet*, vol. 384, no. 9956, pp. 1756–1765, 2014.

[94] I. M. Jacobson, S. C. Gordon, K. V. Kowdley et al., "Sofosbuvir for hepatitis C genotype 2 or 3 in patients without treatment options," *The New England Journal of Medicine*, vol. 368, no. 20, pp. 1867–1877, 2013.

[95] S. Zeuzem, G. M. Dusheiko, R. Salupere et al., "Sofosbuvir and Ribavirin in HCV genotypes 2 and 3," *The New England Journal of Medicine*, vol. 370, no. 21, pp. 1993–2001, 2014.

[96] D. R. Nelson, J. N. Cooper, J. P. Lalezari et al., "All-oral 12-week treatment with daclatasvir plus sofosbuvir in patients with hepatitis C virus genotype 3 infection: ALLY-3 phase III study," *Hepatology*, vol. 61, no. 4, pp. 1127–1135, 2015.

[97] E. J. Gane, R. H. Hyland, D. An et al., "Sofosbuvir/ledipasvir fixed dose combination is safe and effective in difficult-to-treat populations including genotype-3 patients, decompensated genotype-1 patients, and genotype-1 patients with prior sofosbuvir treatment experience," *Journal of Hepatology*, vol. 60, no. 1, pp. S3–S4, 2014.

[98] P. J. Ruane, D. Ain, J. Riad et al., "Sofosbuvir plus ribavirin in the treatment of chronic HCV genotype 4 infection in patients of Egyptian ancestry," in *Proceedings of the 64rd Annual Meeting of the American Association for the Study of Liver Diseases*, Washington, DC, USA, November 2013.

[99] C. Hezode, P. Marcellin, S. Pol et al., "Results from the phase 2 PEARL-I study: interferon-free regimens of ABT-450/R + ABT-267 with or without ribavirin in patients with HCV genotype 4

infection," *Journal of Hepatology*, vol. 60, no. 1, supplement, p. S24, 2014.

[100] R. P. Myers, H. Shah, K. W. Burak, C. Cooper, and J. J. Feld, "An update on the management of chronic hepatitis C: 2015 Consensus guidelines from the Canadian Association for the Study of the Liver," *Canadian Journal of Gastroenterology and Hepatology*, vol. 29, no. 1, pp. 19–34, 2015.

[101] AASLD/IDSA HCV Guidance Panel, "Hepatitis C guidance: AASLD-IDSA recommendations for testing, managing, and treating adults infected with hepatitis C virus," *Hepatology*, vol. 62, no. 3, pp. 932–954, 2015.

[102] L. Hoffmann, J. A. Ramos, E. V. de Souza et al., "Dynamics of resistance mutations to NS3 protease inhibitors in a cohort of Brazilian patients chronically infected with hepatitis C virus (genotype 1) treated with pegylated interferon and ribavirin: a prospective longitudinal study," *Virology Journal*, vol. 10, no. 1, p. 57, 2013.

[103] L. B. Zeminian, J. L. Padovani, S. M. Corvino, G. F. Silva, M. I. D. M. C. Pardini, and R. M. T. Grotto, "Variability and resistance mutations in the hepatitis C virus NS3 protease in patients not treated with protease inhibitors," *Memórias do Instituto Oswaldo Cruz*, vol. 108, no. 1, pp. 13–17, 2013.

[104] C. Sarrazin, "The importance of resistance to direct antiviral drugs in HCV infection in clinical practice," *Journal of Hepatology*, 2015.

[105] S. Bansal, A. K. Singal, B. M. McGuire, and B. S. Anand, "Impact of all oral anti-hepatitis C virus therapy: a meta-analysis," *World Journal of Hepatology*, vol. 7, no. 5, pp. 806–813, 2015.

[106] V. Soriano, E. Vispo, E. Poveda et al., "Directly acting antivirals against hepatitis C virus," *Journal of Antimicrobial Chemotherapy*, vol. 66, no. 8, Article ID dkr215, pp. 1673–1686, 2011.

[107] J. C. Booth, J. O'Grady, J. Neuberger, and Thr Royal College of Physicians of London and the British Society of Gastroenterology, "Clinical guidelines on the management of hepatitis C," *Gut*, vol. 49, supplement 1, pp. I1–I21, 2001.

# 28

# Relationship between Serum Cytokeratin-18, Control Attenuation Parameter, NAFLD Fibrosis Score, and Liver Steatosis in Nonalcoholic Fatty Liver Disease

**Sumitro Kosasih,[1] Wong Zhi Qin,[1] Rafiz Abdul Rani,[2] Nazefah Abd Hamid,[3] Ngiu Chai Soon,[1] Shamsul Azhar Shah,[4] Yazmin Yaakob,[5] and Raja Affendi Raja Ali[1]**

[1] *Gastroenterology and Hepatology Unit, Faculty of Medicine, Universiti Kebangsaan Malaysia, Kuala Lumpur, 56000, Malaysia*
[2] *Gastroenterology Unit, Faculty of Medicine, Universiti Teknologi MARA, Shah Alam, Selangor, 40450, Malaysia*
[3] *Department of Medical and Health Science, Universiti Sains Islam Malaysia, Nilai, Negeri Sembilan, 71800, Malaysia*
[4] *Department of Public Health, Faculty of Medicine, Universiti Kebangsaan Malaysia, Kuala Lumpur, 56000, Malaysia*
[5] *Department of Radiology, Faculty of Medicine, Universiti Kebangsaan Malaysia, Kuala Lumpur, 56000, Malaysia*

Correspondence should be addressed to Raja Affendi Raja Ali; draffendi@ppukm.ukm.edu.my

Academic Editor: Heather Francis

*Backgrounds.* The aim of this study was to appraise the relationship between serum fragmented cytokeratin-18(CK-18), controlled attenuation parameter (CAP), and liver steatosis assessed by ultrasound (US) in nonalcoholic fatty liver disease (NAFLD) patients. *Methods.* Patients who underwent abdominal US were recruited, followed with measurement of CAP using Fibroscan[5] and serum fragmented CK-18 using enzyme-linked immunosorbent assay. The degree of liver steatosis assessed by US was categorized into mild (S1), moderate (S2), and severe (S3). *Results.* A total of 109 patients were included in our study. CAP and fragmented CK-18 level were significantly correlated with liver steatosis grade with $r_s$ = 0.56 and 0.68, $p$=0.001, respectively. NAFLD Fibrosis Score was poorly correlated with liver steatosis grade ($r_s$=-0.096, $p$=0.318). Using fragmented CK-18 level, area under receiver operating characteristic (AUROC) curves for S≥2 and S≥3 were excellent (0.82 and 0.84, respectively). Using CAP, AUROC curves for detection of S≥2 and S≥3 were good (0.76, 0.77, respectively). We also proposed cut-off value of CAP to detect S≥2 and S≥3 to be 263 and 319db/m, respectively, and fragmented CK-18 level to detect S≥2 and S≥3 (194 and 294 U/L, respectively). *Conclusions.* Both the fragmented CK-18 level and the CAP, but not NAFLD Fibrosis Score, were well correlated with hepatic steatosis grade as assessed by US.

## 1. Introduction

Nonalcoholic fatty liver disease (NAFLD) is the liver pandemic in this 21st century, affecting 20-45% population around the world [1–5]. NAFLD has been proven to cause liver fibrosis, liver cirrhosis, and hepatocellular carcinoma [6–9]. Not only does it have an adverse outcome to the liver itself but NAFLD also has been associated with increased rate of metabolic syndrome [10], cardiovascular diseases, and chronic kidney disease [11, 12]. Although NAFLD is usually benign, it may be associated with inflammation and hepatocyte apoptosis resulting in nonalcoholic steatohepatitis (NASH) of 20–30% of subjects. One-fifth of these NASH subjects will progress to develop liver cirrhosis [13].

Liver biopsy is still the gold standard to stage liver fibrosis as it provides a multitude of information on the inflammation activity. However, considering its invasive nature, sampling variability, and cost, other noninvasive modalities of imaging and biomarkers have been developed. The NAFLD fibrosis score (NFS) developed by Angulo et al. utilizes six variables (age, body mass index (BMI), diabetes, aspartatetransaminase (AST), alaninetransaminase (ALT), and albumin) which are commonly available in patient's assessment. It has been shown to reduce the need for biopsy in most NAFLD patients [14]. In NASH, liver cell apoptosis and necroinflammation play a major role. Serum caspase-cleaved fragmented cytokeratin-18(CK-18) reflects the degree of apoptosis and has been shown as an independent predictor in diagnosis of

NASH [15–18]. One meta-analysis in 2014 [19] showed area under receiver operating characteristic (AUROC), sensitivity, and specificity of fragmented CK-18 to be 0.84, 0.83, and 0.71, respectively.

For imaging, ultrasound (US) is the first method to be utilized as it is inexpensive, widely available and has a good sensitivity (70-94%) and specificity (70-97%) for liver steatosis [20, 21]. To enhance its sensitivity and specificity, hepatorenal index contrast has been used, resulting in 91% sensitivity and 84% specificity for liver steatosis.

Transient elastography (TE) has been used in several studies to predict steatosis grades in NAFLD patients by using control attenuated parameter (CAP), while stage of fibrosis is measured by liver stiffness measurement (LSM) [22–24]. There are different CAP cut-off values presented by different studies for distinct grades of liver steatosis defined by biopsy (ranging from S0, which indicates no steatosis, to S3, which indicates the highest level of steatosis); for S⩾1(⩾10% of hepatocytes with fat), the CAP cut-off values range from 214 to289dB/m, with a 64%-91% sensitivity range and a 64%-94% specificity range; for S⩾2(⩾33% hepatocytes with fat), the CAP cut-off values range from 255 to 311dB/m, with a 57%-96% sensitivity range and a 62%-94% specificity range; finally, for S3(⩾66% hepatocytes with fat), the CAP cut-off values range from 281 to 310dB/m, with a 64%-100% sensitivity range and a 53%-92% specificity range [23]. A meta-analysis in 2014 [25] showed good pooled sensitivity and specificity for TE in diagnosing fibrosis (F) stage ≥3 (85% sensitivity, 85% specificity) and F4 (92% sensitivity, 92% specificity) and moderate accuracy to predict F≥2 in NAFLD.

The aims of this study are to evaluate the relationship between CAP, LSM, fragmented CK-18, and liver steatosis grade as assessed by US. We also would like to assess the diagnostic performance of CAP and fragmented CK-18 in liver steatosis. Lastly, we aim to compare the level and degree of association of various clinical and laboratory parameters in different liver steatosis grades. This is the first such study in South East Asia.

## 2. Materials and Methods

*2.1. Patient Characteristics.* The study was approved by Universiti Kebangsaan Malaysia (UKM) Ethics Committee and all patients gave written consent prior to participation. We recruited patients, aged more than 18 years old, who underwent ultrasound abdomen between June 2016 and September 2016. Patients with chronic liver disease, pregnancy, malignancy, and excessive alcohol use were excluded.

All recruited patients underwent US abdomen, clinical, laboratory examination, and Fibroscan[5] assessment.

*2.2. Clinical Assessment.* Comorbid illness (hypertension, diabetes, and dyslipidemia) and alcohol intake, together with anthropometric, laboratory, and past medical history, were obtained from all patients on the same day of ultrasound. Body mass index (BMI) was calculated as body weight in kilograms divided by body height in square meters (kg/m$^2$). Waist circumference was measured in a standing position at a level of the umbilicus.

The diagnosis of metabolic syndrome [26–28] was made according to the joint statement of the International Diabetes Federation and World Heart Federation. Excessive alcohol use was defined by an average daily consumption of alcohol of<20g/day for men and <10g/day for women [29].

*2.3. Ultrasonography.* Ultrasound (US) of the abdomen was performed by single experienced consultant radiologist to omit interobserver bias. The degree of liver steatosis on ultrasound was categorized as mild (S1: increased liver echogenicity), moderate (S2: blurring of portal vein branches), or severe (S3: blurring of the diaphragmatic outline) [21, 30–32].

*2.4. Laboratory Examination.* Blood samples were obtained to measure AST, ALT, total cholesterol (TC), triglyceride(TG), high-density lipoprotein cholesterol (HDL-C), low-density lipoprotein cholesterol(LDL-C), fasting blood sugar(FBS), and C-reactive protein(CRP). For measurement of fragmented CK-18, blood as initially processed to plasma and then stored frozen at -80°C. Plasma caspase-3 generated CK-18 fragments were quantitatively measured using the M30 Apoptosense ELISA kit (PEVIVA: Alexis. Grunwald, Germany).

The M30 Apoptosense[5] ELISA is a solid-phase sandwich enzyme immunoassay. Standards, controls, and samples react with a solid phase capture antibody M5 directed against K18 and the HRP-(horseradish peroxidase) conjugated M30 antibody directed against the K18Asp396 neoepitope. Unbound conjugate is removed by a washing step. TMB Substrate is added. The colour development is stopped and the absorbance is read. The resulting colour is directly proportional to the concentration of the analyte. By plotting a standard curve from known concentrations versus measured absorbance in the microplate reader, the amount of antigen in the sample can be calculated. The concentration of the antigen is expressed as Units per Litre (U/L).

*2.5. NAFLD Fibrosis Score.* This score was calculated based on the study by Angulo et al. [14] with formula of -1.675 + 0.037 xage(years) + 0.094 x BMI(kg/m$^2$) +1.13 x diabetes/IFG(yes=1, no=0) + 0.99xAST/ALT ratio – 0.013 x platelet(x 10$^9$/L) – 0.66 x albumin(g/dL). Score below -1.455 signified prediction of no advanced fibrosis while score more than 0.676 signified presence of advanced fibrosis, and the score in between is labeled as indeterminate.

*2.6. Fibroscan.* A Fibroscan 502, manufactured by Echosens (Paris, France), was used in the study. We considered results as reliable if interquartile range/median (IQR/M) is less than 30 percent and success rate is over 60 percent. Ten valid fibroscan readings were necessary for an examination to be deemed successful [33]. Controlled attenuation parameter (CAP) was measured to quantify liver steatosis, while the degree of liver fibrosis was displayed as liver stiffness measurement (LSM).

*2.7. Statistical Analysis.* Descriptive statistics were computed for all factors. These were presented in means (M) ± standard error of means (SEM) for normally distributed data,

Table 1: Patients' characteristics and comorbid conditions. NAFLD: nonalcoholic fatty liver disease; BMI: Body Mass Index; SEM: Standard Error of Means.

| | Non-hepatic steatosis n=41 | NAFLD n = 68 | $p$ value |
|---|---|---|---|
| Gender | 21:20 | 37:31 | |
| (Male: Female) | | | |
| Age, years | | | |
| Mean ±SEM | 50.4±2.3 | 53.1±1.5 | 0.231 |
| BMI, kg/m$^2$ | | | |
| Mean ± SEM | 24.6±0.89 | 29.05±0.60 | 0.000 |
| Diabetes | 11 (26.8%) | 40 (78.4%) | 0.001 |
| Hypertension | 11 (26.8%) | 35 (76%) | 0.009 |
| Dyslipidemia | 12 (29.2%) | 45 (78.9%) | <0.001 |
| Metabolic Syndrome | 12 (29.2%) | 56 (82.4%) | <0.001 |

median (Me) with interquartile range(IQR) for nonnormally distributed data, and percentiles and frequencies for categorical factors. Categorical data analysis was performed using Pearson's Chi-Square. Comparison of continuous variables analysis was performed using One-Way ANOVA or Kruskal Wallis where appropriate. The degrees of correlation between parameters and liver steatosis grades were calculated using Spearman's correlation coefficient ($r_s$). The predictive value of a variable for detection of liver steatosis was evaluated using AUROC curve analysis. A $p$ value of $< 0.05$ was considered significant. All statistical analyses were performed using SPSS software version 20.0(SPSS Inc. Chicago, IL) for Windows.

## 3. Results

*3.1. Patients' Characteristic.* We recruited 109 patients in this study, with 58 (53.2%) patients were male. Median age of patients in the study was 54, with range from 19 to 78 years of age.

Several comorbidities were found to be significantly higher in NAFLD patients compared to healthy subjects (Table 1), such as metabolic syndrome (n=56, 82% vs n=12, 29.2%, $p$<0.001), dyslipidemia (n=45, 79% vs n=23, 44.2%, and $p$<0.001), hypertension (n=35, 76% vs n=33, 52.4%, and $p$=0.009), and diabetes (n=40, 78% vs n=28, 48.2%, and $p$=0.001).

*3.2. Relationship between Liver Biochemistry, CRP, Serum Fragmented CK-18, CAP, LSM and Liver Steatosis Grade.* All liver biochemistry (ALT and AST), as well as apoptotic markers (fragmented CK-18), was significantly higher in NAFLD group compared to healthy subjects ($p$<0.001) (Table 4). Fragmented CK-18 as shown in Figure 1 was significantly different across the healthy subjects, S1, S2, and S3 steatosis at 91(IQR 70-104), 189.5 (IQR 137-227.5), 277 (IQR 189.5-326), and 441(IQR 338-554.5) U/L, respectively.

CAP differed significantly between healthy subjects - 234 (IQR 95-266) dBm and NAFLD group ($p$<0.001) but was not significantly different in between the steatosis grades (S1-310(IQR 277-330), S2 – 331(IQR 279-364), and S3 - 334(IQR 323-374) dB/m).

*3.3. NAFLD Fibrosis Score and Liver Steatosis.* Only two (1.8%) of our patients were categorized as high risk for advanced fibrosis (F3-F4) according to NFS. The remaining were low risk (n=71, 65.1%) and indeterminate (n=36, 33%). We found that NFS was poorly correlated ($r_s$=-0.096, $p$=0.318) with liver steatosis grade.

*3.4. Diagnostic Performance of Fragmented CK-18 and CAP for Assessing Liver Steatosis.* ROC analysis (Figure 2) was performed for all patients (n=109). By using a cut-off value of 194U/L for diagnosis of liver steatosis S≥2, AUROC of fragmented CK-18 was 0.82 [95% Confidence Interval (CI), 0.74-0.91], while sensitivity and specificity were 70% and 82.6%, respectively. By using cut-off value of 294U/L for liver steatosis S≥3, AUROC was 0.84 (95%CI, 0.69-0.99), while sensitivity and specificity were 75%, and 87.6%, respectively.

CAP has demonstrated satisfactory diagnostic performance in detecting liver steatosis. AUROC for liver steatosisS≥2 by using cut-off value of 263dB/m was 0.76(95%CI, 0.65-0.88), with sensitivity of 86.7% and specificity of 47.5%, while AUROC for liver steatosis S≥3 (with a cut-off value of 319 dB/m) was 0.77(95%CI, 0.65-0.88), with sensitivity of 90.9% and specificity of 59.3%.

*3.5. Factors Associated with CAP.* Using univariate linear regression analysis, BMI ($\beta$=5.5, $p$=0.001), FBS ($\beta$=13.07, $p$=0.02), HDL-C ($\beta$=-76.35, $p$=0.004), waist circumference ($\beta$=5.8, $p$=0.001), fragmented CK-18 ($\beta$=0.17, $p$=0.001), LSM($\beta$=10.1, $p$=0.001), and steatosis grade ($\beta$=36.2,$p$=0.001) were associated with CAP in all our patients. Among all these factors, only LSM, TG, and steatosis grade were shown to be independent factors related to CAP in multivariate linear regression analysis (Table 5). With every increment of LSM of 1kPa and 1 mmol/L of TG, CAP score would increase by 7.9dB/m and 21.2dB/m, respectively, while CAP scores would

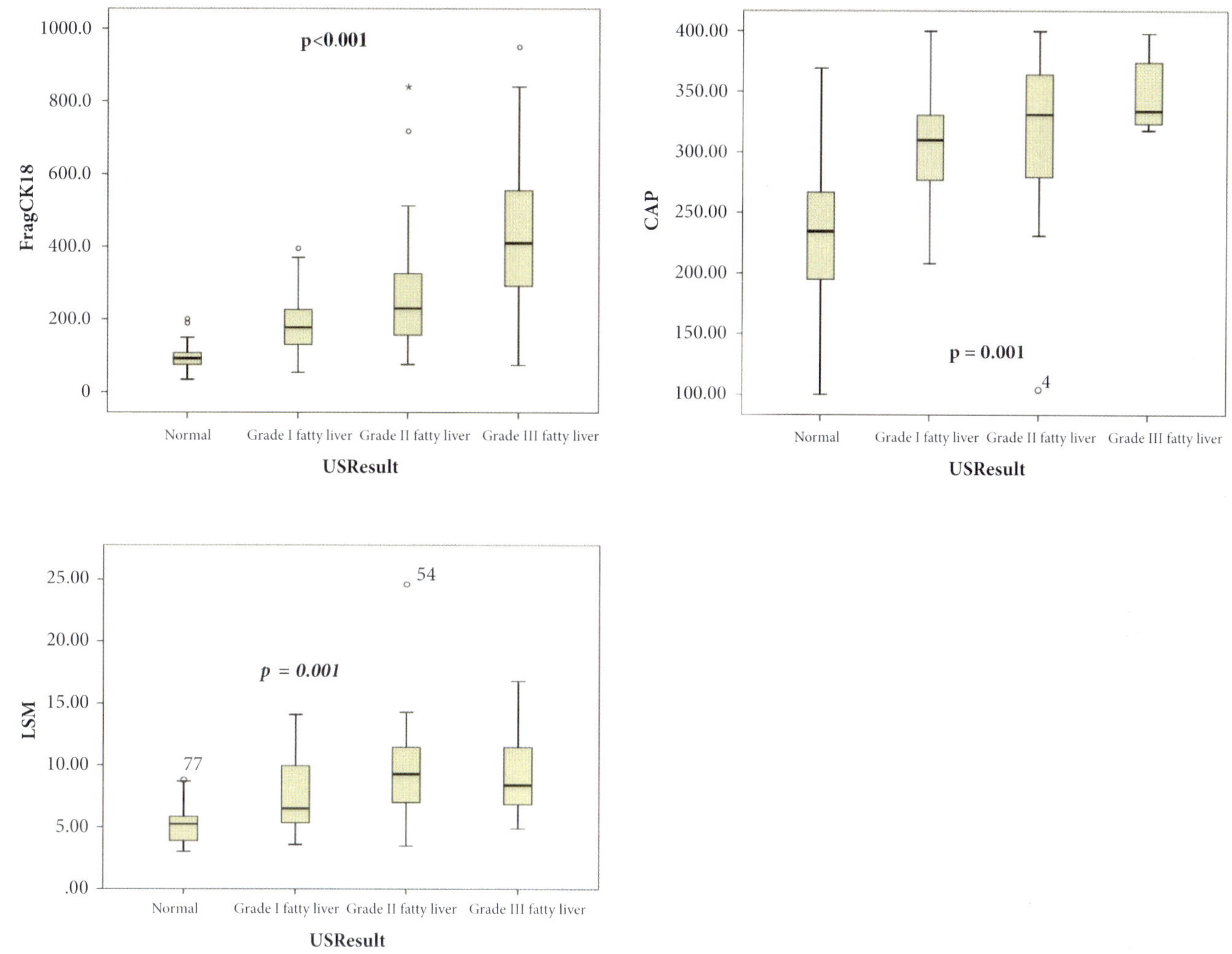


FIGURE 1: The distribution of CAP, LSM, and CK-18 according to steatosis grade assessed by US. Figure 1 showed significant difference in Fragmented CK-18, LSM, and CAP between nonliver steatosis patients and grades I, II, and III liver steatosis patients.

increase by 31.9dB/m with every increment in liver steatosis grade.

## 4. Discussion

Liver biopsy is considered the gold standard for assessing the degree of hepatic steatosis and fibrosis; however, biopsy is rarely done due to its risk and limitation. Liver biopsy has several limitations such as small area of examination (only representing 1/50000 of whole liver), sampling variabilities and error, inter- and intraobserver variability [34–36]. Therefore, steatosis and fibrosis are now being more commonly assessed by using noninvasive modalities like imaging and biomarkers. The short examination time and noninvasiveness make abdominal ultrasonography the best initial screening method for NAFLD. CAP and LSM in fibroscan is a recent, novel way to diagnose NAFLD as well as quantifying hepatic steatosis and fibrosis accurately and in a convenient manner. Fragmented CK-18 is a biomarker that currently under investigation to diagnose NASH and assess the degree of fibrosis [15].

In our study, we found that patient with hypertension, dyslipidemia, diabetes, and metabolic syndrome had higher proportion of suffering from NAFLD, regardless of age and sex. We also found that higher BMI, waist circumference (Table 2), and liver biochemistry (ALT, AST≥35U/L) (Table 3) are associated with increased severity of liver steatosis, as assessed by US. These findings are consistent with previous studies [37, 38]. Chia et al. showed that there was a significant difference in ALT and AST values between mild and significant fatty liver, although they used broader definition of fatty liver population, which included non-NAFLD patients as well.

In a study by Angulo et al. [14], NFS was shown to have a high positive predictive value (90%) of diagnosing advanced fibrosis. However, in our study, we concluded that ultrasonography is not a good tool to differentiate degree of fibrosis, since many of our patients were categorized into low and indeterminate groups, although US showed steatosis grade≥2. This is consistent with previous studies that suggested it is difficult to differentiate steatosis and fibrosis, as

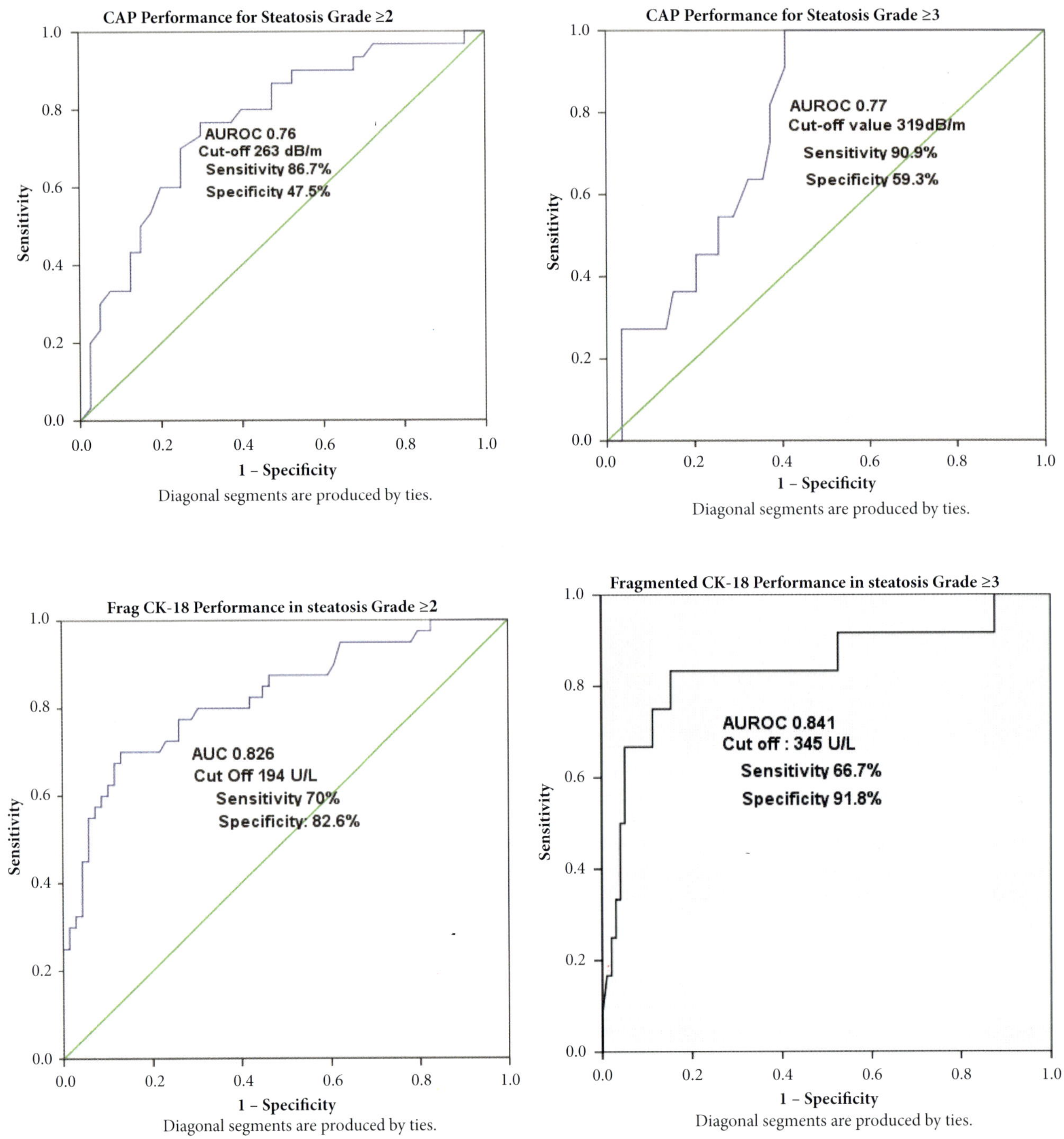


Figure 2: ROC Curve using CAP and Fragmented CK-18, to predict liver steatosis in US. Figure 2 showed CAP value with cutoff value of 263dB/m and 319dB/m had good sensitivity and specificity. FragCK-18 with cut-off value of 194U/L and 345 U/L had a good sensitivity to predict moderate-severe steatosis.

Table 2: Relationship between anthropometric data with liver steatosis as assessed by US. BMI: Body Mass Index; M: means; SEM: standard error or means.$r_s$: Spearman coefficient correlation; ∗: significant.

| | Non Liver steatosis (M±SEM) | LiverSteatosis Grade | | | $p$ value | $r_s$ |
|---|---|---|---|---|---|---|
| | | S1 (M±SEM) | S2 (M±SEM) | S3 (M±SEM) | | |
| BMI, kg/m$^2$ | 24.65±0.88 | 27.73±0.99 | 29.96±0.90 | 29.99±1.02 | <0.001 | 0.46∗ |
| Waist Circumference, inch | 33.40±0.78 | 35.42±0.98 | 37.86±0.86 | 37.95±0.72 | 0.001 | 0.40∗ |

TABLE 3: Relationship between laboratory data and liver steatosis grade as assessed by US. HDL: high-density lipoprotein; FBS: fasting blood sugar; M: mean; SEM: standard error of means; $r_s$, Spearman coefficient correlation; ∗: significant.

| | Non hepatic-steatosis (M±SEM) | Hepatic Steatosis Grade S1 (M±SEM) | S2 (M±SEM) | S3 (M±SEM) | *p* value | $r_s$ |
|---|---|---|---|---|---|---|
| HDL, mmol/L | 1.29±0.05 | 1.31±0.07 | 1.16±0.04 | 1.13±0.06 | 0.181 | -0.14 |
| Triglyceride mmol/L | 1.50±0.13 | 1.50±0.12 | 1.53±0.11 | 1.83±0.19 | 0.574 | 0.15 |
| Total Cholestrol, mmol/L | 4.88±0.16 | 4.95±0.23 | 4.78±0.21 | 5.01±0.30 | 0.920 | -0.05 |
| FBS, mmol/L | 6.52±1.01 | 8.15±1.74 | 6.86±0.43 | 6.49±0.44 | 0.738 | 0.35 |
| Albumin, gr/dL | 40.68±0.58 | 40.8±0.45 | 41.1±0.49 | 40.3±0.82 | 0.875 | 0.01 |
| Platelet, x$10^9$/L | 251.4±10.46 | 245.8±11.8 | 272.9±8.92 | 259.4±10.82 | 0.325 | 0.11 |

TABLE 4: Relationship between inflammatory markers, CK-18, fibroscan findings, and liver steatosis grade as assessed by US. Me, Median; $r_s$: Spearmancoefficient correlation; ∗: significant. ALT: alanine transaminase; AST: aspartate transaminase; CRP: C-reactive protein; CK-18: cytokeratin-18; CAP: controlled attenuated parameter; LSM: liver stiffness measurement.

| | Non hepatic-steatosis Me(IQR) | Hepatic Steatosis Grade S1 Me(IQR) | S2 Me(IQR) | S3 Me(IQR) | *p* value | $r_s$ |
|---|---|---|---|---|---|---|
| ALT, U/L | 18.5(14-27.5) | 31(21.75-65) | 56(31-76) | 68(31-112) | <0.001 | 0.54∗ |
| AST, U/L | 20.5(17-24.5) | 22.5(21-34.5) | 28(24-47.5) | 45(34.5-48.5) | <0.001 | 0.53∗ |
| CRP, mg/dL | 0.08(0.05-0.2) | 0.23(0.06-0.45) | 0.27(0.09-0.73) | 0.33(0.08-0.43) | 0.462 | 0.25 |
| CK-18, U/L | 91(70-104) | 189.5(137-227.5) | 277(189.5-326) | 441(338-554.5) | <0.001 | 0.68∗ |
| CAP, dB/m | 234(95-266) | 310(277-330) | 331(279-364) | 334(323-374) | <0.001 | 0.56∗ |
| LSM, kPa | 5.3(3.9-5.9) | 6.5(5.4-9.9) | 9.3(7-11.5) | 8.4(6.9-11.5) | 0.001 | 0.49∗ |

they may have the same echographic appearance in hepatic US [32].

In our study, fragmented CK-18 level showed a good correlation with steatosis grade as assessed by US with $r_s$ of 0.68. One study by Tsutsui [16] showed correlation of fragmented CK-18 with steatosis assessed by histology activity is 0.482. This discrepancy of result could be explained by possible smaller area of steatosis assessed by liver biopsy. Fragmented CK-18 although was known as a necroinflammatory and apoptotic marker, in our study, we believed that CK-18 has a good predictive value of detecting liver steatosis as assessed by US, especially in liver steatosis grade≥2 and ≥3, with AUROC 0.82, 0.84, respectively.

We had demonstrated a moderate correlation between CAP, LSM, and the degree of liver steatosis ($r_s$=0.56, $r_s$=0.49, respectively). Our CAP correlation coefficient ($r_s$=0.56) was a little bit lower than that of previous study by Carvalhana ($r_s$ = 0.73, $p$<0.001) [31] but comparable to that of the recent study by Ahn JM et al. ($r_s$ =0.58, $p$<0.001) [39, 40]. This discrepancy of results may be explained by differences in both studies populations, by Carvalhana et al. and Ahn JM et al., in which they included chronic viral hepatitis and alcoholic liver disease as well as using the different classification criteria of steatosis grades on US examination.

The predictive value of CAP to detect liver steatosis was compared with previous studies conducted. We demonstrated that optimal cut-off values for detecting S≥2 and S≥3 steatosis by using Youden index were 263 dB/m and 319dB/m, respectively, and these were comparable with previous studies done in Canada and France [40, 41], with cut-off value of 250db/m and 317db/m for S≥2 and S≥3 reported, respectively. However, our cut-off values differed from those in other studies [42–44]. These differences might be explained by different study populations as some studies include not only NAFLD but also chronic viral hepatitis patients.

In our study, predictive value of fragmented CK-18 to detect liver steatosis grade as assessed by US was comparable to studies conducted previously. However, majority of the studies conducted were to detect steatohepatitis (NASH) rather than simple NAFLD on liver biopsy [18, 45, 46].

Our study also showed that liver steatosis grade detected by ultrasound, LSM, and TG was independently associated with CAP. However, study by Ahn et al. showed that only US liver steatosis grade independently affected the CAP score [39]. This could be explained by their different study population which included alcoholic liver disease patients. None of the necroinflammatory markers such as ALT, AST, CRP, and fragmented CK-18 were independently associated with CAP. All these findings were quite consistent with other previous studies. [39, 41].

The strength of this study was its ability to show the relationship of CAP (a convenient but uncommonly used tool), with US (the most commonly available tool) for assessing NAFLD patients. In addition, we compared this relationship with fragmented CK-18, a new biomarker, in the NAFLD patients.

However, our study had several limitations. First, steatosis grade assessed by US has a limitation due to its subjective

Table 5: Factors Influencing CAP (controlled attenuation parameter) in fibroscan. Using Univariate and Multivariate Linear Regression Analysis. B: beta coefficient. Uni: univariate regression analysis; Multi: multivariate regression analysis. BMI: Body Mass Index; FBS: fasting blood sugar; HDL: high-density lipoprotein; TG: triglyceride; TC: total cholesterol; ALT: alanine transaminase; AST: aspartate transaminase; CRP: C-reactive protein; CK18: cytokeratin-18; LSM: liver stiffness measurement; US: ultrasonography; ∗: significant.

| Variable | Uni | | Multi | |
|---|---|---|---|---|
| | $\beta$ | $p$ value | $\beta$ | $p$ value |
| Age | 0.42 | 0.53 | -.505 | 0.442 |
| BMI | 5.5 | 0.001 | -0.811 | 0.834 |
| FBS | 13.07 | 0.02 | 7.54 | 0.064 |
| HDL | -76.35 | 0.004 | -26.3 | 0.337 |
| TG | 16.6 | 0.112 | 21.2 | 0.04∗ |
| TC | -7.3 | 0.339 | -9.4 | 0.215 |
| WaistCircum | 5.8 | 0.001 | 1.9 | 0.612 |
| ALT | 0.47 | 0.07 | -0.17 | 0.588 |
| AST | 0.92 | 0.04 | -0.69 | 0.362 |
| Albumin | -0.69 | 0.81 | -0.06 | 0.98 |
| CRP | 24.9 | 0.228 | -13.4 | 0.533 |
| Platelet | 0.09 | 0.58 | -0.044 | 0.791 |
| CK18 | 0.172 | 0.001 | -0.052 | 0.394 |
| LSM | 10.1 | 0.001 | 7.9 | 0.002∗ |
| USResult | 36.2 | 0.001 | 31.9 | 0.003∗ |

interpretation. Secondly, single operator US may cause a bias in the result. Thirdly, we did not have a comparison against liver biopsy, regarded as gold standard as a reference for our US findings.

## 5. Conclusion

In conclusion, our study showed fragmented CK-18 and CAP were relatively well correlated with steatosis grade as assessed by US. NAFLD fibrosis score, however, did not show any correlation with US. We proposed the cut-off values for fragmented CK-18 and CAP in moderate and severe liver steatosis; fragmented CK-18 for S≥2 and S≥3 were 194U/L and 345U/L, respectively; CAP for S≥2 and S≥3 were 263dB/m and 319dB/m, rspectively. However, larger scale studies are needed to confirm the optimal cut-off values.

## Appendix

See Tables 1–5 and Figures 1 and 2.

## Authors' Contributions

S. Kosasih researched the database, collected samples, and wrote the manuscript. N. A. Hamid, Y. Yaakob and S. Azhar contributed to laboratory, radiology, and statistics work, respectively. R. Abdul Rani, Z. Q. Wong, C. S. Ngiu, and R. A. Raja Ali contributed in reviewing and editing the manuscript.

## Acknowledgments

**The manuscript is supported by** Universiti Kebangsaan Malaysia, no. FF-2014-212.

## References

[1] Z. Li, J. Xue, P. Chen, L. Chen, S. Yan, and L. Liu, "Prevalence of nonalcoholic fatty liver disease in mainland of China: a meta-analysis of published studies," *Journal of Gastroenterology and Hepatology*, vol. 29, no. 1, pp. 42–51, 2014.

[2] E. Magosso, M. A. Ansari, Y. Gopalan et al., "Prevalence of non-alcoholic fatty liver in a hypercholesterolemic population of northwestern peninsular Malaysia," *Southeast Asian Journal of Tropical Medicine and Public Health*, vol. 41, no. 4, pp. 936–942, 2010.

[3] W.-K. Chan, A. T.-B. Tan, S. R. Vethakkan, P.-C. Tah, A. Vijayananthan, and K.-L. Goh, "Non-alcoholic fatty liver disease in diabetics - prevalence and predictive factors in a multiracial hospital clinic population in Malaysia," *Journal of Gastroenterology and Hepatology*, vol. 28, no. 8, pp. 1375–1383, 2013.

[4] C.-H. Chen, M.-H. Huang, J.-C. Yang et al., "Prevalence and risk factors of nonalcoholic fatty liver disease in an adult population of Taiwan: metabolic significance of nonalcoholic fatty liver disease in nonobese adults," *Journal of Clinical Gastroenterology*, vol. 40, no. 8, pp. 745–752, 2006.

[5] E. M. Koehler, J. N. L. Schouten, B. E. Hansen et al., "Prevalence and risk factors of non-alcoholic fatty liver disease in the elderly: results from the Rotterdam study," *Journal of Hepatology*, vol. 57, no. 6, pp. 1305–1311, 2012.

[6] S. Petta and A. Craxì, "Hepatocellular carcinoma and non-alcoholic fatty liver disease: From a clinical to a molecular

association," *Current Pharmaceutical Design*, vol. 16, no. 6, pp. 741–752, 2010.

[7] G. Baffy, E. M. Brunt, and S. H. Caldwell, "Hepatocellular carcinoma in non-alcoholic fatty liver disease: an emerging menace," *Journal of Hepatology*, vol. 56, no. 6, pp. 1384–1391, 2012.

[8] N. Bhala, P. Angulo, D. van der Poorten et al., "The natural history of nonalcoholic fatty liver disease with advanced fibrosis or cirrhosis: an international collaborative study," *Hepatology*, vol. 54, no. 4, pp. 1208–1216, 2011.

[9] C. K. Argo, P. G. Northup, A. M. S. Al-Osaimi, and S. H. Caldwell, "Systematic review of risk factors for fibrosis progression in non-alcoholic steatohepatitis," *Journal of Hepatology*, vol. 51, no. 2, pp. 371–379, 2009.

[10] V. T. Samuel, Z.-X. Liu, X. Qu et al., "Mechanism of hepatic insulin resistance in non-alcoholic fatty liver disease," *The Journal of Biological Chemistry*, vol. 279, no. 31, pp. 32345–32353, 2004.

[11] G. Musso, R. Gambino, and J. H. Tabibian, "Association of non-alcoholic fatty liver disease with chronic kidney disease: a systematic review and meta-analysis," *PLoS Medicine*, vol. 11, no. 7, Article ID e1001680, 2014.

[12] M. R. Ajmal, M. Yaccha, M. A. Malik et al., "Prevalence of nonalcoholic fatty liver disease (NAFLD) in patients of cardiovascular diseases and its association with hs-CRP and TNF-α," *Indian Heart Journal*, vol. 66, no. 6, pp. 574–579, 2014.

[13] P. Angulo, M. V. Machado, and A. M. Diehl, "Fibrosis in nonalcoholic fatty liver disease: Mechanisms and clinical implications," *Seminars in Liver Disease*, vol. 35, no. 2, pp. 132–145, 2015.

[14] P. Angulo, J. M. Hui, G. Marchesini et al., "The NAFLD fibrosis score: a noninvasive system that identifies liver fibrosis in patients with NAFLD," *Hepatology*, vol. 45, no. 4, pp. 846–854, 2007.

[15] N. Alkhouri, C. Carter-Kent, and A. E. Feldstein, "Apoptosis in nonalcoholic fatty liver disease: diagnostic and therapeutic implications," *Expert Review of Gastroenterology & Hepatology*, vol. 5, no. 2, pp. 201–212, 2011.

[16] M. Tsutsui, N. Tanaka, M. Kawakubo et al., "Serum fragmented cytokeratin 18 levels reflect the histologic activity score of nonalcoholic fatty liver disease more accurately than serum alanine aminotransferase levels," *Journal of Clinical Gastroenterology*, vol. 44, no. 6, pp. 440–447, 2010.

[17] M. V. Machado and H. Cortez-Pinto, "Non-invasive diagnosis of non-alcoholic fatty liver disease. A critical appraisal," *Journal of Hepatology*, vol. 58, no. 5, pp. 1007–1019, 2013.

[18] A. E. Feldstein, A. Wieckowska, A. R. Lopez, Y.-C. Liu, N. N. Zein, and A. J. McCullough, "Cytokeratin-18 fragment levels as noninvasive biomarkers for nonalcoholic steatohepatitis: a multicenter validation study," *Hepatology*, vol. 50, no. 4, pp. 1072–1078, 2009.

[19] J. Chen, Y. Y. Zhu, Q. Zheng, and J. J. Jiang, "Serum cytokeratin-18 in the diagnosis of non-alcoholic steatohepatitis: a meta-analysis," *Hepatology Research*, vol. 44, no. 8, pp. 854–862, 2014.

[20] M. Graif, M. Yanuka, M. Baraz et al., "Quantitative estimation of attenuation in ultrasound video images: Correlation with histology in diffuse liver disease," *Investigative Radiology*, vol. 35, no. 5, pp. 319–324, 2000.

[21] S. H. Saverymuttu, A. E. A. Joseph, and J. D. Maxwell, "Ultrasound scanning in the detection of hepatic fibrosis and steatosis," *British Medical Journal*, vol. 292, no. 6512, pp. 13–15, 1986.

[22] N. H. Afdhal, "Fibroscan (transient elastography) for the measurement of liver fibrosis," *Journal of Gastroenterology and Hepatology*, vol. 8, no. 9, pp. 605–607, 2012.

[23] I. Mikolasevic, L. Orlic, N. Franjic, G. Hauser, D. Stimac, and S. Milic, "Transient elastography (FibroScan((R))) with controlled attenuation parameter in the assessment of liver steatosis and fibrosis in patients with nonalcoholic fatty liver disease - Where do we stand?" *World journal of gastroenterology : WJG*, vol. 22, no. 32, pp. 7236–7251, 2016.

[24] V. W.-S. Wong, J. Vergniol, G. L.-H. Wong et al., "Diagnosis of fibrosis and cirrhosis using liver stiffness measurement in nonalcoholic fatty liver disease," *Hepatology*, vol. 51, no. 2, pp. 454–462, 2010.

[25] R. Kwok, Y.-K. Tse, G. L.-H. Wong et al., "Systematic review with meta-analysis: non-invasive assessment of non-alcoholic fatty liver disease-the role of transient elastography and plasma cytokeratin-18 fragments," *Alimentary Pharmacology & Therapeutics*, vol. 39, no. 3, pp. 254–269, 2014.

[26] B. Balkau, T. Drivsholm, K. Borch-Johnsen et al., "Frequency of the WHO metabolic syndrome in European cohorts, and an alternative definition of an insulin resistance syndrome," *Diabetes & Metabolism*, vol. 28, no. 5, pp. 364–376, 2002.

[27] R. J. Molinaro, "Metabolic syndrome: an up prevalence, criteria, and laboratory testing.," *MLO: Medical Laboratory Observer*, vol. 39, no. 11, pp. 24–27, 2007.

[28] C. M. Alexander, P. B. Landsman, S. M. Teutsch, and S. M. Haffner, "NCEP-defined metabolic syndrome, diabetes, and prevalence of coronary heart disease among NHANES III participants age 50 years and older," *Diabetes*, vol. 52, no. 5, pp. 1210–1214, 2003.

[29] T. Gunji, N. Matsuhashi, H. Sato et al., "Alcohol consumption is inversely correlated with insulin resistance, independent of metabolic syndrome factors and fatty liver diseases," *Journal of Clinical Gastroenterology*, vol. 45, no. 9, pp. 808–813, 2011.

[30] N. Khov, A. Sharma, and T. R. Riley, "Bedside ultrasound in the diagnosis of nonalcoholic fatty liver disease," *World Journal of Gastroenterology*, vol. 20, no. 22, pp. 6821–6825, 2014.

[31] S. Carvalhana, J. Leitão, A. C. Alves, M. Bourbon, and H. Cortez-Pinto, "How good is controlled attenuation parameter and fatty liver index for assessing liver steatosis in general population: Correlation with ultrasound," *Official Journal of the International Association for the Study of the Liver*, vol. 34, no. 6, pp. e111–e117, 2014.

[32] M. Lupşor-Platon, H. Stefănescu, D. Mureşçan et al., "Noninvasive assessment of liver steatosis using ultrasound methods," *Medical Ultrasonography*, vol. 16, no. 3, pp. 236–245, 2014.

[33] European Association for Study of Liver and Asociacion Latinoamericana para el Estudio del Higado, "EASL-ALEH Clinical Practice Guidelines: non-invasive tests for evaluation of liver disease severity and prognosis," *Journal of Hepatology*, vol. 63, no. 1, pp. 237–264, 2015.

[34] S. Gawrieh, D. M. Knoedler, K. Saeian, J. R. Wallace, and R. A. Komorowski, "Effects of interventions on intra- and interobserver agreement on interpretation of nonalcoholic fatty liver disease histology," *Annals of Diagnostic Pathology*, vol. 15, no. 1, pp. 19–24, 2011.

[35] Y. Sumida, A. Nakajima, and Y. Itoh, "Limitations of liver biopsy and non-invasive diagnostic tests for the diagnosis of nonalcoholic fatty liver disease/nonalcoholic steatohepatitis," *World Journal of Gastroenterology*, vol. 20, no. 2, pp. 475–485, 2014.

[36] R. Vuppalanchi, A. Ünalp, M. L. Van Natta et al., "Effects of Liver Biopsy Sample Length and Number of Readings on Sampling Variability in Nonalcoholic Fatty Liver Disease," *Clinical Gastroenterology and Hepatology*, vol. 7, no. 4, pp. 481–486, 2009.

[37] C. Wang, T. Tseng, T. Hsieh et al., "Severity of fatty liver on ultrasound correlates with metabolic and cardiovascular risk," *Kaohsiung Journal of Medical Sciences*, vol. 28, no. 3, pp. 151–160, 2012.

[38] M. Hamaguchi, T. Kojima, Y. Itoh et al., "The severity of ultrasonographic findings in nonalcoholic fatty liver disease reflects the metabolic syndrome and visceral fat accumulation," *American Journal of Gastroenterology*, vol. 102, no. 12, pp. 2708–2715, 2007.

[39] J. M. Ahn, Y.-H. Paik, S. Y. Min et al., "Relationship between controlled attenuation parameter and hepatic steatosis as assessed by ultrasound in alcoholic or nonalcoholic fatty liver disease," *Gut and Liver*, vol. 10, no. 2, pp. 295–302, 2016.

[40] R. P. Myers, A. Pollett, R. Kirsch et al., "Controlled Attenuation Parameter (CAP): A noninvasive method for the detection of hepatic steatosis based on transient elastography," *Liver International*, vol. 32, no. 6, pp. 902–910, 2012.

[41] V. de Lédinghen, J. Vergniol, J. Foucher, W. Merrouche, and B. le Bail, "Non-invasive diagnosis of liver steatosis using controlled attenuation parameter (CAP) and transient elastography," *Liver International*, vol. 32, no. 6, pp. 911–918, 2012.

[42] J. K. Kim, K. S. Lee, J. R. Choi et al., "Usefulness of the controlled attenuation parameter for detecting liver steatosis in health checkup examinees," *Gut and Liver*, vol. 9, no. 3, pp. 405–410, 2015.

[43] F. Shen, R. D. Zheng, and Y. Q. Mi, "Controlled attenuation parameter for non-invasive assessment of hepatic steatosis in Chinese patients," *World Journal of Gastroenterology*, vol. 20, no. 16, pp. 4702–4711, 2014.

[44] K. S. Jung, B. K. Kim, S. U. Kim, Y. E. Chon, and K. H. Cheon, "Factors affecting the accuracy of controlled attenuation parameter (CAP) in assessing hepatic steatosis in patients with chronic liver disease," *PLoS ONE*, vol. 9, no. 6, Article ID e98689, 2014.

[45] D. Joka, K. Wahl, S. Moeller et al., "Prospective biopsy-controlled evaluation of cell death biomarkers for prediction of liver fibrosis and nonalcoholic steatohepatitis," *Hepatology*, vol. 55, no. 2, pp. 455–464, 2012.

[46] J. Shen, H. L. Chan, G. L. Wong, A. W. Chan, P. C. Choi, H. Y. Chan et al., "Assessment of non-alcoholic fatty liver disease using serum total cell death and apoptosis markers," *Alimentary Pharmacology & Therapeutics*, vol. 36, no. 11-12, pp. 1057–1066, 2012.

# Different Nodules Identified during Liver Explant Gross Examination: Relevance and Need for Sectioning—Experience from India

**Nalini Bansal,[1] Vivek Vij,[2] and Mukul Rastogi[2]**

[1] *SRL Ltd., Fortis Escorts Heart Institute, New Delhi, India*
[2] *Fortis Hospital, Gurgaon, India*

Correspondence should be addressed to Nalini Bansal; drnalinibansal@yahoo.com

Academic Editor: Daisuke Morioka

*Objective.* The goal of this study was to determine the etiopathological association of various hepatic nodules identified during gross examination of liver explants specimen and the grossing aspects of these abnormal nodules especially those smaller than 1 cm in diameter. Our aim was to analyze whether there is any association of macroregenerative and dysplastic nodule with hepatocellular carcinoma. *Materials and Methods.* Fifty consecutive liver explants specimens were analyzed for the presence of any abnormal nodule (abnormal nodule defined as any nodule different in color, texture, and appearance from adjacent liver tissue). *Results.* Of the total 40 abnormal nodules identified in 50 liver explant specimens, there were 12 (30%) HCC [including 5 small HCC (41% of total HCC) and 1 steatohepatitic HCC (8% of total HCC)], 11 (27%) MRNs, 8 (20%) dysplastic nodules, and 9 (22%) necrotic nodules. Most cases (72%) of MRN are seen in hepatitis C virus related cirrhosis with only 2 cases having associated HCC. Most cases of HCC were seen in cases of HBV associated cirrhosis (60%). The association of MRN was not found to be significantly associated with HCC with a $p$ value of 1.0. Dysplastic nodules were found to be significantly associated with HCC with a $p$ value of 0.02. *Conclusion.* In hepatic carcinogenesis, the role of MRN does not appear to be significant. However, the presence of dysplastic nodules is significantly associated with HCC. The study identified another variant of cirrhotic nodules herein called necrotic nodules that are mostly tan greenish in color and <0.5 cm in diameter. No dysplastic changes were identified in any of these nodules disqualifying the need of sectioning in such nodules.

## 1. Introduction

MRN and dysplastic nodules are increasingly being recognized as important aspects of hepatocellular carcinoma. The results of recent investigations from Japan, America, and Europe have suggested that the old hypothesis of dysplasia-carcinoma sequence in liver needs to be qualified. The identification of this precancerous lesion may aid in prevention and timely management of such patients. Future studies must show whether and if so which immunohistochemical or molecular-genetically detectable changes can be utilized as risk markers in the diagnostic workup of these lesions. With this background, this study was undertaken to identify the distribution of various nodules in explant liver and to analyze their role in hepatic carcinogenesis.

## 2. Material and Methods

From May 2015 to September 2015, 50 liver explant operations were performed at our institution. These explant specimens were analyzed for the presence of any abnormal nodules. Abnormal nodules were defined as nodule of any size, which is different in color, texture, and appearance from surrounding liver parenchyma. These abnormal nodules were histologically classified according to International Working Party classification 1995 as MRN, dysplastic nodule, HCC its variants, and small HCC. The statistical analysis was performed using Fisher's Exact two-tailed tests.

The three major hepatic veins of all explant specimens were opened after inserting a probe and they were thereafter serially sliced at 0.5–1 cm interval; any abnormal nodule identified was sectioned other than the sections taken routinely

Table 1: Etiopathological association of explant liver and HCC.

| Etiology | Number | Percentage | HCC |
|---|---|---|---|
| HCV | 20 | 40% | 5 |
| HBV | 9 | 18% | 5 |
| Alcohol | 7 | 14% | — |
| Cryptogenic | 4 | 8% | 1 |
| PBC | 2 | 4% | — |
| Mixed HBV & HCV | 3 | 6% | — |
| Wilson | 2 | 4% | — |
| NASH | 1 | 2% | 1 |
| PFIC | 1 | 2% | — |
| MLD | 1 | 2% | — |
| Mixed HBV & HCV | 3 | 6% | — |

as three from the right lobe, two from the left lobe, one from the caudate lobe, one from the porta hepatis, and one from the gall bladder. All sections were stained routinely with Haematoxylin and Eosin stain. Special stains including Masson's trichrome, PAS, PAS with diastase, Orcein, Pearl, and reticulin stain were performed as and when required.

Histologically, these nodules were classified according to the International Working Party Classification 1995 as macroregenerative nodules, dysplastic nodules, hepatocellular carcinoma, and small hepatocellular carcinoma.

## 3. Results

A total of 40 nodules were identified in 50 explant liver specimens examined. The ages of patients ranged from 9 to 68 years with a male : female ratio of 5 : 1. Of the total 40 abnormal nodules identified in 50 liver explant specimens, there were 12 (33%) hepatocellular carcinomas [including 5 small HCC (41% of total HCC) and 1 steatohepatitic HCC (8% of total HCC)], 11 (27%) macroregenerative nodules, 8 (20%) dysplastic nodules, and 9 (22%) necrotic nodules. Of the HCC group, there were 5 small HCC measuring <2 cm in size and one was steatohepatitic HCC (SH-HCC).

The commonest etiology of cirrhosis in explant liver specimens in this part of the world was hepatitis C virus (HCV) seen in 40% of all cases followed by hepatitis B virus (18%) and alcohol (14%) (Table 1).

*3.1. Hepatocellular Carcinoma.* HCC were seen in 5/9 cases of hepatitis B virus associated cirrhosis compared to 5/20 cases of hepatitis C virus associated cirrhosis. Only 1 case of HCC was seen in NASH associated cirrhosis and one was cryptogenic. The association of HCC with HBV was significant with a $p$ value of 0.027. Alpha-fetoprotein levels were elevated in 11/12 cases of HCC. Of all HCC cases, there was 1 case of steatohepatitic HCC seen in case of HCV cirrhosis. This patient was a 49-year-old male known to be hypertensive and diabetic for the last 12 years and had been on regular medication. His lipid profile showed serum cholesterol of 230 mg/dL (<200) and triglycerides of 150 mg/dL (35–150), HDL cholesterol of 44 mg/dL (35–85), and LDL cholesterol of 115 mg/dL (<150). The patient had metabolic syndrome with hepatitis C virus associated cirrhosis. Grossly, the nodule measured 2.5 × 2 cm with a yellowish cut surface. Microscopy showed steatohepatitic HCC with prominent ballooning and steatosis and adjacent liver showed cirrhosis with mild steatosis.

*3.1.1. Small Hepatocellular Carcinoma.* Grossly, all cases presented with nodule different in color from adjacent liver tissue measuring 0.8–2 cm in diameter. Diagnosis of small HCC was based on absence of portal tracts, loss of reticulin fibres, and presence of thick trabeculae and pseudoacinar pattern of atypical hepatocytes (Figures 1(a) and 1(b)). AFP was found to be minimally to mildly elevated in all 5 cases of small HCC (9–129 ng/mL) but in none of the cases was it above 500 ng/mL (Table 2). Preoperative triple phase Contrast Enhanced CT has a high diagnostic accuracy (80%) of diagnosing small hepatocellular carcinoma. 80% of cases of small HCC were seen in right lobe and measured 1-2 cm in size. All these cases were diagnosed preoperatively by triple phase CECT. One case in left lobe measuring 0.9 × 0.8 cm could not be diagnosed preoperatively. In one case of small HCC, there were associated dysplastic nodules of both low- and high-grade type. This patient had previous partial hepatectomy for HCC and presented with multiple liver nodules after a year of follow-up in residual liver tissue.

*Another Interesting Finding Was Noted in Few Cases of Small HCC*

*Mushroom Effect.* There was bullous protrusion at one end of the neoplastic nodule probably representing the origin of these small HCC resembling a hand mirror herein called mushrooming phenomenon.

*3.2. Macroregenerative Nodules.* MRNs were observed in 27% of cases of total explant specimens (Figures 2(a) and 2(b)). Most of these nodules were similar in color to surrounding liver with size >1 cm. Microscopy in all showed multiacinar cirrhotic nodules with several portal tracts. In only 2 cases, MRN was seen along with HCC. One of these cases also showed presence of dysplastic nodule along with HCC. No significant association was seen between macroregenerative nodule and HCC and the $p$ value was not significant.

*3.3. Dysplastic Nodules.* There was a significant association of the presence of dysplastic nodules with HCC with a $p$ value of 0.02. The dysplastic nodules grossly were of different color or texture from adjacent liver. Microscopy showed hepatocytes with small or large cell change and scanty portal tracts. Hepatocytes are usually single cell plate thick. Of these 8 dysplastic nodules, there were 6 high-grade dysplastic nodules and 2 low-grade dysplastic nodules showing mild atypia. Five of these nodules (3 of high grade and 2 of low grade) were seen in a single explant with small HCC (Figures 3(a) and 3(b)). Small cell change was seen in 5 of these nodules.

TABLE 2: Etiopathological association of small HCC with AFP level and triple phase CECT.

| S. number | Age | Etiology | AFP (0.2–9 ng/mL) | Histology | Radiology | Concordance |
|---|---|---|---|---|---|---|
| 1 | 46 M | HBV | 9.6 | 2 × 1.5 × 1.5 cm RL | Seg. VIII, 1.8 × 1.5 cm | C |
| 2 | 68 M | Cryptogenic | 13.6 | 1.6 × 1.5 cm RL | Seg. IV A, 15 × 14 mm | C |
| 3 | 49 M | HCV | 12.8 | 0.9 × 0.8 cm LL | No lesion | D |
| 4 | 55 M | HCV | 129 | 2 × 1.8 RL | Seg. VIII, 2 × 2 mm | C |
| 5 | 47 F | HCV | 9.7 | 1.5 × 1.4 cm | Seg. VIII,16 × 13 mm | C |

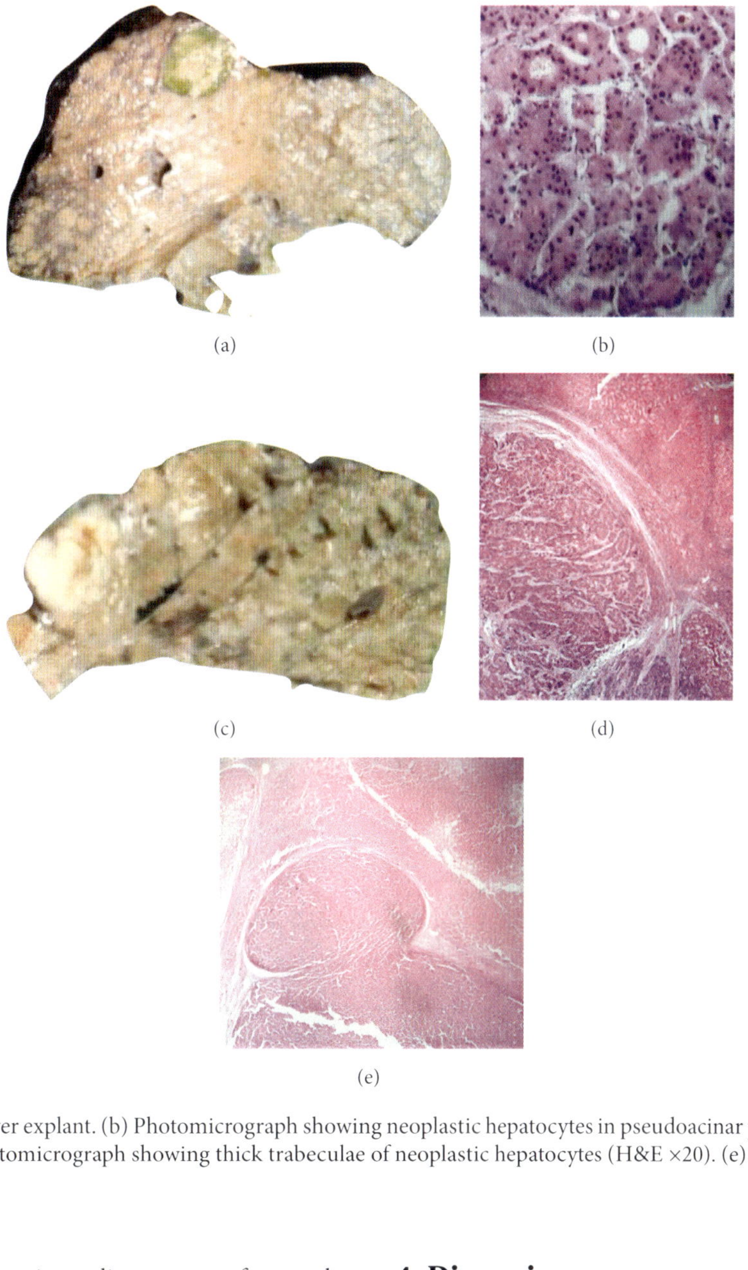

FIGURE 1: (a) Small HCC in liver explant. (b) Photomicrograph showing neoplastic hepatocytes in pseudoacinar pattern (H&E ×40). (c) Small HCC in liver explant. (d) Photomicrograph showing thick trabeculae of neoplastic hepatocytes (H&E ×20). (e) Mushrooming phenomenon of small HCC.

*3.4. Necrotic Nodules.* There is no literature so far on the existence of these nodules. All of these were discolored, greenish yellow, and small (<0.5 cm) in diameter (Figures 4(a), 4(b), 4(c), and 4(d)). Most (87%) of these nodules were identified in HCV related cirrhosis. Microscopy of these nodules showed mainly degenerated hepatocytes with prominence of lipofuscin pigment that is PAS positive. No evidence of dysplasia was identified in any of these nodules.

## 4. Discussion

Distribution of various nodules found on liver explant gross examination has long been a matter of debate especially for evaluating their role in hepatic carcinogenesis. The whole idea is to diagnose these hepatic carcinomas in their precursor stages and treat them early before full-blown malignancy develops. There has been scant literature on etiology and

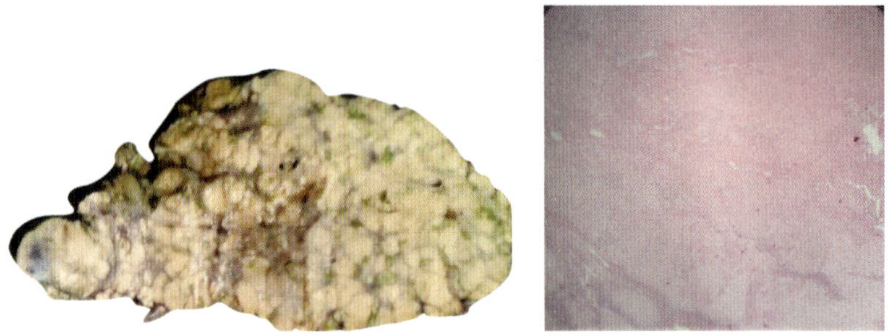

(a) (b)

FIGURE 2: (a) Macroregenerative nodules in explants liver. (b) Photomicrograph showing multiacinar MRN (H&E ×20).

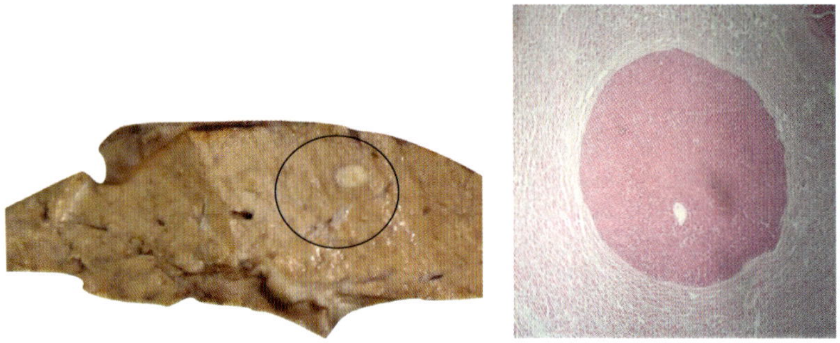

(a) (b)

FIGURE 3: (a) Dysplastic nodule in explant liver. (b) Photomicrograph showing dysplastic nodule with small cell change (H&E ×10).

pathogenesis from South Asia and developing countries mainly because of the lack of registries of liver and other diseases in our population. We found that HCV is the most common etiology of liver cirrhosis in South Asia seen in 40% of cases of explant liver followed by hepatitis B virus and alcohol. A Japanese study on 345 patients states that hepatitis B virus infection appears to be a frequent cause of cirrhosis of the liver and hepatocellular carcinoma in Asia and Africa [1].

Another study from Malaysia on 460 patients also states that the major causes of cirrhosis were chronic hepatitis B (46.1%) followed by chronic hepatitis C (18.5% of cases) [2]. These are in contrast to our group of patients where hepatitis C virus is the major etiological association with liver cirrhosis.

Of these cases of liver cirrhosis, the major etiological association of hepatocellular carcinoma was with hepatitis B virus and the relation was found to be significant with a $p$ value of 0.027.

Chronic HBV infection has been implicated as a dominant risk factor for HCC in most areas of Asia and sub-Saharan Africa with the exception of Japan, where the major risk factor for HCC is chronic HCV infection [3].

Taking a cut-off of 500 ng/mL, the diagnostic accuracy of AFP was very low for small HCC with all cases having AFP < 500 ng/mL. However, in all cases, the value of AFP was higher than normal (>9 ng/mL) ranging from 9 to 129 ng/mL compared to cirrhotics without HCC where AFP was in normal range. In a resource constrained country where people cannot afford to get many tests done, even minor elevation of AFP should be considered to be significant in known cirrhotics and they should undergo radiological evaluation. Other studies have shown that diagnostic accuracy of AFP in small HCC was substantially limited taking a cut-off of >500 ng/mL to be of diagnostic utility. They have emphasized the role of newer markers in early diagnosis of HCC like AFP-L3, prothrombin induced by vitamin K absence-II (PIVKA-II), which is an abnormal prothrombin protein that is present at higher levels in the serum of HCC patients [4].

Relationships of MRN and HCC have been studied extensively in the last decade with major studies coming from the Japanese and American group. The Japanese group initially proposed that MRN could be involved in the morphogenesis of HCC from autopsy studies in patients of chronic liver diseases initially being performed on 345 patients [5].

Also, other studies from Japan [6] on 141 liver explants identified similar large regenerative nodules. They identified 94 large regenerative nodules in 53 cirrhotics. Further studies by Japanese groups [7] on 209 cirrhotics identified ordinary and atypical adenomatous hyperplasia (AAH) in these cirrhotics and concluded that AAH may be an important preneoplastic lesion in cirrhotic livers associated with non-A non-B hepatitis virus (probably hepatitis C virus). They also conducted a follow-up study for these atypical adenomatous nodules, which were resected surgically. They classified these adenomatous hyperplasia nodules as ordinary adenomatous hyperplasia (OAH) lacking hepatocellular atypia, atypical adenomatous hyperplasia with structural and cellular atypia insufficient for carcinoma (AAH), and atypical AH with focal

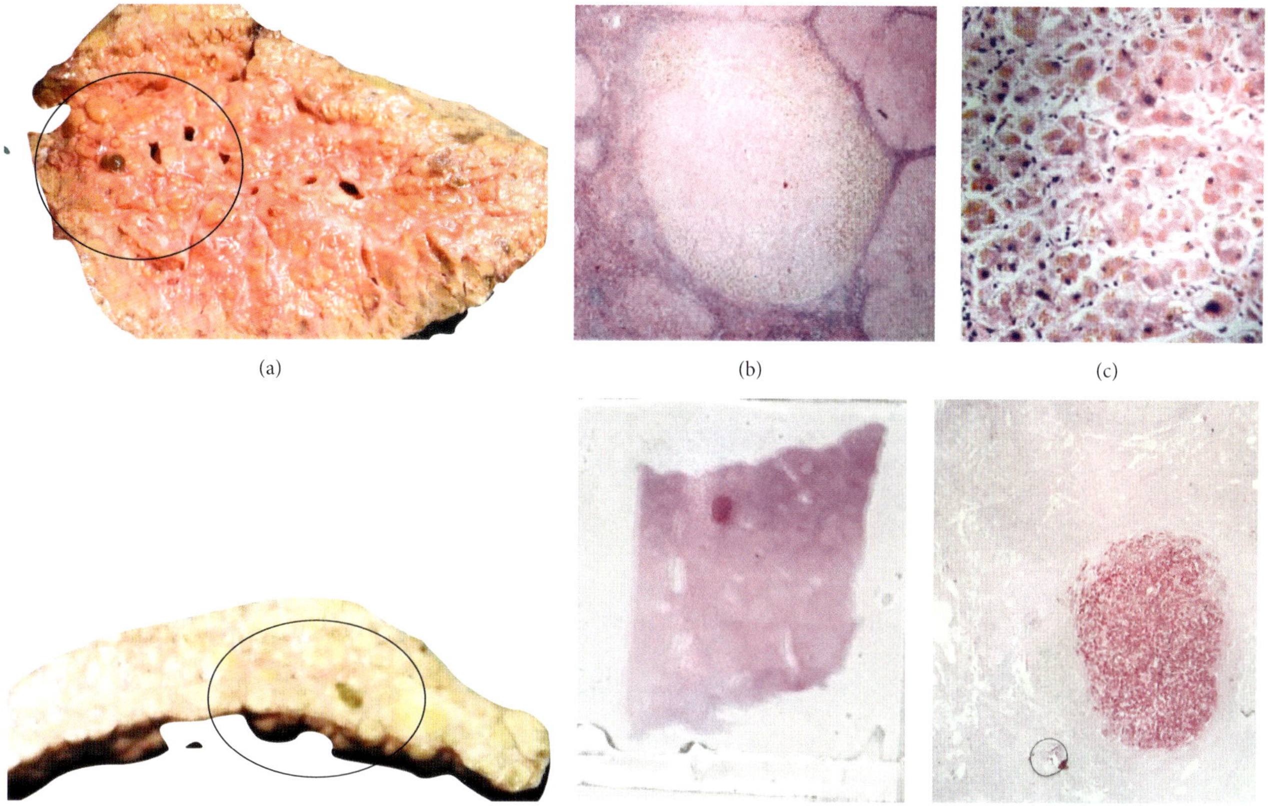

(a) (b) (c)

(d) (e) (f)

FIGURE 4: (a) Necrotic nodule in explant liver (b and c). Photomicrograph showing all degenerated hepatocytes in low and high power (H&E ×10 and 40). (d) Necrotic nodule in explant liver (e and f). Photomicrograph showing PAS positive staining of necrotic nodule in section and low power.

malignancy containing areas of HCC (FM). On follow-up of these patients (follow-up period range: 12–77 months; mean: 31.4 months), HCC was seen in all 3 patients whose resected nodules were classified as FM, in 4 (36%) of 11 with AAH resected nodules, and in none of 10 with OAH resected nodules. The incidence of HCC in the patients with focal malignancy (FM) or AAH nodules was found to be significantly higher than that in those with OAH nodules, thus emphasizing their preneoplastic nature [8].

American groups, mainly the work by Theise et al., in their initial work on 44 explant specimens found 48 MRNs in 11 explants. They concluded that the presence of MRN is more common in non-Japanese cirrhotic patients occurring in several different types of liver diseases and representing precancerous lesions [9].

In the subsequent years, their further study on 155 explant specimens (inclusive of previous study on 44 explants), they again concluded that the presence of either type of MRN (type I: without dysplasia; type II: with dysplasia) was associated with an increased incidence of HCC (all MRNs, $p < 0.00019$; type I MRNs, $p < 0.067$; type II MRNs, $p < 0.012$) compared with cirrhotic livers without MRNs [10].

Another study by Ferrell et al. analyzed 110 liver explant specimens with 28 MRNs with HCC seen in 3 of them. They also proposed a possible role of MRN in HCC [11].

A group from France examined 41 consecutive cirrhotic liver explants from French patients. Thirty-five adenomatous hyperplasias were identified in 10 livers (prevalence: 24%); seven of 10 were HCV positive. Their data also suggest that hepatocarcinogenesis is a multistep process and AAH should be considered as a premalignant lesion whereas OAH had proliferative ability [12].

Studies from African countries have concluded that MRN could not be considered a risk factor for HCC [13].

Our study being the first from the Indian subcontinent also highlighted similar findings with macroregenerative nodules not significantly associated with HCC whereas dysplastic nodules have significant association with HCC with a $p$ value of 0.02 compared to cirrhotic liver without dysplastic nodules, thus emphasizing that dysplastic nodules are involved in tumor carcinogenesis of HCC.

SH-HCC is a recently described variant of HCC with only 3 series and 1 case report reported in the literature. Salomao et al. have proposed histological criteria for diagnosis of SH-HCC. The criteria state that 3 of 5 features are required in >50% of the tumor mass to be diagnosed as SH-HCC. The five features included were steatosis, ballooning degeneration, Mallory Denk Bodies, inflammation, and pericellular fibrosis. Most of these variants are seen to develop in the background of metabolic syndrome or HCV cirrhosis. In our case, the patient had both as reported by other authors [14–17].

*Necrotic Nodules.* These nodules were identified in 9 of 50 liver explant specimens. These nodules were macroscopically seen as greenish yellow nodules mostly <0.5 cm and microscopically composed of lipofuscin pigment containing hepatocytes. None of these nodules showed features of dysplasia or malignancy. Most of these nodules (87%) were seen in HCV related cirrhosis. The literature is quiet on the presence of these nodules in explant liver.

*Mushroom Effect of Small HCC.* Small HCC have been identified to show mushrooming phenomenon seen erupting out from a small bud of neoplastic cells at one of the foci. Similar morphological observations have not been previously reported in the literature.

Recently, several genetic studies have been undertaken to determine whether there are any molecular markers for precarcinogenesis in cirrhotic nodules. Studies by Nault et al. analyzed a series of 268 liver samples for telomerase reverse-transcriptase promoter (TERT) mutations. They found that TERT mutations were highly related to the stepwise hepatocarcinogenesis. They concluded that TERT promoter mutation is the most frequent and also the earliest genetic alteration in early HCC [17, 18].

## 5. Conclusion

Our study from the Indian subcontinent also supports the hypothesis that dysplasia precedes carcinoma and may represent precursor lesion of HCC. MRNs are not significantly associated with HCC. Necrotic nodules identified on explant liver need not be sectioned in explant specimen though the findings need to be substantiated on a larger cohort of patients.

## Competing Interests

The authors declare that they have no competing interests.

## References

[1] K. Iwamura, "Liver cirrhosis in Asia and Africa," *Zeitschrift fur Gastroenterologie*, vol. 21, no. 11, pp. 637–643, 1983.

[2] C.-S. Qua and K.-L. Goh, "Liver cirrhosis in malaysia: peculiar epidemiology in a multiracial asian country," *Journal of Gastroenterology and Hepatology*, vol. 26, no. 8, pp. 1333–1337, 2011.

[3] H. B. El-Serag, "Epidemiology of viral hepatitis and hepatocellular carcinoma," *Gastroenterology*, vol. 142, no. 6, pp. 1264–1273.e1, 2012.

[4] R. Tateishi, H. Yoshida, Y. Matsuyama, N. Mine, Y. Kondo, and M. Omata, "Diagnostic accuracy of tumor markers for hepatocellular carcinoma: a systematic review," *Hepatology International*, vol. 2, no. 1, pp. 17–30, 2008.

[5] K. Furuya, M. Nakamura, Y. Yamamoto, K. Togei, and H. Otsuka, "Macroregenerative nodule of the liver: a clinicopathologic study of 345 autopsy cases of chronic liver disease," *Cancer*, vol. 61, no. 1, pp. 99–105, 1988.

[6] K. Wada, F. Kondo, and Y. Kondo, "Large regenerative nodules and dysplastic nodules in cirrhotic livers: a histopathologic study," *Hepatology*, vol. 8, no. 6, pp. 1684–1688, 1988.

[7] T. Terada, S. Terasaki, and Y. Nakanuma, "A clinicopathologic study of adenomatous hyperplasia of the liver in 209 consecutive cirrhotic livers examined by autopsy," *Cancer*, vol. 72, no. 5, pp. 1551–1556, 1993.

[8] K. Kaji, T. Terada, and Y. Nakanuma, "Frequent occurrence of hepatocellular carcinoma in cirrhotic livers after surgical resection of atypical adenomatous hyperplasia (borderline hepatocellular lesion): a follow-up study," *American Journal of Gastroenterology*, vol. 89, no. 6, pp. 903–908, 1994.

[9] N. D. Theise, M. Schwartz, C. Miller, and S. N. Thung, "Macroregenerative nodules and hepatocellular carcinoma in forty-four sequential adult liver explants with cirrhosis," *Hepatology*, vol. 16, no. 4, pp. 949–955, 1992.

[10] P. Hytiroglou, N. D. Theise, M. Schwartz, E. Mor, C. Miller, and S. N. Thung, "Macroregenerative nodules in a series of adult cirrhotic liver explants: issues of classification and nomenclature," *Hepatology*, vol. 21, no. 3, pp. 703–708, 1995.

[11] L. Ferrell, T. Wright, J. Lake, J. Roberts, and N. Ascher, "Incidence and diagnostic features of macroregenerative nodules vs. small hepatocellular carcinoma in cirrhotic livers," *Hepatology*, vol. 16, no. 6, pp. 1372–1381, 1992.

[12] B. Le Bail, G. Belleannee, P.-H. Bernard, J. Saric, C. Balabaud, and P. Bioulac-Sage, "Adenomatous hyperplasia in cirrhotic livers: histological evaluation, cellular density, and proliferative activity of 35 macronodular lesions in the cirrhotic explants of 10 adult french patients," *Human Pathology*, vol. 26, no. 8, pp. 897–906, 1995.

[13] D. D. R. da Silva and V. H. Leite, "Cirrhotic liver explants: regenerative nodule, dysplasia and hepatocellular carcinoma occurrence," *Jornal Brasileiro de Patologia e Medicina Laboratorial*, vol. 41, no. 6, pp. 437–442, 2005.

[14] M. Salomao, H. Remotti, R. Vaughan, A. B. Siegel, J. H. Lefkowitch, and R. K. Moreira, "The steatohepatitic variant of hepatocellular carcinoma and its association with underlying steatohepatitis," *Human Pathology*, vol. 43, no. 5, pp. 737–746, 2012.

[15] D. Jain, N. C. Nayak, V. Kumaran, and S. Saigal, "Steatohepatitic hepatocellular carcinoma, a morphologic indicator of associated metabolic risk factors: A study from India," *Archives of Pathology and Laboratory Medicine*, vol. 137, no. 7, pp. 961–966, 2013.

[16] N. Gupta, A. Rastogi, and C. Bihari, "Steatohepatitic hepatocellular carcinoma–a case report with literature review," *Indian Journal of Surgical Oncology*, vol. 5, no. 2, pp. 161–163, 2014.

[17] J. C. Nault, J. Calderaro, L. Di Tommaso et al., "Telomerase reverse transcriptase promoter mutation is an early somatic genetic alteration in the transformation of premalignant nodules in hepatocellular carcinoma on cirrhosis," *Hepatology*, vol. 60, no. 6, pp. 1983–1992, 2014.

[18] J. C. Nault, M. Mallet, C. Pilati et al., "High frequency of telomerase reverse-transcriptase promoter somatic mutations in hepatocellular carcinoma and preneoplastic lesions," *Nature Communications*, vol. 4, article 2218, 2013.

# Development of NASH in Obese Mice is Confounded by Adipose Tissue Increase in Inflammatory NOV and Oxidative Stress

**David Sacerdoti,[1,2] Shailendra P. Singh,[1] Joseph Schragenheim,[1] Lars Bellner,[1] Luca Vanella,[3] Marco Raffaele,[3] Aliza Meissner,[1] Ilana Grant,[1] Gaia Favero,[4] Rita Rezzani,[4] Luigi F. Rodella,[4] David Bamshad,[1] Edward Lebovics,[1] and Nader G. Abraham[1,5]**

[1] *Departments of Medicine, Pharmacology and Gastroenterology, New York Medical College, Valhalla, NY 10595, USA*
[2] *Department of Medicine, University of Padova, Padova, Italy*
[3] *Department of Drug Science, University of Catania, Catania, Italy*
[4] *Anatomy and Physiopathology Division, Department of Clinical and Experimental Sciences, University of Brescia, Brescia, Italy*
[5] *Marshall University, Joan C. Edwards School of Medicine, Huntington, WV 25701, USA*

Correspondence should be addressed to Nader G. Abraham; nader_abraham@nymc.edu

Academic Editor: Dirk Uhlmann

*Aim.* Nonalcoholic steatohepatitis (NASH) is the consequence of insulin resistance, fatty acid accumulation, oxidative stress, and lipotoxicity. We hypothesize that an increase in the inflammatory adipokine NOV decreases antioxidant Heme Oxygenase 1 (HO-1) levels in adipose and hepatic tissue, resulting in the development of NASH in obese mice. *Methods.* Mice were fed a high fat diet (HFD) and obese animals were administered an HO-1 inducer with or without an inhibitor of HO activity to examine levels of adipose-derived NOV and possible links between increased synthesis of inflammatory adipokines and hepatic pathology. *Results.* NASH mice displayed decreased HO-1 levels and HO activity, increased levels of hepatic heme, NOV, MMP2, hepcidin, and increased NAS scores and hepatic fibrosis. Increased HO-1 levels are associated with a decrease in NOV, improved hepatic NAS score, ameliorated fibrosis, and increases in mitochondrial integrity and insulin receptor phosphorylation. Adipose tissue function is disrupted in obesity as evidenced by an increase in proinflammatory molecules such as NOV and a decrease in adiponectin. Importantly, increased HO-1 levels are associated with a decrease of NOV, increased adiponectin levels, and increased levels of thermogenic and mitochondrial signaling associated genes in adipose tissue. *Conclusions.* These results suggest that the metabolic abnormalities in NASH are driven by decreased levels of hepatic HO-1 that is associated with an increase in the adipose-derived proinflammatory adipokine NOV in our obese mouse model of NASH. Concurrently, induction of HO-1 provides protection against insulin resistance as seen by increased insulin receptor phosphorylation. Pharmacological increases in HO-1 associated with decreases in NOV may offer a potential therapeutic approach in preventing fibrosis, mitochondrial dysfunction, and the development of NASH.

## 1. Introduction

Metabolic syndrome and its associated pathologies of obesity, insulin resistance (IR), and dyslipidemia are often accompanied by liver involvement, defined as nonalcoholic fatty liver disease (NAFLD) [1]. NAFLD's progression to nonalcoholic steatohepatitis (NASH), characterized by low grade inflammation, cell ballooning, and mitochondrial dysfunction, is a primary risk factor for development of fibrosis and cirrhosis and therefore an important area of clinical research [2]. Chronic, low grade inflammation due to metabolic syndrome is provoked when the capacity for adipocytes to store fat is overwhelmed resulting in the production of inflammatory cytokines leading to metabolic inflammation [3]. Fatty acids released from hypertrophic, dysfunctional, and insulin resistant adipocytes, together with increased hepatic de novo lipogenesis and impaired (FA) fatty acid export, cause an accumulation of triglycerides in the liver leading to lipotoxicity [4]. Increased calorie intake and obesity lead to an increase in tissue fat mass through adipocyte hyperplasia and hypertrophy, subsequently resulting in a decrease in adiponectin and an increase of inflammatory TNF-$\alpha$ causing IR, inflammation, and oxidative stress in the liver [5]. Reactive oxygen species (ROS) can induce lipid peroxidation leading to inflammation and liver damage [6, 7]. Steatotic livers are more sensitive to increased ROS and oxidative stress, leading to mitochondrial dysfunction, decreased levels of hepatocyte antioxidants, and inflammation, and culminating in NASH and fibrosis [8, 9].

Induction of HO-1, an antioxidant gene highly inducible in a range of cells, including erythrocyte phagocytosing Kupffer cells and splenic macrophages and in all organs, including fat tissues, but excluding testes and brain, confers advantageous effects in metabolic syndrome [10, 11]. Cobalt protoporphyrin (CoPP) induction of HO-1 contributes to the phosphorylation of the insulin receptor, thus improving insulin sensitivity [12, 13]. Additionally, HO-1 acts through the degradation products of the prooxidant heme, bilirubin, and biliverdin, antioxidants that increase mitochondrial fusion, while also serving to improve adipocyte function and remodeling by increasing levels of adiponectin expression [14, 15]. Humans with low levels of HO-1 suffer severe oxidative stress and organ failure and demonstrate iron deposits in the liver [16, 17]. CoPP has been used to prevent body weight gain, increase oxygen consumption, and decrease fasting blood glucose in rats and mice [18] (reviewed in [11]). Recently, CoPP decreased expression of proapoptotic protein, abridge percolation of inflammatory cells, and reduced AST and ALT levels in IR induced liver damage [19, 20]. Moreover, HO-1 induction increased mitofusion over fission related proteins and improved mitochondrial quality control [21].

In adipose tissues, induction of HO-1 has been shown to reduce body weight, decrease NOV, and increase PGC-1$\alpha$ mediated thermogenesis, thereby increasing energy uptake and the stimulation of mitochondrial FA oxidation [22]. Adipose PGC-1$\alpha$ serves as a key moderator of energy metabolism and promotes mesenchymal stem cell differentiation into brown fat adipocytes [23] and the browning of white fat to a distinct phenotype known as brite fat, which aids in the prevention of the development of metabolic syndrome and type 2 diabetes mellitus (T2DM) [24].

Another important component of metabolic syndrome is an increase in the levels of the prooxidant heme. Intracellular heme levels play a central role in the regulation of many cell functions [25–27]. Inflammatory increases in IL-6 upregulate hepcidin and iron trapping in Kupffer cell diseases [1]. The resulting increase in cellular heme decreases levels of PGC-1$\alpha$, lipid metabolism, and adipogenesis [28].

The recently discovered inflammatory adipokine, NOV/CCN3 gene (nephroblastoma overexpressed) [29], is also shown to be repressed in conditions of increased HO-1 levels [22]. This protein plays key roles in inflammation, wound healing, fibrosis, and cancers [29]. NOV is involved in the adhesion, migration, proliferation, differentiation, and survival of different cell types [29] and modulates the expression of inflammatory molecules [30, 31].

In adipose tissues, induction of HO-1 has been shown to reduce body weight, decrease NOV, and increase PGC-1$\alpha$ mediated thermogenesis, thereby increasing energy uptake and the stimulation of mitochondrial FA oxidation [22]. Adipose PGC-1$\alpha$ serves as a key moderator of energy metabolism and promotes mesenchymal stem cell differentiation into brown fat adipocytes [23] and the browning of white fat to a distinct phenotype known as brite fat, which aids in the prevention of the development of metabolic syndrome and type 2 diabetes mellitus (T2DM) [24].

A recent study in mice has shown that myeloid-specific depletion of NOV exacerbates liver injury in a mouse model of NAFLD [32]. However, global NOV$^{-/-}$ mice fed a HFD have less steatosis compared to WT mice, and hepatic triacylglycerol content is reduced by approximately threefold [29].

We hypothesize that the development of NASH is the result of the combination of increased NOV and inflammation and a decrease of HO-1 in adipose and hepatic tissues leading to the impairment of mitochondrial function. We further propose that induction of HO-1 in adipose tissues will have positive impact on hepatic tissue and reverse the negative effects on NOV levels, decreasing NASH scores and increasing mitochondrial integrity and function.

## 2. Methods

Eight-week-old C57Bl6 male mice were fed a high fat diet (HFD) for 20 weeks, a time frame in which the manifestations of NASH are present. Mice were divided into four groups of 6 animals each: (1) control normal chow diet; (2) HFD; (3) HFD treated for the last 8 weeks with cobalt protoporphyrin (CoPP) (once/week a dose of 5 mg/100 g, bw); and (4) HFD treated for the last 8 weeks with CoPP and the last 3 weeks with tin mesoporphyrin (SnMP at a dose of 20 mg/100 g BW), an inhibitor of HO activity (twice/week). BW at the end of the 20-week period C57 lean, range; 29-31; HF; 56-59, HF-CoPP; 34-39, CoPP-SnMP; 47-51 gm, blood glucose and alanine aminotransferase (ALT) were measured as described [22, 33]. All animal experiments followed the NYMC IACUC institutionally approved protocol in accordance with the NIH guidelines.

*2.1. Histopathological Examination of Hepatic Tissue, NAS Score Evaluation, and Hepatic Lipid Droplet Analysis.* Liver samples from each experimental group were fixed in 4% paraformaldehyde, dehydrated, embedded in paraffin wax, and sectioned (6 $\mu$m thick). The main liver histopathological features commonly described in NAFLD including steatosis, inflammation, hepatocyte ballooning, and fibrosis were scored according to the NAFLD histologic activity score (NAS) system, and lipid droplet analysis was performed as previously described [33–35]. Briefly, double-blinded analysis identified the degree of steatosis and NASH (grade 0 $\leq$ 5%; 1 = 5–33%; grade 2 = 34%–66%; grade 3 $\geq$ 66%), lobular inflammation (0: no foci, 1 < 2 foci per 200x field, 2: 2 to 4 foci per 200x field, and 3: >4 foci per 200x field), hepatocyte ballooning (0: none; 1: rare or few; 2: many), and fibrosis (0: no fibrosis, 1: perisinusoidal or periportal fibrosis, 2: perisinusoidal and portal/perioral fibrosis, 3: bridging fibrosis, and 4: cirrhosis) [34].

*2.2. Real-Time qPCR, Western Blot Analysis, HO Activity, Heme Measurement, and $O_2$ Consumption.* Total RNA and protein were extracted from liver and visceral adipose tissue and gene expression analysis was performed by RNeasy® Lipid Tissue (Qiagen), as indicated by the manufacturer [24, 33]. RNA was determined by measuring the absorbance at 260 nm (A260) with a Biotek™ plate reader and the Take3™ plate (Biotek, Winooski, VT) and assessed by the A260/A280 ratio. cDNA was synthesized from total RNA (Applied Biosystems) using a High Capacity cDNA Reverse Transcription Kit (Applied Biosystems). Real-time PCR was performed using TaqMan® Fast Universal Master Mix (2x), on a 7500 HT Fast Real-Time PCR System (Applied Biosystems). For western blotting analyses, tissue was lysed in RIPA lysis buffer supplemented with protease and phosphatase inhibitors (Complete™ Mini and PhosSTOP™, Roche Diagnostics, Indianapolis, IN as previously described [35]. Heme levels were determined by ELISA (BioVision, Inc., Milpitas, CA) as described [35].

HO activity was determined as described [36]. Briefly, freshly lysed and homogenized tissue samples were incubated in sealed vials at 37°C for 90 min with 30 $\mu$M heme, and 2 mM NADPH, in the absence or presence of an HO inhibitor, SnMP (50 $\mu$M). After termination of reaction, headspace gas was analyzed for CO with $C^{13}O^{16}$ added as an internal standard. CO measurements were performed using an Agilent 5890 GC-MS. HO activity is calculated by subtracting CO levels obtained in the presence of SnMP from those obtained without. Data are normalized to total protein and are presented as pmol CO/mg protein/h.

Mouse oxygen consumption was assessed as described [22, 24]. Briefly, oxygen consumption ($VO_2$) and carbon dioxide production ($VCO_2$) were measured using the Oxylet gas analyzer and air flow unit (Oxylet; Panlab-Bioseb, Vitrolles, France). Hourly respiratory quotients were measured and performed twice, on individual mice using the $VCO_2$ and $VO_2$ obtained by the gas analyzer. The results are expressed as the consumed $VO_2$ per kilogram body weight per minute (ml/kg/min). The respiratory quota is expressed as $CO_2$ eliminated/$O_2$ consumed.

*2.3. Isolation and Development of NOV Overexpressing Adipocytes.* Viral transduction was performed as previously described [35]. Briefly, $1x10^6$ cells were seeded per well of a 6-well plate 24 h prior to transduction. The cells were incubated with the transduction medium ($1x10^6$ transducing units (TU) of lentiviral particles (Precision LentiORF for NOV (Dharmacon, Lafayette, CO)) in 0.5ml $\alpha$-MEM growth medium supplemented with polybrene (8 $\mu$g/ml) for 3h to maximize the contact between each cell and lentiviral particles. Additional culture medium supplemented with polybrene was then added to each well. After an additional 48 h incubation, antibiotic selection medium was used to kill all the nontransduced cells.

*2.4. Statistical Analyses.* Statistical significance between experimental groups was determined by Student's t-test for pairwise comparison between groups or by ANOVA with Tukey-Kramer post hoc analysis for comparison between multiple groups. The data are presented as means ± SEM and the null hypothesis was rejected at $p<0.05$.

## 3. Results

*3.1. HO-1 Induction Prevents Fibrosis and Decreases NASH Score.* As expected, livers of lean mice showed no significant evidence of steatosis (0.67% of cells positive for intracellular lipid accumulation) with only rare ballooning and no inflammatory foci and no fibrosis. The livers from HF mice revealed a higher NAS score (NAS: 9) with elevated steatosis, moderate lobular inflammatory loci, significant hepatocyte ballooning, and fibrosis (Table 1; Figures 1(a)–1(e)). Increased HO-1 expression with CoPP improved this score (NAS: 3), diminished all the pathological parameters, and resulted in mild steatosis, rare inflammatory loci and ballooning, and no fibrosis. Inhibition of HO activity in HF mice caused perisinusoidal steatosis and ballooning and portal fibrosis (NAS: 8). Furthermore, the adverse effect of hepatosteatosis was confirmed by detailed morphometrical analysis of liver lipid droplet diameter (Figures 1(a)–1(e)). From these results, we conclude that increased levels of HO-1 can prevent lipid droplet formation in the liver, ultimately preventing the development of NAFLD and NASH in obese mice.

*3.2. Induction of HO-1 Decreases NOV and Fibrotic Markers and Improves ALT and AST.* As seen in Figure 2(f), levels of NOV in the lean mouse are significantly ($p<0.05$) higher in visceral adipose tissue (VAT) than in liver tissue. The HF diet increased the expression of hepatic NOV/ CCN3 mRNA and protein content (Figures 2(a), 2(b), and 2(c)) as compared to lean mice ($p<0.05$). An increase in HO-1 expression resulted in a normalization of NOV expression, an effect that was blocked by an inhibitor of HO activity; SnMP ($p<0.05$) (Figures 2(a), 2(b), and 2(c)) ($p<0.05$). Similarly, FAS protein expression was significantly ($p<0.05$) elevated in HF fed mice and normalized by CoPP (Figures 2(b) and 2(d)). Fibrotic protein signaling in hepatic tissue of obese mice as measured by the expression of MMP2 was reduced by increased HO-1 levels ($p<0.05$), an effect that was prevented by inhibition of HO activity (Figures 2(b) and 2(e)). Obese mice developed impaired liver function as indicated by increased levels of serum AST ($p < 0.05$) and ALT ($p < 0.05$), all of which were normalized by HO-1 induction ($p<0.05$) (Figures 2(g) and 2(h)). HO-1 reduction in AST and ALT levels was eliminated by SnMP (Figures 2(g) and 2(h)). Taking all of these findings together, it can be concluded that a decrease in levels of the proinflammatory adipokine NOV in conjunction with increased levels of HO-1 mitigates the development of fibrotic markers that contribute to the NASH phenotype.

*3.3. Induction of HO-1 Decreases Heme and Hepcidin Expression.* In accordance with our hypothesis, our results indicate that NASH livers have significantly ($p<0.01$) increased heme

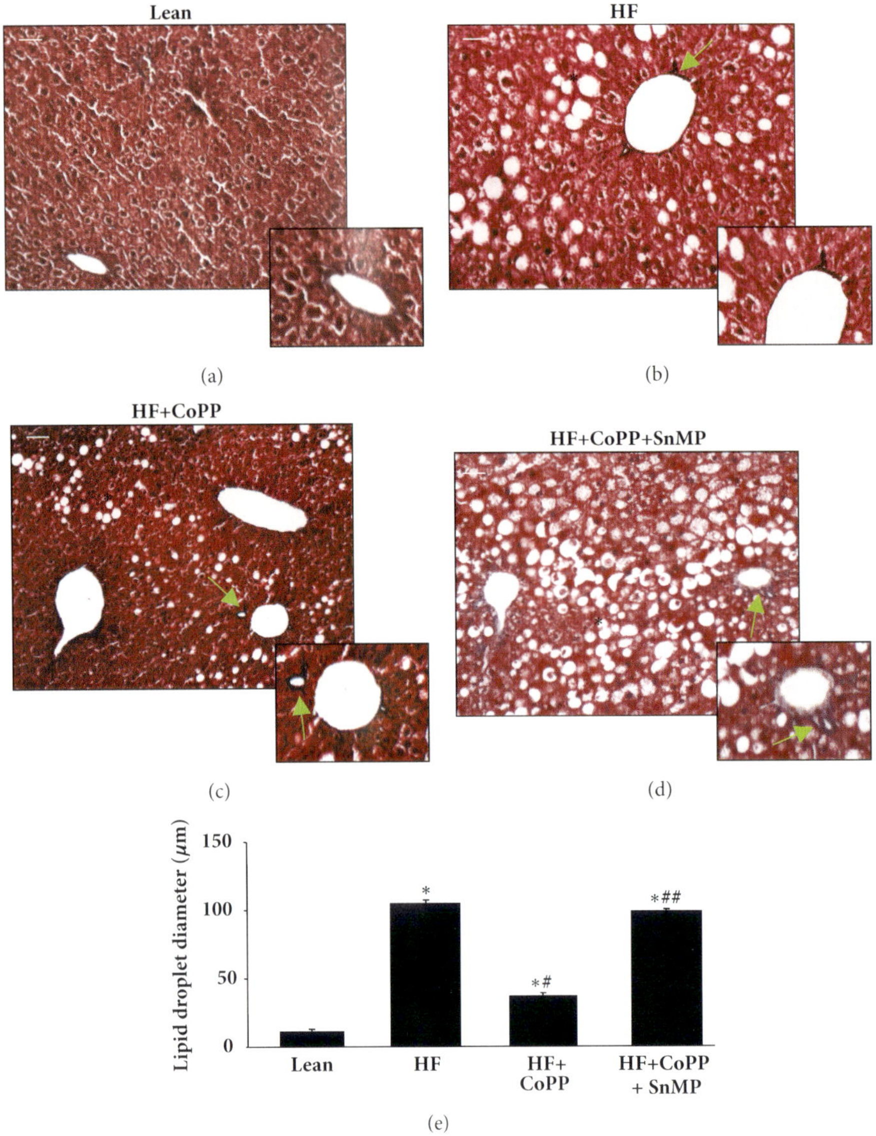


FIGURE 1: HO-1 induction prevents fibrosis and decreases NASH score. Liver of lean (a), HF fed (b), HF fed treated with CoPP (c), and HF fed treated with CoPP and SnMP (d) in mice and (e) graph summarizes the morphometrical analysis of liver lipid droplet diameter. * $p < 0.05$ versus lean; # $p < 0.05$ versus HF fed; and + $p < 0.05$ versus HF fed mice + CoPP. Masson's trichrome staining. Bar 20 μm. The arrow shows hepatic perivascular fibrosis and (*) indicates the steatosis of control lean mice, HF fed mice, HF fed mice + CoPP, and HF fed mice + CoPP + SnMP.

TABLE 1: **Histopathological NAS score evaluation.** Degree of steatosis and NASH (grade 0 ≤ 5%; 1 = 5–33%; grade 2 = 34%–66%; grade 3 ≥ 66%), lobular inflammation (0: no foci, 1 < 2 foci per 200x field, 2: 2 to 4 foci per 200x field, and 3: foci per 200x field), hepatocyte ballooning (0: none; 1: rare or few; 2: many), and fibrosis (0: no fibrosis, 1: perisinusoidal or periportal fibrosis, 2: perisinusoidal and portal/perioral fibrosis, 3: bridging fibrosis, and 4: cirrhosis).

| NAS pathological score factors | Control | HF | HF + CoPP | HF + CoPP + SnMP |
|---|---|---|---|---|
| Steatosis | 0 (0.67%) | 2 (42.24%) | 1 (10.28%) | 2 (33.05%) |
| Inflammation | 0 (no foci) | 2 (2-4 foci/field) | 1 (<2 foci/field) | 2 (2-4 foci/field) |
| Ballooning | 1 (rare) | 2 (many) | 1 (rare) | 2 (many) |
| Fibrosis | 0 (no fibrosis) | 3 (bridging fibrosis) | 0 (no fibrosis) | 2 (perisinusoidal and portal fibrosis) |
| NAS value | 1 | 9 NASH | 3 | 8 NASH |

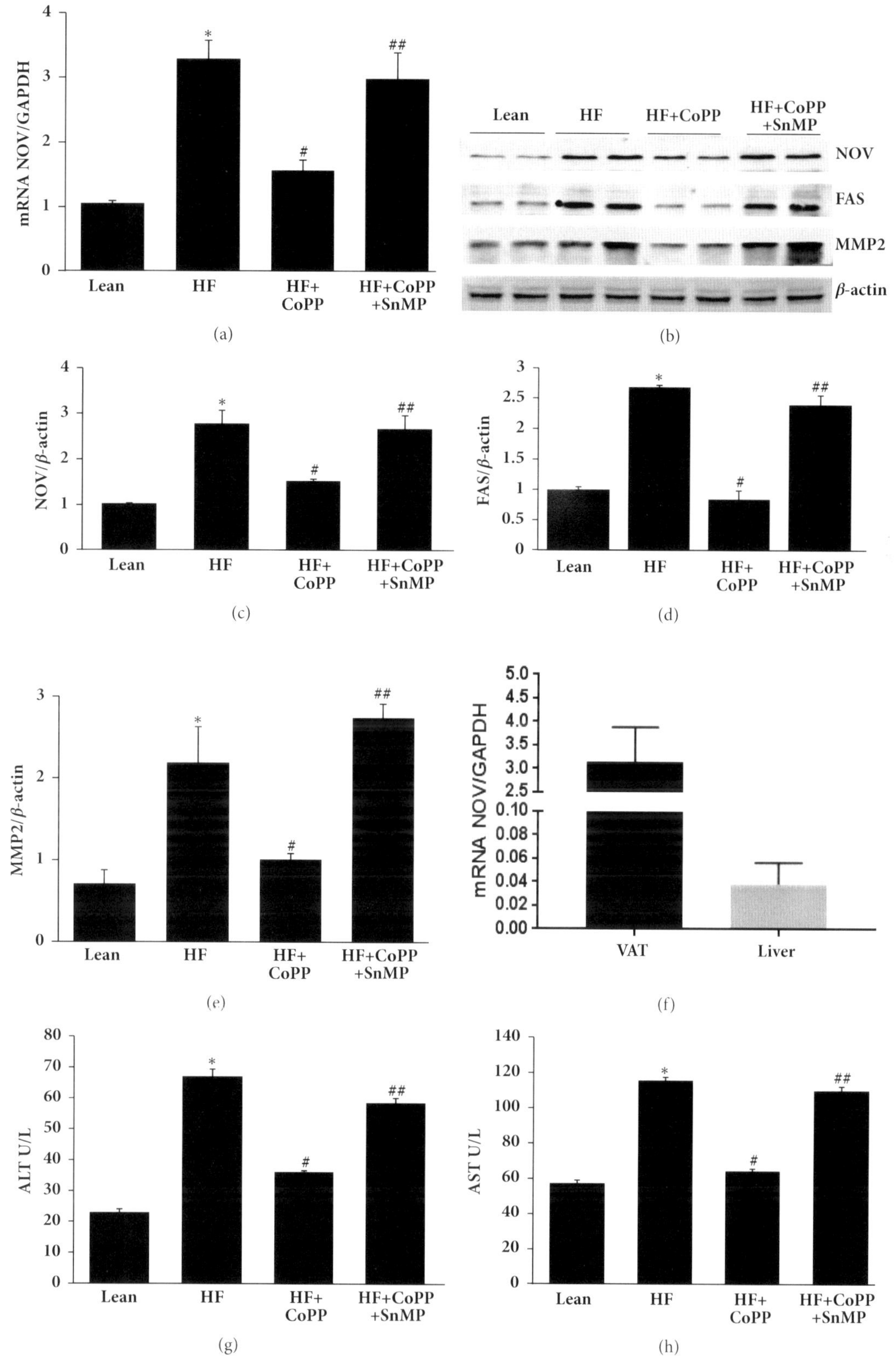


FIGURE 2: Induction of HO-1 decreases NOV and fibrotic markers and improves ALT and AST. (a) The mRNA expression of NOV, (b) representative western blots and densitometry analysis of (c) NOV, (d) FAS, and (e) MMP2 and levels of (f) AST(U/L), and (g) ALT(U/L) in hepatic tissues of control lean mice, HF fed mice, HF fed + with CoPP, and HF fed mice + CoPP + SnMP. (h) NOV mRNA levels in visceral adipose tissue (VAT) and liver of lean mice. Results are mean ± SE, n=6, ∗p<0.05 versus lean mice, #p<0.05 versus HF fed mice, and ##p<0.05 versus HF fed mice + CoPP.

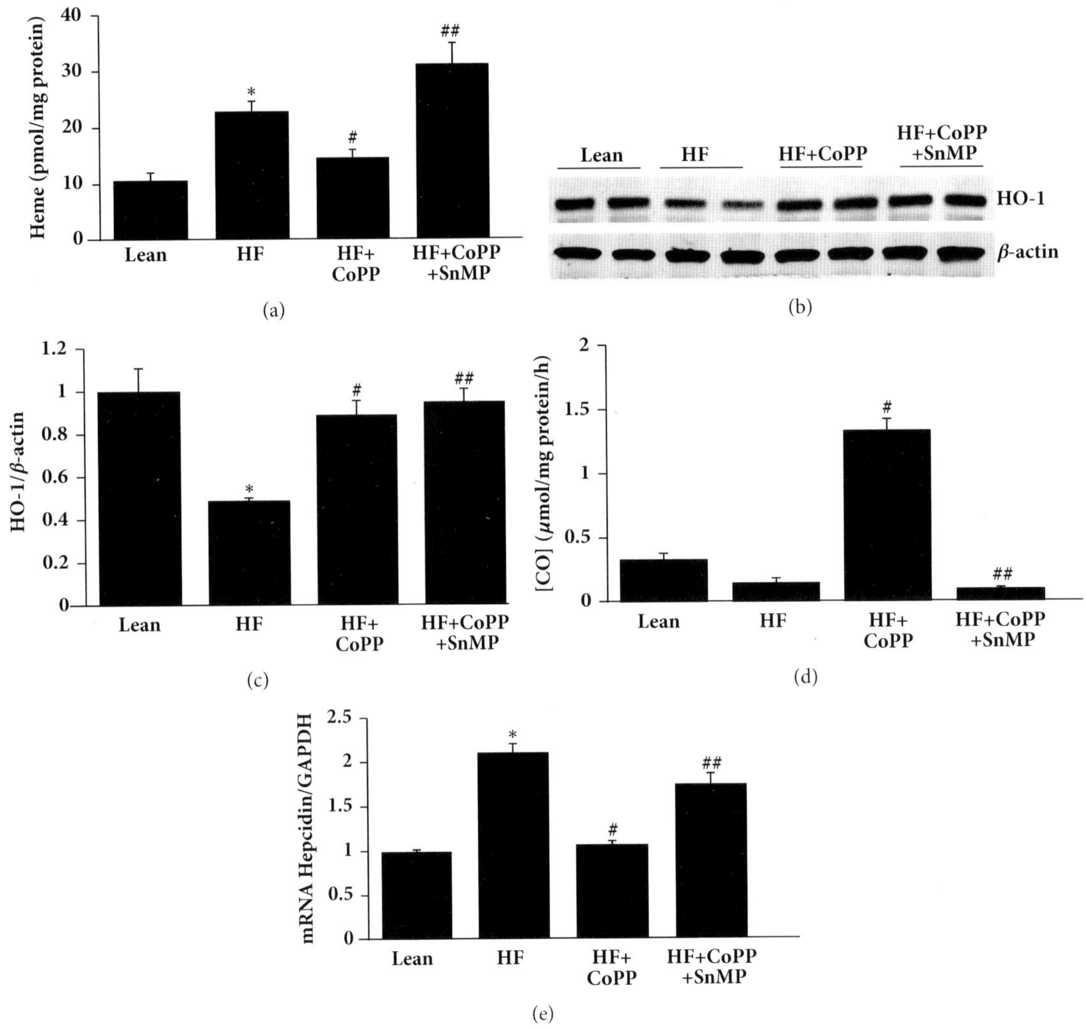


FIGURE 3: Increase of HO-1 decreases heme levels and hepcidin expression. (a) Heme (pmol/mg protein) content, (b) representative western blots of HO-1, (c) densitometry analysis of HO-1 and (d) CO production (μmol/mg protein/h), and (e) mRNA expression of hepcidin in hepatic tissues of control lean mice, HF fed mice, HF fed mice + CoPP, and HF fed mice + CoPP + SnMP. Results are mean ± SE, n=6, ∗p<0.05 versus lean mice, #p<0.05 versus HF fed mice, and ##p<0.05 versus HF fed mice treated with CoPP.

levels as compared to control lean mice fed a normal chow diet. Induction of HO-1 decreased heme levels as compared to the HF diet group (p<0.01). The favorable effects of induction of HO-1 were reversed by SnMP (Figure 3(a)). Western blot analysis demonstrated that hepatic tissues of mice fed a HF diet for 20 weeks had significantly (P<0.05) decreased levels of HO-1 protein as compared to hepatic tissues of mice fed a normal chow diet (Figures 3(b) and 3(c)). CoPP treatment for 8 weeks increased liver levels of HO-1 as compared to mice fed a HF diet alone, p<0.01 (Figures 3(b) and 3(c)). The positive effects of increased HO-1 levels were reversed by SnMP (Figures 3(b)–3(d)). Of note is the fact that SnMP does not prevent an increase in HO-1 protein expression but rather inhibits HO activity [37]. HO activity in hepatic tissue was increased by CoPP and decreased by SnMP in HF fed mice, p<0.05 (Figure 3(d)). As seen in Figure 3(e), hepcidin mRNA level was increased in NASH livers of HF fed mice, as compared to lean mice. Increased HO-1 expression significantly, p<0.05, reduced the expression of hepcidin, an effect which was reversed by SnMP (p<0.05).

*3.4. Increase of HO-1 Expression Augments Mitochondrial Integrity.* MFN1, MFN2, and OPA1 expression levels were increased, while FIS1 mRNA was decreased by HO-1 induction (p <0.05) an effect that was reversed by SnMP (p<0.05) (Figures 4(a)–4(d)). These results indicate that HO-1 is a powerful inducer of mitochondrial fusion (the merge of dysfunctional to functional) and an inhibitor of mitochondrial fission. This increase in fusion (MFN1 and MFN2) and decrease in fission (FIS1) contribute to an increase in overall mitochondrial function, leading to a decrease in adiposity in HF fed mice, a consequent reduction in obesity, and a concurrent reduction in the development of NASH. Mitochondrial expression of COX2 and COX4 as well as ATP synthase were reduced in obese mice as compared to lean mice (p<0.05), effects that were reversed by increased levels

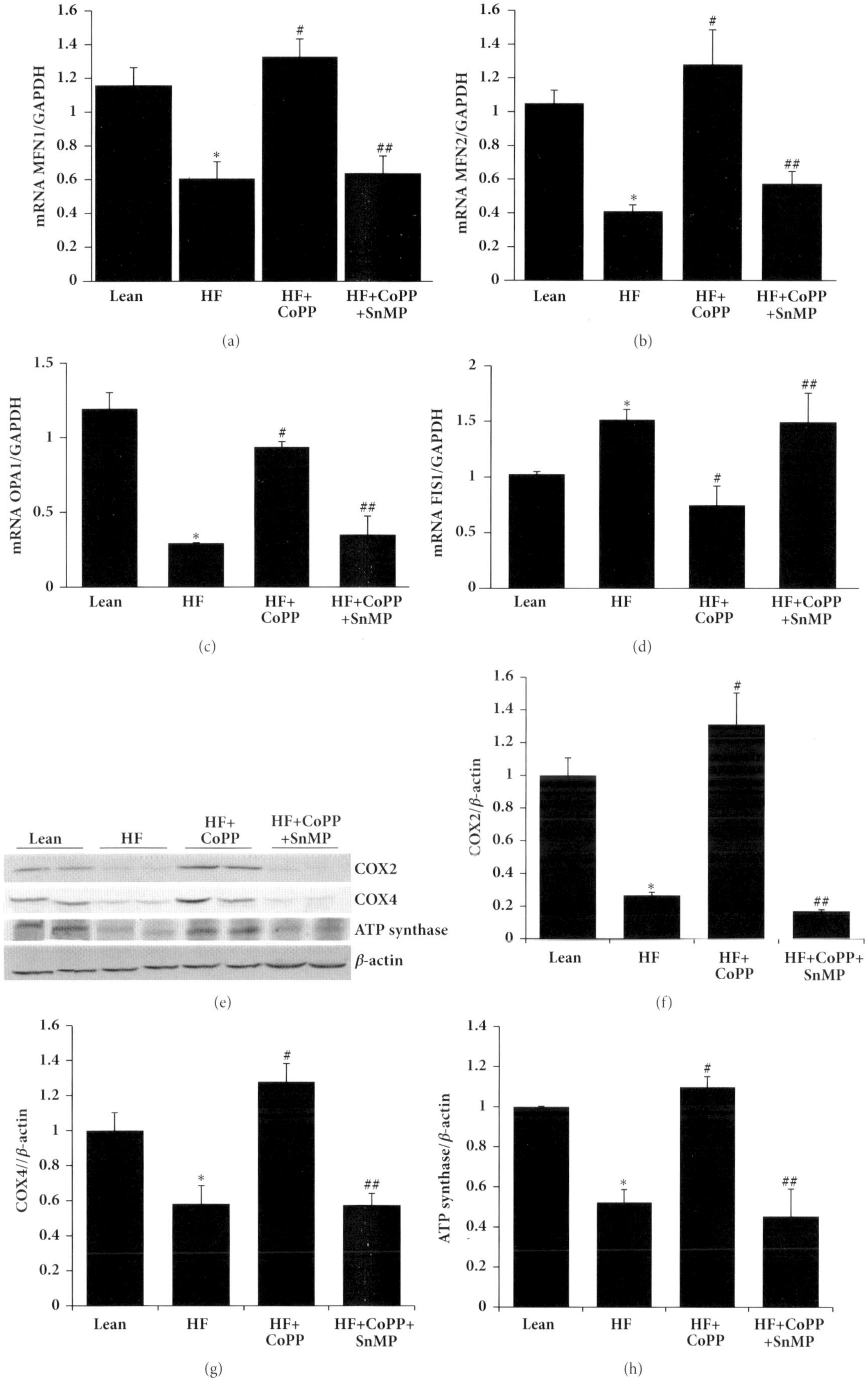


Figure 4: Continued.

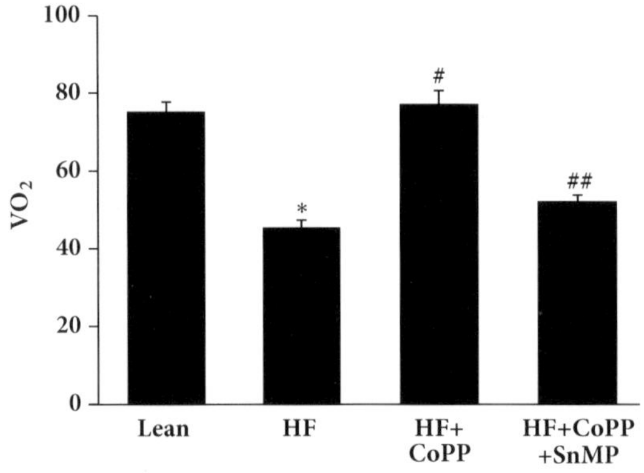


(i)

Figure 4: Increase of HO-1 expression augments mitochondrial integrity. mRNA expression of (a) MFN1, (b) MFN2, (c) OPA1, and (d) FIS1. (e) Representative western blots and densitometric analysis of (f) COX2, (g) COX4, and (h) ATP synthase. (i) Total body oxygen consumption ($VO_2$) of mice, in hepatic tissues of control lean mice, HF fed mice, HF fed mice + CoPP, and HF fed mice + CoPP + SnMP. Results are mean ± SE, n=6, ∗p<0.05 versus lean mice, #p<0.05 versus HF fed mice, and ##p<0.05 versus HF fed mice + CoPP.

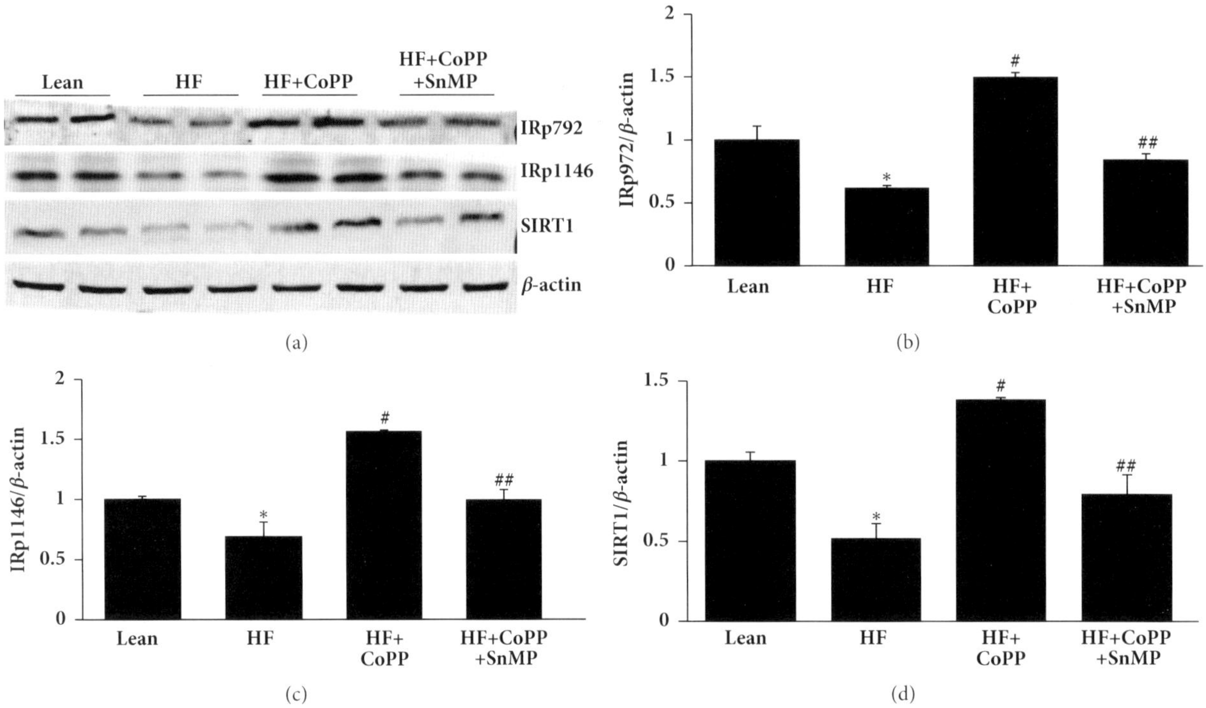


Figure 5: HO-1 upregulation increases hepatic pAKT, pAMPK, and insulin receptor phosphorylation levels. Representative western blots (a) and densitometry analysis of (b) IRp972, (c) IRp1146, and (d) SIRT1 in hepatic tissues of control lean mice, HF fed mice, HF fed mice + CoPP, and HF fed mice + CoPP + SnMP. Results are mean ± SE, n=4, ∗p<0.05 versus lean mice, #p<0.05 versus HF fed mice, and ##p<0.05 versus HF fed mice + CoPP.

of HO-1 (p<0.05) (Figures 4(e)–4(h)). Oxygen consumption in obese mice was decreased as compared to lean mice (p<0.05) (Figure 4(i)). However, CoPP treatment of obese mice normalized $O_2$ consumption (p<0.05), an effect blocked by SnMP (Figure 4(i)).

*3.5. HO-1 Upregulation Increases Phosphorylation of the Insulin Receptor in the Liver of Obese Mice.* Obese mice had decreased expression levels of IRp-Tyr 972 and IRp-Tyr 1146 (p<0.05), as well as levels of SIRT1, as compared to control lean mice. HO-1 induction ameliorated the effect of HFD on insulin receptor phosphorylation and significantly increased IRp-Tyr 972 and IRp-Tyr 1146, as well as SIRT1 levels (p<0.05) (Figures 5(a)–5(d)). These effects were reversed by SnMP (Figures 5(a)–5(d)). The reversal of these beneficial effects corroborates the role of HO-1 expression and HO activity in mediating the beneficial effects of CoPP.

*3.6. Adipose Tissue HO-1 Upregulation Increases Phosphorylation of Both the Insulin Receptor and Acetyl-CoA-Carboxylase (ACC).* To test the possibility that NOV-mediated increases in adipose inflammation in turn decreases insulin receptor phosphorylation in an obese mouse model, we examined the effects of HO-1 on insulin receptor phosphorylation in adipose tissue. Adipose tissue of obese mice had decreased phosphorylation levels of IRp-Tyr 1146, IRp-Tyr 972, AMPK, and ACC and reduced expression of HO-1 as compared to control lean mice ($p<0.05$) (Figures 6(a)–6(f)). The negative effects associated with obesity were normalized in obese mice following induction of HO-1 ($p<0.05$) (Figures 6(a)–6(f)) and reversed by inhibition of HO activity ($p<0.05$) (Figures 6(a)–6(f)).

*3.7. Adipose Tissue HO-1 Upregulation Increases Anti-Inflammatory Adiponectin and Mitochondrial Fusion-Associated Proteins, While Decreasing Proinflammatory NOV and the Mitochondrial Fission-Associated Protein, FIS1.* To further test the possibility of potential crosstalk between adipose and hepatic tissue we examined the effects of HO-1 on adipose mitochondrial function as it is related to the proinflammatory adipokine NOV. Inflamed adipose tissue from untreated obese mice expressed elevated levels of NOV. As seen in Figures 7(a) and 7(b), the NOV level in visceral adipose tissues of HF diet fed mice was elevated as compared to the levels in lean mice ($p<0.05$). HO-1 induction decreased visceral adipose tissue NOV levels ($p<0.05$), suggesting that induction of HO-1 reprograms white adipose tissue to beige, resulting in less inflammation (Figures 7(a) and 7(b)).

More importantly, as mitochondrial integrity in liver tissue of HF diet fed mice was increased by HO-1 induction and as mitochondrial function is very important also for the health of adipose tissue, we assessed the levels of mitochondrial fusion and fission proteins in the visceral adipose tissue. As seen in Figure 7(a), 7(c)–7(e), the levels of MFN1 and MFN2 were decreased, while FIS1 was increased in obese mice as compared to lean mice, $p<0.05$. HO-1 induction normalized these levels, an effect reversed by concomitant SnMP-treatment ($p<0.05$) (Figure 7(a), 7(c)–7(e)). Healthy adipocytes express the anti-inflammatory adipokine, adiponectin. As seen in Figures 7(a) and 7(f), the adiponectin levels in visceral adipose tissues of HF diet fed mice were decreased as compared to the levels in lean mice ($p<0.05$). CoPP-mediated HO-1 induction normalized visceral adipose tissue adiponectin levels, an effect that was prevented by SnMP-treatment ($p<0.05$) (Figures 7(a) and 7(f)).

As induction of HO-1 in adipocytes decreased NOV levels, we wondered whether overexpression of NOV would cause a decrease of HO-1 levels. As seen in Figure 7(g), overexpression of NOV in cultured adipocytes led to a reduction in the HO-1 mRNA levels ($p<0.05$). Successful transduction of cells with the NOV ORF lentiviral particles was confirmed by measuring mRNA levels of NOV in transduced and control adipocytes. The NOV mRNA level was upregulated more than 100-fold ($p<0.05$) in the NOV overexpressing cells as compared to control cells (data not shown).

## 4. Discussion

The primary findings of this study are the following. (1) The increase of the proinflammatory adipokine NOV and decrease of HO-1 in hepatic and adipose tissue of obese mice is associated with mitochondrial dysfunction and the development and progression of obesity-induced NASH. (2) Fat expansion is associated with remodeling marked by an increase in proinflammatory molecules and oxidative stress and a decrease in PGC-1$\alpha$ and insulin receptor phosphorylation with the eventual development of metabolic abnormalities. (3) TNF-$\alpha$ and NOV are increased while adiponectin is decreased in obese mice. (4) Reduction of levels of heme through the pharmacological induction of HO-1 reduces the severity of steatosis, inflammation, and fibrosis through the improvement of hepatic mitochondrial function. We and others have shown that heme levels are elevated in lipid laden, unhealthy, terminal differentiated adipocyte, and increase of HO-1; i.e., increase of heme degradation decreases adiposity [38, 39]. Diminishing HO-1 levels are seen in maturing inflamed adipocyte in hepatic tissues [35, 39, 40].

Increased levels of HO-1 shown to play a critical role in the amelioration of oxidative stress, and, in both humans and mice, low levels of HO-1 lead to organ damage [16, 41]. Moreover, overexpression of HO-1 lowers levels of the inflammatory mediators TNF-$\alpha$ and IL-6 in the liver of mice [42]. A decrease in HO activity exacerbates mitochondrial lipid peroxidation and mitochondrial dysfunction, while induction of HO-1 upregulates mitochondrial transcription factor [21], all of which support the hypothesis that a reduction in HO activity results in mitochondrial dysfunction and increased insulin resistance [22, 24]. Mitochondrial dysfunction leads to a decrease in beta oxidation in the liver which allows fat to accumulate resulting in a "fatty liver" [43, 44].

The potential beneficial role of decreasing NOV in obesity and metabolic syndrome has been recently described [22]. Increased levels of NOV appear to be a key component of the inflammatory and fibrotic response in the liver of obese mice, and adiposity mediated increase of NOV appears to be involved in hepatic IR and in the pathophysiology of the inflammation and resulting fibrosis. In NOV$^{-/-}$ obese mice, there is a reduction in body weight, a decrease in expression of proinflammatory cytokines and chemokines, and increase in the levels of PGC-1$\alpha$ and UCP1. In our obese mouse model, increased levels of HO-1 led to a concomitant reduction in NOV mRNA, as inflammation and markers of fibrosis to the levels of lean animals. This effect was reversed by inhibiting HO activity, not HO-1 protein, by SnMP, a well-known effect for SnMP [37] indicating the pivotal role of HO-1 and HO activity in the regulation of obesity and metabolic syndrome. We speculate that a crosstalk exists between adipose dysfunction and the development of fibrosis and NASH.

Mitochondrial dysfunction is also a key player in the generation of ROS [45], which results in abnormal respiration [43]. Oxidative stress in NAFLD/NASH is associated with the reduced expression of PGC-1$\alpha$ in adipose tissue, negatively affecting mitochondrial biogenesis, thereby resulting in the mitochondrial dysfunction that is seen in the development of

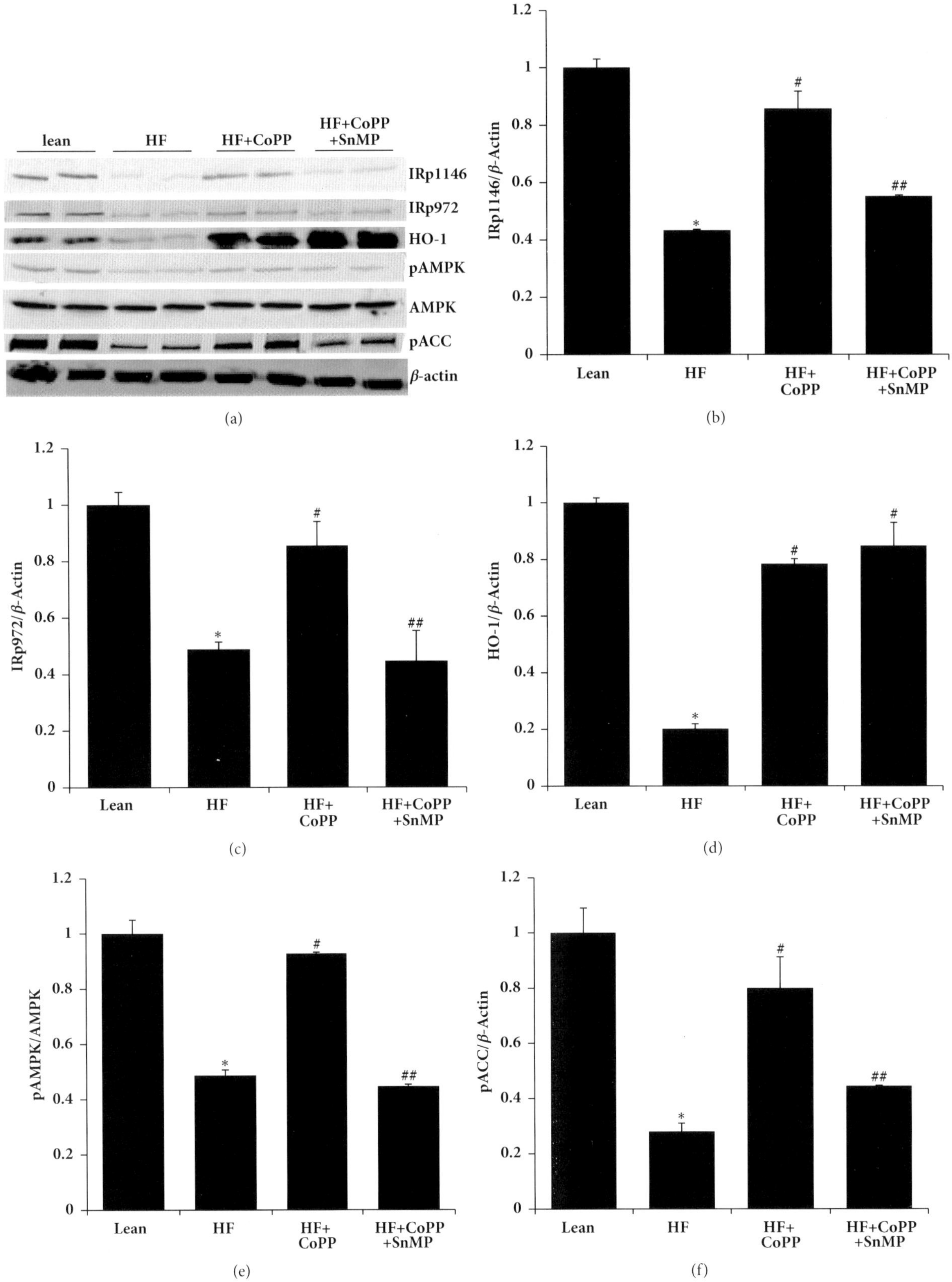


Figure 6: Adipose tissue HO-1 upregulation increases phosphorylation of both insulin receptor and ACC. Representative western blot (a) and densitometry analysis of (b) IRp1146, (c) IRp972, (d) HO-1, (e) pAMPK, and (f) pACC. Results are mean ± SE, n=4, ∗$p<0.05$ versus lean mice, #$p<0.05$ versus HF fed mice, and ##$p<0.05$ versus HF fed mice + CoPP.

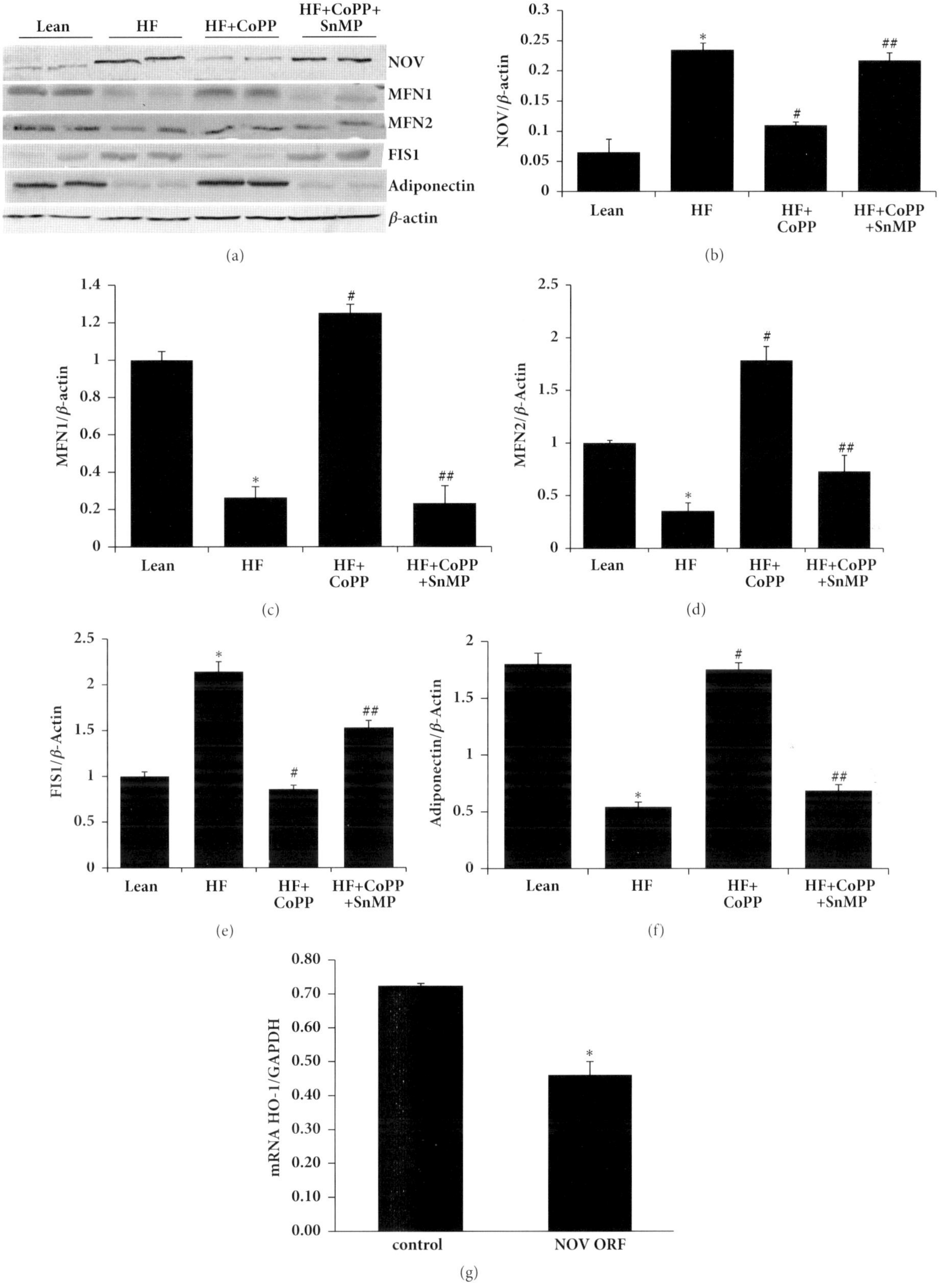


FIGURE 7: Adipose tissue HO-1 upregulation increases anti-inflammatory adiponectin and mitochondrial fusion-associated proteins, while decreasing proinflammatory NOV and the mitochondrial fission-associated protein, FIS1. (a) Representative western blots, and densitometry analysis of (b) NOV, (c) MFN1, (d) MFN2, (e) FIS1, and (f) adiponectin. (g) HO-1 mRNA levels in NOV overexpressing 3T3-L1 derived adipocytes. Results are mean ± SE, n=4, ∗p<0.05 versus lean mice/control, #p<0.05 versus HF fed mice, and ##p<0.05 versus HF fed mice + CoPP.

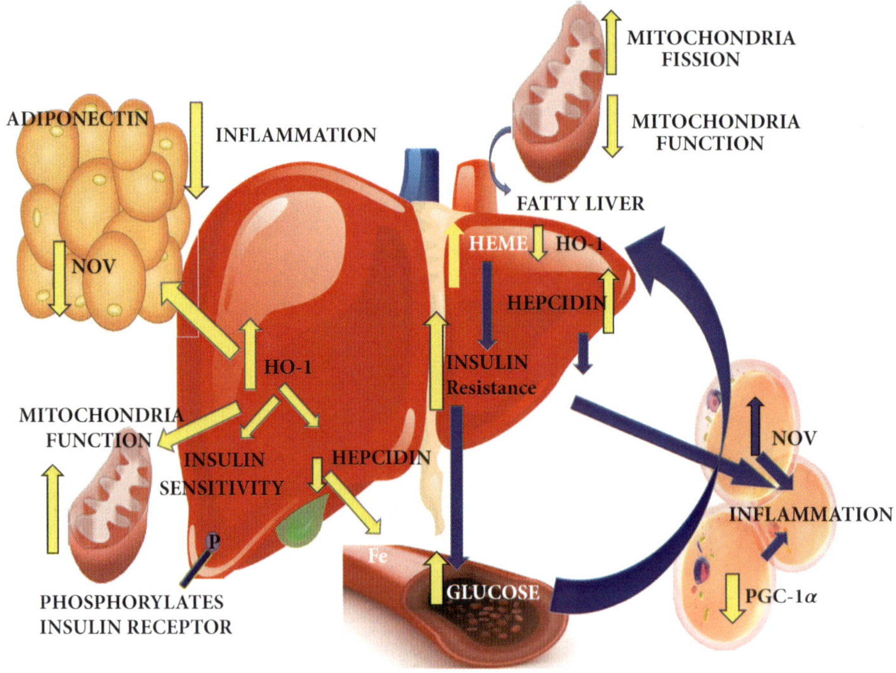


Figure 8: Schematic description of the HO-1 mediated induction of adipose tissue of HF fed mice. As seen in right side panel, decreased HO-1 resulted in an increase of hepatic heme, hepcidin, which is associated with the development and progression of obesity-induced NASH, fibrosis via mitochondrial dysfunction (fission and decreases in COX 2 and 4). Fat expansion was associated with remodeling marked by an increase in adipocyte hyperplasia and hypertrophy leading to proinflammatory molecule NOV, which is associated with a decrease of PGC-1$\alpha$ and insulin receptor phosphorylation and eventually development of fibrosis and NAS. In the left panel, induction of HO-1 reduced the severity of steatosis, inflammation, and fibrosis through decrease in NOV and an increase of adiponectin that resulted in the improvement of hepatic mitochondrial integrity, pAMPK-pAKT, and insulin receptor phosphorylation that all in concert leads to an improvement in hepatic function and steatosis.

IR [45]. PGC-1$\alpha$ targets SIRT3, a mitochondrial deacetylase, which promotes mitochondrial biogenesis, suppression of ROS [46], and mitochondrial FA oxidation [47]. PGC-1$\alpha$ adipocyte knockout mice develop IR and glucose intolerance and consequently elevated levels of circulating lipids and cholesterol [48]. This demonstrates the existence of PGC-1$\alpha$ crosstalk between adipocytes and the liver, thereby correlating adipocyte mediated release of inflammatory cytokines with hepatic insulin resistance and steatosis. With HO-1 induction, levels of PGC-1$\alpha$ and markers of mitochondrial fusion increase in adipose tissue, oxidative stress decreases, and lipogenesis and liver function in obese mice improve.

A HFD increases the expression of the FIS1 gene, which regulates mitochondrial fission, while concomitantly reducing the expression of those genes responsible for mitochondrial quality control and fusion processes, fueling ROS generation, and causing tissue inflammation [49]. An inverse relationship exists between Mfn2 mRNA levels in skeletal muscles and BMI. Consistent with these observations, skeletal muscle from obese subjects presents an altered, fragmented mitochondrial network, associated with nutrient oxidation, respiratory chain defects, and IR [50]. Additionally, liver MFN2 levels are decreased in obesity, but increased by increasing HO-1 levels, thereby reducing the severity of NASH. In particular, increased levels of HO-1 decrease steatosis and abolish fibrosis, and the NAS score is reduced. In agreement with our data, NASH and fatty liver are both associated with IR, but NASH alone is associated with mitochondrial structural defects [51]. Finally, since hepcidin is released from adipose tissue and is upregulated by NOV, it follows that there would be increased hepcidin in individuals with higher BMI and metabolic abnormalities who would be more likely to develop NASH [1]. Thus, considering only a small percentage of patients with NAFLD progress to NASH, an increase in hepcidin might explain the conversion and associated mitochondrial dysfunction and inflammation. Additionally, differences may exist in patients with fatty liver based on different genetic backgrounds of these individuals (increased heme-NOV and a decrease in HO-1 expression).

In conclusion, these data identify that a decrease in adipose and hepatic HO-1 is associated with an increase in adipose-derived NOV activation and that these perturbations can be regarded as key mediators in the development and progression of obesity-induced fibrosis and NASH. Decreased heme levels result in improved mitochondrial function and decreased FAS with an overall reduction in NOV-inflammation, fibrosis, and NASH scores (summarized in Figure 8). As the pursuit of a reliable surrogate marker of inflammation and fibrosis continues, liver histopathology is reflected by the NAFLD Activity Score, which remains the gold standard end-point of therapeutic efficacy. However, future pharmacologic targeting of the NOV/HO-1 axis may prove fruitful in reducing the severity of a disease process that is increasing significantly in prevalence.

## Authors' Contributions

David Sacerdoti and Shailendra P. Singh contributed equally to this work.

## Acknowledgments

All authors had full access to the data and take responsibility for its integrity. All authors have read and agree with the manuscript as written. The content is solely the responsibility of the authors and does not necessarily represent the official views of the National Institutes of Health.

## References

[1] J. E. Nelson, L. Wilson, E. M. Brunt et al., "Relationship between the pattern of hepatic iron deposition and histological severity in nonalcoholic fatty liver disease," *Hepatology*, vol. 53, no. 2, pp. 448–457, 2011.

[2] J. E. Nelson, R. Bhattacharya, K. D. Lindor et al., "HFE C282Y mutations are associated with advanced hepatic fibrosis in caucasians with nonalcoholic steatohepatitis," *Hepatology*, vol. 46, pp. 723–729, 2007.

[3] K. V. Kowdley, P. Belt, L. A. Wilson et al., "Serum ferritin is an independent predictor of histologic severity and advanced fibrosis in patients with nonalcoholic fatty liver disease," *Hepatology*, vol. 55, no. 1, pp. 77–85, 2012.

[4] D. F. Vatner, S. K. Majumdar, N. Kumashiro et al., "Insulin-independent regulation of hepatic triglyceride synthesis by fatty acids," *Proceedings of the National Academy of Sciences of the United States of America*, vol. 112, no. 4, pp. 1143–1148, 2015.

[5] Y. Li, L. Ding, W. Hassan, D. Abdelkader, and J. Shang, "Adipokines and hepatic insulin resistance," *Journal of Diabetes Research*, vol. 2013, Article ID 170532, 8 pages, 2013.

[6] G. V. Jayashree, K. Krupashree, P. Rachitha, and F. Khanum, "Patulin Induced Oxidative Stress Mediated Apoptotic Damage in Mice, and its Modulation by Green Tea Leaves," *Journal of Clinical and Experimental Hepatology*, vol. 7, no. 2, pp. 127–134, 2017.

[7] R. Krithika, R. J. Verma, P. S. Shrivastav, and L. Suguna, "Phyllanthin of Standardized Phyllanthus amarus Extract Attenuates Liver Oxidative Stress in Mice and Exerts Cytoprotective Activity on Human Hepatoma Cell Line," *Journal of Clinical and Experimental Hepatology*, vol. 1, no. 2, pp. 57–67, 2011.

[8] P.-C. Lee, L.-Y. Yang, Y.-W. Wang et al., "Mechanisms of the prevention and inhibition of the progression and development of non-alcoholic steatohepatitis by genetic and pharmacological decoy receptor 3 supplementation," *Hepatology Research*, vol. 47, no. 12, pp. 1260–1271, 2017.

[9] Y. Okura, T. Namisaki, K. Moriya et al., "Combined treatment with dipeptidyl peptidase-4 inhibitor (sitagliptin) and angiotensin-II type 1 receptor blocker (losartan) suppresses progression in a non-diabetic rat model of steatohepatitis," *Hepatology Research*, vol. 47, no. 12, pp. 1317–1328, 2017.

[10] N. Goda, K. Suzuki, M. Naito, S. Takeoka, E. Tsuchida, Y. Ishimura et al., "Distribution of heme oxygenase isoforms in rat liver. Topographic basis for carbon monoxide-mediated microvascular relaxation," *Journal of Clinical Investigation*, vol. 101, pp. 604–612, 1998.

[11] N. G. Abraham, J. M. Junge, and G. S. Drummond, "Translational significance of heme oxygenase in obesity and metabolic syndrome," *Trends in Pharmacological Sciences*, vol. 37, no. 1, pp. 17–36, 2016.

[12] D. H. Kim, A. P. Burgess, and M. Li, "Heme oxygenase-mediated increases in adiponectin decrease fat content and inflammatory cytokines tumor necrosis factor-$\alpha$ and interleukin-6 in Zucker rats and reduce adipogenesis in human mesenchymal stem cells," *The Journal of Pharmacology and Experimental Therapeutics*, vol. 325, no. 3, pp. 833–840, 2008.

[13] A. Nicolai, M. Li, D. H. Kim et al., "Heme oxygenase-1 induction remodels adipose tissue and improves insulin sensitivity in obesity-induced diabetic rats," *Hypertension*, vol. 53, no. 3, pp. 508–515, 2009.

[14] J. Cao, S. J. Peterson, K. Sodhi et al., "Heme oxygenase gene targeting to adipocytes attenuates adiposity and vascular dysfunction in mice fed a high-fat diet," *Hypertension*, vol. 60, no. 2, pp. 467–475, 2012.

[15] N. Puri, Y. Arefiev, R. Chao et al., "Heme Oxygenase Induction Suppresses Hepatic Hepcidin and Rescues Ferroportin and Ferritin Expression in Obese Mice," *Journal of Nutrition and Metabolism*, vol. 2017, pp. 1–11, 2017.

[16] A. Kawashima, Y. Oda, A. Yachie, S. Koizumi, and I. Nakanishi, "Heme oxygenase-1 deficiency: the first autopsy case," *Human Pathology*, vol. 33, no. 1, pp. 125–130, 2002.

[17] A. Yachie, Y. Niida, T. Wada et al., "Oxidative stress causes enhanced endothelial cell injury in human heme oxygenase-1 deficiency," *The Journal of Clinical Investigation*, vol. 103, no. 1, pp. 129–135, 1999.

[18] E. Csongradi, J. M. Docarmo, J. H. Dubinion, T. Vera, and D. E. Stec, "Chronic HO-1 induction with cobalt protoporphyrin (CoPP) treatment increases oxygen consumption, activity, heat production and lowers body weight in obese melanocortin-4 receptor-deficient mice," *International Journal of Obesity*, vol. 36, no. 2, pp. 244–253, 2012.

[19] J. Li, B. Wu, D. Teng et al., "Cobalt-protoporphyrin enhances heme oxygenase 1 expression and attenuates liver ischemia/reperfusion injury by inhibiting apoptosis," *Molecular Medicine Reports*, 2018.

[20] X. Zhan, Z. Zhang, H. Huang, Y. Zhang, and Z. Zeng, "Effect of heme oxygenase-1 on the protection of ischemia reperfusion injury of bile duct in rats after liver transplantation," *Clinics and Research in Hepatology and Gastroenterology*, 2017.

[21] J. Park, H. Choi, S. Yim, and S. Lee, "Heme Oxygenase-1 Protects the Liver from Septic Injury by Modulating TLR4-Mediated Mitochondrial Quality Control in Mice," *Shock*, p. 1, 2018.

[22] J. Cao, S. P. Singh, J. A. McClung et al., "EET intervention on Wnt1, NOV, and HO-1 signaling prevents obesity-induced

cardiomyopathy in obese mice," *American Journal of Physiology-Heart and Circulatory Physiology*, vol. 313, no. 2, pp. H368–H380, 2017.

[23] P. I. Huang, Y. C. Chen, L. H. Chen, C. C. Juan, K. u. HH, S. T. Wang et al., "PGC-1alpha mediates differentiation of mesenchymal stem cells to brown adipose cells," *Journal of Atherosclerosis and Thrombosis*, vol. 18, pp. 966–980, 2011.

[24] S. P. Singh, J. Schragenheim, J. Cao, J. R. Falck, N. G. Abraham, and L. Bellner, "PGC-1 alpha regulates HO-1 expression, mitochondrial dynamics and biogenesis: Role of epoxyeicosatrienoic acid," *Prostaglandins & Other Lipid Mediators*, vol. 125, pp. 8–18, 2016.

[25] A. L. Kruger, S. J. Peterson, M. L. Schwartzman et al., "Up-regulation of heme oxygenase provides vascular protection in an animal model of diabetes through its antioxidant and antiapoptotic effects," *The Journal of Pharmacology and Experimental Therapeutics*, vol. 319, no. 3, pp. 1144–1152, 2006.

[26] S. J. Peterson, D. Husney, A. L. Kruger et al., "Long-term treatment with the apolipoprotein A1 mimetic peptide increases antioxidants and vascular repair in type I diabetic rats," *The Journal of Pharmacology and Experimental Therapeutics*, vol. 322, no. 2, pp. 514–520, 2007.

[27] C. K. Fujihara, C. R. Sena, D. M. A. C. Malheiros, A. L. Mattar, and R. Zatz, "Short-term nitric oxide inhibition induces progressive nephropathy after regression of initial renal injury," *American Journal of Physiology-Renal Physiology*, vol. 290, no. 3, pp. F632–F640, 2006.

[28] N. Kumar, L. A. Solt, Y. Wang et al., "Regulation of adipogenesis by natural and synthetic REV-ERB ligands," *Endocrinology*, vol. 151, no. 7, pp. 3015–3025, 2010.

[29] C. Martinerie, M. Garcia, T. T. H. Do et al., "NOV/CCN3: A new adipocytokine involved in obesity-associated insulin resistance," *Diabetes*, vol. 65, no. 9, pp. 2502–2515, 2016.

[30] B. L. Riser, F. Najmabadi, B. Perbal et al., "CCN3 (NOV) is a negative regulator of CCN2 (CTGF) and a novel endogenous inhibitor of the fibrotic pathway in an in vitro model of renal disease," *The American Journal of Pathology*, vol. 174, no. 5, pp. 1725–1734, 2009.

[31] G. Le Dréau, L. Kular, A. B. Nicot et al., "NOV/CCN3 upregulates CCL2 and CXCL1 expression in astrocytes through beta1 and beta5 integrins," *Glia*, vol. 58, pp. 1510–1521, 2010.

[32] W. Wu, X. Hu, X. Zhou, P. A. Klenotic, Q. Zhou, and Z. Lin, "Myeloid deficiency of CCN3 exacerbates liver injury in a mouse model of nonalcoholic fatty liver disease," *Journal of Cell Communication and Signaling*, pp. 1–11, 2017.

[33] S. P. Singh, I. Grant, A. Meissner, A. Kappas, and N. G. Abraham, "Ablation of adipose-HO-1 expression increases white fat over beige fat through inhibition of mitochondrial fusion and of PGC1$\alpha$ in female mice," *Hormone Molecular Biology and Clinical Investigation*, vol. 31, no. 1, 2017.

[34] P. Bedossa, C. Poitou, N. Veyrie et al., "Histopathological algorithm and scoring system for evaluation of liver lesions in morbidly obese patients," *Hepatology*, vol. 56, no. 5, pp. 1751–1759, 2012.

[35] M. Waldman, L. Bellner, L. Vanella et al., "Epoxyeicosatrienoic Acids Regulate Adipocyte Differentiation of Mouse 3T3 Cells, Via PGC-1alpha Activation, Which Is Required for HO-1 Expression and Increased Mitochondrial Function," *Stem Cells and Development*, vol. 25, pp. 1084–1094, 2016.

[36] N. Puri, F. Zhang, S. R. Monu et al., "Antioxidants condition pleiotropic vascular responses to exogenous H 2O2: Role of modulation of vascular TP receptors and the heme oxygenase system," *Antioxidants & Redox Signaling*, vol. 18, pp. 471–480, 2013.

[37] M. K. Sardana and A. Kappas, "Dual control mechanism for heme oxygenase: Tin(IV)-protoporphyrin potently inhibits enzyme activity while markedly increasing content of enzyme protein in liver," *Proceedings of the National Academy of Sciences of the United States of America*, vol. 84, pp. 2464–2468, 1987.

[38] P. A. Hosick and D. E. Stec, "Heme oxygenase, a novel target for the treatment of hypertension and obesity?" *American Journal of Physiology-Regulatory, Integrative and Comparative Physiology*, vol. 302, pp. R207–R214, 2012.

[39] T. N. Salley, M. Mishra, S. Tiwari, A. Jadhav, and J. F. Ndisang, "The heme oxygenase system rescues hepatic deterioration in the condition of obesity co-morbid with type-2 diabetes," *PLoS ONE*, vol. 8, no. 11, Article ID e79270, 2013.

[40] T. D. Hinds Jr., K. Sodhi, C. Meadows et al., "Increased HO-1 levels ameliorate fatty liver development through a reduction of heme and recruitment of FGF21," *Obesity*, vol. 22, no. 3, pp. 705–712, 2014.

[41] N. Radhakrishnan, S. P. Yadav, A. Sachdeva et al., "Human heme oxygenase-1 deficiency presenting with hemolysis, nephritis, and asplenia," *Journal of Pediatric Hematology/Oncology*, vol. 33, no. 1, pp. 74–78, 2011.

[42] S. Qu, B. Yuan, H. Zhang et al., "Heme Oxygenase 1 Attenuates Hypoxia-Reoxygenation Injury in Mice Liver Sinusoidal Endothelial Cells," *Transplantation*, p. 1, 2018.

[43] S. Spahis, E. Delvin, J. M. Borys, and E. Levy, "Oxidative Stress as a Critical Factor in Nonalcoholic Fatty Liver Disease Pathogenesis," *Antioxid Redox Signal*, vol. 26, pp. 519–541, 2017.

[44] K. Cusi, "Role of obesity and lipotoxicity in the development of nonalcoholic steatohepatitis: pathophysiology and clinical implications," *Gastroenterology*, vol. 142, no. 4, pp. 711.e6–725.e6, 2012.

[45] D. D. Gutterman, "Mitochondria and reactive oxygen species: an evolution in function," *Circulation Research*, vol. 97, no. 4, pp. 302–304, 2005.

[46] M. Aharoni-Simon, M. Hann-Obercyger, S. Pen, Z. Madar, and O. Tirosh, "Fatty liver is associated with impaired activity of PPAR$\gamma$-coactivator 1$\alpha$ (PGC1$\alpha$) and mitochondrial biogenesis in mice," *Laboratory Investigation*, vol. 91, no. 7, pp. 1018–1028, 2011.

[47] M. D. Hirschey, T. Shimazu, E. Goetzman et al., "SIRT3 regulates mitochondrial fatty-acid oxidation by reversible enzyme deacetylation," *Nature*, vol. 464, no. 7285, pp. 121–125, 2010.

[48] B. Spiegelman, P. Puigserver, and Z. Wu, "Regulation of adipogenesis and energy balance by PPAR$\gamma$ and PGC-1," *International Journal of Obesity*, vol. 24, no. S4, pp. S8–S10, 2000.

[49] S. Satapati, B. Kucejova, J. A. Duarte et al., "Mitochondrial metabolism mediates oxidative stress and inflammation in fatty liver," *The Journal of Clinical Investigation*, vol. 125, no. 12, pp. 4447–4462, 2015.

[50] D. Bach, D. Naon, S. Pich et al., "Expression of *Mfn2*, the Charcot-Marie-Tooth neuropathy type 2A gene, in human skeletal muscle: effects of type 2 diabetes, obesity, weight loss, and the regulatory role of tumor necrosis factor $\alpha$ and interleukin-6," *Diabetes*, vol. 54, no. 9, pp. 2685–2693, 2005.

[51] A. J. Sanyal, C. Campbell-Sargent, F. Mirshahi et al., "Nonalcoholic steatohepatitis: association of insulin resistance and mitochondrial abnormalities," *Gastroenterology*, vol. 120, no. 5, pp. 1183–1192, 2001.

# A Comprehensive Review of Portosystemic Collaterals in Cirrhosis: Historical Aspects, Anatomy, and Classifications

**Cyriac Abby Philips,[1] Ankur Arora,[2] Rajesh Shetty,[2] and Vivek Kasana[2]**

[1]*Department of Hepatology and Transplant Medicine, Institute of Liver and Biliary Sciences, D-1, Vasant Kunj, New Delhi 110070, India*
[2]*Department of Radiodiagnosis, Institute of Liver and Biliary Sciences, D-1, Vasant Kunj, New Delhi 110070, India*

Correspondence should be addressed to Cyriac Abby Philips; abbyphilips@gmail.com

Academic Editor: Pierluigi Toniutto

Portosystemic collateral formation in cirrhosis plays an important part in events that define the natural history in affected patients. A detailed understanding of collateral anatomy and hemodynamics in cirrhotics is essential to envisage diagnosis, management, and outcomes of portal hypertension. In this review, we provide detailed insights into the historical, anatomical, and hemodynamic aspects to portal hypertension and collateral pathways in cirrhosis with emphasis on the various classification systems.

## 1. Introduction

*Historical Aspects.* Portosystemic pathways form secondary to angioarchitectural changes in the liver in which the blood bypasses an occlusion or a distortion, flowing from high pressure to low pressure areas of vascular beds. Recanalization of embryonic channels and/or reversal of flow in venous systems lead to portosystemic collateral formation [1–3] In 1906, Gilbert and Villaret coined the term "Portal Hypertension" (PHT) to describe a condition characterized by increment in portal pressures, at least 5 mm of Hg above inferior vena caval (IVC) pressure, which was associated with portal circulatory structural changes and gastrointestinal bleeding [4]. The portal venous system and its pathological Roentgen anatomy were initially beautifully delineated by Doenher and colleagues in 1956 [5]. Johns and Evans in 1962 gave the first true anatomical account of natural portosystemic collaterals in a young man who had liver abscess that subsequently lead to development of portal vein (PV) thrombosis [6]. Ruzicka and Rossi demonstrated portal venous pathways using arterioportography techniques in 1969 [7]. The use of computed tomography (CT) for demonstration of caput medusae and paraumbilical collaterals was done by Stanley and colleagues in 1977. Ishikawa and coworkers demonstrated the complete abnormal portosystemic collateral pathway by CT imaging in 1979 and gave descriptions of the anatomical sites of collaterals and compared modalities of CT with that of endoscopy and barium imaging [8]. In 1981, Dokmeci and coworkers evaluated portosystemic collaterals by way of ultrasonography (USG). The standard of diagnosis for collaterals in PHT at the time was splenoportography, abdominal angiography, or percutaneous transhepatic portography which were quite invasive. The frequency of collateral detection using USG was 85% for coronary, 100% for paraumbilical, and 10% for short gastric veins (SGV). The authors concluded that real time sonography needs to be the first-choice procedure in demonstration of collateral veins and diagnosis of portal hypertension [9]. Patriquin et al. in 1987 assessed PHT using qualitative Doppler Sonography and discovered that portal collateral pathways could be easily delineated using techniques that assessed portal blood flow volume, selective flow-velocity measurements, direction, and change in abdominal anatomy. They found that there was a significant association between upper gastrointestinal bleeding and size of left gastric vein (LGV) and esophagogastroscopy was important in such patients, where sclera-therapeutic procedures could be offered [10]. Identification of portal systemic collaterals using blood-spool single photon emission CT (SPECT) was done in

1989 by Kashiwagi and coworkers. The use of direct portosystemic collateral evaluation using scintiphotosplenoportography was found to be inferior to noninvasive use of SPECT in patients of PHT in this study [11]. Computed tomography and angiography could demonstrate more variceal types than endoscopy could and CT was found to be superior to angiography even in detection of paraumbilical and retroperitoneal varices. In 1995, Cho and coworkers improved CT imaging using dynamicity and bolus contrast administration to delineate collateral pathways much better. This modality showed presence of esophageal, paraumbilical, abdominal wall, perisplenic, retrogastric, paraesophageal, omental, retroperitoneal-paravertebral, and mesenteric varices exquisitely and also presence of splenorenal and gastrorenal shunts [12]. In the current review, we provide detailed descriptions on anatomy, classifications, and imaging of portosystemic collaterals in cirrhosis.

## 2. Portosystemic Collaterals in Cirrhosis

*2.1. Esophageal Varices.* The venous blood from the esophagus drains into the submucosal plexus which in turn drains into the periesophageal venous plexus. From this second plexus, esophageal veins arise in a segmental manner, following the arterial supply. Ultimately the dense submucosal plexus drains into the superior vena cava (SVC) [13]. With regard to esophageal variceal anatomy, 4 distinct zones of venous drainage have been defined around gastroesophageal region: the gastric zone, containing the longitudinal venous distribution; the palisade zone with parallel vessels arranged in groups that lie within the lamina propria; the perforating zone with "treble clef" shaped vasculature which drains blood into the extrinsic veins; and the truncal zone which contains 4 to 5 deep descending veins. This distribution is mainly seen within the esophageal mucosa and the bidirectional venous flow at the palisade zone produces a high resistance water shed area between portal and systemic circulation leading to high accommodation of blood volume in the presence of PHT leading to variceal development [14–16]. Esophageal varices are dilated veins located within lower esophageal wall in contrast to paraesophageal varices that are located outside the wall. The former is usually supplied by the anterior branch of LGV (which dilates >7 mm in diameter in presence of PHT with retrograde flow within) whereas posterior branch takes part in formation of the paraesophageal collateral system. Esophageal varices usually drain into the left subclavian vein and/or brachiocephalic vein, while paraoesophageal varices commonly drain into the azygos or hemiazygos system (Figures 1(a) and 1(b)). Sometimes, only paraesophageal collaterals form without formation of esophageal varices. Portosystemic pathways are normally present embryonic channels that open up in presence of PHT [13]. The common and uncommon portosystemic pathways in cirrhosis and portal hypertension are shown in Table 1 [17–19]. In odd cases, tracheal and bronchial varices also form through efferents of esophageal varices that drain into the bronchial and pulmonary veins connected through bronchial plexus venous system [20].

*2.2. Gastric Varices.* Gastric varices (GV) are defined according to their location and also to their relationship with the esophageal varices. Gastric varices at the hepatofugal collateral pathways can drain into the systemic circulation through two types of collateral systems: the gastrophrenic system or the gastroesophageal system (which eventually drains into the azygous vein). Apart from this, gastric variceal formation in a hepatopetal collateral circulation pathway can develop in case of isolated splenic vein (SV) occlusion. The most commonly used classification is the Sarin classification which does not account for the underlying vascular anatomy. However, the Japanese Society for Portal Hypertension classified GV into cardiac, fundal, or cardiofundal varices which is more refined from an anatomical point of view. In this system, Type 1 gastric (fundal) varices have a single feeding channel that arise from the SV and drain into the left renal vein (LRV) through the gastric cardia and/or fundus and Type 2 gastric varices follow a similar course to the LRV with multiple feeding tributaries [21–24]. In Sarin classification, Type 1 GOV (Figure 1(c)) drains through esophageal and paraesophageal varices, IGV1 (Figure 1(d)) through left inferior phrenic vein, and GOV 2 through both esophageal and inferior phrenic veins. In sinistral (left sided) PHT, in the hepatopetal collateral circulation, drainage is through gastric veins (IGV2). Gastric varices can also drain into azygous vein through the ascending lumbar vein and vertebral plexus of veins. In IGV, the efferent is mainly through the gastric or splenorenal shunt and inferior phrenic vein to the IVC. Gastric varices can also drain from SV to LRV through gonadal vein. Most common drainage routes of IGVs are gastrorenal shunt (GRS; hypertrophied inferior phrenic vein connected to the left renal vein and draining point of left adrenal vein 85%), followed by gastrophrenic shunts (GPS) in 10% and lastly, gastropericardiac shunt in 5%. Another common pathway is the gastrocaval shunt (GCS), where drainage of GV occurs through inferior phrenic or pericardiophrenic vein (which can also drain into the brachiocephalic vein) into the IVC [25–28].

Collateral pathways associated with gastric varices can also be simply divided into those associated with gastroesophageal system or gastrophrenic system. In the former, varices develop between the LGV and azygous system in PHT and in the latter, gastric veins in and around posterosuperior part of gastric wall anastomose with left inferior phrenic vein at the region of gastrophrenic ligament, near the bare area of stomach [29]. In majority of cases (85%) the gastric varices are connected to the SVC through the esophageal varices. Apart from these, the left inferior phrenic vein can also drain into the subcostal, intercostals, right inferior phrenic vein, adrenal vein, or azygous vein thereby providing drainage through these routes also. Isolated gastric varices form due to large portosystemic venous shunts due to anastomoses between gastric vein and left inferior phrenic vein in the presence of PHT [21, 30–33].

## 3. Spontaneous Portosystemic Shunts

Spontaneous portosystemic shunts (SPSS, Figures 2(a)–2(c)) develop between the portal and systemic venous circulation and grow in relevance to enable large amounts of flow within

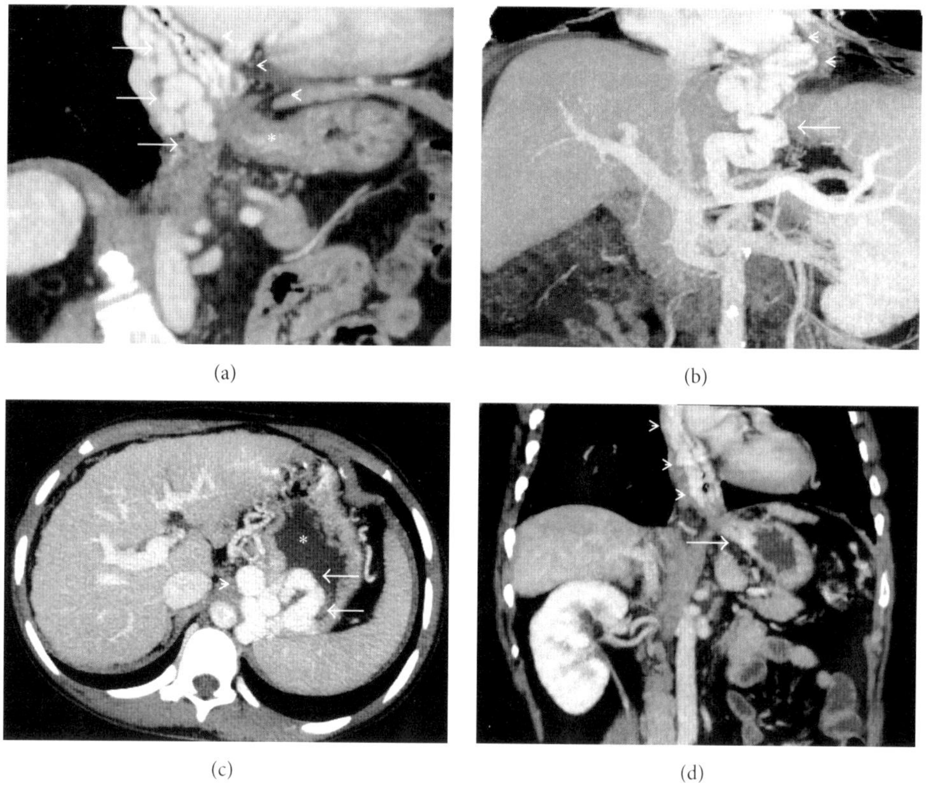

FIGURE 1: (a) Coronal-oblique MIP image demonstrating multiple collaterals in the esophagus (arrowheads) as well as paraesophageal region (arrow). Asterisk denotes the gastroesophageal junction; (b) coronal-oblique maximum-intensity-projection (MIP) CECT image showing a dilated left gastric vein (arrow) which is serving as an afferent for multiple paraesophageal collaterals (arrowheads); (c) axial MIP image showing multiple gastric fundal collaterals (arrows) being drained by a tortuous gastrorenal shunt (arrowheads) into the left renal vein (not shown). Asterisk denotes the gastric lumen. This corresponds to IGV-1 in Sarin classification of gastric varices; (d) coronal MIP image showing multiple esophageal collaterals (arrowheads) continuing along the cardia to form collaterals in the lesser curvature of stomach. This corresponds to GOV-1 in Sarin classification of gastric varices.

them. This flow stabilizes and increases when either the portal or systemic venous circulations develop high pressure or is obstructed or both occur. Spontaneous shunts develop in an attempt to reduce high pressures or bypass an obstruction.

Spontaneous portosystemic shunts can be divided into left and right (or central) sided shunts. Left sided shunts are described based on their location (left of midline or left of the confluence of splenic and mesenteric vein). These shunts have hemodynamic involvement directly or indirectly with the SV or its branches, namely, the LGV, SGV, or PGVs. Left sided SPSS include the GRS occurring in 80 to 85% of patients in gastric varices, GCS, the least frequent type of left sided PSS, but associated with gastric varices and SRS which is not uncommon in cirrhosis patients and has no association with gastric varices. Gastrorenal shunts occur in 10% of patients with PHT. The communication is between GV and LRV, but in reality, it is a small part of the larger PSS communication that involves the SV along with LRV and GV. Hence, hemodynamically, this is a SRS. This whole complex is termed the gastric variceal system. Hence, the part of this complex, which encompasses the GRS, should be ideally called the splenogastrorenal shunt.

Splenorenal shunt is not in true terms a hemodynamically described shunt. This shunt is more likely a morphologic or anatomical shunt and is not associated with gastric varices. It is tortuous, meandering direct communication between SV and the LRV without involvement of the gastrointestinal tract and is a vascular channel without variceal formation and without spontaneous bleeding risk.

## 4. Descriptive Classifications of Gastric Variceal System and Gastric Varices and Importance of Portosystemic Shunts

The gastric variceal system includes GRS and central part of GV with or without the afferent portal venous feeding collaterals. It is important to keep in mind that GRS is hemodynamically a part of a larger complex that is SRS and that morphologically the SRS is not associated with GV (absence of shunt extension into the gastric wall). It is also important to note that gastric varices may have a direct component that is part of the SRS but does not contribute to gastric varices formation, but, in reality, bypassing the stomach wall.

Table 1: Common portosystemic collaterals [17–19].

| Collaterals | Afferent | Efferent |
|---|---|---|
| | *Common pathways* | |
| Esophageal varices | Left gastric vein | Azygos-hemiazygos veins |
| Gastric varices | Anterior branch of the left gastric vein (gastroesophageal varices Type 1)<br>Short gastric and posterior gastric veins (gastroesophageal varices Type 2) | Esophageal or paraesophageal veins |
| Paraumbilical vein | Left portal vein | Anterior abdominal wall veins and iliofemoral veins |
| Perisplenic, splenoiliac | Splenic vein | Iliac vein |
| Internal-external mammary | Branches of portal veins, posterior or short gastric veins | Superior epigastric, inferior epigastric veins, and superficial veins of the thorax |
| Internal hemorrhoids | Inferior mesenteric vein | Iliac vein |
| Rectal varices | Superior rectal veins | Middle and inferior rectal veins, tributaries of internal iliac and pudendal veins |
| Gastrorenal shunt | Gastric varices or posterior or short gastric veins | Left renal vein |
| Splenorenal shunt | Splenic vein | Left renal vein |
| Pericholecystic varices | Cystic vein or a branch of the right portal vein | Hepatic vein, intrahepatic portal vein, or anterior abdominal wall collaterals |
| Mesenteric collaterals | Superior mesenteric vein and inferior mesenteric vein | Inferior vena cava through the retroperitoneal or pelvic veins (veins of Retzius) |
| Retroperitoneal collaterals | Colic or mesenteric branches (veins of Retzius) | Retrogastric varices or inferior phrenic veins to left renal vein or directly into the inferior vena cava |
| Omental varices | Superior or inferior mesenteric veins | Retroperitoneal or pelvic veins or gastroesophageal veins |
| | *Uncommon pathways* | |
| Tracheal and bronchial varices | Tracheobronchial plexus of veins | Pulmonary veins<br>Bronchial veins<br>Esophageal/paraesophageal varices |
| Aberrant left gastric collateral | Left portal vein | Hepatogastric ligament |
| Colonic varices | Ileocolic, right, middle colic, or sigmoid colic vein | Right gonadal vein, right renal vein, and systemic lumbar veins |
| Jejunal or ileal varices | Jejunal and ileal veins | Abdominal wall veins or the veins of Retzius |
| Duodenal varices | Superior and inferior pancreaticoduodenal veins, cystic branches of the superior mesenteric veins, gastroduodenal vein, and pyloric vein | Veins of Retzius into the inferior vena cava |
| Pancreatic varices | Ventral and dorsal pancreatic veins, pancreaticoduodenal veins | Inferior vena cava |
| Uterovaginal varices | Superior hemorrhoidal plexus | Uterine and hypogastric veins to inferior vena cava |
| Vesical varices | Mesenteric veins (commonly root of mesentery) | Internal and external iliac veins |
| Bare area of the liver | Portal venous branches | Inferior phrenic and right internal thoracic vein |
| Vertebral collaterals | Innominate, vertebral, intercostal, lumbar, and sacral veins | Azygos and internal mammary pathways |
| Lateral thoracic | Lateral thoracic, thoracoepigastric, superficial circumflex, long saphenous, and femoral veins | Inferior vena cava |
| Sub-hepatic-porto-iliac | Main portal vein | Iliac veins |
| Gastrocaval shunt | Gastric varices or posterior gastric vein | Left inferior phrenic and pericardiophrenic vein to inferior vena cava |
| Transsplenic shunt | Splenic veins | Intercostal veins |
| Transhepatic shunt | Intrahepatic branches of the portal vein | Inferior vena cava, coronary vein, vertebral plexus, and hemiazygos vein |

Table 1: Continued.

| Collaterals | Afferent | Efferent |
|---|---|---|
| Right infradiaphragmatic shunt/apex type shunt | Peripheral branch of left portal vein | Internal thoracic vein and intercostal vein |
| Left infradiaphragmatic shunt/left triangular ligament shunt | Peripheral portal branch of the left lateral segment of liver | Intercostal vein or left pericardiophrenic vein to left inferior phrenic vein to inferior vena cava or left triangular ligament to inferior vena cava |
| Indirect gastrocaval shunt | Gastric varices or posterior or short gastric veins | Inferior phrenic vein |
| Mesentericorenal shunt | Mesenteric veins | Capsular renal veins or left renal vein |
| Mesenteric-gonadal shunt | Mesenteric veins | Right gonadal vein |
| Splenocaval/phrenic/azygos shunt | Splenic vein or perisplenic collaterals | Hypogastric vein into inferior vena cava |

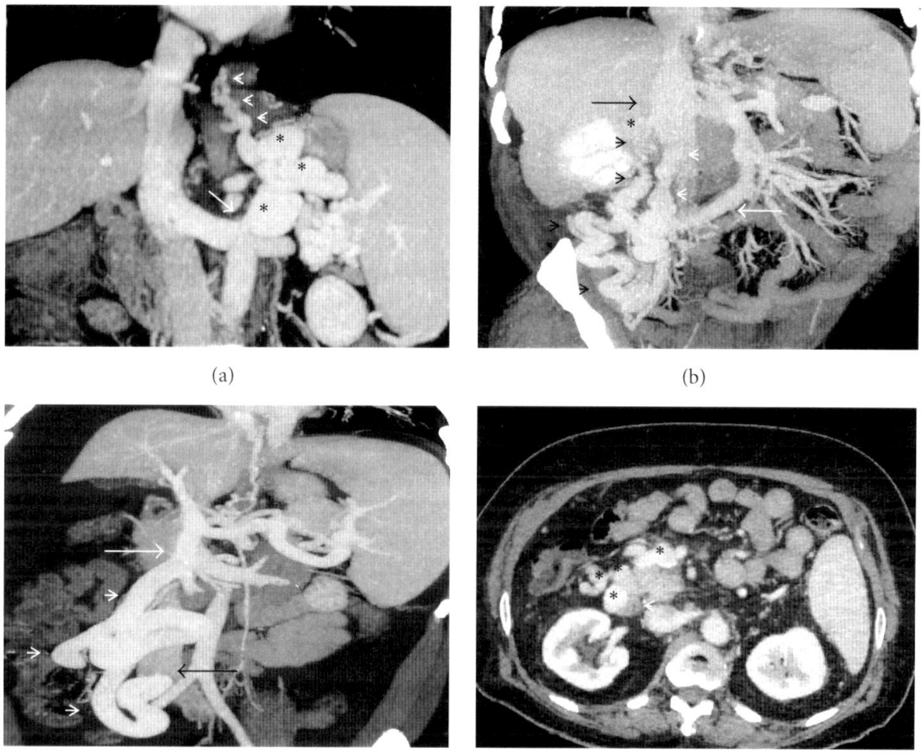

(a) (b) (c) (d)

Figure 2: (a) Coronal-oblique MIP image showing a tortuous gastro-lieno-renal shunt (asterisks) draining multiple gastroesophageal collaterals (arrowheads) into the superior aspect of the left renal vein (arrow); (b) coronal MIP image demonstrating a mesentericorenal and a mesentericocaval shunt in the same patient (black and white arrowheads, resp.). Asterisk: right renal vein, black arrow: IVC, and white arrow: superior mesenteric vein (double portosystemic shunts); (c) coronal-oblique MIP image demonstrating a dilated and tortuous mesentericocaval shunt (arrowheads) communicating between the superior mesenteric vein (white arrow) and the inferior vena cava (black arrow); (d) axial CECT image showing multiple duodenal and paraduodenal collaterals (asterisks). Arrowhead denotes the duodenum.

The GV have an afferent limb (portal inflow), central part, and efferent limb (systemic venous outflow) portions. The portal inflow or afferent feeders supply GV. These feeders do not directly communicate with true GV (intragastric, submucosal) but do so with GVs outside the gastric wall and form the extragastric or false GVs (Figure 3).

The feeders include LGV (or coronary vein), PGV, and SGVs. The PGV, which is usually single, can have a duplication and early bifurcation leading to multiple feeder profile, making it difficult to identify a laterally lying PGV from a medially lying SGV that could be acting as an afferent and is an important technical implication in interventional treatment.

Left gastric vein is the right sided component of SPSS because it comes off from the PV near the midline. Posterior and SGVs are also left sided parts of the portosystemic system. The SGVs traverse forward medially towards the GVs from the splenic hilum and enter the varix at a level higher,

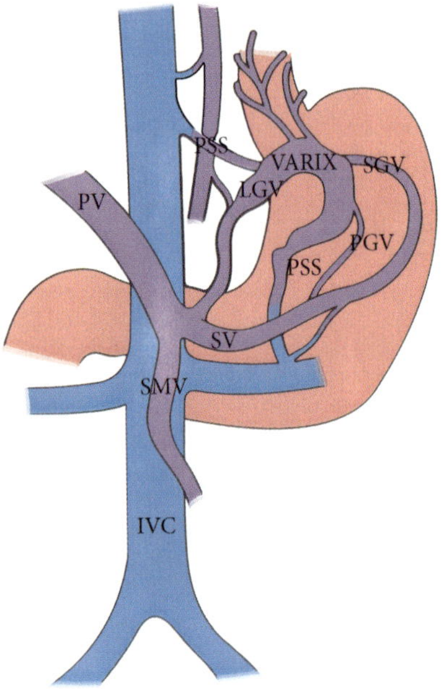


Figure 3: The basic portosystemic venous anatomy of gastric varices. PV: portal vein, SV: splenic vein, SMV: superior mesenteric vein, IVC: inferior vena cava, PSS: portosystemic shunt, SGV: short gastric vein, LGV: left gastric vein, and PGV: posterior gastric vein. Modified from [34].

anterior or ventral, than the PGVs. The dominance of portal inflow feeders is important. In some, the dominant feeder is the LGV, but PGV or SGVs can also act dominant. If the gastric variceal system is very complex, then all three feeders become equally dominant. The only condition in which the SGVs become the only dominant feeder is in presence of SV or PV thrombosis. If SGVs become the dominant feeder in portal hypertensive gastric variceal complex formation, the gastric varices extend over fundus, cardia, and also body, antrum, and gastric outlets. The central part of the gastric variceal system consists of true submucosal intragastric and false extragastric varices. Sometimes these also communicate with each other through a singular perforator vein. Gastric varices are also seen between prominent folds in the stomach, but they can also be confused with prominent gastric rugal folds or self-thrombosed GVs. Regarding extragastric varices that do not have an intragastric submucosal component, the afferent feeders usually drain into these and perforators commence from them to penetrate the gastric wall to form true GVs. The efferent or outflow system of GVs may be simple (only GRS) but can also be very complex, involving the inferior phrenic or pericardiophrenic veins. To understand the outflow system, it is important to understand the GRS and the pericardiophrenic collateral pathways. The GRS commences from false gastric (extragastric) varices and starts as small convolutions intraperitoneally in the lesser sac. It travels caudally and posteriorly and becomes retroperitoneal as the flow increases and it grows in size. This initial convoluted portion is termed the intraperitoneal transition zone. In the retroperitoneal region, the shunt becomes less convoluted and reaches the left adrenal vein (area of common stump). The entrance of the retroperitoneal portion of the shunt with the left adrenal vein occurs at different angles. The commonest angular relation of the shunt with the stump is between 10 and 12 o' clock positions. Less commonly, the angle between the shunt and the stump occurs at 12 and 1 o' clock positions. In rare situations, the retroperitoneal portion of the shunt joins the left gonadal vein instead of the left adrenal vein. More in rarity is the duplication of the GRS in which the LRV supply the shunt, forming anterior and posterior GRS. The phrenic vein or inferior phrenic vein has two parts, the infradiaphragmatic horizontal position and the vertical part (composed of ascending and descending regions). It is the descending part that forms a component of GRS by anastomosing with the left adrenal or left gonadal vein. The phrenic venous system can become complex in the presence of duplication, ecstatic trunk, or multiple isolated veins which then form a complicated system of collaterals. The pericardial vein traverses the left heart border and after travelling along the left hemidiaphragm, it anastomoses with the transverse part of inferior phrenic vein. The pericardial vein and the inferior phrenic vein are collectively called the pericardiophrenic vein [21, 36, 37].

## 5. Hemodynamic Classification of Gastric Variceal Systems

The new classification systems for GVs are descriptive for hemodynamics (based on efferent inflow or afferent outflow) of variceal system rather than just their location. These include the Saad-Caldwell Classification for gastric varices (inflow and outflow) and the Saad Classification for gastroduodenal and mesenteric variceal systems (dealt with later on, under ectopic varices). Also important are the Kiyosue Efferent Classification System, Hirota-BORV Classification, Fukuda-Hirota Classification, and the Matsumoto Hemodynamic Classification Systems.

### *5.1. Classifications Based on Draining Venous Anatomy (Efferent Outflow)*

(I) *The Kiyosue classification of gastric variceal system* (Figure 4(a)) is a simple way based on hemodynamic classification. In this classification, they are divided into 4 types. In Type A, the varices are in continuation with a single draining shunt (most commonly a GRS shunt or, seldom, GCS) draining through hypertrophied inferior phrenic vein into IVC directly. In Type B, the GVs are contiguous commonly with a GRS and one or multiple collateral veins. This drains through a plexus of vessels back into the right atrium or IVC but there is no distinguished shunt formation. The draining veins can include pericardiophrenic, intercostal, perivertebral, ascending lumbar, and, rarely, azygous veins. Type B is further divided into three types: B1, small collateral veins; B2, medium sized collateral veins; and B3, large collateral veins with high flow but without shunt. Type C varices are contiguous with both GRS and GCS and this is also subdivided into C1, representing small sized second shunt that cannot be

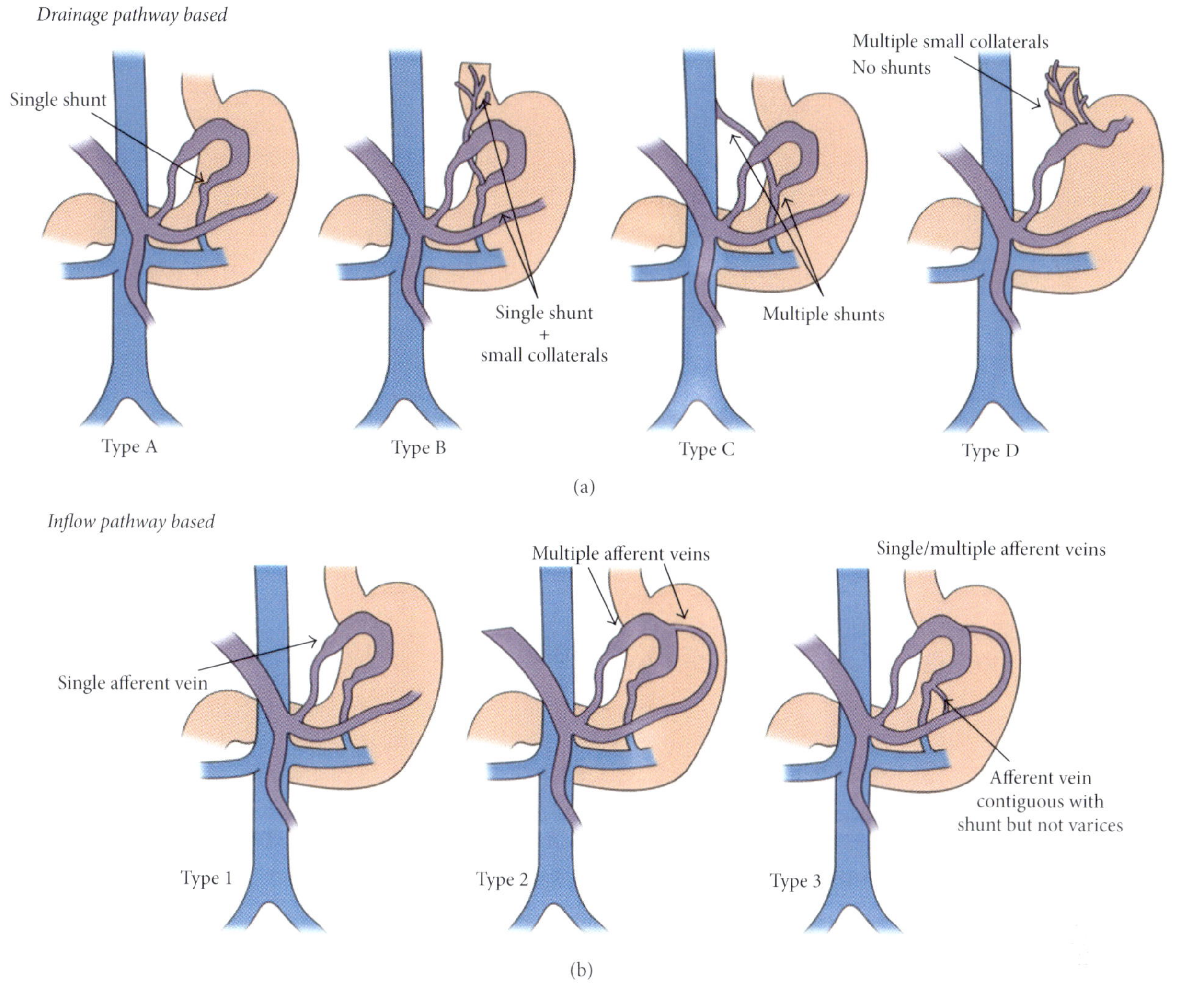


FIGURE 4: The Kiyosue classification of gastric varices. (a) Classification based on drainage pathway. Type A consists of a portosystemic shunt as the only drainage; Type B portosystemic shunts along with additional small portosystemic collaterals; in Type C, there is presence of multiple large portosystemic shunts; and Type D consists of multiple small portosystemic collaterals as the drainage pathways without proper shunt formation. (b) Classification based on the inflow pathway: Type 1 consists of single afferent vein for the varices; Type 2 has multiple afferent vessels contributing to the variceal formation; Type 3 is similar to Type 2 but with additional small collateral/shunts directly communicating with outflow tract. Modified and redrawn from [17].

catheterized, and C2, large sized second shunt which is large enough to be catheterized. Finally in Type D, a shunt is not present and the varices drain through small collaterals and do not drain directly into IVC or renal vein.

(II) In the original *Saad Classification* the characterization of collaterals and shunts is similar to that in Kiyosue, except for subclassification in Type D, as Types D1 and D2. In Type D1 of Saad modification, the predominance of systemic vein drainage is not obvious and any vein, out of inferior phrenic, hemiazygos tributaries, and intercostals veins or adrenal veins, can become predominant. In Type D2, the morphology is similar to D1, but predominant systemic venous draining vein is usually 4.3 mm in diameter through unconventional systemic veins.

(III) *The Hirota Classification* follows similar descriptions as the Kiyosue classification (for efferent pathway), except for Hirota-BORV Type V in which a gastrorenal shunt is too large for balloon occlusion procedures (no catheter size available) and maybe a cause of technical failure during BRTO treatment. For such shunts, Balloon Antegrade Transvenous Occlusion has been proposed.

*5.2. Classifications Based on Portal Afferent Inflow*

(I) Based on portal venous *afferent inflow* (Figure 4(b)), *according to Kiyosue*, gastric varices are classified into three types, with regard to pattern of afferent veins. In Type 1, the varices are supplied by a single afferent gastric vein, which is the commonest and easiest type to treat. In Type 2, multiple afferent gastric veins supply the varices and in Type 3, single or multiple gastric veins supply the varices in presence of other gastric veins that are directly in continuation with a shunt, which do not significantly contribute to variceal formation. In Type 1, the afferent is most commonly the LGV or PGV. In Type 2, it is both LGV and PGV and in Type 3, a separate afferent vein drains directly into a shunt that does not communicate with the GVs [38, 39]. Clinical implications of Types 1 to 3 GVs with regard to venous inflow are that, because of simplicity of anatomy in Type 1, during occlusion procedures of collateral pathways, the administered sclerosant refluxes into the gastric variceal complex and stays there because of high pressure from the portal system allowing for minimal reflux into afferent vein and better chances at complete occlusion. In Type 2, since two pathways act simultaneously, one of the low pressure efferent veins functions as a draining vein once outflow is obstructed with sclerosant, resulting in efflux of material into portal circulation. In Type 3, since the separate vein does not supply the GVs, during occlusion procedures, the sclerosant can reflux into the portal circulation rather than the gastric variceal complex. Hence, separate embolization of this noncommunicating shunt will be required for complete variceal occlusion [40–45].

(II) *The Saad-Caldwell Classification* (Table 2) can be used uniformly in all splanchnic varices (i.e., gastric duodenal and mesenteric). It is mainly applicable in the management of duodenal and mesenteric varices. Saad modified the gastroesophageal varices system proposed by Al-Osaimi and Caldwell which was a revamped version of Sarin classification of gastric varices, to include management modality. In Saad Type 1, the dominant portal venous feeder is the left gastric vein, commencing from either the main PV, splenoportal junction, or the distal SV. This can be associated with presence (Type 1b) or absence (Type 1a) of gastrorenal shunt. In Type 2, the dominant portal venous feeder is the PGVs or SGVs. In Saad Type 3 all feeders that are involved have dominance that is variable. Type 4 Saad gastric varices are more similar to Type 3 but occur in the presence of SV thrombosis [46, 47].

### 5.3. *Other Hemodynamics Based Classifications of Gastric Variceal Systems*

(I) *Hirota* and coworkers classified GVs based on balloon retrograde transvenography (BRTO). They classified the degree of progression of gastric varices and collateral veins into five grades: Grade 1: gastric varices well opacified without any collateral vein evidence; Grade 2: contrast opacification in gastric varices for ≥3 minutes, in the presence of small and few collateral veins; Grade 3: contrast opacification of gastric varices partial and disappeared within 3 minutes with medium to large collateral veins which were few in number; Grade 4: noncontrast opacification of gastric varices and presence of many large collaterals; and Grade 5: in which shunt could not be occluded because of very large size of shunt and rapid blood flow [48].

Table 2: The Saad-Caldwell Classification of gastroesophageal varices.

| | | |
|---|---|---|
| Type 1 | Isolated cardiogastric varices without fundic varices<br>Type 1b – GRS +<br>Type 1a – GRS – | Correlate with endoscopic Sarin classification: gastroesophageal varices Type 1 (GOV1) |
| Type 2 | Isolated fundal gastric varices without cardiac extension<br>Type 2b – GRS+<br>Type 2a – GRS – | Correlated endoscopic Sarin classification: isolated gastric varices Type 1 (IGV 1) |
| Type 3 | High association with esophageal varices<br>3b – GRS +<br>3a – GRS – | Correlate with endoscopic Sarin classification: gastroesophageal varices Type 2 (GOV 2)<br>Usually complex and large variceal systems |
| Type 4 | Like Type 2 or Type 3 (more likely to be similar to Type 3) | Presence of splenic and/or portal venous thrombosis |

(II) *The Fukuda Classification System* of gastric varices is different from the Hirota Classification [49] because it is based on hemodynamic features involving the superior mesenteric and celiac angiography findings. In this classification, Type 1 refers to LGV dominant gastric variceal complex and Type 2 refers to the separation between the esophageal varices (LGV dominant) and the GVs (PGV/SGV dominant). In Type 4, there is right sided dominance of gastric variceal system and Type 3 is a very complex system consisting of both right and left sided feeding vessels.

(III) *Matsumoto* et al. described a *classification system* for gastric varices for predicting the aggravation of esophageal varices after BRTO procedure [50]. This is based on left gastric angiography. The classification includes Type 1 which has portosystemic flow in the gastrorenal shunt and Type 2 which has no portosystemic flow in the gastrorenal shunt. In both, subtypes have been described, in which Subtype A has hepatopetal flow and Subtype B has hepatofugal flow in the LGV. Aggravation of grade of esophageal varices occurred after BRTO in Type 1b varices, which had portosystemic flow in the GRS (the occlusion of shunt causes back flow and worsening of variceal grade).

Gastric varices can also be differentiated as *primary* (naturally developed) and *secondary* (developing after endotherapy for esophageal varices, seen in 9%) [51].

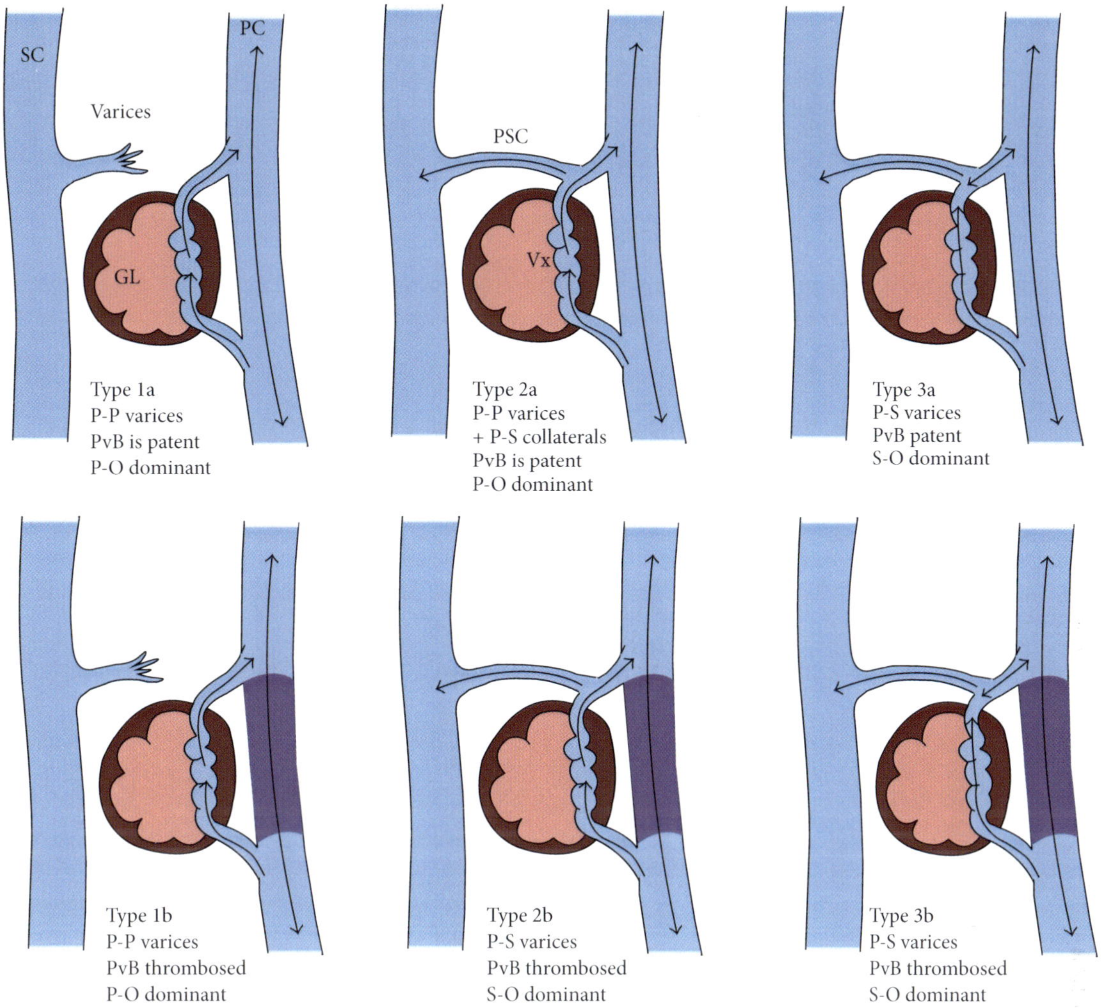


FIGURE 5: Classification of ectopic varices. SC: systemic circulation; PC: portal circulation; P-P: portoportal collaterals, P-S: portosystemic collaterals; PvB: portal venous branch; P-O: portal outflow; S-O: systemic outflow. Modified and redrawn from [35].

## 6. Ectopic Varices

These are dilated splanchnic or mesoportal varicosities and/ or portosystemic collaterals that are present along the gastrointestinal tract outside of the common variceal sites. These can be broadly divided into Type a (nonocclusive or oncotic) and Type b (occlusive) subdivided into Type 1 (purely portoportal collaterals), Type 2 (predominantly portoportal collaterals with some portosystemic branches), and Type 3 (predominantly portosystemic collaterals with some portoportal branches) as per Saad-Caldwell Classification (Figure 5). The portal venous branch can be any vein (location or size) in the portal circulation which includes mesenteric vein and tributaries and PV tributaries as well as the main portal and splenic veins. The importance of this classification lies mainly from therapy point of view. For example, balloon-occluded retrograde transvenous obliteration (BRTO) of Type 1 varices is not feasible because, by definition, BRTO is through the portosystemic collaterals from the systemic venous side and in Type 1, there are no portosystemic collaterals. Hence, obliteration from the portal venous side (BATO: balloon-occluded antegrade transvenous obliteration) is more feasible in this scenario.

## 7. Duodenal Varices (Figure 2(d))

The first 2.5 cm (duodenal bulb) is drained by the prepyloric vein which drains into the PV and the rest of duodenum is drained by the superior pancreaticoduodenal veins that drain into the PV and the inferior pancreaticoduodenal veins that drain into the SMV (which is present to the right of superior mesenteric artery in front of third part of duodenum). The pancreaticoduodenal veins are four small veins that also drain the head of pancreas and adjacent second and third parts of the duodenum, forming a venous arcade (anterior and posterior) between the superior and inferior veins. It is the posterior superior pancreaticoduodenal vein that drains into the PV and the anterior superior pancreaticoduodenal and posterior inferior pancreaticoduodenal veins that drain into superior mesenteric vein. Duodenal varices (DV) were first reported in 1931 by Alberti. Duodenal variceal bleeding represents only 1/3rd of all ectopic variceal bleeding sources, even though in some studies, the prevalence of paraduodenal varices by angiography demonstration was as high as 40% [52]. Duodenal varices make up 1 to 3% of all varices in patients of PHT. These varices are smaller in diameter and shorter in length and found in deeper locations or over paraduodenal areas and enter through the perforators in the submucosal region. Duodenal varices can occur on the serosal surface as well as in the muscular layer, but bleeding manifestation is evident only when they expand onto the submucosal surface. In a study by Amin and coworkers, the commonest site of DV was found to be at the duodenal bulb [53]. There have been studies on association of DVs with GEVs and it has been shown in two different studies that DV were more commonly associated with intrahepatic as well as extrahepatic PHT [54]. Further studies on this association were confirmed in a study by Stephan and colleagues wherein they found that 40% of patients had an extrahepatic source of PHT [55]. Unlike colonic and jejunal varices, DVs have never been associated with previous surgical adhesions and it has also been shown to be associated with postsclerotherapy for esophageal varices.

Duodenal varices are portoportal or portosystemic retroperitoneal collaterals or a combination of both (see classification of ectopic varices below). The afferent (portal venous feeders) includes inferior and superior pancreaticoduodenal veins, cystic branches of superior mesenteric veins, pyloric vein, and gastroduodenal vein. The efferent or systemic drainage channels include gonadal vein (mostly the right) and capsular renal veins that ultimately drain into the inferior vena cava. The left gonadal vein, when involved, produces ectopic duodenal varices at third and fourth parts of the duodenum and is very rare. Rarely, direct drainage into inferior vena cava is also seen as is efferent drainage through paravertebral or innominate retroperitoneal veins. The pathways associated with DV differ in cirrhosis and in patients with extrahepatic portal hypertension. In cirrhosis, the efferents are formed in descending or transverse parts of duodenum, flowing hepatofugal through retroperitoneal veins of Retzius (small shunts), finally into the IVC and also through subcostal and ascending lumbar vein into vertebral-lumbar azygous system and ultimately draining into the SVC. In patients with extrahepatic portal hypertension (commonest cause of duodenal varices), the efferents are formed mostly in first 2.5 cm of the duodenum (bulb region) with a blood flow that is hepatopetal through portoportal collaterals into liver. These portoportal collaterals form from venous plexus around common bile duct or tributaries of PV that are patent above obstructed portion of the portal venous system. Next most common site of duodenal varices is the second part of duodenum and rarely in third and fourth parts [53, 55].

## 8. Varices of Jejunum and Ileum (Figure 6(a))

The jejunal and ileal veins eventually drain into the SMV which drains into the IVC through the pelvic or retroperitoneal veins. There are many veins on the dorsal wall of the abdomen, called veins of Retzius that form anastomosis between the IVC and the SMV/IMV. This anastomosis can occur normally in the absence of PHT. The veins of Retzius group gives rise to various portosystemic pathways, such as mesenteric-caval, mesenteric-iliac, mesenteric-gonadal, or mesenteric-renal. Out of these, the commonest is an ileocolic vein draining into IVC or the right renal vein by way of the right gonadal vein, the mesenteric-gonadal pathway. Jejunoileal varices develop mainly at sites of prior surgeries or adhesions after surgery, mostly between the jejunum and the abdominal wall. The afferents of jejunoileal varices are mainly the tributaries of the superior mesenteric vein and the efferents are veins of the abdominal wall and also through the veins of Retzius [56–58].

## 9. Varices of the Colon (Figure 6(b))

The venous supply of colon mirrors arterial supply. The ileocolic, right (draining ascending colon), and middle colic veins (draining transverse colon) are tributaries of the SMV and the superior and inferior left colic veins are tributaries of inferior mesenteric vein. The IMV drains into the SV and the SMV joins the SV to form the PV. The cecum is drained by the anterior and posterior cecal veins which arise from the ileocolic veins which are tributaries of the SMV. Colonic ectopic varices are normally seen in the cecal and rectosigmoid regions, found in a segmental distribution. The afferents to colonic varices include ileocolic vein, right colic and middle colic vein, and sigmoid colic vein while the efferents include right gonadal vein, right renal vein, and systemic lumbar veins that drain into the veins of Retzius and veins of the ascending colon that drain through renal capsular vein into IVC [59–61].

## 10. Varices of Rectum and Anal Canal (Figure 6(c))

The pectinate line (or dentate or mucocutaneous line) is an important landmark in defining certain anatomic points in the rectum and anal canal anatomy. It is present at the inferior most level of anal columns and defines the junction of superior part of anal canal and the inferior part of anal canal, both of which have different embryonic origins. The vascular supply to rectum and anal canal is defined by making pectinate line a landmark. The superior rectal vein divides into two branches, which enter the lateral wall of rectum, about 10 cm above the dentate line. The middle and inferior rectal veins drain into the caval system. The rectal veins form two plexuses, one lying in the submucosa (intrinsic) and the other lying outside the muscular wall of the bowel below the level of the peritoneal reflection (extrinsic). Above the pectinate line, the intrinsic rectal plexus drains into the superior rectal vein and below the pectinate line it drains into the inferior rectal veins. The intrinsic rectal venous plexus consists of two groups of veins draining in opposite direction. The inferior group passes down to form the inferior rectal veins, dilation of which leads to formation of external hemorrhoids. The vessels of the superior group in the anal columns dilate to form internal hemorrhoids and those in the rectum form rectal varices. Rectal varices (RV) were first reported in 1954. Rectal

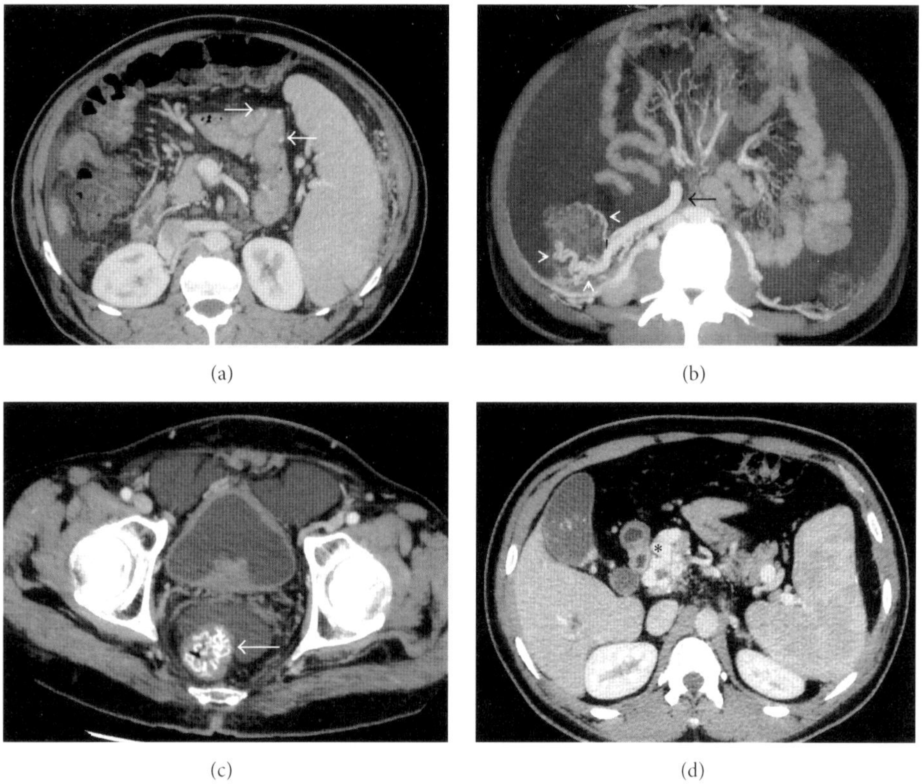

FIGURE 6: (a) Axial MIP image demonstrating multiple jejunal collaterals (arrows); (b) axial-oblique MIP CECT image showing multiple pericolonic collaterals (arrowheads) arising from the superior mesenteric vein (arrow); (c) axial MIP CECT image showing multiple rectal collaterals (arrow); (d) axial CECT image showing multiple paracholedochal collaterals (asterisks) encircling the common bile duct (arrow) in a patient with EHPVO.

varices are dilated submucosal portosystemic collaterals that extend from midrectum to the anorectal junction and are considered distinct from internal hemorrhoids (submucosal arteriovenous communications of the anorectal vascular plexus). Four distinct zones of mucosal circulation similar to those seen in esophagus occur in the rectum also: an inflow area analogous to the gastric zone, the downflow area analogous to the palisade zone, outflow area in the rectum which is analogous to the perforating zone, and the outflow area in anal canal which is analogous to the truncal zone of esophageal varices. The submucosal portosystemic communications of rectal varices have hepatofugal inflow. The flow to the intrinsic rectal venous plexus occurs through the wall of rectum by branches of superior rectal vein, a tributary of inferior mesenteric vein.

From both the plexuses, the portal hemorrhoidal blood drains into systemic circulation through two portosystemic shunts (rectogenital and interrectal). The rectogenital communication connects the rectal venous plexus with vesicoprostatic or vaginal venous plexus. Theinterrectal communications occur between the three rectal veins. Hemorrhoids occur independent of rectal varices. In a large series of cirrhotics, it was shown that RV were present in 44% and bleeding from rectal varices occurs in 8% and that the prevalence increased with increase in severity of PHT: 19% more in patients with cirrhosis and without esophageal varices, 39% in patients with esophageal without prior bleeding, and 59% in patients with prior bleeding. Thirty percent of patients can have concomitant hemorrhoids with RV and it is very important to differentiate rectal varices from hemorrhoids. Table 3 shows important characteristics of RV and their differentiating points from hemorrhoids [62–64].

TABLE 3: Differentiating features on endoscopy between hemorrhoids and rectal varices.

| Rectal varices | Hemorrhoids |
|---|---|
| Extend superior to levator ani | Extension above levator ani not seen |
| Usually originate more than 4 cm above anal verge, distinct from hemorrhoids | Usually originated less than 4 cm below level of anal verge |
| Not contiguous with anal column or pectinate line | Maybe contiguous |
| Dilated, tortuous, submucosal vein, 3 to 6 mm in diameter and dark blue in color | Less dilated, nontortuous, paler, smaller in size |
| Do not prolapse into the proctoscope during examination | Prolapse into proctoscope commonly seen with higher grade |

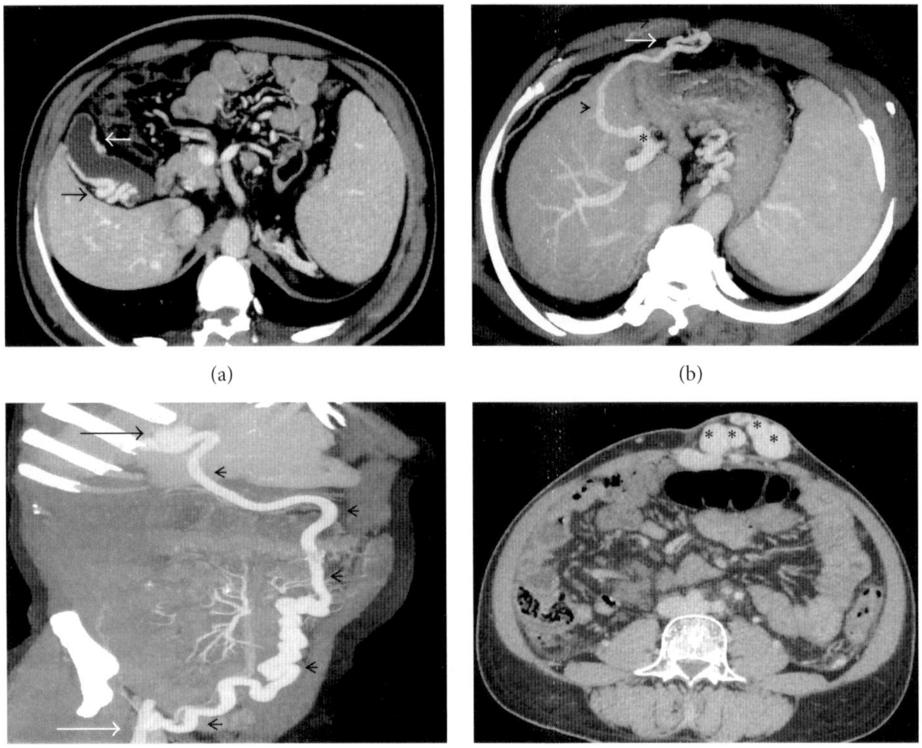

(a) (b) (c) (d)

Figure 7: (a) Axial CECT image showing multiple pericholecystic collaterals (arrows); (b) axial-oblique MIP image showing a right infradiaphragmatic type of shunt (arrowhead) arising from the left portal vein branch (asterisk) and draining into the intercostal vein; (c) coronal-oblique MIP image demonstrating a prominent recanalized paraumbilical vein (arrowheads) arising from the left branch of portal vein (black arrow) and draining into the right internal iliac vein (white arrow); (d) caput medusa, multiple periumbilical abdominal wall varices (asterisks).

## 11. Biliary Varices and Portal Hypertensive Biliopathy (Figures 6(d) and 7(a))

These are most commonly seen in extrahepatic obstruction of PV (EHPVO) and can cause extensive collateral venous circulation at porta hepatis. The description of portal biliopathy was first given in 1944 by Fraser and later on by Gibson in 1965. The term portal biliopathy or pseudosclerosing cholangitis was first coined in early 90s and used to describe abnormalities of extra- and intrahepatic biliary tract, gall bladder, and cystic ducts in patients of PHT. Even though biliary tract changes occur in 80 to 100% of EHPVO patients, symptomatic obstruction occurs in only 5 to 30% patients. Anatomical understanding of varices in the biliary tract stems from pristine description provided by Petren and Saint in 1932 and 1971, respectively. There are two venous systems that run along the biliary tract: the paracholedochal veins (of Petren) that run parallel to the common bile duct and the epicholedochal plexus (of Saint) forming a fine reticular network over the common bile duct. The former is a separate system from the bile duct, so much that variceal formation within this group produces extrinsic compression whereas dilatation of the latter group causes only mild to moderate irregularities of the biliary ductal system. The venous plexus of Petren is connected with the gastric, pancreaticoduodenal, and portal venous system and also to the liver directly. The right sided biliary plexus communicates with gastrocolic vein and pancreaticoduodenal vein to cystic vein or directly to liver. Left side biliary venous plexus communicates with jejunal veins, left and right gastric vein, and the left PV with flow moving towards branches of PV [65, 66]. Endoscopic retrograde cholangiography (ERCP) and endoscopic ultrasonography have helped in identifying these biliary varices and map their anatomy well. On ERCP, the biliary abnormalities secondary to biliary varices include smooth strictures, luminal irregularity, segmental dilations, indentations, ectasias, angular deviations of ducts, and pruning and clustering of intrahepatic ducts. Left hepatic duct is more involved than the right probably because collateral veins are more frequently formed between the paraumbilical veins and the left branch of PV compared to the right system. ERCP grading of biliary varices/portal biliopathy has been divided into 4 types: Type 1 in which there is involvement of extrahepatic bile duct only, Type 2 with intrahepatic bile ducts only, Type 3a with extrahepatic and unilateral intrahepatic bile duct involvement, and Type 3b with extrahepatic and bilateral intrahepatic ductal involvement [67, 68]. On EUS evaluation, the collaterals enter subepithelial layer of CBD after perforating the fibromuscular layer of CBD wall forming intracholedochal varices. Perforators from the paracholedochal collaterals act as link between veins outside and inside the muscular wall of CBD. Currently EUS could be the investigation of choice in evaluation of origin, caliber, entry, and course of intracholedochal varices throughout the CBD. Early on, changes occur in the paracholedochal vein of Petren which later involve those of Saint [69–72].

## 12. Other Ectopic Varices and Their Afferent and Efferent Pathways Including Veins of Sappey and Burrow: Umbilical and Paraumbilical Veins in Portosystemic Collaterals

Burrow in 1838 described a pair of veins ascending from inferior epigastric veins along the umbilical vein and uniting into a single channel, draining into the upper part of umbilical vein. Sappey in 1883 noted that paraumbilical veins were distended in patients of PHT on postmortem studies. He referred to these veins as accessory PVs, which had superior and inferior divisions. The superior group drains the median part of diaphragm and traverses the falciform ligament in its upper part to reach the convex surface of liver, entering the sublobular branches of PV. The tributaries of the inferior group run alongside inferior part of falciform ligament, entering the hepatic fissure. Inferiorly they communicate with epigastric and cutaneous veins and become dilated in presence of PHT: one channel gets selectively dilated to connect the right epigastric vein with the liver [73, 74]. Later on, it was shown that umbilical vein and the veins of Burrow also become dilated in the presence of PHT and that the dilated veins of Burrow communicate with dilated deep epigastric veins after piercing the rectus sheath. Veins of Burrow can also enter the portal system directly and correspond to the inferior veins of Sappey. On the contrary, Sappey's veins when they drain into the umbilical vein came to be known as intercalary veins of Baumgarten. Sappey's veins enter the portal system through the liver capsule from different directions and form transhepatic portosystemic shunts in the liver. The common locations of occurrence of Sappey's veins are shown in the following list. The superior veins of Sappey connect the convex anterosuperior part of the liver surface to the diaphragm and connect with internal thoracic veins. The paraumbilical veins (inferior veins of Sappey) in PHT connect the anterior parietal veins like the superior and inferior epigastric veins in rectus sheath and thoracoepigastric vein in subcutaneous tissue at the umbilicus with the left branch of PV. These connections can also occur in the anterior abdominal wall, around the umbilical regions, forming "caput medusae." Portosystemic collaterals also occur through the bare area of liver (right inferior phrenic vein) and the left triangular ligament (through left intercostal, pericardiophrenic, and inferior phrenic veins). Caput medusae is also responsible for varicosities in the anterior right thigh and is also associated with varicose veins in legs [75–77] (Figures 7(b)–7(d)).

Sappey's veins and their anatomical considerations are as follows:

Upper and lower part of falciform ligament.

Left triangular ligament: left inferior phrenic vein and intercostal vein regions.

Ligamentum teres, central portion of falciform ligament, and recanalized umbilical vein.

Right triangular ligament: right inferior phrenic vein region.

Diaphragmatic veins (near bare area of liver).

Ligamentum venosum: patent ductus venosus.

Gastrohepatic omentum: cystic veins and branches of left gastric vein region.

## 13. Conclusions

The current review describes various portosystemic collateral pathways pertinent to portal hypertension and their current classifications beyond traditional, with special emphasis on hemodynamics. It is very important that the Hepatologist and the interventional Radiologist know and understand the various patterns of portosystemic collateral channels for accurate diagnosis, sensible management, and prevention of accidental vascular injury during intervention.

## Competing Interests

The authors declare that they have no competing interests.

## References

[1] A. Cárdenas and P. Ginès, "Portal hypertension," *Current Opinion in Gastroenterology*, vol. 25, no. 3, pp. 195–201, 2009.

[2] H. Cichoz-Lach, K. Celiński, M. Słomka, and B. Kasztelan-Szczerbińska, "Pathophysiology of portal hypertension," *Journal of Physiology and Pharmacology*, vol. 59, no. 2, pp. 231–238, 2008.

[3] R. Moreau, "VEGF-induced angiogenesis drives collateral circulation in portal hypertension," *Journal of Hepatology*, vol. 43, no. 1, pp. 6–8, 2005.

[4] A. Gilbert and M. Villaret, "Contribution al'etude du syndrome d'hypertension portale; Cytologie des liquides d'ascite dans less cirrhoses," *Comptes Rendus Societe de Biologie*, vol. 60, pp. 820–823, 1906.

[5] G. A. Doehner, F. F. Ruzicka Jr., L. M. Rousselot, and G. Hoffman, "The portal venous system: on its pathological roentgen anatomy," *Radiology*, vol. 66, no. 2, pp. 206–217, 1956.

[6] T. N. Johns and B. B. Evans, "Collateral pathways in portal hypertension," *Annals of Surgery*, vol. 155, no. 6, pp. 838–845, 1962.

[7] F. F. Ruzicka Jr. and P. Rossi, "Arterial portography: patterns of venous flow," *Radiology*, vol. 92, no. 4, pp. 777–787, 1969.

[8] T. Ishikawa, Y. Tsukune, Y. Ohyama, M. Fujikawa, K. Sakuyama, and M. Fujii, "Venous abnormalities in portal hypertension demonstrated by CT," *American Journal of Roentgenology*, vol. 134, no. 2, pp. 271–276, 1980.

[9] A. K. Dokmeci, K. Kimura, S. Matsutani et al., "Collateral veins in portal hypertension: demonstration by sonography," *American Journal of Roentgenology*, vol. 137, no. 6, pp. 1173–1177, 1981.

[10] T. Kashiwagi, K. Kimura, T. Kozuka et al., "Portosystemic collaterals in portal hypertension: visualization by using blood-pool

SPECT imaging," *American Journal of Roentgenology*, vol. 153, no. 2, pp. 281–285, 1989.

[11] K. C. Cho, Y. D. Patel, R. H. Wachsberg, and J. Seeff, "Varices in portal hypertension: evaluation with CT," *Radiographics : a review publication of the Radiological Society of North America, Inc*, vol. 15, no. 3, pp. 609–622, 1995.

[12] H. K. Kang, Y. Y. Jeong, J. H. Choi et al., "Three-dimensional multi-detector row CT portal venography in the evaluation of portosystemic collateral vessels in liver cirrhosis," *Radiographics*, vol. 22, no. 5, pp. 1053–1061, 2002.

[13] G. N. Postma, M. W. Seybt, and C. J. Rees, "Esophagology," in *Ballinger's Otolaryngology Head & Neck Surgery*, J. B. Snow and P. A. Wackym, Eds., pp. 975–995, BC Decker, Shelton, Conn, USA, 17th edition, 2009.

[14] J. F. Vollweiler and M. F. Vaezi, "The esophagus: anatomy, physiology, and diseases," in *Otolaryngology Head and Neck Surgery*, C. W. Cummings, P. W. Flint, L. A. Harker et al., Eds., vol. 2, Mosby-Elsevier, Philadelphia, Pa, USA, 4th edition, 2005.

[15] A. Vianna, P. C. Hayes, G. Moscoso et al., "Normal venous circulation of the gastroesophageal junction. A route to understanding varices," *Gastroenterology*, vol. 93, no. 4, pp. 876–889, 1987.

[16] B. Kuo and D. Urma, "Esophagus—anatomy and development," *GI Motility Online, Nature*, 2006, http://www.nature.com/gimo/contents/pt1/full/gimo6.html.

[17] A. Arora, S. Rajesh, Y. S. Meenakshi, B. Sureka, K. Bansal, and S. K. Sarin, "Spectrum of hepatofugal collateral pathways in portal hypertension: an illustrated radiological review," *Insights into Imaging*, vol. 6, no. 5, pp. 559–572, 2015.

[18] M. Sharma and C. S. Rameshbabu, "Collateral pathways in portal hypertension," *Journal of Clinical and Experimental Hepatology*, vol. 2, no. 4, pp. 338–352, 2012.

[19] Z. A. Wani, R. A. Bhat, A. S. Bhadoria, R. Maiwall, and A. Choudhury, "Gastric varices: classification, endoscopic and ultrasonographic management," *Journal of Research in Medical Sciences*, vol. 20, no. 12, pp. 1200–1207, 2015.

[20] A. I. Youssef, S. Escalante-Glorsky, R. B. Bonnet, and Y. K. Chen, "Hemoptysis secondary to bronchial varices associated with alcoholic liver cirrhosis and portal hypertension," *American Journal of Gastroenterology*, vol. 89, no. 9, pp. 1562–1563, 1994.

[21] B. M. Ryan, R. W. Stockbrugger, and J. M. Ryan, "A pathophysiologic, gastroenterologic, and radiologic approach to the management of gastric varices," *Gastroenterology*, vol. 126, no. 4, pp. 1175–1189, 2004.

[22] H. Kiyosue, H. Mori, S. Matsumoto, Y. Yamada, Y. Hori, and Y. Okino, "Transcatheter obliteration of gastric varices: part 1. Anatomic classification," *Radiographics*, vol. 23, no. 4, pp. 911–920, 2003.

[23] S. Hayashi, S. Saeki, and T. Ushini, "Gastric fundic varices: hemodynamics and non-surgical treatment," *Digestive Endoscopy*, vol. 17, no. 3, pp. 198–202, 2005.

[24] M. Arakawa, T. Masuzaki, and K. Okuda, "Pathomorphology of esophageal and gastric varices," *Seminars in Liver Disease*, vol. 22, no. 1, pp. 73–82, 2002.

[25] V. A. Luketic and A. J. Sanyal, "Esophageal varices. I. Clinical presentation, medical therapy, and endoscopic therapy," *Gastroenterology Clinics of North America*, vol. 29, no. 2, pp. 337–385, 2000.

[26] A. I. Sharara and D. C. Rockey, "Gastroesophageal variceal hemorrhage," *The New England Journal of Medicine*, vol. 345, no. 9, pp. 669–681, 2001.

[27] F. Chikamori, N. Kuniyoshi, S. Shibuya, and Y. Takase, "Correlation between endoscopic and angiographic findings in patients with esophageal and isolated gastric varices," *Digestive Surgery*, vol. 18, no. 3, pp. 176–181, 2001.

[28] W. Widrich, M. Srinivasan, M. Semine, and A. Robbins, "Collateral pathways of the left gastric vein in portal hypertension," *American Journal of Roentgenology*, vol. 142, no. 2, pp. 375–382, 1984.

[29] S. K. Sarin and S. R. Agarwal, "Gastric varices and portal hypertensive gastropathy," *Clinics in Liver Disease*, vol. 5, no. 3, pp. 727–767, 2001.

[30] E. Moubarak, A. Bouvier, J. Boursier et al., "Portosystemic collateral vessels in liver cirrhosis: a three-dimensional MDCT pictorial review," *Abdominal Imaging*, vol. 37, no. 5, pp. 746–766, 2012.

[31] J. An, K. W. Kim, S. Han, J. Lee, and Y.-S. Lim, "Improvement in survival associated with embolisation of spontaneous portosystemic shunt in patients with recurrent hepatic encephalopathy," *Alimentary Pharmacology and Therapeutics*, vol. 39, no. 12, pp. 1418–1426, 2014.

[32] W. Laleman, M. Simon-Talero, G. Maleux et al., "Embolization of large spontaneous portosystemic shunts for refractory hepatic encephalopathy: a multicenter survey on safety and efficacy," *Hepatology*, vol. 57, no. 6, pp. 2448–2457, 2013.

[33] C. A. Philips, L. Anand, K. N. Kumar, V. Kasana, and A. Arora, "Rare, spontaneous trans-splenic shunt and intra-splenic collaterals with attendant splenic artery aneurysms in an adult patient with compensated cirrhosis and portal hypertension," *Gastroenterology Report*, vol. 3, no. 2, pp. 162–166, 2015.

[34] W. E. Saad, P. O. Simon, and S. C. Rose, "Balloon-occluded retrograde transvenous obliteration of gastric varices," *CardioVascular and Interventional Radiology*, vol. 37, no. 2, pp. 299–315, 2014.

[35] W. E. A. Saad, A. Lippert, N. E. Saad, and S. Caldwell, "Ectopic varices: anatomical classification, hemodynamic classification, and hemodynamic-based management," *Techniques in Vascular and Interventional Radiology*, vol. 16, no. 2, pp. 158–175, 2013.

[36] J. C. Garcia-Pagán, M. Barrufet, A. Cardenas, and À. Escorsell, "Management of gastric varices," *Clinical Gastroenterology and Hepatology*, vol. 12, no. 6, pp. 919.e1–928.e1, 2014.

[37] W. E. Saad, "Endovascular management of gastric varices," *Clinics in Liver Disease*, vol. 18, no. 4, pp. 829–851, 2014.

[38] H. Kiyosue, H. Mori, S. Matsumoto, Y. Yamada, Y. Hori, and Y. Okino, "Transcatheter obliteration of gastric varices: part 2. Strategy and techniques based on hemodynamic features," *Radiographics*, vol. 23, no. 4, pp. 921–937, 2003.

[39] H. Kiyosue, H. Mori, S. Matsumoto, Y. Yamada, Y. Hori, and Y. Okino, "Transcatheter obliteration of gastric varices: part-2: strategy and techniques based on hemodynamic features," *Radiographics*, vol. 23, no. 4, pp. 921–937, 2003.

[40] M. Kitamoto, M. Imamura, K. Kamada et al., "Balloon-occluded retrograde transvenous obliteration of gastric fundal varices with hemorrhage," *American Journal of Roentgenology*, vol. 178, no. 5, pp. 1167–1174, 2002.

[41] K. C. Sung, S. W. Shin, H. L. In et al., "Balloon-occluded retrograde transvenous obliteration of gastric varices: outcomes and complications in 49 patients," *American Journal of Roentgenology*, vol. 189, no. 6, 2007.

[42] H. Arai, T. Abe, R. Shimoda, H. Takagi, T. Yamada, and M. Mori, "Emergency balloon-occluded retrograde transvenous obliteration for gastric varices," *Journal of Gastroenterology*, vol. 40, no. 10, pp. 964–971, 2005.

[43] M. Girotra, S. Raghavapuram, R. R. Abraham, M. Pahwa, A. R. Pahwa, and R. F. Rego, "Management of gastric variceal bleeding: role of endoscopy and endoscopic ultrasound," *World Journal of Hepatology*, vol. 6, no. 3, pp. 130–136, 2014.

[44] M. Triantafyllou and A. J. Stanley, "Update on gastric varices," *World Journal of Gastrointestinal Endoscopy*, vol. 6, no. 5, pp. 168–175, 2014.

[45] L. L. Fujii-Lau, R. Law, L. M. Wong Kee Song, and M. J. Levy, "Novel techniques for gastric variceal obliteration," *Digestive Endoscopy*, vol. 27, no. 2, pp. 189–196, 2015.

[46] A. M. S. Al-Osaimi and S. H. Caldwell, "Medical and endoscopic management of gastric varices," *Seminars in Interventional Radiology*, vol. 28, no. 3, pp. 273–282, 2011.

[47] W. E. A. Saad, A. M. S. Al-Osaimi, and S. H. Caldwell, "Pre- and post-balloon-occluded retrograde transvenous obliteration clinical evaluation, management, and imaging: indications, management protocols, and follow-up," *Techniques in Vascular and Interventional Radiology*, vol. 15, no. 3, pp. 165–202, 2012.

[48] S. Hirota, S. Matsumoto, M. Tomita, M. Sako, and M. Kono, "Retrograde transvenous obliteration of gastric varices," *Radiology*, vol. 211, no. 2, pp. 349–356, 1999.

[49] T. Fukuda, S. Hirota, K. Sugimoto, S. Matsumoto, C. A. Zamora, and K. Sugimura, "'Downgrading' of gastric varices with multiple collateral veins in balloon-occluded retrograde transvenous obliteration," *Journal of Vascular and Interventional Radiology*, vol. 16, no. 10, pp. 1379–1383, 2005.

[50] A. Matsumoto, N. Hamamoto, T. Nomura et al., "Balloon-occluded retrograde transvenous obliteration of high risk gastric fundal varices," *American Journal of Gastroenterology*, vol. 94, no. 3, pp. 643–649, 1999.

[51] D. Crisan, M. Tantau, and A. Tantau, "Endoscopic management of bleeding gastric varices—an updated overview," *Current gastroenterology reports*, vol. 16, no. 10, p. 413, 2014.

[52] G. Stephen and R. Miething, "Roentgendiagnostik varicoser duodenal-veranderungen bei portaler hypertension," *Radiologie*, vol. 8, article 90, 1968.

[53] R. Amin, R. Alexix, and J. Kowzis, "Fatal ruptured duodenal Varis: a case report and review of literature," *The American Journal of Gastroenterology*, vol. 80, pp. 13–18, 1985.

[54] F. Khouqeer, C. Morrow, and P. Jordan, "Duodenal varices as a cause of massive upper gastrointestinal bleeding," *Surgery*, vol. 102, no. 3, pp. 548–552, 1987.

[55] D. Lebrec and J. Behamou, "Ectopic varices in portal hypertension," *Journal of Clinical Gastroenterology*, vol. 14, pp. 105–119, 1985.

[56] T. Sato, "Transabdominal color Doppler ultrasonography for the diagnosis of small intestinal and vesical varices in a patient successfully treated with Percutaneous transhepatic obliteration," *Clinical Journal of Gastroenterology*, vol. 3, no. 4, pp. 214–218, 2010.

[57] K. Ibukuro, T. Tsukiyama, K. Mori, and Y. Inoue, "Veins of retzius at CT during arterial portography: anatomy and clinical importance," *Radiology*, vol. 209, no. 3, pp. 793–800, 1998.

[58] V. C. McAlister and N. A. Al-Saleh, "Duodenal dearterialization and stapling for severe hemorrhage from duodenal varices with portal vein thrombosis," *American Journal of Surgery*, vol. 189, no. 1, pp. 49–52, 2005.

[59] M. Feldman, V. M. Smith, and C. G. Warner, "Varices of the colon. Report of three cases," *JAMA*, vol. 179, pp. 729–730, 1962.

[60] J. Weingart, W. Hochter, and R. Ottenjann, "Varices of the entire colon: an unusual cause of recurrent intestinal bleeding," *Endoscopy*, vol. 14, no. 2, pp. 69–70, 1982.

[61] F. Francois, C. Tadros, and D. Diehl, "Pan-colonic varices and Idiopathicportal hypertension," *Journal of Gastrointestinal and Liver Diseases*, vol. 16, pp. 325–328, 2007.

[62] R. K. Dhiman, V. A. Saraswat, G. Choudhuri, B. C. Sharma, R. Pandey, and S. R. Naik, "Endosonographic, endoscopic, and histologic evaluation of alterations in the rectal venous system in patients with portal hypertension," *Gastrointestinal Endoscopy*, vol. 49, no. 2, pp. 218–227, 1999.

[63] R. Shudo, Y. Yazaki, S. Sakurai et al., "Combined endoscopic variceal ligation and sclerotherapy for bleeding rectal varices associated with primary biliary cirrhosis: a case showing a long-lasting favorable response," *Gastrointestinal Endoscopy*, vol. 53, no. 6, pp. 661–665, 2001.

[64] J.-S. Hsieh, C.-J. Huang, Y.-S. Huang, and T.-J. Huang, "Demonstration of rectal varices by transhepatic inferior mesenteric venography," *Diseases of the Colon & Rectum*, vol. 29, no. 7, pp. 459–461, 1986.

[65] T. Petren, "The veins of the extrahepatic biliary system and their pathologic anatomic significance," *Verhandlungen der Anatomischen Gesellschaft*, vol. 41, pp. 139–143, 1932.

[66] J. H. Saint, "The epicholedochal venous plexus and its importance as a means of identifying the common duct during operations on the extrahepatic biliary tract," *The British journal of surgery*, vol. 48, no. 211, pp. 489–498, 1961.

[67] R. Chandra, D. Kapoor, A. Tharakan, A. Chaudhary, and S. K. Sarin, "Portal biliopathy," *Journal of Gastroenterology and Hepatology*, vol. 16, no. 10, pp. 1086–1092, 2001.

[68] I. D. Vellar, "Preliminary study of the anatomy of the venous drainage of the intrahepatic and extrahepatic bile ducts and its relevance to the practice of hepatobiliary surgery," *ANZ Journal of Surgery*, vol. 71, no. 7, pp. 418–422, 2001.

[69] M. Sharma and A. Pathak, "Perforators of common bile duct wall in portal hypertensive biliopathy (with videos)," *Gastrointestinal Endoscopy*, vol. 70, no. 5, pp. 1041–1043, 2009.

[70] S. Kim and F. S. Chew, "Choledochal varices," *American Journal of Roentgenology*, vol. 150, no. 3, pp. 578–580, 1988.

[71] M. Sharma and A. Pathak, "Intracholedochal varices in portal hypertensive biliopathy," *European Journal of Radiology Extra*, vol. 72, no. 3, pp. e119–e123, 2009.

[72] Y. Chawla, J. B. Dilawari, and S. Katariya, "Gallbladder varices in portal vein thrombosis," *American Journal of Roentgenology*, vol. 162, no. 3, pp. 643–645, 1994.

[73] K. A. Burrow, "Beitrag zur gefasslehre des fotus," *Archiv fur Anatomie und Physiologie*, pp. 44–45, 1838.

[74] M. C. Sappey, "Memoire sur les veines portes accessoires," *Journal de L'anatomie et de la Physiologie Normales et Pathologiques de L'homme et des Animaux*, vol. 19, pp. 517–525, 1883.

[75] O. C. Gonzales, "Portography; A preliminary report of a new technique via the umbilical vein," *Clinical Proceedings. Childrens Hospital*, vol. 15, pp. 120–122, 1959.

[76] B. F. Martin and R. G. Tudor, "The umbilical and paraumbilical veins of man," *Journal of Anatomy*, vol. 130, pp. 305–322, 1980.

[77] Y. Itai, T. Kokubo, K. Ohtomo et al., "Collaterals of portal hypertension running through the liver. Part 1. Paraumbilical vein," *Rinsho Hoshasen*, vol. 34, no. 8, pp. 865–870, 1989.

# 32

# The Effect of Artichoke Leaf Extract on Alanine Aminotransferase and Aspartate Aminotransferase in the Patients with Nonalcoholic Steatohepatitis

**Vajiheh Rangboo,[1] Mostafa Noroozi,[2] Roza Zavoshy,[3] Seyed Amirmansoor Rezadoost,[4] and Asghar Mohammadpoorasl[5]**

[1] *Department of Nutrition, Faculty of Health, Qazvin University of Medical Sciences, Qazvin, Iran*
[2] *Children Growth Research Center, Qazvin University of Medical Sciences, Qazvin, Iran*
[3] *Department of Nutrition, Faculty of Nutrition, Qazvin University of Medical Sciences, Qazvin, Iran*
[4] *Shahid Chamran Hospital, Shahid Beheshti University of Medical Sciences, Tehran, Iran*
[5] *Department of Epidemiology, Tabriz University of Medical Sciences, Tabriz, Iran*

Correspondence should be addressed to Mostafa Noroozi; mnoroozi@ymail.com

Academic Editor: Roberto Lupi

*Background.* Based on recent basic and clinical investigations, the extract of artichoke (*Cynara scolymus*) leaf has been revealed to be used for hepatoprotective and cholesterol reducing purposes. We aimed to assess the therapeutic effects of artichoke on biochemical and liver biomarkers in patients with nonalcoholic steatohepatitis (NASH). *Methods.* In a randomized double blind clinical trial, 60 consecutive patients suffering NASH were randomly assigned to receive *Cynara scolymus* extract (as 6 tablets per day consisting of 2700 mg extract of the herb) as the intervention group or placebo as the control group for two months. *Results.* Comparing changes in study markers following interventions showed improvement in liver enzymes. The levels of triglycerides and cholesterol were significantly reduced in the group treated with *Cynara scolymus* when compared to placebo group. To compare the role of *Cynara scolymus* use with placebo in changes in study parameters, multivariate linear regression models were employed indicating higher improvement in liver enzymes and also lipid profile particularly triglycerides and total cholesterol following administration of *Cynara scolymus* in comparison with placebo use. *Conclusion.* This study sheds light on the potential hepatoprotective activity and hypolipidemic effect of *Cynara scolymus* in management of NASH. This clinical trial is registered in the IRCT, Iranian Registry of Clinical Trials, by number IRCT2014070218321N1.

## 1. Introduction

Nonalcoholic fatty liver disease (NAFLD) refers to a wide spectrum of disorders characterized by fatty infiltration in the liver and steatosis [1]. By developing oxidative stress, hepatocellular inflammation, and steatosis, the term was replaced by nonalcoholic steatohepatitis (NASH) that may culminate in cirrhosis and hepatocellular carcinoma [2, 3]. Within the last decade, prevalence of NASH has interestingly doubled especially in the Middle East, Far East, Africa, the Caribbean, and Latin America due to its close association with lifestyle disorders such as diabetes and obesity [4]. In this regard, the best treatment approaches for this phenomenon include weight loss, changes in dietary regimens, and lifestyle modifications. Also, in cases with documented hyperlipidemia or diabetes, use of insulin sensitizing and lipid lowering drugs can be also considered [5]. However, since NASH is a multifactorial disorder, single target based therapy has limited implications. Hence, the use of herbal medicine approach can be a promising alternative due to its multipronged mechanisms of action [6–8].

Artichoke (*Cynara scolymus*) is a plant frequently grown in Mediterranean countries that is rich in natural antioxidants and thus is used as a herbal drug [9]. Based on recent basic and clinical investigations, the extract of artichoke leaf has been revealed to be used for hepatoprotective [10–12], antimicrobial [13], and cholesterol reducing purposes [14].

Artichoke has been found to decrease the production of reactive oxygen species, the oxidation of low-density lipoproteins [15], lipid peroxidation [11], and protein oxidation and increase the activity of glutathione peroxidase [16]. In this regard, it seems that the use of this herb may be promising to treat NASH. The present study aimed to assess the therapeutic effects of artichoke on biochemical and liver biomarkers in patients with NASH.

## 2. Subjects and Methods

*2.1. Study Population.* In a randomized double blind clinical trial, 60 consecutive patients who suffered NASH (based on changes in liver enzymes and sonographic evidences) were included in the study. The main inclusion criteria were elevation of liver enzymes (>30 $\mu$/L), any evidences of fatty liver in abdominal sonography, and the existence of at least one of these characteristics: total cholesterol > 200 mg/dL, high density lipoprotein (HDL) < 40 mg/dL for men and <50 mg/dL for women, serum triglycerides level > 150 mg/dL, fasting blood sugar > 100 mg/dL, obesity defined as body mass index > 30 kg/m$^2$, or blood pressure > 130/85 mmHg. In this regard, the main exclusion criteria were daily alcohol consumption, diabetes mellitus type I, the existence of concomitant liver diseases such as hepatitis B or C, autoimmune hepatitis, Wilson, hemochromatosis, alpha-1 antitrypsin deficiency, or biliary obstruction, the use of vitamin C, livergol, hepatotoxic drugs, NASH inducing drugs such as amiodarone, calcium-channel blockers, or tamoxifen, pregnancy or breastfeeding, sensitivity to artichoke species, or any life-threatening disorders.

The two groups were matched in terms of sex distribution (21 male and 9 female in both groups) and mean age (47.27 ± 8.12 years in intervention group and 49.83 ± 12.79 years in placebo group, $P = 0.357$). The two groups were also similar in other baseline characteristics including weight, levels of liver enzymes, lipid profile, and fasting blood sugar on initial assessment.

*2.2. Study Intervention.* The baseline characteristics of patients were collected by interviewing and the study questionnaires were recorded. The patients were then randomly assigned to receive *Cynara scolymus* extract (as 6 tablets per day consisting of 2700 mg extract of the herb prepared in Dineh company, Qazvin, Iran) as the intervention group or placebo as the control group for two months (placebo was prepared from the same ingredient as treatment except *Cynara scolymus* extract). The randomization was done using computer generated random number tables. Both groups were advised to maintain regular physical activity (20 min walking within 5 days a week) and an appropriate dietary regimen (calculated based on patients' weight, height, age, and percentage of activity using the Mifflin formula to gradually reduce body weight).

*2.3. Measurement of Biomarkers.* Serum alanine transaminase (ALT) and aspartate transaminase (AST) activity was estimated colorimetrically using an especial kit (Pars Azmoon company, Iran) according to the method of Reitman and Frankel [17]. Serum cholesterol (Chol) concentration was determined colorimetrically using an especial kit (Pars Man company, Iran) according to the method of Allain et al. [18]. Serum LDL-cholesterol (LDL) concentration was assayed colorimetrically using an especial kit (Pars Azmoon company, Iran) according to the method of Assmann et al. [19]. Serum HDL-cholesterol (HDL) concentration was measured colorimetrically using an especial kit (Pars Man company, Iran) according to the method of Lopez-Virella et al. [20]. Serum triglycerides (TG) level was determined colorimetrically using an especial kit (Pars Azmoon company, Iran) according to the method of Fassati and Prencipe [21]. The biomarkers were measured at the two time points: admission time and 2 months after the initial assessment (completing treatment protocols).

*2.4. Statistical Analysis.* Results were presented as mean ± standard deviation (SD). Continuous variables were compared using $t$-test or nonparametric Mann-Whitney $U$ test. The changes in study biomarkers after interventions were assessed using the Paired $t$-test or nonparametric Wilcoxon test. The multivariate linear regression analysis was used for assessing study outcomes following different employed protocols as follows. First, the baseline variables as probable confounders with a $P$ value <0.20 in univariate analyses were taken in a multivariate logistic regression model to assess the difference between the treatment groups receiving *Cynara scolymus* extract or placebo with the presence of these confounders. For the statistical analysis, the statistical software SPSS version 21.0 for windows (SPSS Inc., Chicago, IL) was used.

## 3. Results

As shown in Table 1, following administration of *Cynara scolymus*, significant reduction was observed in mean weight, as well as in serum levels of ALT, AST, blood sugar, total cholesterol, LDL, and triglycerides. Also, mean systolic blood pressure was significantly reduced using *Cynara scolymus*. In contrast, using placebo resulted in significant reduction in mean weight, as well as in serum levels of ALT and AST; however, among other biomarkers, blood sugar and lipid profile remained unchanged. Comparing changes in study markers following interventions showed the changes in liver enzymes, and also levels of triglycerides and cholesterol were significantly more in group treated with *Cynara scolymus* when compared to placebo group (Table 2). To compare the role of *Cynara scolymus* use with placebo in changes in study parameters, multivariate linear regression models were employed (Table 2) indicating higher improvement in liver enzymes and also lipid profiles of triglycerides and total cholesterol following administration of *Cynara scolymus* in comparison with placebo use.

TABLE 1: Changes in study biomarkers in intervention and placebo groups.

| Marker | Intervention group | | | Placebo group | | | Intergroup difference |
|---|---|---|---|---|---|---|---|
| | Before | After | *P* value | Before | After | *P* value | |
| Weight (kg) | 83.90 ± 15.83 | 79.28 ± 14.25 | <0.001 | 81.81 ± 14.25 | 77.05 ± 14.83 | <0.001 | 0.859 |
| ALT (mg/dL) | 81.77 ± 38.73 | 38.40 ± 14.15 | <0.001 | 74.13 ± 23.61 | 64.07 ± 20.36 | <0.001 | <0.001 |
| AST (mg/dL) | 45.53 ± 13.78 | 24.60 ± 7.43 | <0.001 | 44.50 ± 9.82 | 39.60 ± 10.41 | <0.001 | <0.001 |
| FBS (mg/dL) | 108.07 ± 28.90 | 97.60 ± 14.50 | 0.029 | 107.43 ± 18.48 | 102.57 ± 10.78 | 0.096 | 0.302 |
| Chol (mg/dL) | 206.47 ± 31.20 | 182.87 ± 34.64 | 0.001 | 213.67 ± 48.48 | 211.63 ± 48.96 | 0.686 | 0.008 |
| LDL (mg/dL) | 122.14 ± 30.42 | 108.12 ± 32.36 | 0.039 | 116.09 ± 29.38 | 113.23 ± 31.79 | 0.659 | 0.120 |
| HDL (mg/dL) | 45.87 ± 10.46 | 43.33 ± 8.20 | 0.129 | 45.50 ± 7.50 | 44.87 ± 6.10 | 0.689 | 0.403 |
| TG (mg/dL) | 193.37 ± 86.03 | 154.50 ± 84.93 | 0.011 | 179.87 ± 45.67 | 184.23 ± 57.83 | 0.659 | 0.016 |
| SBP (mg/dL) | 132.70 ± 13.55 | 126.57 ± 8.54 | 0.004 | 130.23 ± 10.34 | 128.20 ± 6.62 | 0.044 | 0.070 |
| DBP (mg/dL) | 80.00 ± 9.21 | 79.03 ± 6.89 | 0.578 | 80.87 ± 8.52 | 81.63 ± 7.31 | 0.504 | 0.403 |

TABLE 2: Multivariate linear regression models for determining the role of *Cynara scolymus* use on changes in liver enzymes and lipid profile.

| Marker | Variable | Beta | 95% confidence interval | *P* value |
|---|---|---|---|---|
| ALT change | Artichoke use | −31.365 | −45.201 to −17.528 | <0.001 |
| | Male sex | −0.634 | −16.252 to 14.983 | 0.935 |
| | Age | −0.754 | −1.434 to −0.074 | 0.030 |
| AST change | Artichoke use | −16.041 | −21.405 to −10.677 | <0.001 |
| | Male sex | −2.995 | −9.049 to 3.060 | 0.326 |
| | Age | 0.003 | −0.261 to 0.266 | 0.983 |
| Chol change | Artichoke use | −21.673 | −37.245 to −6.101 | 0.007 |
| | Male sex | −17.072 | −34.648 to 0.505 | 0.057 |
| | Age | 0.041 | −0.723 to 0.806 | 0.914 |
| TG change | Artichoke use | −41.960 | −76.613 to −7.307 | 0.019 |
| | Male sex | −28.315 | −67.428 to 10.798 | 0.153 |
| | Age | −0.496 | −2.198 to 1.206 | 0.562 |

## 4. Discussion

Our study aimed to assess the beneficial effects of *Cynara scolymus*, a herb with antioxidant compounds, on liver function and also lipid profile and fasting blood glucose. On the other hand, we aimed to demonstrate therapeutic effects of this herb on liver functional biomarkers and also hemodynamic parameters in patients with NASH. In this double blind clinical trial, patients in intervention group received *Cynara scolymus* extract for two months and changes in study biomarkers were reassessed.

Serum ALT and AST are effective biomarkers in the diagnosis of hepatic damage. Sever liver damage was demonstrated by remarkable elevation of serum ALT and AST levels. This elevation may be attributed to the release of these enzymes from the cytoplasm in to the blood circulation after rupture of the plasma membrane and cellular damage [22].

The result of the present study showed significant changes in serum ALT and AST levels in intervention group in comparison with the placebo group ($P < 0.001$). This effect could be attributed to the antioxidant ingredients in *Cynara scolymus* extract such as mono- and dicaffeoylquinic acid (cynarin and chlorogenic acid), caffeic acid and flavonoids including the glycosides luteolin-7-$\beta$-rutinoside (scolymoside), luteolin-7-$\beta$-D-glucoside, and luteolin-4-$\beta$-D-glucoside that are mainly compounds in *Cynara scolymus* extract [23–25]. And chlorogenic acid is the most active antioxidant in *Cynara scolymus* extract [26]. Antioxidants are components that prevent oxidative reactions often by scavenging free radicals before they can damage cells [27, 28]. Several in vitro and animal studies assessed the antioxidative and free radical scavenging potential of artichoke extracts in protection hepatocytes from oxidative stress [29–32], but there are a few human and clinical studies in this regard. The result of the present study in reduction of serum ALT and AST levels is in agreement with Saffa et al. They investigate the efficacy of *Cynara scolymus* total methanolic extract (CSM) and its fraction (CSF) in rat. Their result showed that CSF is more active in comparison with CSM. Perhaps it is because of high concentration of monocaffeoylquinic acid derivatives (chlorogenic acid) in CSF [33]. In Huber's study although the used doses of *Cynara scolymus* extract and duration of study were more than the present study, remarkable reduction in serum ALT and AST levels was not seen in patients with hepatitis C, which is not in agreement with our study. It appears that because of microbial agent and sever damage of hepatocytes uneffectiveness of *Cynara scolymus* extract on ALT and AST was caused [34]. Also, in present study, improvement of lipid profile was significantly observed in the group receiving *Cynara scolymus* extract not in placebo group. These effects could be attributed to active ingredients in *Cynara scolymus* extract which are known as caffeoylquinic acid derivatives (cynarin and chlorogenic acid). Some previous studies showed that these compounds can reduce cholesterol by inhibiting HMG-COA reductase and having a hypolipidemic influence lowering blood cholesterol [26].

Our result on hypocholesterolemic effect of *Cynara scolymus* extract is in agreement with Pittler et al. [35]. Some studies suggest that *Cynara scolymus* extract reduces blood lipids by directly influencing biosynthesis of cholesterol and also by production and secretion of bile from the liver [36, 37]. Reduction in triglycerides level is attributed to improvement in glycemic control and reduction of glucose instead of fat. Acetyl COA yield from pyruvic acid enters Krebs cycle and leads to metabolism of glucose completely instead of triglycerides biosynthesis.

In present study improvement in fasting blood sugar was significantly observed in group receiving *Cynara scolymus* extract not in placebo group. This beneficial effect could be attributed to high antioxidant capacity of this herb. Phenolic compounds, specially, such as caffeic acid and flavonoids, are representative of this effect.

Another mechanism for reducing glucose level by *Cynara scolymus* extract is affecting glucose absorption. Antioxidant compounds delay depletion of stomach and bowels and they inhibited $\alpha$-amylase and $\alpha$-glucosidase enzymes in bowels and blocked glucose transportation to blood. On the other hand antioxidants have insulin-like effect and increase glucose absorption in peripheral tissue. Another probable mechanism is influencing $\beta$-cells, repairing damage cells, and stimulating these cells to secrete insulin. Studies show that chlorogenic acid has antidiabetic effect [38, 39] and reduction glucose by reason of this compound.

Another point of this study was the parallel improvement in liver enzymes and also lipid profile by administrating *Cynara scolymus* that was not simultaneously in placebo group. Cholesterol metabolism is associated with liver fat content independent of body weight, implying that the more the fat the liver contains, the higher the cholesterol synthesis is [40]. Cellular cholesterol synthesis is regulated by activation of membrane bound transcription factors, designated sterol regulatory element-binding proteins (SREBPs) which are the most abundant in the liver [41], and the excess of cellular cholesterol is esterified by the acyl CoA-cholesterol acyltransferase (ACAT) [42]. The high level of cholesterol synthesis and the increased SREBP-2 activity have paradoxically been shown in subjects with NASH [43]. It is thus suggested that the effects of *Cynara scolymus* may appear by inducing and involving these metabolic pathways in the liver.

The main strength of the study was to shed light on the potential role of artichoke on biochemical and liver biomarkers in patients with NASH in a controlled trial. Although, in previous studies, the role of this herb to treat NASH has been assessed, a few studies focused directly on the improvement of liver enzymes *via* administrating this herbal drug. Another strength of the current study was to assess the simultaneous changes in liver enzymes, blood sugar, and lipid profile. This concomitant assessment is important because the central role of liver leads to metabolic pathways regulating the level of these metabolic biomarkers. However, our study had some potential limitations including small sample size leading to partially low study power as well as ignoring other baseline clinical and pharmacological confounders affecting the employed regression models used for assessing the effects of artichoke on biochemical and liver biomarkers in NASH.

## 5. Conclusion

In conclusion, the current study sheds light on the potential role of *Cynara scolymus* in management of NASH. The active constituents of this herb such as flavonoids and caffeoylquinic acid may be responsible for this effect. These compounds have been proven to have hepatoprotective activity and hypolipidemic effect.

## Competing Interests

The authors have no competing interests.

## Acknowledgments

The authors would like to thank Children Growth Research Center, Qazvin University of Medical Sciences, Qazvin, Iran, and Deputy of Research, Qazvin University of Medical and Health Sciences, Qazvin, Iran, for financial support (Grant no. D.44.7929). Thanks are due to the mothers who participated in their study. They would also like to thank the health care staff for cooperation in collecting the data and thank Dineh company for providing the extract of artichoke leaf and placebo.

## References

[1] N. Chalasani, Z. Younossi, J. E. Lavine et al., "The diagnosis and management of non-alcoholic fatty liver disease: practice guideline by the American Gastroenterological Association, American Association for the Study of Liver Diseases, and American College of Gastroenterology," *Gastroenterology*, vol. 142, no. 7, pp. 1592–1609, 2012.

[2] J. K. Dyson, Q. M. Anstee, and S. McPherson, "Non-alcoholic fatty liver disease: a practical approach to treatment," *Frontline Gastroenterology*, vol. 5, no. 4, pp. 277–286, 2014.

[3] M. V. Machado and H. Cortez-Pinto, "Non-alcoholic fatty liver disease: what the clinician needs to know," *World Journal of Gastroenterology*, vol. 20, no. 36, pp. 12956–12980, 2014.

[4] R. L. Corrado, D. M. Torres, and S. A. Harrison, "Review of treatment options for nonalcoholic fatty liver disease," *Medical Clinics of North America*, vol. 98, no. 1, pp. 55–72, 2014.

[5] A. Eguchi, D. Povero, N. Alkhouri, and A. E. Feldstein, "Novel therapeutic targets for nonalcoholic fatty liver disease," *Expert Opinion on Therapeutic Targets*, vol. 17, no. 7, pp. 773–779, 2013.

[6] P. Uhl, G. Fricker, U. Haberkorn, and W. Mier, "Current status in the therapy of liver diseases," *International Journal of Molecular Sciences*, vol. 15, no. 5, pp. 7500–7512, 2014.

[7] M. Mouzaki and J. Allard, "Non-alcoholic steatohepatitis: the therapeutic challenge of a global epidemic," *Annals of Gastroenterology*, vol. 25, no. 3, pp. 207–217, 2012.

[8] R. Jadeja, R. V. Devkar, and S. Nammi, "Herbal medicines for the treatment of nonalcoholic steatohepatitis: current scenario and future prospects," *Evidence-Based Complementary and Alternative Medicine*, vol. 2014, Article ID 648308, 18 pages, 2014.

[9] N. Mulinacci, D. Prucher, M. Peruzzi et al., "Commercial and laboratory extracts from artichoke leaves: estimation of caffeoyl esters and flavonoidic compounds content," *Journal of Pharmaceutical and Biomedical Analysis*, vol. 34, no. 2, pp. 349–357, 2004.

[10] A. Y. Leung and S. Foster, *Encyclopedia of Common Natural Ingredients Used in Food. Drugs and Cosmetics*, John Wiley & Sons, New York, NY, USA, 2nd edition, 1996.

[11] C. A. Newall, L. A. Anderson, and J. D. Phillipson, *Herbal Medicines: A Guide for Health-Care Professionals*, The Pharmaceutical Press, London, UK, 1996.

[12] E. Speroni, R. Cervellati, P. Govoni, S. Guizzardi, C. Renzulli, and M. C. Guerra, "Efficacy of different *Cynara scolymus* preparations on liver complaints," *Journal of Ethnopharmacology*, vol. 86, no. 2-3, pp. 203–211, 2003.

[13] X. Zhu, H. Zhang, and R. Lo, "Phenolic compounds from the leaf extract of artichoke (*Cynara scolymus* L.) and their antimicrobial activities," *Journal of Agricultural and Food Chemistry*, vol. 52, no. 24, pp. 7272–7278, 2004.

[14] Z. Küskü-Kiraz, G. Mehmetçik, S. Dogru-Abbasoglu, and M. Uysal, "Artichoke leaf extract reduces oxidative stress and lipoprotein dyshomeostasis in rats fed on high cholesterol diet," *Phytotherapy Research*, vol. 24, no. 4, pp. 565–570, 2010.

[15] D. Zapolska-Downar, A. Zapolski-Downar, M. Naruszewicz, A. Siennicka, B. Krasnodbska, and B. Kolodziej, "Protective properties of artichoke (*Cynara scolymus*) against oxidative stress induced in cultured endothelial cells and monocytes," *Life Sciences*, vol. 71, no. 24, pp. 2897–2908, 2002.

[16] A. Jiménez-Escrig, L. O. Dragsted, B. Daneshvar, R. Pulido, and F. Saura-Calixto, "In vitro antioxidant activities of edible artichoke (*Cynara scolymus* L.) and effect on biomarkers of antioxidants in rats," *Journal of Agricultural and Food Chemistry*, vol. 51, no. 18, pp. 5540–5545, 2003.

[17] S. Reitman and S. Frankel, "Colorimetric method for the determination of serum glutamic oxalacetic and glutamic pyruvic transaminases," *American Journal of Clinical Pathology*, vol. 28, no. 1, pp. 56–63, 1957.

[18] C. C. Allain, L. S. Poon, C. S. Chan, W. Richmond, and P. C. Fu, "Enzymatic determination of total serum cholesterol," *Clinical Chemistry*, vol. 20, pp. 470–475, 1974.

[19] G. Assmann, H.-U. Jabs, U. Kohnert, W. Nolte, and H. Schriewer, "LDL-cholesterol determination in blood serum following precipitation of LDL with polyvinylsulfate," *Clinica Chimica Acta*, vol. 140, no. 1, pp. 77–83, 1984.

[20] M. F. Lopez-Virella, P. Stone, S. Elli, and J. A. Golwell, "Cholesterol determination in HDL-chol separated by three different methods," *Clinical Chemistry*, vol. 23, no. 5, pp. 882–884, 1977.

[21] P. Fossati and L. Prencipe, "Serum triglycerides determined colorimetrically with an enzyme that produces hydrogen peroxide," *Clinical Chemistry*, vol. 28, no. 10, pp. 2077–2080, 1982.

[22] S. R. Naik and V. S. Panda, "Antioxidant and hepatoprotective effects of Ginkgo biloba phytosomes in carbon tetrachloride-induced liver injury in rodents," *Liver International*, vol. 27, no. 3, pp. 393–399, 2007.

[23] E. Azzini, R. Bugianesi, F. Romano et al., "Absorption and metabolism of bioactive molecules after oral consumption of cooked edible heads of *Cynara scolymus* L. (Cultivar Violetto di Provenza) in human subjects: a pilot study," *The British Journal of Nutrition*, vol. 97, no. 5, pp. 963–969, 2007.

[24] S. M. Wittemer, M. Ploch, T. Windeck et al., "Bioavailability and pharmacokinetics of caffeoylquinic acids and flavonoids after oral administration of Artichoke leaf extracts in humans," *Phytomedicine*, vol. 12, no. 1-2, pp. 28–38, 2005.

[25] K. Schütz, D. Kammerer, R. Carle, and A. Schieber, "Identification and quantification of caffeoylquinic acids and flavonoids from artichoke (*Cynara scolymus* L.) heads, juice, and pomace by HPLC-DAD-ESI/MSn," *Journal of Agricultural and Food Chemistry*, vol. 52, no. 13, pp. 4090–4096, 2004.

[26] R. Gebhardt, "Inhibition of cholesterol biosynthesis in primary cultured rat hepatocytes by artichoke (*Cynara scolymus* L) extracts," *Journal of Pharmacology and Experimental Therapeutics*, vol. 286, no. 3, pp. 1122–1128, 1998.

[27] J. Vaya and M. Aviram, "Nutritional antioxidants mechanisms of action, analyses of activities and medical applications," *Current Medicinal Chemistry-Immunology, Endocrine & Metabolic Agents*, vol. 1, no. 1, pp. 99–117, 2001.

[28] I. Urquiaga and F. Leighton, "Plant polyphenol antioxidants and oxidative stress," *Biological Research*, vol. 33, no. 2, pp. 55–64, 2000.

[29] E. Heidarian, Y. Soofiniya, and R. Hajihosseini, "The effect of aerial part of *Cynara scolymus* extract on the hyperlipidemia, plasma antioxidant capacity, and superoxide dismutase activity in diabetic rats," *Journal of Shahrekord University of Medical Sciences*, vol. 13, no. 5, pp. 1–10, 2013.

[30] N. S. Metwally, T. E. Kholeif, K. Z. Ghanem, A. R. H. Farrag, N. M. Ammar, and A. H. Z. Abdel-Hamid, "The protective effects of fish oil and artichoke on hepatocellular carcinoma in rats," *European Review for Medical and Pharmacological Sciences*, vol. 15, no. 12, pp. 1429–1444, 2011.

[31] G. Mehmetçik, G. Özdemirler, N. Koçak-Toker, U. Çevikbaş, and M. Uysal, "Effect of pretreatment with artichoke extract on carbon tetrachloride-induced liver injury and oxidative stress," *Experimental and Toxicologic Pathology*, vol. 60, no. 6, pp. 475–480, 2008.

[32] S. Miccadei, D. D. Venere, A. Cardinali et al., "Antioxidative and apoptotic properties of polyphenolic extracts from edible part of artichoke (*Cynara scolymus* L.) on cultured rat hepatocytes and on human hepatoma cells," *Nutrition and Cancer*, vol. 60, no. 2, pp. 276–283, 2008.

[33] M. Safaa, A. Hanaa, F. Abdel, A. Nahila, and S. Abdelaaty, "Cynara scolymus for relieving on nonalcoholic steatohepatitis

induced in rat," *International Journal of Pharmacy and Pharmaceutical Sciences*, vol. 5, no. 1, pp. 57–66, 2013.

[34] R. Huber, M. Müller, J. Naumann, T. Schenk, and R. Lüdtke, "Artichoke leave extract for chronic hepatitis C—a pilot study," *Phytomedicine*, vol. 16, no. 9, pp. 801–804, 2009.

[35] M. H. Pittler, C. J. Thompson, and E. Ernst, "Artichoke leaf extract for treating hypercholesterolaemia," *The Cochrane Database of Systematic Reviews*, no. 4, Article ID CD003335, 2009.

[36] H. Shimoda, K. Ninomiya, N. Nishida et al., "Anti-hyperlipidemic sesquiterpenes and new sesquiterpene glycosides from the leaves of artichoke (*Cynara scolymus* L.): structure requirement and mode of action," *Bioorganic and Medicinal Chemistry Letters*, vol. 13, no. 2, pp. 223–228, 2003.

[37] Z. Qiang, S.-O. Lee, Z. Ye, X. Wu, and S. Hendrich, "Artichoke extract lowered plasma cholesterol and increased fecal bile acids in Golden Syrian hamsters," *Phytotherapy Research*, vol. 26, no. 7, pp. 1048–1052, 2012.

[38] W. J. Arion, W. K. Canfield, F. C. Ramos et al., "Chlorogenic acid and hydroxynitrobenzaldehyde: new inhibitors of hepatic glucose 6-phosphatase," *Archives of Biochemistry and Biophysics*, vol. 339, no. 2, pp. 315–322, 1997.

[39] A. A. Cetto and H. Wiedenfeld, "Hypoglycemic effect of *Cecropia obtusifolia* on streptozotocin diabetic rats," *Ethnopharmacology*, vol. 78, no. 2-3, pp. 145–149, 2001.

[40] P. Simonen, A. Kotronen, M. Hallikainen et al., "Cholesterol synthesis is increased and absorption decreased in non-alcoholic fatty liver disease independent of obesity," *Journal of Hepatology*, vol. 54, no. 1, pp. 153–159, 2011.

[41] M. S. Brown and J. L. Goldstein, "The SREBP pathway: regulation of cholesterol metabolism by proteolysis of a membrane-bound transcription factor," *Cell*, vol. 89, no. 3, pp. 331–340, 1997.

[42] E. Ikonen, "Cellular cholesterol trafficking and compartmentalization," *Nature Reviews Molecular Cell Biology*, vol. 9, no. 2, pp. 125–138, 2008.

[43] F. Caballero, A. Fernandez, A. M. De Lacy, J. C. Fernandez-Checa, J. Caballeria, and C. Garcia-Ruiz, "Enhanced free cholesterol SREBP-2 and StAR expression in human NASH," *Journal of Hepatology*, vol. 50, no. 4, pp. 789–796, 2009.

# 33

# Sofosbuvir Plus Daclatasvir in Treatment of Chronic Hepatitis C Genotype 4 Infection in a Cohort of Egyptian Patients: An Experiment the Size of Egyptian Village

**Ossama Ashraf Ahmed,[1] Eslam Safwat,[1] Mohamed Omar Khalifa,[2] Ahmed I. Elshafie,[1] Mohamed Hassan Ahmed Fouad,[1] Mohamed Magdy Salama,[1] Gina Gamal Naguib,[1] Mohamed Mahmoud Eltabbakh,[2] Ahmed Fouad Sherief,[2] and Sherief Abd-Elsalam[3]**

[1]*Internal Medicine Department, Gastroenterology and Hepatology Unit, Ain Shams University, Cairo, Egypt*
[2]*Tropical Medicine Department, Ain Shams University, Cairo, Egypt*
[3]*Tropical Medicine & Infectious Diseases Department, Tanta University, Tanta, Egypt*

Correspondence should be addressed to Sherief Abd-Elsalam; sherif_tropical@yahoo.com

Academic Editor: Daisuke Morioka

*Background and Aims.* As indicated by the World Health Organization (WHO), Egypt is positioned as the country with the world's highest prevalence of Hepatitis C virus (HCV). HCV is transmitted through unexamined blood transfusions, different employments of syringes, and poor cleansing, as per the WHO. Our study aimed at screening and management of chronic hepatitis C genotype 4 infected patients in Bardeen village, Sharkeya Governorate, Egypt, with Sofosbuvir plus Daclatasvir, as well as estimating the safety and efficacy of that regimen. *Methods.* Screening of adult patients in Bardeen village was done from March 2016 till November 2016 using hepatitis C virus antibodies by third-generation ELISA testing. Positive results were confirmed by PCR. Patients eligible for treatment received Sofosbuvir 400 mg and Daclatasvir 60 mg daily for 12 weeks and were assessed for sustained virologic response at 12 weeks following the end of treatment (SVR 12). *Results.* Out of 2047 subjects screened for hepatitis C virus, 249 (12.2%) showed positive results. 221 out of those 249 subjects (88.7%) had detectable RNA by PCR. Treatment of eligible patients (183 patients) with Sofosbuvir plus Daclatasvir for 12 weeks resulted in 96% achievement of sustained virologic response at week 12. Adverse events were tolerable. *Conclusion.* Sofosbuvir plus Daclatasvir regimen is safe and effective for treatment of chronic hepatitis C Genotype 4 infected patients with minimal adverse events. HCV eradication program implemented in Egypt can be a model for other countries with HCV and limited resources. The availability of generic drugs in Egypt will help much in eradication of the virus.

## 1. Introduction

Several recent studies discussed the epidemiology of HCV infection worldwide. It is estimated that 10.4 million patients are infected with HCV genotype 4 which accounts for 13% of all HCV infections worldwide. HCV genotype 4 infection is common in the Middle East, Northern Africa, and Sub-Saharan Africa. In Egypt, 15% of an estimated population of 80 million is HCV positive, of which 93% are infected with genotype 4 [1–5].

During the past few years, there have been enormous efforts to understand the structure and life cycle of hepatitis C virus (HCV) and to develop specific medications targeting different viral proteins such as NS3/4A protease, NS5B polymerase, and NS5A replication complex. The discovery of direct acting antiviral agents (DAAs) represented a revolution in the management of chronic hepatitis C virus infection [6].

The pipeline of treatment regimens included combining interferon with DAAs with or without Ribavirin. Later on, interferon-free regimens were introduced through combining different classes of DAAs together. A need has arisen for a DAA based regimen that is pangenotypic, is well tolerated with minimal adverse effects, has low pill burden, and shows minimal drug interactions [7].

Daclatasvir is an NS5A inhibitor with pangenotypic activity that is effective against the six major HCV genotypes with a pharmacokinetic profile permitting once-daily dosing. Daclatasvir is well tolerated. Headache is the most frequently encountered adverse event. Daclatasvir is a weak inducer of cytochrome P450 and thus it has minimal drug interactions. In addition, its metabolism is mainly hepatic, which permits its use without dose adjustments in patients with chronic kidney disease. For prevention of emergence of resistant infections, an appropriate dose of Daclatasvir in combination with other suitable DAAs is recommended [8].

Sofosbuvir is another pangenotypic oral NS5B inhibitor with once-daily dosing that is both effective and tolerable. It has few drug interactions. Sofosbuvir/Daclatasvir combination is associated with a high rate of SVR in genotype 1 or 4 patients who are assumed to be difficult to treat. Adding Ribavirin increases the SVR rate in treatment-experienced and cirrhotic patients [4, 8].

Both agents have proven effectiveness against HCV genotype 4 infections in phase III ALLY-1, ALLY-2, and ALLY-3 studies that evaluate the role of this combination among different HCV genotypes. Phase II IMPACT study evaluates this combination in addition to Simeprevir in treatment of HCV genotypes 1 and 4 DAA-naïve patients with portal hypertension or decompensated cirrhosis. All patients achieved SVR12 regardless of the presence of baseline detectable resistance-associated mutations in 83% of patients [9].

Our study aimed at screening and management of chronic hepatitis C genotype 4 infected patients in Bardeen village, Sharkeya Governorate, Egypt, with Sofosbuvir plus Daclatasvir, as well as estimating the safety and efficacy of that regimen.

## 2. Subjects and Methods

This study was a prospective observational study conducted in Bardeen village (Sharkeya Governorate, Egypt) between March 2016 and November 2016. Adult patients (≥18 years) underwent HCV screening using HCV antibodies by third-generation ELISA. Those with positive HCV antibodies were submitted to clinical, laboratory, and imaging assessment prior to treatment.

Before treatment, all patients were subjected to a full medical history including history of previous treatment for HCV and any features of decompensated cirrhosis and a thorough clinical examination. Baseline laboratory studies were done including liver function tests, kidney function tests with estimation of glomerular filtration rate (eGFR), complete blood count, alpha fetoprotein, HBsAg, pregnancy test for females at child bearing age, and abdominal ultrasonography. Blood samples were obtained from all patients, centrifuged, and then stored at −20°C until measurements. A quantitative measurement serum load of HCV was performed by real-time PCR (Cobas Ampliprep/Taqman HCV Monitor version 2.0, with a detection limit of 15 IU/ml; Roche Diagnostic Systems, Pleasanton, California, USA), and it was repeated at the end of treatment, and 12 weeks after treatment to detect SVR 12. All included patients were assumed to have HCV genotype 4.

Treatment-experienced patients and patients with hepatitis B virus coinfection, advanced liver disease (decompensated cirrhosis) or HCC, eGFR < 30 ml/min, haemoglobin less than 10 g/dl, or platelet count less than 50,000/mm$^3$ were referred for further pretreatment assessment and were excluded from the current study.

Treatment eligible patients received Sofosbuvir 400 mg and Daclatasvir 60 mg daily for 12 weeks. During treatment, they were closely monitored at week 2, week 4, week 8, and week 12 by laboratory studies including CBC, creatinine, AST, ALT, and total bilirubin.

The primary end point of our study was detecting the percentage of genotype 4 hepatitis C virus infected treatment-naïve participants with sustained virologic response at follow-up week 12 (SVR12). The secondary end point of our study was detection of any adverse events with treatment.

All patients signed a written informed consent prior to inclusion into this study and institutional ethical committee in Tanta University Faculty of Medicine approved the study. The study protocol conforms to the ethical guidelines of the 1975 Declaration of Helsinki (6th revision, 2008).

All collected data were analysed and correlated. Statistical analysis was performed using the Statistical Package for Social Sciences (SPSS) version 24. Basic descriptive statistics including means and standard deviations were performed. Comparison of qualitative data between groups was performed using Chi-square test. Independent *t*-test or Mann–Whitney *U* test were used to compare quantitative data between groups with parametric distribution or nonparametric distribution, respectively. The continuous variables across time were compared using paired *t*-test or Wilcoxon Signed-Rank Test. Differences were considered statistically significant if the *P* value was less than 0.05.

## 3. Results

This study was conducted between March 2016 and November 2016 in Bardeen Village from Sharkeya Governorate, Egypt. 2047 adult Egyptians were screened for HCV antibodies by ELISA. 249 subjects (12.2%) showed positive results. Real-time PCR for detection of HCV RNA was done for antibody positive patients where 28 subjects (11.3%) were found to have undetectable level of HCV RNA, whereas 221 subjects (88.7%) had detectable HCV RNA by PCR.

Further assessment of the 221 patients that had detectable PCR for HCV RNA yielded 183 patients (82.8%) that were eligible for treatment, while 38 patients (17.2%) were deferred from the study according to our exclusion criteria. 19 of those patients suffered advanced liver disease (decompensated cirrhosis and HCC) (50%), 3 patients were pregnant (7.9%), another 3 patients were coinfected with hepatitis B virus (7.9%), and 13 more patients had hematologic problems (platelet count below 50000/mm$^3$ or haemoglobin level below 10 gm/dl) (34.2%%).

Treatment eligible group included 183 patients who started Sofosbuvir 400 mg daily plus Daclatasvir 60 mg daily for 3 months. After starting treatment, 6 patients (3.3%) were lost during follow-up, while 177 patients (96.7%) completed their treatment course. Their mean age was 48.53 ± 12.93. 75

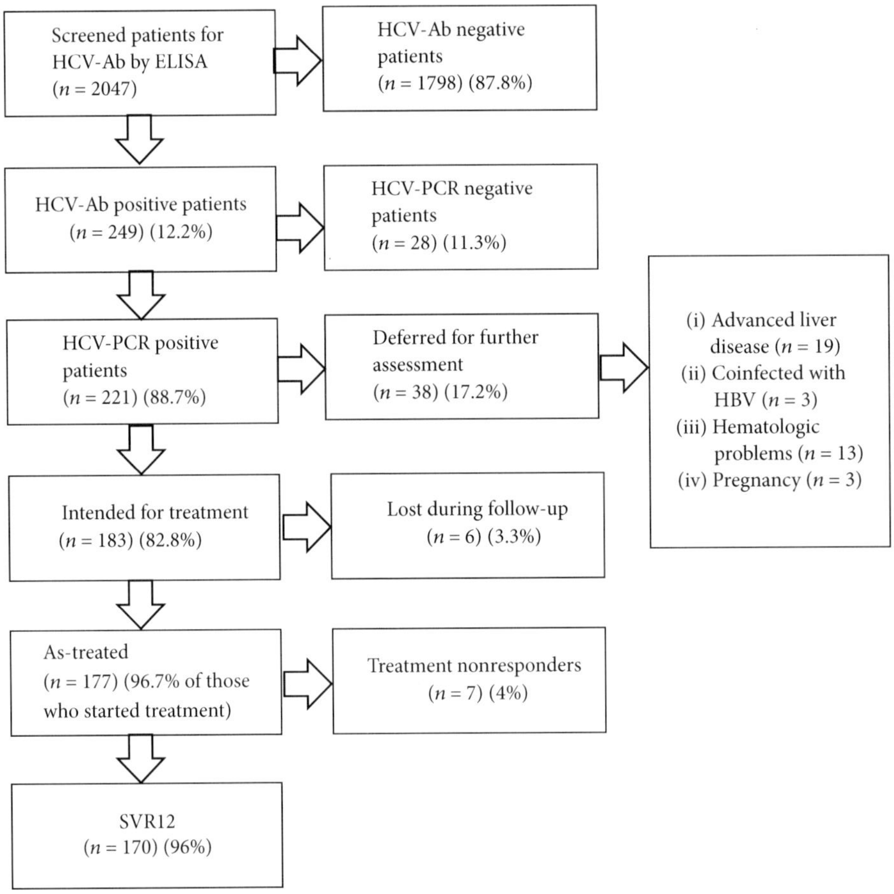


Figure 1: Study design.

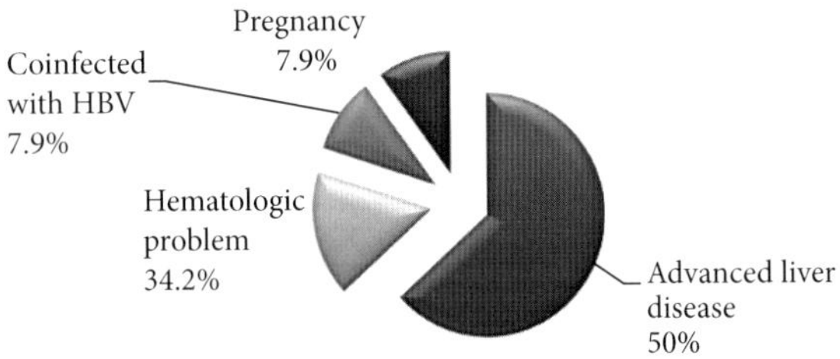


Figure 2: Analysis of causes of deferral from the current study.

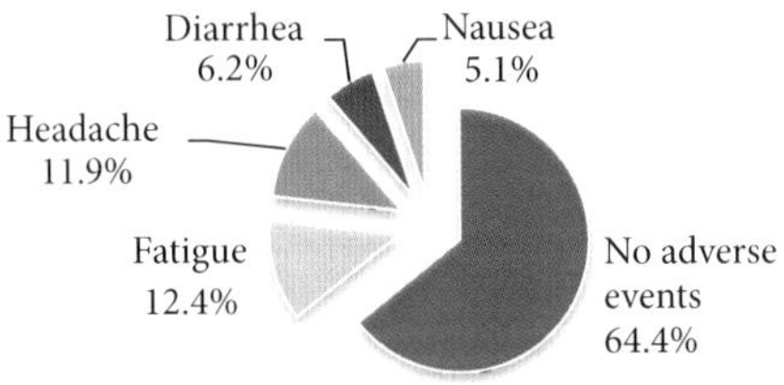


Figure 3: Adverse events for Sofosbuvir/Daclatasvir regimen.

patients were males (42.4%) and 102 patients were females (57.6%) (Figures 1 and 2).

Neither age nor gender nor pretreatment biochemical profile showed any statistically significant correlation with treatment outcome (Table 1).

114 of the as-treated group (64.4%) tolerated medications with no notable adverse events. 22 patients (12.4%) experienced fatigue, 21 patients (11.9%) experienced headache, 11 patients (6.2%) experienced diarrhea, and 9 patients (5.1%) experienced nausea (Figure 3).

Within the 177 patients who completed 12 weeks of treatment, 170 patients (96%) achieved SVR12 (negative PCR at week 12 following end of treatment). 7 patients (4%) were treatment nonresponders and were scheduled for retreatment in the nonresponders clinic.

Regarding treatment responders, pretreatment ALT showed a median value of 40 IU/L, while posttreatment ALT showed a median of 24 IU/L. Pretreatment AST showed a median value of 40 IU/L, while posttreatment AST showed a median value of 25 IU/L. Statistically significant reductions in ALT and AST were observed in responders following 12 weeks of treatment ($P < 0.001$).

## 4. Discussion

Chronic hepatitis C virus infection is a major health issue worldwide. It is the leading cause of liver-related morbidity

TABLE 1: Relation between patients' age and baseline biochemical parameters and achievement of SVR.

| Baseline data | Response to Treatment Nonresponder ($n$ = 7) Mean ± SD/median (IQR) | Responder ($n$ = 177) Mean ± SD/median (IQR) | $P$ |
|---|---|---|---|
| Age | 48.86 ± 9.17 | 48.57 ± 13.09 | 0.95* |
| ALT (IU/l) | 24 (21–41) | 40 (26.75–60.25) | 0.2** |
| AST (IU/l) | 35 (20–56) | 40 (27–67) | 0.39** |
| S. albumin (g/dl) | 3.7 (3.3–4.2) | 4.1 (3.87–4.4) | 0.056** |
| Total bil. (mg/dl) | 0.7 (0.45–1) | 0.7 (0.5–0.9) | 0.69** |
| INR | 1.05 (1–1.19) | 1.05 (1–1.13) | 0.96** |
| HCV-RNA | 266591 (110000–3800000) | 220500 (45000–864307.25) | 0.95** |
| TLC ($\times10^3$/mm$^3$) | 5.9 (4.5–8.3) | 7 (4.85–8.35) | 0.51** |
| HGB (gm/l) | 12.63 ± 0.64 | 12.94 ± 1.75 | 0.72* |
| PLT ($\times10^3$/mm$^3$) | 186.29 ± 85.35 | 233.61 ± 66.91 | 0.07* |
| Creatinine (mg/dl) | 0.94 ± 0.21 | 0.87 ± 0.22 | 0.44* |

*Independent $t$-test; **Mann–Whitney $U$ test; ALT: alanine transaminase, AST: aspartate transaminase, bil.: bilirubin, HGB: haemoglobin, INR: international normalized ratio, IQR: interquartile range, TLC: total leucocytic count, PLT: platelet.

and mortality in Egypt and one of the most common indications for liver transplantation. The introduction of direct acting antiviral agents shifted the management of chronic HCV infection to a new level. The combination of Sofosbuvir plus Daclatasvir proved to be very effective in treating hepatitis C virus infection, particularly genotype 1. However, data on genotype 4 are still deficient.

This observational study was conducted on a cohort of patients from Bardeen village, Sharkeya Governorate, Egypt. The prevalence of HCV antibody positive subjects and that of RNA positive subjects were 12.2% and 10.8%, respectively. This goes in agreement with CDC statistics which estimates the prevalence of chronic HCV infection in Egypt as 10%.

More than 2000 individuals were screened where 12% of them were anti-HCV positive. The majority of these were HCV RNA positive, and only 11% had spontaneously cleared their HCV infection. In the current study, 96% of as-treated population showed SVR12.

Only 177 of the screened patients were directly managed by our team. Only 7 of them were nonresponders. They were referred to "nonresponders clinic" where they started receiving Sofosbuvir/Daclatasvir/Simeprevir/Ribavirin regimen and were managed separately.

Sulkowski et al. studied the effect of Sofosbuvir plus Daclatasvir on treatment naïve genotype 1 chronic hepatitis C infected patients in one arm of their study which showed that 100% of patients in that arm ($N$ = 41) achieved SVR12 after completing 12 weeks of treatment [10].

In a study by Fontaine et al. in 2015, 82 genotype 4 infected patients were treated with Sofosbuvir plus Daclatasvir with or without Ribavirin and with or without Simeprevir. The 33 patients who received Sofosbuvir plus Daclatasvir only were subjected to statistical analysis. SVR12 was achieved in 88.9% of those patients. However, this could be explained by the fact that the studied group included patients who were difficult to treat, whether because they were treatment-experienced or with advanced liver disease [11]. Another large study in Egypt documented the high SVR12 in patients receiving generic Sofosbuvir and Daclatasvir [12].

Regarding the patients who were excluded from the study, 19 patients with advanced liver disease were referred as part of our protocol to "Advanced Cirrhosis Clinic" where they receive assessment for liver transplantation and possible preemptive therapy. However, we did not include them in our study. Thirteen patients with hematological problems including anemia, thrombocytopenia, and other suspected blood disorders were routinely referred to "Hematology Clinic" where they were investigated for the cause of the hematologic disorder and then referred back for comanagement of hepatitis C in specialized HCV treatment unit with hematology. Three coinfected HBV/HCV patients were referred as part of our protocol to "Coinfection Clinic" in specialized hepatitis C treatment center where they had undergone further assessment for combined HBV/HCV treatment with Sofosbuvir/Daclatasvir/tenofovir. However, we did not include them in our study. Three pregnant ladies were listed for treatment after delivery. However, we did not include them in our study. This real life experiment describes the challenges which we face in our attempt for complete eradication of hepatitis C virus.

In the current study, 114 of the as-treated group (64.4%) tolerated Sofosbuvir plus Daclatasvir with no notable adverse events. None of our patients died during treatment and none of them stopped treatment due to significant adverse events. 22 patients of the as-treated population (12.4%) experienced fatigue, 21 patients (11.9%) experienced headache, 11 patients (6.2%) experienced diarrhea, and 9 patients (5.1%) experienced nausea. This came in accordance with Babatin et al. who studied 96 patients with chronic HCV genotype 4 who were treated by Sofosbuvir plus Daclatasvir or Sofosbuvir plus Simeprevir. The Sofosbuvir plus Daclatasvir arm included 40 patients. 42.5% of those patients developed adverse events where 27.5% suffered fatigue, 25% suffered headache, 7.5% suffered nausea, 10% suffered insomnia, 3% suffered nausea, and 4% suffered diarrhea [13].

There was significant reduction in AST and ALT level ($P$ < 0.001 for both) after completion of the antiviral treatment which came in accordance with one previous study by Mehta et al. in 2017 who studied the safety and efficacy of Sofosbuvir and Daclatasvir for treatment of chronic hepatitis C infection in a group of patients with B-Thalassemia major. Treatment responders showed significant improvement in transaminases compared to pretreatment values after 12 weeks of treatment with Sofosbuvir plus Daclatasvir indicating their role in improving necroinflammation in patients with chronic HCV. However, the study was carried on genotype 3 thalassemic patients [14].

In the current study, neither age nor any of the pretreatment biochemical markers including haemoglobin, leukocytic count, platelet count, ALT, AST, albumin, INR, bilirubin, and PCR for HCV RNA showed significant correlation with treatment outcome. To our knowledge, this is one of the first studies to assess the pretreatment laboratory results as predictors for HCV genotype 4 response to Sofosbuvir plus Daclatasvir regimen.

A more interesting part is the epidemiology and the actual percentage of persons that were reached and treated in this study. The introduction of novel direct acting antiretroviral drugs in treating hepatitis C in Egypt has led to widespread treatment to become the largest program to treat hepatitis C virus worldwide [15]. Thanks to novel drugs, we are now talking of the possibility of eradicate hepatitis C virus. Also, the availability of generic drugs reduced costs, and will help in achieving complete eradication of HCV.

Finally, we can conclude that Sofosbuvir and Daclatasvir are effective in treatment of chronic HCV genotype 4 infections with minimal adverse events. Pretreatment liver chemistry does not seem to correlate with treatment outcome.

## Authors' Contributions

All authors contributed equally to this work. All the authors participated sufficiently in the work and approved the final version of the manuscript.

## References


[1] E. Gower, C. C. Estes, S. Hindman, K. Razavi-Shearer, and H. Razavi, "Global epidemiology and genotype distribution of the hepatitis C virus," *Journal of Hepatology*, vol. 61, supplement 1, pp. S45–S57, 2014.

[2] A. E. M. Aly Abd Elrazek, S. E. Bilasy, A. E. M. Elbanna, and A. E. A. Elsherif, "Prior to the oral therapy, what do we know about HCV-4 in Egypt: a randomized survey of prevalence and risks using data mining computed analysis," *Medicine (United States)*, vol. 93, no. 28, p. e204, 2014.

[3] N. Elwan, A. Elfert, S. Abd-Elsalam et al., "Study of hepatic steatosis index in patients with chronic HCV infection," *International Journal of Current Microbiology and Applied Sciences*, vol. 5, no. 5, pp. 266–279, 2016.

[4] S. Abd-Elsalam, M. Sharaf-Eldin, S. Soliman, A. Elfert, R. Badawi, and Y. K. Ahmad, "Efficacy and safety of sofosbuvir plus ribavirin for treatment of cirrhotic patients with genotype 4 hepatitis C virus in real-life clinical practice," *Archives of Virology*, pp. 1–6, 2017.

[5] O. A. Ahmed, H. H. Kaisar, N. Hawash et al., "Efficacy of sofosbuvir plus ribavirin with or without peginterferon-alfa in treatment of a cohort of egyptian patients with hepatitis C virus infection," *Infectious Disorders—Drug Targets*, vol. 17, no. 2, pp. 95–100, 2017.

[6] G. Bertino, A. Ardiri, M. Proiti et al., "Chronic hepatitis C: this and the new era of treatment," *World Journal of Hepatology*, vol. 8, no. 2, pp. 92–106, 2016.

[7] D. Banerjee and K. R. Reddy, "Review article: Safety and tolerability of direct-acting anti-viral agents in the new era of hepatitis C therapy," *Alimentary Pharmacology & Therapeutics*, vol. 43, no. 6, pp. 674–696, 2016.

[8] S. Pol, A. Vallet-Pichard, and M. Corouge, "Daclatasvir-sofosbuvir combination therapy with or without ribavirin for hepatitis C virus infection: from the clinical trials to real life," *Hepatic Medicine: Evidence and Research*, vol. 8, pp. 21–26, 2016.

[9] E. Hathorn and A. M. Elsharkawy, "Management of hepatitis C genotype 4 in the directly acting antivirals era," *BMJ Open Gastroenterology*, vol. 3, no. 1, Article ID e000112, 2016.

[10] M. S. Sulkowski, D. F. Gardiner, M. Rodriguez-Torres et al., "Daclatasvir plus sofosbuvir for previously treated or untreated chronic HCV infection," *The New England Journal of Medicine*, vol. 370, no. 15, pp. 1469-1469, 2014.

[11] H. Fontaine, C. Hezode, F. Zoulim et al., "Efficacy of the oral sofosbuvir-based combinations in HCV genotype 4-monoinfected patients from the french observational cohort ANRS CO22 Hepather," in *Proceedings of the 50th Annual Meeting of European Association for the Study of thel Liver*, Vienna, Austria, April 2015.

[12] H. Omar, W. El Akel, T. Elbaz et al., "Generic daclatasvir plus sofosbuvir, with or without ribavirin, in treatment of chronic hepatitis C: real-world results from 18 378 patients in Egypt," *Alimentary Pharmacology & Therapeutics*, vol. 47, no. 3, pp. 421–431, 2018.

[13] M. A. Babatin, A. S. Alghamdi, A. Albenmousa et al., "Efficacy and safety of simeprevir or daclatasvir in combination with sofosbuvir for the treatment of hepatitis C genotype 4 infection," *Journal of Clinical Gastroenterology*, Article ID 28767462, 2017.

[14] R. Mehta, M. Kabrawala, S. Nandwani et al., "Safety and efficacy of sofosbuvir and daclatasvir for hepatitis C virus infection in patients with $\beta$-thalassemia major," *Journal of Clinical and Experimental Hepatology*, 2017.

[15] A. Elsharkawy, M. El-Raziky, W. El-Akel et al., "Planning and prioritizing direct-acting antivirals treatment for HCV patients in countries with limited resources: lessons from the egyptian experience," *Journal of Hepatology*, 2017.

# Permissions

All chapters in this book were first published in IJH, by Hindawi Publishing Corporation; hereby published with permission under the Creative Commons Attribution License or equivalent. Every chapter published in this book has been scrutinized by our experts. Their significance has been extensively debated. The topics covered herein carry significant findings which will fuel the growth of the discipline. They may even be implemented as practical applications or may be referred to as a beginning point for another development.

The contributors of this book come from diverse backgrounds, making this book a truly international effort. This book will bring forth new frontiers with its revolutionizing research information and detailed analysis of the nascent developments around the world.

We would like to thank all the contributing authors for lending their expertise to make the book truly unique. They have played a crucial role in the development of this book. Without their invaluable contributions this book wouldn't have been possible. They have made vital efforts to compile up to date information on the varied aspects of this subject to make this book a valuable addition to the collection of many professionals and students.

This book was conceptualized with the vision of imparting up-to-date information and advanced data in this field. To ensure the same, a matchless editorial board was set up. Every individual on the board went through rigorous rounds of assessment to prove their worth. After which they invested a large part of their time researching and compiling the most relevant data for our readers.

The editorial board has been involved in producing this book since its inception. They have spent rigorous hours researching and exploring the diverse topics which have resulted in the successful publishing of this book. They have passed on their knowledge of decades through this book. To expedite this challenging task, the publisher supported the team at every step. A small team of assistant editors was also appointed to further simplify the editing procedure and attain best results for the readers.

Apart from the editorial board, the designing team has also invested a significant amount of their time in understanding the subject and creating the most relevant covers. They scrutinized every image to scout for the most suitable representation of the subject and create an appropriate cover for the book.

The publishing team has been an ardent support to the editorial, designing and production team. Their endless efforts to recruit the best for this project, has resulted in the accomplishment of this book. They are a veteran in the field of academics and their pool of knowledge is as vast as their experience in printing. Their expertise and guidance has proved useful at every step. Their uncompromising quality standards have made this book an exceptional effort. Their encouragement from time to time has been an inspiration for everyone.

The publisher and the editorial board hope that this book will prove to be a valuable piece of knowledge for researchers, students, practitioners and scholars across the globe.

# Contributors

**Yi-Hsin Liang**
Department of Hemato-Oncology, E-Da Hospital, No. 1, Yi-da Road, Jiaosu Village, Yanchao, Kaohsiung 82445, Taiwan
Department of Oncology, National Taiwan University Hospital, No. 7, Chung-Shan South Road, Taipei City 10002, Taiwan

**Jia-Yi Chen**
Department of Oncology, National Taiwan University Hospital, No. 7, Chung-Shan South Road, Taipei City 10002, Taiwan

**Yu-Yun Shao**
Department of Oncology, National Taiwan University Hospital, No. 7, Chung-Shan South Road, Taipei City 10002, Taiwan
Graduate Institute of Oncology, College of Medicine, National Taiwan University, No. 1, Section 1, Ren-Ai Road, Taipei City 10051, Taiwan

**Po Ann-Lii Cheng**
Department of Oncology, National Taiwan University Hospital, No. 7, Chung-Shan South Road, Taipei City 10002, Taiwan
Graduate Institute of Oncology, College of Medicine, National Taiwan University, No. 1, Section 1, Ren-Ai Road, Taipei City 10051, Taiwan
Department of Internal Medicine, National Taiwan University Hospital, No. 7, Chung-Shan South Road, Taipei City 10002, Taiwan

**Zhong-Zhe Lin**
Department of Oncology, National Taiwan University Hospital, No. 7, Chung-Shan South Road, Taipei City 10002, Taiwan
Department of Internal Medicine, National Taiwan University Hospital, No. 7, Chung-Shan South Road, Taipei City 10002, Taiwan

**Chin Liang**
Department ofMedical Imaging, National Taiwan University Hospital, No. 7, Chung-Shan South Road, Taipei City 10002, Taiwan

**Sona Chandra**
Department of Biomedical Engineering, Georgia Institute of Technology, Atlanta, GA 30332, USA

**Shannon Luetkemeyer**
Children's Healthcare of Atlanta, Transplant Services, Atlanta, GA 30322, USA

**Rene Romero and Nitika Arora Gupta**
Children's Healthcare of Atlanta, Transplant Services, Atlanta, GA 30322, USA
Department of Pediatrics, Emory University School of Medicine, Health Science Research Building (HSRB), Suite No. E200, Office No. 216, Atlanta, GA 30322, USA

**M. Pitchaimuthu, G. Aidoo-Micah, C. Coldham, R. Sutcliffe, J. K. Roberts, P. Muiesan, J. Isaac, D. Mirza, andR. Marudanayagam**
Liver and HPB Unit, Queen Elizabeth Hospital, University Hospitals Birmingham NHS Foundation Trust, Birmingham B15 2TH, UK

**Toru Yanagawa and Hiroki Bukawa**
Department of Oral and Maxillofacial Surgery, Clinical Sciences, University of Tsukuba, Ibaraki 305-8575, Japan

**Kahori Seto**
Department of Oral and Maxillofacial Surgery, Clinical Sciences, University of Tsukuba, Ibaraki 305-8575, Japan
Department of Pharmacoepidemiology, Graduate School of Medicine and Public Health, Kyoto University, Yoshida Konoe-cho, Sakyo-ku, Kyoto 606-8501, Japan

**Tomohisa Horibe, Masayuki Kohno and Koji Kawakami**
Department of Pharmacoepidemiology, Graduate School of Medicine and Public Health, Kyoto University, Yoshida Konoe-cho, Sakyo-ku, Kyoto 606-8501, Japan

**Junichi Shoda**
Medical Science, Faculty of Medicine, University of Tsukuba, Ibaraki 305-8575, Japan

**Eiji Warabi**
Division of Biomedical Science, Faculty of Medicine, University of Tsukuba, Ibaraki 305-8575, Japan

**Yasuni Nakanuma**
Department of Human Pathology, Graduate School of Medical Science, Kanazawa University, Kanazawa 920-1192, Japan

**Manuela Scorza, Renato Liguori, Felice Amato and Giuseppe Castaldo**
CEINGE—Biotecnologie Avanzate Scarl, Via Gaetano Salvatore 486, 80145 Napoli, Italy
Dipartimento di Medicina Molecolare e Biotecnologie Mediche, Universit`a di Napoli Federico II, Via Sergio Pansini 5, 80131 Napoli, Italy

**Ausilia Elce**
CEINGE—Biotecnologie Avanzate Scarl, Via Gaetano Salvatore 486, 80145 Napoli, Italy
Dipartimento di Medicina Molecolare e Biotecnologie Mediche, Università di Napoli Federico II, Via Sergio Pansini 5, 80131 Napoli, Italy
Università Telematica Pegaso, Piazza Trieste e Trento 48, 80132Napoli, Italy

**Federica Zarrilli**
CEINGE—Biotecnologie Avanzate Scarl, Via Gaetano Salvatore 486, 80145 Napoli, Italy

Dipartimento di Bioscienze e Territorio, Università del Molise, Contrada Fonte Lappone, Pesche, 86090 Isernia, Italy

**Kazuya Shiogama, Ken-ichi Inada, YasuyoshiMizutani, Takanori Onouchi and Yutaka Tsutsumi**
Department of Pathology, Fujita Health University School of Medicine, Toyoake, Aichi 470-1192, Japan

**Michinori Kohara**
Department of Microbiology and Cell Biology, Tokyo Metropolitan Institute of Medical Science, Tokyo 156-8506, Japan

**Hidemi Teramoto**
Department of Internal Medicine, Kojin Hospital, Nagoya 463-8530, Japan

**Ida Louise Heiberg and Birthe Hogh**
Department of Paediatrics, Hvidovre Hospital, University of Copenhagen, Kettegaard All´e 30, 2650Hvidovre, Denmark

**Thilde NordmannWinther and Kari Stougaard Jacobsen**
Department of Paediatrics, Hvidovre Hospital, University of Copenhagen, Kettegaard Allé 30, 2650Hvidovre, Denmark
Department of Paediatrics and Center for Non-Coding RNA in Technology and Health, Herlev Hospital, University of Copenhagen, Arkaden, 2730 Herlev, Denmark

**Aashiq Hussain Mirza, Claus Heiner Bang-Berthelsen and Flemming Pociot**
Department of Paediatrics and Center for Non-Coding RNA in Technology and Health, Herlev Hospital, University of Copenhagen, Arkaden, 2730 Herlev, Denmark

**Hirayuki Enomoto and Shuhei Nishiguchi**
Division of Hepatobiliary and Pancreatic Disease, Department of Internal Medicine, Hyogo College of Medicine, Mukogawacho 1-1, Nishinomiya, Hyogo 663-8501, Japan

**Shin-ichi Inoue and Akio Matsuhisa**
Research and Development Center, Fuso Pharmaceutical Industries, Ltd., Morinomiya 2-3-30, Joto-ku, Osaka 536-8523, Japan

**Masaki Maruyama**
Division of Gastroenterology and Hepatology, Department of Internal Medicine, Kashiwazaki Central Hospital, 2-1-25 Ekimae, Niigata, Kashiwazaki 9450055, Japan

**Osamu Isokawa**
Division of Gastroenterology and Hepatology, Kashiwazaki General Hospital and Medical Center, 2-11-3 Kitahanda, Kashiwazaki, Niigata, 9458535, Japan

**Koki Hoshiyama**
Division of Cardiology, Department of Internal Medicine, Kashiwazaki Central Hospital, 2-1-25 Ekimae, Niigata, Kashiwazaki 9450055, Japan

**Ayako Hoshiyama and Mari Hoshiyama**
Division of Endocrinology and Metabolism, Department of Internal Medicine, Kashiwazaki Central Hospital, 2-1-25 Ekimae, Niigata, Kashiwazaki 9450055, Japan

**Yoshihiro Hoshiyama**
Department of Surgery, Kashiwazaki Central Hospital, 2-1-25 Ekimae, Niigata, Kashiwazaki 9450055, Japan

**Roberto Galuppo, Angie McCall and Roberto Gedaly**
Department of Surgery, College of Medicine, University of Kentucky, Lexington, KY 40536-0293, USA

**Feng Chen and Ann-Marie T. Baine**
Department of Neuroscience, Mayo Clinic, Jacksonville, FL 32224, USA

**Tomohide Hori and Toshiyuki Hata**
Department of Neuroscience, Mayo Clinic, Jacksonville, FL 32224, USA
Division of Hepato-Biliary-Pancreatic and Transplant Surgery, Department of Surgery, KyotoUniversity Graduate School of Medicine, 54 Shogoinkawara-cho, Sakyo-ku, Kyoto 606-8507, Japan

**Lindsay B.Walden**
Department of Neuroscience, Mayo Clinic, Jacksonville, FL 32224, USA
Division of Transplant Surgery, Department of Transplantation, Mayo Clinic, Jacksonville, FL 32224, USA

**Shinji Uemoto**
Division ofHepato-Biliary-Pancreatic and Transplant Surgery, Department of Surgery, KyotoUniversity Graduate School of Medicine, 54 Shogoinkawara-cho, Sakyo-ku, Kyoto 606-8507, Japan

**Justin H. Nguyen**
Division of Transplant Surgery, Department of Transplantation, Mayo Clinic, Jacksonville, FL 32224, USA

**Andreas L. Koutsoumpas**
Division of Medicine, School of Health Sciences, University of Thessaly, Thessaly, Viopolis, 40500 Larissa, Greece

**Dimitrios P. Bogdanos**
Division of Medicine, School of Health Sciences, University of Thessaly, Thessaly, Viopolis, 40500 Larissa, Greece
Institute of Liver Studies, King's College London School of Medicine at King's College Hospital, Denmark Hill Campus, London SE5 9RS, UK
Cellular Immunotherapy and Molecular Immunodiagnostics, Biomedical Section, Institute of Research and Technology-Thessaly (IRETETH), 41222 Larissa, Greece

**Daniel S. Smyk**
Institute of Liver Studies, King's College London School of Medicine at King's College Hospital, Denmark Hill Campus, London SE5 9RS, UK

**Saurav Das and Sajjadh M. J. Ali**
Department of Medical Gastroenterology, Stanley Medical College and Hospital, Chennai 600001, India

**James Seward**
Banner Alzheimer's Institute, EWilletta Street, Phoenix, AZ 85006, USA

**Jayanthi Venkataraman**
Global Health City, Perumbakkam, Chennai, Tamil Nadu 600100, India

**Mahmoud Omar, Wael Abdel-Razek, Gamal Medhat Assem and Gasser El-Azab**
Department of Hepatology, National Liver Institute, Menoufia University, Shebeen El-Kom, Egypt

**Abo-Raia**
Department of Clinical Pathology, National Liver Institute, Menoufia University, Shebeen El-Kom, Egypt

**TatsuoMiyamura, Tatsuo Kanda, Makoto Arai, Masato Nakamura, Shuang Wu, Xia Jiang, Reina Sasaki, Yuki Haga, Shin Yasui, Yoshihiko Ooka, Tetsuhiro Chiba, Fumio Imazeki and Osamu Yokosuka**
Departments of Gastroenterology and Nephrology, Graduate School of Medicine, Chiba University,
1-8-1 Inohana, Chuo-ku, Chiba 260-8677, Japan

**Shingo Nakamoto**
Department of Molecular Virology, Graduate School of Medicine, Chiba University, Chiba 260-8677, Japan

**ShigeruMikami**
Department of Gastroenterology, Kikkoman General Hospital, Noda 278-0005, Japan

**Sanaz Ainechi**
Anatomic Pathology, Albany Medical College, 47 New Scotland Avenue, MC81, Albany, NY 12208, USA

**Hwajeong Lee**
Anatomic Pathology, Albany Medical College, 47 New Scotland Avenue, MC81, Albany, NY 12208, USA
Anatomic Pathology, University of Massachusetts, 1 Innovation Drive, Biotech 3, Worcester, MA 01605, USA

**Karen Dresser**
Anatomic Pathology, University of Massachusetts, 1 Innovation Drive, Biotech 3, Worcester, MA 01605, USA

**Elizabeth M. Kurian**
Anatomic Pathology, University of Massachusetts, 1 Innovation Drive, Biotech 3, Worcester, MA 01605, USA
Anatomic Pathology, University of Texas Southwestern Medical Center, 5323 Harry Hines Boulevard, Dallas, TX 75390-9234, USA

**Fugui Bai, Nungki Anggorowati, Hanggoro Tri Rinonce, Dewiyani IndahWidasari and Yoshitake Hayashi**
Center for Infectious Diseases, Kobe University Graduate School of Medicine, Kobe 650-0017, Japan

**Yoshihiko Yano**
Center for Infectious Diseases, Kobe University Graduate School of Medicine, Kobe 650-0017, Japan
Department of Gastroenterology, Kobe University Graduate School of Medicine, Kobe 650-0017, Japan

**Masaya Saito, Hirotaka Hirano, Takanobu Hayakumo, Yasushi Seo and Takeshi Azuma**
Department of Gastroenterology, Kobe University Graduate School of Medicine, Kobe 650-0017, Japan

**Takumi Fukumoto, Atsushi Takebe, Motofumi Tanaka, Kaori Kuramitsu and Yonson Ku**
Department of Hepato-Biliary-Pancreatic Surgery, Kobe University Graduate School of Medicine, Kobe 650-0017, Japan

**P. Priyanka**
Department of Medicine, West Virginia University Hospitals, Morgantown, WV, USA

**J. T. Kupec, M. Krafft and G. J. Reynolds**
Department of Medicine, Section of Digestive Diseases, West Virginia University Hospitals, Morgantown, WV, USA

**N. A. Shah**
Department of Medicine, Section of Hematology, West Virginia University Hospitals, Morgantown, WV, USA

**Vijay Gayam, Amrendra KumarMandal, Mazin Khalid, OsamaMukhtar, Arshpal Gill, Pavani Garlapati and Mohammed Mansour**
Department of Medicine and Gastroenterology, Interfaith Medical Center, 1545 Atlantic Avenue, Brooklyn, NY 11213, USA

**Mowyad Khalid**
Department of Medicine, Wayne State University/Detroit Medical Center, Detroit, Michigan, USA

**Yasir Al-Azzawi**
University of Massachusetts School of Medicine, 55 North Lake Ave, Worcester, MA 01606, USA

**Lidia Spaho, MohammedMahmoud, Joan Kheder, Anne Foley and David Cave**
University of Massachusetts School of Medicine, USA

**Erik J. Groessl, Lin Liu, Marisa Sklar and Samuel B. Ho**
VA San Diego Healthcare System, San Diego, CA, USA
University of California, San Diego, San Diego, CA, USA

**Kamran Qureshi**
Department of Medicine, Section of Gastroenterology, Temple University Lewis Katz School of Medicine, Philadelphia, PA, USA

**Shyam Patel and AndrewMeillier**
Department of Medicine, Internal Medicine Residency Program, Temple University Hospital, Philadelphia, PA, USA

**Sameh Abdelkhalik Ahmed**
Department of Anesthesia, Tanta University, Tanta, Egypt

**Amal Selim**
Internal Medicine Department, Tanta University, Tanta, Egypt

**Nehad Hawash, Ahmed Khaled Tawfik, Mohamed Yousef, Abdelrahman Kobtan, Rehab Badawi, Sally Elnawasany, Reham Abdelkader Elkhouly, Loai Mansour and Sherief Abd-Elsalam**
Tropical Medicine Department, Tanta University, Tanta, Egypt

**Amr Shaaban Hanafy**
Internal Medicine Department, Zagazig University, Zagazig, Egypt

**Fatma H. Rizk**
Department of Physiology, Tanta University, Tanta, Egypt

**Mavidi Sunil Kumar, Piyush Ranjan and Naval K. Vikram**
Department of Internal Medicine, All India Institute of Medical Sciences, New Delhi 110029, India

**Akanksha Singh, Ashok Kumar Jaryal and K. K. Deepak**
Department of Physiology, All India Institute of Medical Sciences, New Delhi 110029, India

**Sanjay Sharma**
Department of Radiodiagnosis, All India Institute of Medical Sciences, New Delhi 110029, India

**R. Lakshmy**
Department of Cardiac Biochemistry, All India Institute of Medical Sciences, New Delhi 110029, India

**R. M. Pandey**
Department of Biostatistics, All India Institute of Medical Sciences, New Delhi 110029, India

**Ayane A. Rodrigues**
Postgraduate Program in Biomedical Sciences, Federal University of Piaui, Parnaiba, PI, Brazil

**Daniel F. P. Vasconcelos**
Postgraduate Program in Biomedical Sciences, Federal University of Piaui, Parnaiba, PI, Brazil
Postgraduate Program in Biotechnology, Federal University of Piaui, Parniba, PI, Brazil
Department of Biomedicine, Federal University of Piaui, Parnaiba, PI, Brazil

**Ra-ssa S. B. Andrade**
Postgraduate Program in Biotechnology, Federal University of Piaui, Parniba, PI, Brazil

**Apichet Sirinawasatien, Thanaya Techasirioangkun and Siriporn Thongsri**
Division of Gastroenterology, Department ofMedicine, Rajavithi Hospital, College ofMedicine, Rangsit University, Bangkok, Thailand

**Rodolfo Castro, Hugo Perazzo, Beatriz Grinsztejn and Valdilea G. Veloso**
Evandro Chagas National Institute of Infectious Diseases, Oswaldo Cruz Foundation, Laboratory of Clinical Research on STD/AIDS, Avenida Brasil 4365, 21040-900 Manguinhos, RJ, Brazil

**Chris Hyde**
Institute of Health Research, Peninsula Technology Assessment Group (PenTAG), Evidence Synthesis and Modelling for Health Improvement (ESMI), University of Exeter Medical School, University of Exeter, St Luke's Campus, South Cloisters, Exeter EX1 2LU, UK

**Sumitro Kosasih, Wong Zhi Qin, Ngiu Chai Soon and Raja Affendi Raja Ali**
Gastroenterology and Hepatology Unit, Faculty of Medicine, Universiti KebangsaanMalaysia, Kuala Lumpur, 56000, Malaysia

**Rafiz Abdul Rani**
Gastroenterology Unit, Faculty of Medicine, Universiti Teknologi MARA, Shah Alam, Selangor, 40450, Malaysia

**Nazefah Abd Hamid**
Department of Medical and Health Science, Universiti Sains IslamMalaysia, Nilai, Negeri Sembilan, 71800, Malaysia

**Shamsul Azhar Shah**
Department of Public Health, Faculty of Medicine, Universiti KebangsaanMalaysia, Kuala Lumpur, 56000, Malaysia

**Yazmin Yaakob**
Department of Radiology, Faculty of Medicine, Universiti KebangsaanMalaysia, Kuala Lumpur, 56000, Malaysia

**Nalini Bansal**
SRL Ltd., Fortis Escorts Heart Institute, New Delhi, India

**Vivek Vij and Mukul Rastogi**
FortisHospital, Gurgaon, India

**Shailendra P. Singh, Joseph Schragenheim, Lars Bellner, Aliza Meissner, Ilana Grant, David Bamshad and Edward Lebovics**
Departments of Medicine, Pharmacology and Gastroenterology, New York Medical College, Valhalla, NY 10595, USA

**David Sacerdoti**
Departments of Medicine, Pharmacology and Gastroenterology, New York Medical College, Valhalla, NY 10595, USA
Department of Medicine, University of Padova, Padova, Italy

**Nader G. Abraham**
Departments of Medicine, Pharmacology and Gastroenterology, New York Medical College, Valhalla, NY 10595, USA
Marshall University, Joan C. Edwards School of Medicine, Huntington, WV 25701, USA

**Luca Vanella and Marco Raffaele**
Department of Drug Science, University of Catania, Catania, Italy

**Gaia Favero, Rita Rezzani and Luigi F. Rodella**
Anatomy and Physiopathology Division, Department of Clinical and Experimental Sciences, University of Brescia, Brescia, Italy

**Cyriac Abby Philips**
Department of Hepatology and Transplant Medicine, Institute of Liver and Biliary Sciences, D-1, Vasant Kunj, New Delhi 110070, India

**Ankur Arora, Rajesh Shetty and Vivek Kasana**
Department of Radiodiagnosis, Institute of Liver and Biliary Sciences, D-1, Vasant Kunj, New Delhi 110070, India

**Vajiheh Rangboo**
Department of Nutrition, Faculty of Health, Qazvin University of Medical Sciences, Qazvin, Iran

**Mostafa Noroozi**
Children Growth Research Center, Qazvin University of Medical Sciences, Qazvin, Iran

**Roza Zavoshy**
Department of Nutrition, Faculty of Nutrition, Qazvin University of Medical Sciences, Qazvin, Iran

**Seyed Amirmansoor Rezadoost**
Shahid Chamran Hospital, Shahid Beheshti University of Medical Sciences, Tehran, Iran

**AsgharMohammadpoorasl**
Department of Epidemiology, Tabriz University of Medical Sciences, Tabriz, Iran

**Ossama Ashraf Ahmed, Eslam Safwat, Ahmed I. Elshafie, Mohamed Hassan Ahmed Fouad, Mohamed Magdy Salama and Gina Gamal Naguib**
Internal Medicine Department, Gastroenterology and Hepatology Unit, Ain Shams University, Cairo, Egypt

**Mohamed Mahmoud Eltabbakh, Ahmed Fouad Sherief and Mohamed Omar Khalifa**
Tropical Medicine Department, Ain Shams University, Cairo, Egypt

**Sherief Abd-Elsalam**
Tropical Medicine and Infectious Diseases Department, Tanta University, Tanta, Egypt

# Index